NUTRIENT REQUIREMENTS OF HORSES

SIXTH REVISED EDITION

Committee on Nutrient Requirements of Horses

Board on Agriculture and Natural Resources

Division on Earth and Life Studies

NATIONAL RESEARCH COUNCIL
OF THE NATIONAL ACADEMIES

THE NATIONAL ACADEMIES PRESS
Washington, D.C.
www.nap.edu

THE NATIONAL ACADEMIES PRESS • 500 Fifth Street, N.W. • Washington, DC 20001

NOTICE: The project that is the subject of this report was approved by the Governing Board of the National Research Council, whose members are drawn from the councils of the National Academy of Sciences, the National Academy of Engineering, and the Institute of Medicine. The members of the committee responsible for the report were chosen for their special competences and with regard for appropriate balance.

This study was supported by grants from the American Feed Industry Association, the American Paint Horse Association, the American Quarter Horse Association, the Equine Science Society, the North American Equine Ranching Information Council, general support of The Animal Nutrition Series provided by The Department of Health and Human Services (U.S. Food and Drug Administration) under Award No. 223-01-01-2460, and internal National Research Council funds. Any opinions, findings, conclusions, or recommendations expressed in this publication are those of the author(s) and do not necessarily reflect the views of the organizations or agencies that provided support for the project.

Library of Congress Cataloging-in-Publication Data

Nutrient requirements of horses / Committee on Nutrient Requirements of Horses,
Board on Agriculture and Natural Resources, Division on Earth and Life Studies,
National Research Council of the National Academies. — 6th rev. ed.
    p. cm.
 Includes bibliographical references and index.
 ISBN-10: 0-309-10212-X (cloth)
 ISBN-10: 0-309-66096-3 (pdf)
 ISBN-13: 978-0-309-10212-4 (cloth)
 ISBN-13: 978-0-309-66096-9 (pdf)
 1. Horses—Nutrition—Requirements. 2. Horses—Feeding and feeds. I. National
Research Council (U.S.). Committee on Nutrient Requirements of Horses.
SF285.5.N37 2007
636.1′0852—dc22
                              2006030795

Additional copies of this report are available from the National Academies Press, 500 Fifth Street, N.W., Lockbox 285, Washington, DC 20055; (800) 624-6242 or (202) 334-3313 (in the Washington metropolitan area); Internet, http://www.nap.edu.

Copyright 2007 by the National Academy of Sciences. All rights reserved.

Printed in the United States of America

First Printing, March 2007
Second Printing, November 2007
Third Printing, October 2009
Fourth Printing, August 2012
Fifth Printing, September 2013
Sixth Printing, September 2015
Seventh Printing, January 2017
Eighth Printing, January 2018

THE NATIONAL ACADEMIES
Advisers to the Nation on Science, Engineering, and Medicine

The **National Academy of Sciences** is a private, nonprofit, self-perpetuating society of distinguished scholars engaged in scientific and engineering research, dedicated to the furtherance of science and technology and to their use for the general welfare. Upon the authority of the charter granted to it by the Congress in 1863, the Academy has a mandate that requires it to advise the federal government on scientific and technical matters. Dr. Ralph J. Cicerone is president of the National Academy of Sciences.

The **National Academy of Engineering** was established in 1964, under the charter of the National Academy of Sciences, as a parallel organization of outstanding engineers. It is autonomous in its administration and in the selection of its members, sharing with the National Academy of Sciences the responsibility for advising the federal government. The National Academy of Engineering also sponsors engineering programs aimed at meeting national needs, encourages education and research, and recognizes the superior achievements of engineers. Dr. Wm. A. Wulf is president of the National Academy of Engineering.

The **Institute of Medicine** was established in 1970 by the National Academy of Sciences to secure the services of eminent members of appropriate professions in the examination of policy matters pertaining to the health of the public. The Institute acts under the responsibility given to the National Academy of Sciences by its congressional charter to be an adviser to the federal government and, upon its own initiative, to identify issues of medical care, research, and education. Dr. Harvey V. Fineberg is president of the Institute of Medicine.

The **National Research Council** was organized by the National Academy of Sciences in 1916 to associate the broad community of science and technology with the Academy's purposes of furthering knowledge and advising the federal government. Functioning in accordance with general policies determined by the Academy, the Council has become the principal operating agency of both the National Academy of Sciences and the National Academy of Engineering in providing services to the government, the public, and the scientific and engineering communities. The Council is administered jointly by both Academies and the Institute of Medicine. Dr. Ralph J. Cicerone and Dr. Wm. A. Wulf are chair and vice chair, respectively, of the National Research Council.

www.national-academies.org

COMMITTEE ON NUTRIENT REQUIREMENTS OF HORSES

LAURIE M. LAWRENCE, *Chair*, University of Kentucky, Lexington
NADIA F. CYMBALUK, Linwood Equine Ranch, Brandon, Manitoba, Canada
DAVID W. FREEMAN, Oklahoma State University, Stillwater
RAYMOND J. GEOR, Virginia Polytechnic and State University, Middleburg
PATRICIA M. GRAHAM-THIERS, Virginia Intermont College, Bristol
ANNETTE C. LONGLAND, Institute of Grassland and Environmental Research, Ceredigion, Wales, United Kingdom
BRIAN D. NIELSEN, Michigan State University, East Lansing
PAUL D. SICILIANO, North Carolina State University, Raleigh
DONALD R. TOPLIFF, West Texas A&M University, Canyon
EDUARDO V. VALDES, Disney's Animal Kingdom, East Bay Lake, Florida
ROBERT J. VAN SAUN, The Pennsylvania State University, University Park

Staff

AUSTIN J. LEWIS, Study Director
JAMIE S. JONKER, Study Director*
DONNA LEE JAMEISON, Senior Program Assistant**
RUTH S. ARIETI, Project Assistant

External Support

MICHAEL C. BARRY (AgModels, LLC), Computer Programmer
PAULA T. WHITACRE (Full Circle Communications), Editor

*Through June 2004
**Through January 2006

BOARD ON AGRICULTURE AND NATURAL RESOURCES

W. REG GOMES, *Chair*, University of California, Oakland
SANDRA J. BARTHOLMEY, University of Illinois at Chicago
ROGER N. BEACHY, Donald Danforth Plant Science Center, St. Louis, Missouri
H. H. CHENG, University of Minnesota, St. Paul
BRUCE L. GARDNER, University of Maryland, College Park
JEAN HALLORAN, Consumer Policy Institute/Consumers Union, Yonkers, New York
HANS R. HERREN, Millennium Institute, Arlington, Virginia
KIRK C. KLASING, University of California, Davis
BRIAN W. MCBRIDE, University of Guelph, Guelph, Canada
TERRY L. MEDLEY, E. I. duPont de Nemours & Co., Wilmington, Delaware
ROBERT PAARLBERG, Wellesley College, Watertown, Massachusetts
ALICE N. PELL, Cornell University, Ithaca, New York
BOBBY PHILLS, Florida A&M University, Tallahassee
SONYA B. SALAMON, University of Illinois, Urbana-Champaign
HAL SALWASSER, Oregon State University, Corvallis
PEDRO A. SANCHEZ, The Earth Institute at Columbia University, Palisades, New York
B. L. TURNER, II, Clark University, Worcester, Massachusetts
LAURIAN UNNEVEHR, University of Illinois, Urbana-Champaign
TILAHUN D. YILMA, University of California, Davis
JAW-KAI WANG, University of Hawaii, Honolulu

Staff

ROBIN A. SCHOEN, Director
KAREN L. IMHOF, Administrative Assistant
AUSTIN J. LEWIS, Program Officer
PEGGY TSAI, Research Associate
RUTH S. ARIETI, Project Assistant

Preface

The domesticated members of the genus *Equus* (horses, ponies, donkeys, mules) are used for many purposes including competition, recreation, entertainment, transportation, farm and ranch work, and even therapy. Several nondomesticated species of *Equus* are maintained in zoological parks or are the focus of conservation efforts. The demand for information relating to the nutrition and feeding management of horses, ponies, and their relatives has grown with the popularity of these animals and with the increased interest in nutrition in general.

The Sixth Revised Edition of the Nutrient Requirements of Horses is a project of the Board on Agriculture and Natural Resources of the National Academies. This document was produced from the work of a committee appointed in February 2004. The committee accepted input from stakeholders and sponsors during several public information sessions and from a public website. The purpose of this publication is to review the existing scientific literature relating to the nutrition and feeding of horses and to summarize the information relating to nutrient requirements of horses of various physiological classes. The publication is accompanied by a web-based computer program. The computer program will calculate nutrient requirements of domestic horses and ponies of specific weights and physiological classes. Included in this edition of this publication is a discussion of the nutrition and feeding of donkeys, mules, and captive equids.

A complete review of information pertaining to the digestive physiology of the horse was outside of the charge given to this committee for this report. However, an understanding of the anatomy and physiology of the equine digestive tract will be helpful in interpreting and applying many of the recommendations contained in this publication. Reviews of various aspects of equine digestive physiology may be found in veterinary and animal science texts cited in this publication.

A great deal of new information has appeared in the scientific literature on topics related to the nutrition and feeding of horses since the publication of the previous edition in 1989. New information, previously existing information, and previous recommendations have been considered in the process of determining requirements. In some cases, authors of papers on specific subjects were contacted for clarification. In addition a few data sets were obtained for some areas (growth) to augment existing values. In most cases these data sets were from a graduate thesis so were published in some format. Some areas of equine nutrition have received little study from the scientific community. Therefore, data from other animals were reviewed for applicability when studies using horses were not available. Most recent research has used horses of light horse breeding (such as Thoroughbreds, Quarter horses, Standardbreds, and Arabians). Several older studies used ponies. Very little recent information is available for draft breeds, and, similarly, few studies have compared draft breeds, light horse breeds, and pony breeds. Users should recognize that many recommendations for ponies and draft horses have been extrapolated from data obtained using light horses. Therefore, it is suggested that the recommendations for ponies and draft horses be applied with discretion. Several sections of the text provide information on how body size might affect requirements for specific nutrients.

A central purpose of this publication was to evaluate the recommendations in the previous edition in light of new information about the nutrient requirements of horses and to revise nutrient requirements when appropriate. Several mathematical equations have been derived to provide more dynamic estimates of requirements for some physiological states including growth, gestation, and exercise. The requirements shown in the tables provide recommendations for broad classifications of horses, whereas the computer program allows some flexibility in calculating the nutrient requirements for a specific animal. The values listed in this document represent the committee's best estimates of the nutrient requirements of horses of different physiological states. The required amounts of many nutrients have been determined using average values for nutrient availability in common horse feeds. Users of the document and the associated computer program may choose to recalculate requirements when they possess specific information on nutrient availability for the rations being fed in practice. The committee recognizes that the values suggested here may not meet the need for all horses in all situations and that adjustments may be needed for individual horses or to meet specific production goals. Users of this document will find a more detailed review of the literature on equine nutrition than in previous editions. The committee has attempted to summarize information on the factors that might modify a requirement, such as individual variation, breed, feed composition, and environment. It is not possible for the committee to predict every combination of variables that could influence the nutrient requirements of a specific animal. Therefore, it is incumbent upon the user to accurately assess the factors that could alter requirements and then apply appropriate adjustments accordingly.

Laurie M. Lawrence
Chair, Committee on Nutrient
Requirements of Horses

Acknowledgments

This report has been reviewed in draft form by persons chosen for their diverse perspectives and technical expertise in accordance with procedures approved by the National Research Council's Report Review Committee. The purpose of this independent review is to provide candid and critical comments that will assist the institution in making its published report as sound as possible and to ensure that the report meets institutional standards of objectivity, evidence, and responsiveness to the study charge. The review comments and draft manuscript remain confidential to protect the integrity of the deliberative process. We wish to thank the following for their review of this report:

Joseph J. Bertone, Western University of Health Sciences, Pomona, CA
Manfred Coenen, University of Leipzig, Leipzig, Germany
Patricia A. Harris, Waltham Centre for Pet Nutrition, Leicestershire, United Kingdom
Kenneth W. Hinchcliff, Ohio State University, Columbus, OH
Rhonda M. Hoffman, Middle Tennessee State University, Murfreesboro, TN
James H. Jones, University of California, Davis, CA
Edgar A. Ott, University of Florida, Gainesville, FL (retired)
Joe D. Pagan, Kentucky Equine Research, Versailles, KY
Sarah L. Ralston, Rutgers University, New Brunswick, NJ
Judith A. Reynolds, ADM Alliance Nutrition, Quincy, IL
Virginia Rich, Rich Equine Nutritional Consulting, Eads, TN
Ronald E. Rompala, Blue Seal Feeds, Londonderry, NH

Although the reviewers listed above have provided many constructive comments and suggestions, they were not asked to endorse the conclusions or recommendations, nor did they see the final draft of the report before its release. The review of this report was overseen by R. L. Baldwin, Jr., University of California, Davis. Appointed by the National Research Council, he was responsible for making certain that an independent examination of this report was carried out in accordance with institutional procedures and that all review comments were carefully considered. Responsibility for the final content of this report rests entirely with the author committee and the institution.

The committee on Nutrient Requirements of Horses would like to express deep appreciation to all of the sponsors that contributed the funds to support this effort. Sponsors for the Sixth Revised Edition of the Nutrient Requirements of Horses included the American Feed Industry Association (www.afia.org), American Paint Horse Association (www.apha.com), American Quarter Horse Association (www.aqha.com), Equine Science Society (www.enps.org), general support of The Animal Nutrition Series provided by the Department of Health and Human Services (U.S. Food and Drug Administration) under Award No. 223-01-01-2460 (www.fda.gov/cvm/), and North American Equine Ranching Information Council (www.naeric.org). The funding for this project was necessary to support the travel and communications costs of the committee during the course of its work, as well as the work of the National Research Council staff who organized meetings, maintained the website, and compiled the draft and final documents.

The committee would also like to thank all of the individuals who helped to make this project a reality. Charlotte Kirk Baer, former Board on Agriculture and Natural Resources (BANR) director, was instrumental in developing the original proposal that received approval from the Board on Agriculture and Natural Resources in August of 2003. Ms. Baer was also integrally involved in developing the funding for this project, as were Dr. Donald Topliff, West Texas A&M University, and Dr. Randy Robbins, chairman of the American Feed Industry Association (AFIA) Specialty Committee. Austin Lewis was a tireless manager as the program officer assigned to this committee. The committee sincerely appreciates the wealth of experience and perpetual optimism that Dr. Lewis brought to this project. The work of this committee could not have been completed without the able assistance of Donna Jameison, senior program assistant and Ruthie Arieti, project assistant. Finally, we would like to thank Robin Schoen, who replaced Ms. Baer as BANR director in 2004.

In the process of planning, researching, and writing this document, the committee obtained input and advice from several sources. We would like to thank Kentucky Equine Research, Inc. and the American Society of Animal Science for allowing us to present public information sessions at their annual meetings in 2004. The committee also thanks Dr. Mary Beth Hall and Dr. George Fahey, who provided advice on topics related to carbohydrate classification and analysis. We would also like to thank the American Feed Industry Association for providing input at an open session of the initial meeting of our committee. The committee is indebted to Michael Barry, who compiled the computer program that accompanies this report and provided invaluable advice to the committee. Finally the committee would like to thank their families, students, colleagues, and home institutions. Without their patience and willingness to accept additional responsibilities, this project would not have been accomplished. This list of acknowledgements would not be complete without the recognition of the work of previous committees. We hope that our efforts will do justice to the tradition of excellence established by those who came before us.

Contents

SUMMARY	1
1 ENERGY	3
2 CARBOHYDRATES	34
3 FATS AND FATTY ACIDS	44
4 PROTEINS AND AMINO ACIDS	54
5 MINERALS	69
6 VITAMINS	109
7 WATER AND WATER QUALITY	128
8 FEEDS AND FEED PROCESSING	141
9 FEED ADDITIVES	183
10 FEED ANALYSIS	203
11 FEEDING BEHAVIOR AND GENERAL CONSIDERATIONS FOR FEEDING MANAGEMENT	211
12 UNIQUE ASPECTS OF EQUINE NUTRITION	235
13 DONKEYS AND OTHER EQUIDS	268
14 RATION FORMULATION AND EVALUATION	280
15 COMPUTER MODEL TO ESTIMATE REQUIREMENTS	285
16 TABLES	293
NUTRIENT REQUIREMENT TABLES	294
FEED COMPOSITION TABLES	304

	COMPOSITION OF MARE'S MILK TABLES	311
	TABLE OF CONVERSIONS	315

APPENDIXES

A	COMMITTEE STATEMENT OF TASK	317
B	ABBREVIATONS AND ACRONYMS	319
C	COMMITTEE MEMBER BIOGRAPHIES	323
D	BOARD ON AGRICULTURE AND NATURAL RESOURCES PUBLICATIONS	325
	INDEX	327

Tables and Figures

TABLES

1-1	Summary of Studies that Measured Heat Production in Horses at Maintenance	8
1-2	Three Proposed Levels of Digestible Energy Intake for Maintenance Mcal/d in Adult Horses as Compared to the Previous Recommendation	9
1-3	Lower and Upper Critical Temperatures in Horses	11
1-4	Effect of Age on the Amount of Digestible Energy (DE) Required per Kilogram of Gain for Growing Horses	14
1-5	Summary of Estimates of the Relationship Between Age and Percentage of Mature Body Weight in Growing Horses	14
1-6	Body Weight Predicted by Equation 1-3 and Expected Mature Body Weight and Body Weight Estimated in the Previous NRC (1989) for Growing Horses	15
1-7	A Condition Scoring System for Horses	21
1-8	Estimated Oxygen Consumption and Net Energy Utilization of a 500-kg Horse Ridden by a 50-kg Rider at Various Heart Rates	24
1-9	Hypothetical Weekly Net Energy Expenditure (above maintenance) of a 500-kg Horse Used for Recreational Riding	25
1-10	Example Weekly Workloads of Horses in the Light, Moderate, Heavy, and Very Heavy Exercise Categories	26
1-11	Estimated Increase in Digestible Energy (DE) Intake Necessary to Change the Condition Score of a 500-kg Horse from 4 to 5	28
2-1	Neutral Detergent Fiber (NDF), Nonfiber Carbohydrate (NFC), and Nonstructural Carbohydrate (NSC) Composition of Selected Feedstuffs on a Dry Matter Basis	35
2-2	Carbohydrate Composition (dry matter basis) of Selected Feed Ingredients	36
7-1	Estimated Water Needs of Horses	131
7-2	Guidelines for Total Dissolved Solids (TDS) or Total Soluble Salts (TSS)	135
7-3	Water Hardness Guidelines	136
7-4	Generally Considered Safe Upper Level Concentrations (mg/L) of Some Potentially Toxic Nutrients and Contaminants in Water for Horses	137
8-1	Estimated Voluntary Fresh Matter Intake (VFMI) and Voluntary Dry Matter Intake (VDMI) of Fresh Herbage	145
8-2	Contents of Digestible Energy and Protein and Apparent Dry Matter and Protein Digestibilities of Various Fresh Forages by Horses	146
8-3	Estimated Voluntary Dry Matter Intake of Various Hays by Horses and Ponies	151
8-4	Apparent Dry Matter, Organic Matter, Energy, Protein, and Fiber Digestibilities of Various Hays in Horses	153
8-5	Voluntary Dry Matter Intakes (VDMI) of Ensiled Forages by Ponies and Horses	155

8-6	Apparent Dry Matter, Organic Matter, Protein, and Energy Digestibility of Ensiled Forages by Ponies	155
8-7	Fatty Acid Composition of Some Fats and Oils Available for Use in Equine Feeds	163
8-8	Amino Acid Contents of Some Horse Feed Ingredients and Forages	164
8-9	Supplemental Vitamin Sources: Chemical Form, Vitamin Activity, Physical Form, and Applications	168
8-10	Comparison of Small Intestinal Starch Digestibility of Processed Corn	169
8-11	Comparison of Small Intestinal Starch Digestibility of Processed Oats	170
8-12	Comparison of Small Intestinal Starch Digestibility of Processed Oats and Barley	170
8-13	Comparison of Small Intestinal Starch Digestibility of Grains	171
8-14	Comparison of Small Intestinal Starch Digestibility of Grains Fed at Moderate Intakes	171
8-15	Comparison of Small Intestinal Nitrogen Digestibility of Diets Containing Micronized and Crimped Oats and Sorghum	172
8-1A	Selected Terminology Related to Feed Identification and Processing	173
9-1	AAFCO Feed Ingredient Definitions for Organic Mineral Products	195
11-1	Summary of Ranges of Reported Average Voluntary Dry Matter Intakes (AVDMI) of Selected Feedstuffs	214
11-2	Foraging Criteria by Horses Provided Various Feeds	215
12-1	Guidelines for Feeding Horses during Cold Weather	238
12-2	Guidelines for Feeding Horses during Hot Weather	239
12-3	Grasses That May Contain Excessive Amounts of Oxalates	251
13-1	Comparative Energy Expenditures in Horses and Donkeys	271
13-2	Chemical Composition (g/100 ml) of Milk of Donkeys and Other Animal Species	273
13-3	Daily Rations for Adult Donkeys	273
13-4	Estimated Nutrient Intakes for Adult Donkeys Consuming Diets Based on Poor or Good Quality Forage (dry matter basis)	273
13-5	Wild Equids Found in Zoological Parks	274
13-6	Diet Ingredients and Nutrient Composition (dry matter basis) of Typical Diets Fed to Wild Equids in Zoological Parks	275
13-7	Digestibility Coefficients, Organic Matter (OM) Intake, OM Extraction, and Cell Wall Extraction by Wild Equids	276
14-1	Feed Ingredient Nutrient Composition (dry matter basis)	281
14-2	Example Estimates of Nutrient Requirements	281
14-3	Comparison of Nutrient Intake and Estimated Requirements	282
14-4	Feed Ingredient Nutrient Composition	282
14-5	Example Intake Limit (as-fed basis) and Estimated Nutrient Requirements	282
14-6	Comparison of Nutrient Intake and Estimated Requirements	282
14-7	Targeted Nutrient Concentration of the Example Concentrate (dry matter)	282
14-8	Nutrient Composition of Feedstuffs (100% dry matter basis)	283
14-9	Nutrient Concentration of an 80:20 Mix of Grain One and Grain Two	283
14-10	Comparison of the Grain Mix and Protein Supplement with the Targeted Nutrient Densities for the Concentrate	283
14-11	Comparison of the Grain Mix, Protein Supplement, and Mineral One with the Targeted Nutrient Densities for the Concentrate	283
14-12	Comparison of the Final Formulation with the Targeted Nutrient Densities for the Concentrate	284
14-13	Formulated Concentrate Constituents on a Dry Matter and As-Fed Basis	284

16-1	Daily Nutrient Requirements of Horses (Mature Body Weight of 200 kg)	294
16-2	Daily Nutrient Requirements of Horses (Mature Body Weight of 400 kg)	296
16-3	Daily Nutrient Requirements of Horses (Mature Body Weight of 500 kg)	298
16-4	Daily Nutrient Requirements of Horses (Mature Body Weight of 600 kg)	300
16-5	Daily Nutrient Requirements of Horses (Mature Body Weight of 900 kg)	302
16-6	Nutrient Composition of Selected Feedstuffs	304
16-7	Compositions of Inorganic Mineral Sources on a 100% Dry Matter Basis	308
16-8	Research Findings on Composition of Mare's Milk (1989 NRC)	311
16-9	Research Findings on Composition of Mare's Milk (Since 1989 NRC)	313
16-10	Conversion Factors	315

FIGURES

1-1	Energy flow diagram	3
1-2	Comparison of digestible energy (DE) intakes of growing horses as predicated by NRC (1989) and actual intakes reported in the literature	11
1-3	Effect of age on digestible energy for maintenance (DE_m) (Kcal/Kg BW) in growing horses	12
1-4	Relationship between age (in months) and the amount of digestible energy (DE) required above maintenance per kilogram of gain in growing horses	13
1-5	Digestible energy (DE) intakes of growing horses as predicted by equation 1-4 and actual intakes reported in the literature	16
1-6	Fetal weight during gestation as a percentage of birth weight	17
1-7	Comparison of two equations (1-5b and 1-5d) that predict fetal weight as a percentage of birth weight	18
4-1	Regression of means from nitrogen digestibility studies for sedentary horses	56
4-2	Regression of means from nitrogen digestibility studies evaluating foregut vs. total tract digestibility of nitrogen	56
4-3	Relationship between calculated available protein (AP) intake and digestible protein (DP) intake	57
4-4	Linear and nonlinear regression for nitrogen balance for horses at maintenance	58
10-1	Fractionation of plant carbohydrates and related compounds	206

Summary

The National Research Council has published five previous editions of *Nutrient Requirements of Horses*. A great deal of research on the nutrition and feeding of horses has been conducted since the fifth edition was published in 1989. The Sixth Revised Edition contains updated information on the nutrient requirements of domestic horses and ponies, as well as expanded information on general considerations for equine feeding management. This report includes a discussion of feeding management of other equids, such as donkeys and wild equids kept in captivity. One chapter provides information on the feeding management of horses with nutritionally related disorders. A new web-based computer program has been developed that will assist users in determining the nutrient requirements of domestic horses and ponies of specific physiological classes.

In 2005, the American Horse Council estimated that the number of horses in the United States exceeded 9 million and that more than 2 million people were involved in horse ownership. The economic impact of the U.S. horse industry was estimated to be more than $100 billion. Horses are used for recreational purposes, sport (e.g., racing, polo, and Olympic events), exhibition, breeding, ranch and farm work, and even therapy. Type of use, age, and physiological state affect the nutrient requirements of horses. Horses are distributed broadly across the United States and the world, where they are subjected to a variety of climates and housing conditions. Effective feeding management practices must consider many factors, including nutrient requirements, environmental conditions, and available feeds. This report addresses not only the nutrient requirements of horses, but also provides information on feeds, feed processing, and feeding behavior of horses. It is expected that professional nutritionists, veterinarians, feed manufacturers, researchers, teachers, students, and horse owners will use the information.

Energy systems and energy requirements of horses are discussed in Chapter 1. The energy needs of horses for maintenance, reproduction, lactation, growth, and exercise are expressed in units of digestible energy. Maintenance requirements have been related to body weight, and guidelines for adjusting the energy intake to meet the needs of adult horses with various levels of voluntary activity are given. A method that enables users to estimate expected body weight of growing horses at any age from expected mature body weight has been proposed. The effect of exercise on energy requirements is discussed in this chapter, as are the effects of excessive and deficient energy intakes on horses.

Chapters 2 (Carbohydrates) and 3 (Fats and Fatty Acids) address the main energy-containing compounds used by horses. These chapters include information on the metabolism of carbohydrates and fats during exercise. Chapter 2 discusses the classification of carbohydrates in horse feeds, and Chapter 3 provides extensive review of the effects of feeding fat-supplemented diets to horses.

A comprehensive review of protein and amino acid nutrition of horses is presented in Chapter 4. Protein requirements are expressed in grams of crude protein, and lysine requirements are estimated. This chapter includes a discussion of protein digestibility and protein quality.

The requirements of horses for macrominerals and microminerals are found in Chapter 5. There has been a substantial amount of research on the mineral nutrition of horses since the previous edition of this document was published in 1989. This chapter includes an expanded discussion on several topics in mineral nutrition, including the effect of exercise on mineral requirements, and the addition of chromium and silicon to equine diets.

Chapter 6 addresses the vitamin requirements of horses. A review of the literature revealed that previous recommendations for several vitamins were based on extremely limited data. There have been a few new studies on vitamin nutrition in horses since 1989, and these studies were used to evaluate previous vitamin requirements. However, the committee relied on previous recommendations as a basis for the current estimates of requirements for several vitamins.

The section of the publication dealing with water requirements of horses has been significantly expanded.

Chapter 7 discusses water requirements, factors affecting water requirements, and water quality.

Feeds and feed processing are covered in Chapter 8. This chapter includes an extensive discussion of forages and the factors affecting forage composition. Grains, byproduct feeds, protein supplements, vitamin supplements, and mineral supplements are also discussed. The effect of feed processing on nutrient digestibility and site of nutrient absorption is also reviewed. Chapter 9 describes feed additives that affect feed characteristics (such as colors, antioxidants, flavors, and pellet-binders), as well as additives that are intended to affect animal health.

The implementation of a successful feeding program depends on an accurate assessment of the nutritional value of the feed, as well as an understanding of the nutrient requirements of an animal. Therefore, Chapter 10 addresses feed analysis. This chapter reviews many of the analytical procedures currently available for feed analysis, with particular emphasis on carbohydrates and proteins. Chapter 10 includes a schematic that compares several systems used to classify carbohydrates in animal nutrition.

Chapter 11 reviews the existing literature pertaining to feeding behavior in horses and also provides guidelines for general considerations relating to feeding management. Included in this chapter is a discussion of factors affecting voluntary feed intake. This chapter also addresses the relationship between dietary management of horses and the excretion of nutrients into the environment. Chapter 12 covers several unique aspects of equine nutrition, such as feeding the orphan foal and feeding horses in very hot or very cold weather. Chapter 12 also addresses the interactions between feeding management and several disorders such as colic, laminitis, recurrent airway obstruction, polysaccharide storage myopathy, and gastric ulcer syndrome. The interaction between nutrition and developmental orthopedic disease is also discussed. A new addition to this publication is Chapter 13, which summarizes the existing information related to the feeding management of wild equids in captivity as well as donkeys.

The sixth revised edition of *Nutrient Requirements of Horses* concludes with Chapters 14 and 15, which cover ration formulation and the equations used to develop the computer program that accompanies this document. In addition, the document contains sample tables that list the nutrient requirements of selected types of horses, feed composition tables, and a table summarizing the composition of mare's milk. Users should recognize that many recommendations for ponies and draft horses have been extrapolated from data obtained using light horses. Therefore, it is suggested that the recommendations for ponies and draft horses be applied with discretion.

1

Energy

ENERGY SYSTEMS

Conceptual energy systems have been developed to partition and quantify the energy utilized by animals and the energy contained in feeds. The chemical energy in feeds may be partitioned into the portion that is recovered in product or tissue and the portion that is lost (Figure 1-1). Energy requirements of animals and the energy content of animal foods are expressed in calories in the United States. The energy requirements of horses are often expressed in terms of kilocalories (kcal) or megacalories (Mcal). Energy requirements may also be expressed in joules. One megacalorie is equivalent to 4.184 megajoules (MJ).

Gross Energy

The gross energy of a feed represents the amount of heat produced from the total combustion of that feed, as measured in a bomb calorimeter (NRC, 1998). The chemical composition of a feed will affect its gross energy. Lipids are higher in gross energy per unit weight than proteins or carbohydrates. The type of carbohydrate in a feed has minimal effect on the gross energy of a feed because the gross energy of a nonstructural carbohydrate such as starch is similar to the gross energy of a structural carbohydrate such as cellulose. Feeds that are composed mostly of minerals are very low in gross energy. The total amount of gross energy consumed by an animal is termed the intake energy (IE), as shown in Figure 1-1 (NRC, 1981).

Digestible Energy

The apparent digestible energy (DE) content of a ration is calculated by subtracting the gross energy in the feces from the gross energy (intake energy) consumed by an animal. The term "apparent" is used because some of the material excreted in the feces does not originate from the feed but from cells sloughed from the gastrointestinal tract and digestive secretions. The true DE of a feed may be calculated if fecal endogenous losses are known. Endogenous fecal energy losses are not routinely determined in studies with horses and thus most DE values represent apparent DE, not true DE.

Two factors that impact the amount of DE in a feed are the gross energy content of the feed and the digestibility of the energy-containing components. A feeding trial is the most accurate method of estimating the DE content of feeds. Digestible energy values for some common horse feeds have been determined using feeding trials, but the number of equine studies is limited compared to studies with other species. Prior to 1989, it was common to estimate the DE value of horse feeds from data compiled in other species (NRC, 1978). Because digestive processes vary among species of animals, the DE value of a feed also varies among species. For example, when fed to dairy cattle, alfalfa meal has a DE value of 2.6 Mcal/kg (NRC, 2001), but when fed to swine, the value is 1.83 Mcal/kg (NRC, 1998).

The NRC (1989) adopted the following equations for estimating DE content of horse feeds from the chemical composition of the feeds.

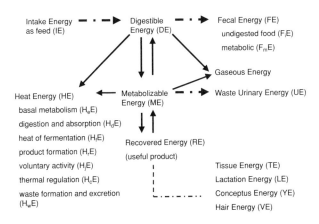

FIGURE 1-1 Energy flow diagram (NRC, 1981).

Dry Forages and Roughages, Pasture, Range Plants, and Forages Fed Fresh:
DE × (Mcal/kg) = 4.22 − 0.11 × (%ADF) + 0.0332 × (%CP) + 0.00112 × (%ADF^2)

Energy Feeds and Protein Supplements:
DE × (Mcal/kg) = 4.07 − 0.055 × (%ADF)

where ADF = acid detergent fiber and CP = crude protein. These equations were based on work by Fonnesbeck (1981) that summarized chemical and biological data from 108 digestion trials conducted with horses. Fonnesbeck (1981) did not report any of the characteristics of the specific feeds used in the digestion trials.

Using data from 30 different diets (120 observations), Pagan (1998) reported that DE could be estimated from the following equation:

DE × (kcal/kg DM) = 2,118 + 12.18 × (%CP) − 9.37 × (%ADF) − 3.83 × (%hemicellulose) + 47.18 × (%fat) + 20.35 × (%non-structural carbohydrate) − 26.3 (%ash); R^2 = 0.88

where hemicellulose = ADF − neutral detergent fiber (NDF) and nonstructural carbohydrate = (100 − %NDF − %Fat − %Ash − %CP).

DE content predicted by the equations from NRC (1989) and Pagan (1998) were reported to be similar for many feeds (Pagan, 1998). However, Pagan (1998) suggested that neither equation accurately predicted the DE content of some high-fiber feeds, and feeds that were high in fat. The DE of rice bran was measured to be 3.17 Mcal/kg (as fed basis), whereas the values estimated by the NRC (1989) and Pagan (1998) equations were 2.62 and 2.71 Mcal/kg (as fed basis), respectively (Pagan, 1998). Pagan (1998) suggested that DE values for feeds containing more than 5 percent fat could be adjusted by increasing the DE (as fed basis) by 0.044 Mcal/kg for each 1 percent fat above 5 percent. The measured DE value for beet pulp was approximately 20 percent higher than the value estimated from chemical composition (Pagan, 1998). The measured value for soybean hulls was approximately 42 percent higher than the value predicted by the Pagan (1998) equation and 52 percent higher than predicted by the NRC (1989) equation (Pagan, 1998). The Pagan (1998) and NRC (1989) equations overestimated the DE content of oat hulls by 55 and 27 percent, respectively. Zeyner and Kienzle (2002) have also developed an equation to estimate the DE content of horse feeds, using data from 170 digestion trials. The diets used to develop the equation ranged in composition from 5.7–28.7 percent crude protein, 4.2–34.7 percent crude fiber (CF), 33.8–69.8 percent nitrogen-free extract (NFE), and 1.6–7.9 percent acid ether extract (AEE). The equation derived by Zeyner and Kienzle (2002) to predict DE of horse feeds was:

DE (MJ/kg DM) = −3.6 + 0.211 × (%CP) + 0.421 × (%AEE) + 0.015 × (%CF) + 0.189 × (%NFE)

When the equation was tested using an additional set of observations not included in the original data set, there was no systematic deviation between the actual and predicted values for feeds containing less than 35 percent crude fiber and less than 8 percent AEE (DM basis). The relationship between predicted and actual values was given as r = 0.626 with a standard error (SE) of the regression equation of 1.012 (Zeyner and Kienzle, 2002). The authors stated that the DE content of feeds high in fat or highly fermentable fiber was somewhat underestimated, but specific values were not given.

For most cereal grains, cereal grain byproducts, and some other byproduct feeds (such as pulps), the equations developed by Pagan (1998) and by Zeyner and Kienzle (2002) to predict DE content do not appear to have any advantages over the equation previously used by the NRC (1989). However, the equation developed by Zeyner and Kienzle (2002) may predict DE content more accurately than the equations in the previous NRC (1989) edition for feeds high in fat. However, the equation derived by Zeyner and Kienzle (2002) utilizes chemical components of the diet that may not be available in current feed databases, such as acid ether extract, crude fiber, and nitrogen free extract.

The DE content of a ration or particular feed may not be constant across all situations. Diet digestibility may be affected by individual variation, exercise, and diet form (processing) (Hintz et al., 1985; Pagan et al., 1998). There is also potential for one feed component to affect the digestibility of another feed component. Kienzle et al. (2002) reported that the addition of concentrate to a diet consisting of poor quality roughage (straw) could increase the digestibility of the roughage. It was suggested that this associative effect was due to a positive effect of the concentrate on the ability of the microbial population to digest fiber. However, Martin-Rosset (2000) suggested that the ratio of forage to concentrate does not affect organic matter digestibility in horses. Adding fat to equine diets has been reported to reduce fiber digestibility in some experiments (Jansen et al., 2000, 2002), but not in others (Rich et al., 1981; Bush et al., 2001). A complete discussion of the effects of dietary fat can be found in Chapter 3. Energy digestibility of a specific feed may also be affected by differences among horses. Pagan and Hintz (1986a) reported that energy digestibility of a pelleted alfalfa-oat diet ranged from 58.8 percent to 65.8 percent among individual horses.

Metabolizable Energy

Metabolizable energy (ME) is calculated by subtracting urinary energy losses and gaseous losses from DE. Urinary and gaseous losses in the horse are smaller than fecal losses. When horses were fed a pelleted diet, approximately 87 percent of the DE was converted to ME (Pagan and Hintz, 1986a). The efficiency of DE conversion to ME will be influenced by the composition of the diet consumed (Vermorel et al., 1997a). Gaseous losses will be higher when feeds are digested in the large intestine. Vermorel et al. (1991) reported that the efficiency of DE conversion to ME was 90 percent for a mixed diet and 87 percent for a hay diet. When ponies were fed diets consisting primarily of oats, the efficiency of DE use for ME was greater than 90 percent (Kane et al., 1979).

Net Energy

Metabolizable energy is the starting point for net energy (NE) systems (Ferrell, 1988). Metabolizable energy may be transformed to recovered energy (RE) or to heat (Figure 1-1). Recovered energy includes energy stored in tissues (during pregnancy or weight gain) or secreted in a product (such as milk). Recovered energy may be designated as NE_r and may be further partitioned according to its specific type (lactation, growth, conceptus). Total heat production (HE) is the amount of energy lost to the environment. Total heat production may be partitioned into several components (NRC, 1981). The components of HE include:

H_eE = the heat associated with basal metabolism;
H_jE = the heat associated with voluntary activity;
H_cE = the heat of thermal regulation;
H_rE = the heat associated with product formation;
H_dE = the heat of digestion and absorption;
H_wE = the heat associated with waste formation and excretion;
H_fE = the heat of fermentation.

The term "heat increment" (H_iE) encompasses H_rE, H_dE, H_wE, and H_fE (NRC, 1981). In thermoneutral environments, when H_cE is zero, the metabolizable energy for maintenance (ME_m) includes H_jE, H_eE, and H_iE.

Because specific losses can be partitioned, NE systems have the potential to predict more accurately the ability of specific diets to meet the true energy needs of an animal. However, NE systems require more information and are more complicated than DE systems. The losses described above do not constitute a consistent proportion of the ME in feeds. For example, the energy costs associated with obtaining and chewing food can vary. The energy cost of eating various feeds has been reported to range from 1–28 percent of ME (Vermorel et al., 1997b). These losses might be accounted for as either H_jE or H_dE. The chemical composition of the energy-yielding components of ME will also influence the magnitude of the various losses from individual feeds. H_fE would be expected to be larger for feeds that are digested by microbial fermentation than for feeds assimilated through enzymatic digestion. Therefore, the NE value of a feed containing starch could vary depending upon whether the starch was digested and absorbed in the small intestine, or if it was fermented and absorbed as volatile fatty acids (VFAs). The NE value of a feed may also vary with its ultimate use in the body (maintenance, exercise, lactation). For example, in the NE system currently in use for dairy cattle, an individual feed may be assigned four different NE values (NRC, 2001). Information relating to the NE value of each feed for each specific function is considered one of the requirements of a useful NE system (NRC, 1981).

In the United States, NE systems have been developed for cattle (NRC, 2000, 2001), but the DE system has been used for horses (NRC, 1989). Work on an NE system for horses was initiated in France in the early 1980s. Kronfeld (1996) also proposed an approach to modeling NE that focuses primarily on the exercising horse. Although the two systems share some common characteristics, Harris (1997) pointed out that they make different assumptions about the efficiency of ME use of various fuels during exercise. In addition, the system proposed by Kronfeld (1996) did not encompass all physiological classes of horses or define NE values for horse feeds. At this time, the French system is the most fully developed NE system for horses. French horse-feeding standards are based on the Unite Fourragere Cheval (UFC; or horse feed unit) (Martin-Rosset et al., 1994; Vermorel and Martin-Rosset, 1997; Martin-Rosset, 2000; Martin-Rosset and Vermorel, 2004). The UFC system relates the NE requirements and the NE value of feeds to a standard unit derived from the NE value of 1 kg of barley (1 UFC = NE of 1 kg standard barley). The UFC system utilizes information about the gross energy and digestibility of horse feeds, the efficiency of DE conversion to ME (determined in horses), the expected proportions of energy supplied by absorbed nutrients, and estimates of the efficiency of ME utilization for those nutrients (Martin-Rosset et al., 1994; Vermorel and Martin-Rosset, 1997). In the French system the efficiency of converting ME to NE is estimated at 85 percent for glucose, 80 percent for long-chain fatty acids, 70 percent for amino acids, and 63–68 percent for VFAs. The French system also accounts for the energy cost of eating (Martin-Rosset, 2000) in assessing the efficiency of ME use for NE for various feeds. The French system has NE values for many common horse feeds, but it does not currently assign different values to feeds based on their efficiency of use for different physiological functions.

The advantages and disadvantages of applying NE or DE systems in equine nutrition have been discussed elsewhere (Hintz and Cymbaluk, 1994; Harris, 1997; Martin-Rosset, 2000; Cuddeford, 2004). Net energy systems provide a more complete theoretical basis for matching the energy content of feeds to the energy requirements of specific animals. Harris (1997) concluded that NE systems better explain the values of various feeds for exercising horses, as a DE system may overestimate the value of forage compared to grains or fats. However, a system based on NE would be more complex than a system based on DE as it accounts for more losses, many of which are interrelated. Cuddeford (2004) has suggested that because of its complexity, a NE system may not offer a major advantage over the DE system used in the NRC (1989) system. In France, the NE values of common feeds were related to the NE value of a standard, well-accepted feed (barley), creating a system where users can compare feeds on a substitution basis rather than on an absolute energy basis (Vermorel and Martin-Rosset, 1997). This substitution system may be more easily understood and applied in practical situations. Barley was chosen as the reference feed in the French system, but it might not be as widely accepted as the standard horse feed elsewhere in the world. In addition, the French system does not currently account for differences among feeds in their efficiency of use for different purposes. This concern may not be significant for situations in which maintenance requirements represent the majority of the daily energy needs. However, failure to account for differences in the efficiency of energy use for various physiological functions may induce errors into the estimates for certain types of horses, such as horses in heavy work or rapidly growing horses. Few studies have compared the two systems in practice, although several authors made comparisons based on theoretical diets. Hintz and Cymbaluk (1994) found that the estimated amount of feed required by broodmares as calculated using the UFC system was similar to the amount calculated using the DE system in the 1989 NRC system. Martin-Rosset and Vermorel (2004) calculated that a diet of hay, barley, and soybean meal that met the DE requirements (NRC, 1989) of growing horses exceeded the NE requirement estimated by the UFC system by about 19 percent. Many feeding trials with different classes of horses and different types of feeds will be necessary to completely compare the effectiveness of the two systems.

Even though NE systems are more complex, they offer an opportunity to partition energy more completely in individual situations. NE systems have been well accepted and applied with success in other sectors of the livestock industry. The most fully developed NE system for horses has been created in France. However, the system still lacks information about the NE values of all feeds of all classes of horses. In addition, more information is needed to verify that diets based on UFC units meet the requirements for horses for different activities and physiological states. The DE system is retained in this document as the method for expressing the energy requirements of horses. The DE system is retained, in part, because the French UFC system is considered to be somewhat incomplete and because the use of barley as a reference unit is potentially confusing to individuals who do not use it as a common horse feed. This should not be taken as a criticism of the French UFC system, as it has many positive attributes and has advanced the understanding of energy use by horses. However, the DE system has a few practical advantages over the French UFC system. More is known about estimating the DE content of horse feeds from chemical composition. Most feeding experiments with horses in the United States (and perhaps the world) have expressed the dietary energy content on a DE basis. The DE system is more familiar to equine nutritionists, veterinarians, feed manufacturers, and horse owners.

ENERGY SOURCES

The following section provides a brief overview of energy sources used by the horse. More detailed discussions of carbohydrate, fat, and protein metabolism in horses can be found in Chapters 2, 3, and 4. A discussion of energy-yielding feedstuffs and information on the effect of feed processing on energy availability can be found in Chapter 8.

Adenosine triphosphate (ATP) is the major source of readily available chemical energy in cells. Cells generate ATP from the catabolism of carbohydrates, fats, and proteins. Carbohydrates and fats are the predominant sources of ATP under normal circumstances. The balance between carbohydrate and fat utilization may be influenced by the physiological status of the horse, feeding state, physical conditioning, and type of diet being consumed.

Glucose is the primary form of carbohydrate used for ATP production. Cells may obtain glucose from the circulation or from intracellular stores of glycogen. Glucose in the circulation may originate from hepatic gluconeogenesis, from hepatic glycogenolysis, or from food consumed and digested by the horse. Red blood cells and brain cells depend almost entirely on glucose as an energy source under normal circumstances. Other tissues may use fat as an energy source and, in some cases, amino acids. Amino acid catabolism may be accelerated during starvation, but in most other cases, amino acids are a relatively minor component of the energy used by the body.

Fat is the most abundant energy source in the body. The long-chain fatty acids utilized by cells may originate from recently consumed food, but most of the long-chain fatty acids that are oxidized for energy probably come from either intracellular stores or adipose tissue. The triglycerides in adipose tissue are broken down to long-chain fatty acids and glycerol that are released into the blood.

Short-chain (volatile) fatty acids can also be used for energy production. Most short-chain fatty acids originate from the large intestinal fermentation of carbohydrates. VFA production in the cecum may be sufficient to meet up to 30 percent of a horse's energy needs at maintenance (Glinsky et al., 1976). Additional VFAs are produced in the colon. It has been estimated that horses consuming a diet composed primarily of hay will meet more than 80 percent of their energy needs from VFAs (Vermorel et al., 1997a). VFAs may be available as energy sources to cells or they may be metabolized to long-chain fatty acids or glucose. After measuring blood acetate concentrations and estimating blood flow, Pethick et al. (1993) suggested that acetate oxidation might contribute about 30 percent of the energy utilized by the hind limb at rest. Acetate that is not oxidized for energy could be converted to long-chain fatty acids and stored in adipose tissue, or converted to long-chain fatty acids for secretion into milk. Acetate is the predominant VFA produced in the large intestine, but significant amounts of propionate are also generated. Lieb (1971) demonstrated that a large portion of propionate infused into the cecum does not pass the liver. In addition, Argenzio and Hintz (1970) demonstrated that propionate infusion can elevate blood glucose levels in fasted ponies. More recent work has suggested that up to 50–60 percent of circulating glucose in forage-fed ponies originates from absorbed propionate (Simmons and Ford, 1991).

Excess energy consumed by horses can be stored as glycogen or as triglyceride. It is most efficient to immediately utilize absorbed energy sources because there is an energetic cost of storing, and then mobilizing, endogenous energy sources. These energy costs are included in H_dE—the heat production associated with digestion and absorption. It has been estimated that the energy cost of incorporating glucose into glycogen for later use is about 5 percent (Blaxter, 1989). However, if glucose is metabolized for the synthesis of long-chain fatty acids and then the long-chain fatty acids are oxidized, the energy cost is greater (Blaxter, 1989). McMiken (1983) estimated that a 500-kg horse with 5 percent body fat would have almost 10 times more calories stored in fat than in glycogen. However, several studies have reported the body fat of horses to be greater than 10 percent of body weight (Robb et al., 1972; Schryver et al., 1974; Westervelt et al., 1976; Lawrence et al., 1986; Kane et al., 1987). Therefore the amount of energy stored as fat can vary among individuals. Several indirect methods have been used to estimate body fat percentage in horses. Westervelt et al. (1976) reported that rump fat thickness as determined by ultrasound was related to percent extractable fat in the carcass. Kane et al. (1987) also reported a relationship between ultrasonically determined rump fat thickness and percent body fat in horses. These studies used small numbers of animals, and effects due to breed, gender, and age were not investigated. However, in the absence of more comprehensive studies validating indirect estimates of body fat in horses, many subsequent studies have utilized the methods described by Westervelt et al. (1976) or Kane et al. (1987) to estimate body fat in sedentary and athletic horses. These indirect estimates indicate body fat in mature, sedentary horses in moderate or fleshy body condition may exceed 15 percent (Kubiak et al., 1987; Kearns et al., 2002a), while the body fat of competitive endurance horses was estimated at less than 11 percent (Lawrence et al., 1992b). Similarly, Kearns et al. (2002b) estimated that the body fat of elite harness racing horses was approximately 8 percent, and Webb et al. (1987) reported an estimated body fat in cutting horses of 12 percent.

ENERGY REQUIREMENTS

Maintenance

Animals that are not pregnant, lactating, growing, or performing work are often considered to be in a physiological state of maintenance. The amount of dietary energy needed to prevent a change in the total energy contained in the body of these animals can be considered the maintenance requirement.

Maintenance energy requirements have been estimated in mature horses using a variety of methods, including indirect calorimetry, metabolic balance trials, and simple feeding trials. In addition, maintenance energy requirements have been expressed on a body weight basis and on a metabolically scaled basis, usually $BW^{0.75}$ or $BW^{0.67}$. The convention of expressing energy requirements on a metabolically scaled basis was established to account for differences in the relationship of surface area to body weight in animals of widely differing sizes. However, because many other nutrient requirements are expressed on a body weight basis, it is convenient to express energy requirements on a body weight basis as well. In addition, Pagan and Hintz (1986a) concluded that maintenance energy requirements varied linearly with body weight for equids weighing 125 to 856 kg. The previous edition of this document used the results of Pagan and Hintz (1986a) as a reason to express daily energy requirements on a body weight basis. It is recognized that their study utilized a small number of horses. However, in the absence of a study illustrating the benefits of using a metabolically scaled body weight, energy requirements calculated in this document will be calculated on a body weight basis.

A number of studies have estimated the amount of ME required by adult horses or ponies at maintenance by measuring daily heat production. The components of daily heat production are shown in Figure 1-1. Studies that have measured heat production in horses have utilized a variety of methods. These studies have used all forage as well as mixed diets and results have been reported on either a metabolically scaled basis or on a body weight basis. Data from several studies are summarized in Table 1-1 (Wooden et al., 1970; Pagan and Hintz, 1986a; Martin-Rosset and Vermorel, 1991; Vermorel et al., 1991; Vermorel et al., 1997a). When studies reported results on a metabolic body weight basis, these values were converted to a body weight basis using the body weights reported in the study. When data were reported for individual horses, the values were averaged to provide a mean value for a particular diet or feeding level. The average heat production ranged from 22.2 to 30.6 kcal/kg BW across treatments and studies. The digestible energy for maintenance (DE_m) was calculated using the efficiency of DE use for ME reported for each diet within each study. The DE_m estimated across studies ranged from 25.7 to 35.1 kcal/kg BW.

It is not surprising that variation exists in the estimated values of DE_m that are reported by different studies. Coenen (2000) suggested that the DE requirements for maintenance range from 0.48 to 0.62 MJ/kg $BW^{0.75}$/day (d) (approximately 24.3 to 31.4 kcal/kg BW/d for a 500-kg horse). Some of the factors that can affect maintenance requirements are discussed below. Within a study, heat production is often higher when the diet consists of hay than when mixed diets are fed (Table 1-1). Higher fiber diets would increase H_fE; it

TABLE 1-1 Summary of Studies that Measured Heat Production in Horses at Maintenance[a]

Author	Number of Animals	Type of Diet	Level of Feeding	BW (kg)	Heat Production kcal/kg BW	Efficiency DE/ME	DE_m
Pagan and Hintz, 1986a	4	Alfalfa and oats	Near maintenance	421.8 (125–856)	22.3	86.3	25.8
Pagan and Hintz, 1986a	4	Alfalfa and oats	Above maintenance	421.8 (125–856)	27.0	87.6	30.8
Pagan and Hintz, 1986a	4	Alfalfa and oats	Above maintenance	421.8 (125–856)	24.5	86.6	28.3
Wooden et al., 1970	2	Alfalfa and concentrate	Near maintenance	454.5 (413–496)	27.2	90.0	30.2
Wooden et al., 1970	2	Alfalfa and concentrate	Above maintenance	463.5 (417–510)	28.7	90.8	31.6
Vermorel et al., 1991	4	Meadow hay	Maintenance and above maintenance	490	29.7	87.2	34.1
Vermorel et al., 1991	4	Meadow hay and concentrate	Maintenance and above maintenance	470	28.6	90.0	31.8
Vermorel et al., 1997a	6	Grass hay and protein supplement	Below maintenance	475	30.6	87.2	35.1
Vermorel et al., 1997a	6	Grass hay and barley	Maintenance	475	28.3	90.1	31.4
Vermorel et al., 1997a	6	Grass hay	Maintenance	475	27.8	87.2	31.9
Vermorel et al., 1997a	6	Grass hay	Above maintenance	475	29.4	88.2	33.3
Vermorel et al., 1997a	6	Grass hay and barley	Maintenance	475	25.3	89.5	28.3
Vermorel et al., 1997a	6	Grass hay and barley	Above maintenance	475	25.4	90.5	28.1
Vermorel et al., 1997a	6	Grass hay	Above maintenance	475	27.6	89.1	31.0
Vermorel et al., 1997a	6	Grass hay and corn	Above maintenance	475	25.7	90.2	28.5
Vermorel et al., 1997a	6	Grass hay and beet pulp	Above maintenance	475	27.6	89.1	31.0
Vermorel et al., 1997a	6	Straw and concentrate	Above maintenance	475	26.1	89.9	29.0
Vermorel et al., 1997a	8	Alfalfa hay	Above maintenance	475	27.8	87.1	31.9
Vermorel et al., 1997a	8	Grass hay	Above maintenance	475	27.0	84.6	31.9
Vermorel et al., 1997a	8	Grass hay and corn	Above maintenance	475	26.3	89.7	29.3
Vermorel et al., 1997b	8	Grass hay and corn	Above maintenance	475	25.1	87.7	28.6
Vermorel et al., 1997b	6	Grass hay	Near maintenance	208	26.3	85.2	30.9
Vermorel et al., 1997b	6	Grass hay	Near maintenance	208	27.3	85.2	32.0
Vermorel et al., 1997b	6	Grass hay and corn	Near maintenance	208	22.2	86.4	25.7
Vermorel et al., 1997b	6	Grass hay and corn	Maintenance	208	23.5	87.7	26.8

[a]For several studies, values expressed as kcal/kg $BW^{0.75}$ were converted to a body weight basis.

is also possible that high-forage diets could increase tissue mass in the gastrointestinal tract, which would impact other components of HE. McLeod and Baldwin (2000) reported that lambs fed a high-forage diet at 2-times maintenance had heavier gut tissues than lambs fed an isocaloric high-concentrate diet. The gastrointestinal tract has a high metabolic rate, and, thus, an increase in gut size could account for elevated maintenance requirements in forage-fed animals. Potter et al. (1989) reported that less DE was needed to maintain body weight when horses were fed a fat-supplemented diet than when they were fed a diet with no supplemental fat. As noted previously, individual differences can exist among horses in their ability to digest energy; therefore, the horse-to-horse variation for DE_m could be relatively high. Differences may exist due to age and breed as well. Martin-Rosset and Vermorel (1991) found that ME_m requirements were lower for horses approximately 11 years old than for horses approximately 4 years old. Vermorel et al. (1997b) later reported that ME_m requirements of ponies were lower per unit of metabolic body size ($BW^{0.75}$) than for horses. Another source of variation could be body composition. Oxygen consumption is more closely related to lean body mass than to total body mass (Blaxter, 1989; Kearns et al., 2002a). Therefore, the energy cost of maintaining a 500-kg horse with a higher lean body mass may be different than the energy cost of maintaining a 500-kg horse with a lower lean body mass. The effect of body composition on maintenance requirements has been demonstrated in dairy cattle, where fasting heat production was inversely related to body condition score (Birnie et al., 2000).

It has been suggested that equations used to estimate maintenance requirements should be applied with considerations for factors such horse-to-horse variation, environment, and diet composition (NRC, 1989). Pagan and Hintz (1986a) noted that their estimates of maintenance requirements were based on measurements made while horses were confined to metabolism stalls in a thermoneutral environment. They suggested that estimates of maintenance requirements for horses kept in typical environments should include an adjustment for normal activity and proposed that the maintenance requirement could be estimated by DE (kcal/d) = 1,375 + (30 × BW). This equation was later modified by the NRC (1989) to DE (Mcal/d) = 1.4 + (0.03 × BW) for horses weighing 600 kg or less. For horses weighing more than 600 kg, maintenance DE was estimated from the equation (NRC, 1989): DE (Mcal/d) = 1.82 + (0.0383 × BW) − (0.000015 × BW^2).

The equations developed by Pagan and Hintz (1986a) and NRC (1989) provide estimates of the average maintenance requirements of horses of different body weights. They do not, however, give guidance on how to adjust the requirement for horses with needs above or below the average requirement.

When the studies in Table 1-1 are summarized, the mean estimate for DE_m is 30.3 kcal/kg BW/d. Stillions and Nelson (1972) estimated the daily DE_m of mature geldings at 33.8 kcal/kg BW, which was similar to the value determined by Anderson et al. (1983). Barth et al. (1977) estimated the daily DE_m for pony stallions at 39.6 kcal/kg BW. These studies used BW maintenance to estimate the DE requirement, and the estimates are higher than the mean value (30.3 kcal/kg BW) obtained from Table 1-1.

The mean daily DE_m derived from Table 1-1 (30.3 kcal DE/kg BW) was calculated from pooled data from horses and ponies that were confined during the experiments. Therefore, this value (30.3 kcal DE/kg BW) may be considered to represent the average minimum requirement for horses at maintenance. This average minimum maintenance requirement may be appropriate for horses that have a very sedentary lifestyle, either due to confinement or due to a docile, nonreactive temperament. Horses in this group might include older animals that live in stables or small pens with limited turnout, or horses that engage in limited voluntary activity even when kept in larger paddocks or pastures.

An estimate for DE_m for horses with average voluntary activity was obtained by increasing the minimum value by 10 percent to 33.3 kcal/kg BW. The average daily maintenance requirement of 33.3 kcal DE/kg (16.7 Mcal/500 kg BW horse/d) represents the needs of adult horses with alert temperaments and moderate voluntary activity. Horses in this group would probably be turned out for several hours per day but could include stabled horses that are active in their stalls. Examples of horses in this group might be open broodmares and some performance horses that are being rested.

A third estimate of DE_m was derived for adult horses with nervous temperaments or high levels of voluntary activity. Members of this group might include stallions or young adult horses that are noticeably active in their stalls or during periods of turnout. An elevated daily maintenance requirement of 36.3 Mcal DE/kg BW (18.2 Mcal DE/500 kg horse/d) was estimated by increasing the minimal requirement by approximately 20 percent.

The daily DE intakes of horses as determined using the estimates for minimum, average, and elevated maintenance are compared to the recommendations from NRC (1989) in Table 1-2. The average maintenance requirement of 33.3 kcal/kg BW results in a daily DE requirement that is very similar to the previous requirement for 500-kg horses (NRC, 1989). The average daily requirement of 33.3 kcal/kg BW results in a lower daily requirement for ponies than the previous recommendation (NRC, 1989), which appears to be consistent with work of Vermorel et al. (1997a). However, the requirement of 33.3 kcal/kg BW/d is higher than the previous estimate for draft horses (NRC, 1989) and is not consistent with Potter et al. (1987), who estimated the maintenance DE requirement of draft horses to be 24.6 kcal/kg BW. This estimate was derived from the relationship of weight gain to DE intake (Potter et al., 1987), and the authors noted that their methodology could have underestimated DE intake of some horses. Morrison (1961) recommended that idle draft horses (818 kg) receive 11 to 13.4 lb (5 to 6.1 kg) of total digestible nutrients (TDN) per day. If 1 kg of TDN contains 4.4 Mcal DE (NRC, 1978), then the Morrison (1961) recommendation for 818-kg horses would be equivalent to 22 to 26.8 Mcal DE/d or 26.9 to 32.8 kcal/kg BW. It is possible that the minimum maintenance estimate (30.3 kcal/kg BW) should be applied to idle draft horses.

The minimum and elevated values given here should not be considered to be the absolute minimum or maximum that would be appropriate for a specific animal. Many studies estimated DE_m to be lower than 30.3 kcal/kg BW (Table 1-1). Several of the values in Table 1-1 were obtained with diets fed above maintenance. However, other values were obtained with diets containing more concentrate than would commonly be fed to maintenance horses. Therefore, it is suggested that the minimum, average, and elevated values be used as guides in formulating diets for maintenance horses and that adjustments be made to meet individual situations.

TABLE 1-2 Three Proposed Levels of Digestible Energy Intake for Maintenance (Mcal/d) in Adult Horses as Compared to the Previous Recommendation (NRC, 1989)

Body weight (kg)	Minimum (30.3 kcal/kg BW)	Average (33.3 kcal/kg BW)	Elevated (36.3 kcal/kg BW)	NRC (1989)
200	6.1	6.7	7.3	7.4
400	12.1	13.3	14.5	13.3
500	15.2	16.7	18.2	16.4
600	18.2	20.0	21.8	19.4
800	24.2	26.6	29.0	22.9

Effect of Environment on Maintenance Requirements

Horses are adaptable to wide temperature ranges and thrive in many diverse climatic conditions. The five climatic variables that affect horses are ambient temperature, wind velocity, global solar radiation, precipitation, and relative humidity. The main climatic factor affecting thermoregulation is ambient temperature, which affects insensible (evaporative) and sensible heat (convection, conduction, and radiation) exchange. However, the impact of climate on horse productivity is not a one-factor model but is the combined effect of all climatic factors, often called the effective ambient temperature. A model has been proposed that integrates the effect of the climatic factors on heat balance of exercised horses (Mostert et al., 1996), but to date no useful five-factor index has been developed that will predict nutritional needs created by climatic influences. The two-factor index of ambient temperature and wind velocity called windchill was highly correlated to weight gain of young horses (Cymbaluk and Christison, 1989).

Horses are homeotherms and must maintain a nearly constant body core temperature. Cold or hot weather can cause body core temperature to decrease or increase, respectively. The horse responds to cold or heat through acute or chronic physiologic, metabolic, and behavioral responses. During sudden cold spells, horses respond by eating more to increase metabolic heat production and by postural changes to reduce heat loss (Booth, 1998). Chronic metabolic responses to cold involve longer feeding periods, increased hair coat, decreased rectal temperature, and decreased respiratory rate (Cymbaluk, 1990; Cymbaluk and Christison, 1993; Booth, 1998). Weanling horses housed at temperatures of about 1°C had 27 percent lower respiratory frequency, slightly lower heart rates, 20 percent more dense haircoats, and peripheral skin temperatures that were 8–15°C degrees lower than cohorts housed at 17°C (Cymbaluk and Christison, 1993). Metabolic responses by horses to acute heat exposure include an increased sweating rate, increased respiratory rate, decreased feed intake, and increased water intake (Geor et al., 1996; Morgan, 1997; Morgan et al., 1997; Marlin et al., 2001).

Cold and heat stress occur at temperatures below and above (respectively) the thermoneutral zone (TNZ). The TNZ is the temperature range when metabolic heat production does not need to be increased to maintain thermostability (NRC, 1981). The TNZ itself consists of three divisions: cool, optimal, and warm. The lowest temperature of the TNZ is termed the lower critical temperature (LCT) and is the temperature below which metabolic heat production is increased to maintain body core temperature. The upper critical temperature (UCT) is the high temperature end of the TNZ and is the temperature above which evaporative heat loss must be increased to control body temperature. The TNZ, LCT, and UCT for horses vary with age, body condition, breed, season, adaptation, and climate (Table 1-3).

The ambient temperature to which the horse is accustomed determines its TNZ. The TNZ for Standardbred horses adapted to moderate (10°C) outdoor temperatures ranged from 5 to 25°C (Morgan et al., 1997; Morgan, 1998), whereas the TNZ for maintenance-fed adult horses acclimatized to cold outdoor winter temperatures was −15 to 10°C (McBride et al., 1985). Thus the LCT for adults can be 5°C in mild climates or as low as −15°C in mature horses adapted to very cold outdoor temperatures.

Young horses may be cold-stressed at milder temperatures than adult horses. The TNZ for cold-adapted yearling Quarter horses fed highly digestible diets was estimated at −10 to 10°C (Cymbaluk and Christison, 1989). However, in a subsequent study, an LCT of 0°C was estimated for Standardbred yearlings (Cymbaluk, 1990). An LCT of about 20°C was determined for 2- to 9-day-old foals, but individual variability was wide. Below the LCT, foals had an increased metabolic rate, shivering, and piloerection (Ousey et al., 1992). However, neonates kept at temperatures well below 20°C gained weight normally and remained healthy when shelter, bedding, and feed were plentiful (Cymbaluk et al., 1993). The UCT for newborn foals was determined to be about 36–40°C (Ousey et al., 1992). The UCT for adult horses is harder to establish because various indices can be used to define this criterion but each index has a different temperature threshold (Morgan, 1998). In Table 1-3, the UCT is based on an increase in evaporative heat loss. Unlike other species, idle horses exposed to temperatures above UCT thermoregulate principally through evaporative heat loss, i.e., by sweating and/or by breathing more rapidly.

Full acclimation by horses to either hot or cold ambient temperatures appears to take about 21 days, although considerable acclimation has occurred by 10–14 days after heat or cold exposure. Acclimation of exercised horses to hot weather occurred largely within 14–15 days with minor improvement in response over the next week (Geor et al., 1996; Marlin et al., 1999; Geor et al., 2000). However, the retention time of heat (or cold) acclimation is uncertain. Based on data collected from a small number of grazing horses, acclimation to short-term thermal stress (cold or warm) was cyclic occurring in a time series manner over 10–11 days (Senft and Rittenhouse, 1985). Thus, the temperature values for the LCT and UCT are dynamic.

Temperature stress or exposure to ambient temperatures at which the horse is unacclimated will alter the resting metabolic rate. Adult horses with an LCT of −15°C that were acclimated to winter temperatures had an average hourly metabolic rate of about 102.9 kcal/100 kg BW at temperatures in their TNZ (McBride et al., 1985). As ambient temperatures decreased below −10°C, hourly metabolic rates increased linearly to 117.9 kcal/100 kg BW at −20°C, to 146.9 kcal/100 kg BW at −30°C, and to 181.6 kcal/kg BW at −40°C. It was concluded that DE intakes of adult horses at maintenance should be raised 2.5 percent for each degree

TABLE 1-3 Lower and Upper Critical Temperatures in Horses[a]

Life Stage	Lower Critical Temperature (°C) Average	Range	Upper Critical Temperature (°C)	Feed Intake Level	Exposure Type	Reference
2–4 days	22	16–26	36	Suckle; limited	Acute cold	Ousey et al., 1992
7–9 days	19	13–23	~40	Suckle	Acute cold	Ousey et al., 1992
Yearling	0	Unknown	Not determined	2 × maintenance	Acclimated	Cymbaluk, 1990
Yearling	–11	Unknown	Not determined	2–2.5 × maintenance	Acclimated	Cymbaluk and Christison, 1993
Mature	–15	–20 to –9.4	Not determined	Maintenance	Acute or acclimated	McBride et al., 1985
Mature	5	Unknown	25	Maintenance	Acute cold or heat	Morgan et al., 1997; Morgan, 1998

[a]SOURCE: Adapted from Cymbaluk (1994).

Celsius below the LCT (McBride et al., 1985). Cymbaluk and Christison (1990) suggested that the maintenance requirement of growing horses was increased by about 33 percent in cold housing conditions (–15°C) and by more than 50 percent in severely cold conditions (–25°C). Therefore, it may be appropriate to increase the total DE intake of growing horses by 1.3 percent for each degree Celsius below the LCT (Cymbaluk, 1990). As noted previously, the entire climatic effect on horses encompasses more than just temperature and includes other conditions such as rain or wind. Horses exposed to cold and wet conditions have been reported to have DE requirements elevated as much as 50 percent above maintenance (Kubiak et al., 1987). Maintenance energy needs are expected to increase when horses are exposed to conditions above the UCT. However, the magnitude of this increase has not been quantified.

Because heat production can be affected by feed intake and feed composition, the type and amount of feed may assist the horse in coping with cold or heat stress. Pagan and Hintz (1986a) reported that heat production increased with increased feed intake. However, in that study, increased DE intake was coupled with increased feed intake, so it is not clear whether heat production increased as a result of increased dry matter intake or increased DE intake. In another study, feeding at 1.3 times maintenance increased heat output by 0.39-fold (Vernet et al., 1995). Ponies fed a 70:30 hay-grain diet at maintenance feeding levels had a lower daily maintenance heat production compared to an all-hay diet (Vermorel et al., 1997b). However, weanling horses fed high-hay or high-grain diets and kept at either warm (17°C) or cold (0°C) temperatures showed no difference in energy utilization or gain (Cymbaluk and Christison, 1993). Similarly, heat production did not differ when horses were fed either hay or hay-grain diets at maintenance levels (Vernet et al., 1995).

In hot weather conditions, the feeding program for idle horses should be designed to minimize heat load. Although high-fat diets may prove potentially useful in reducing heat load in hot weather (Kronfeld, 1996; Ott, 2005), few studies have critically examined the metabolic effects of high-fat diets on thermoregulation of idle horses in hot weather conditions. Less DE may be needed to maintain body weight when horses are fed a fat-supplemented diet than when they are fed a diet with no supplemental fat (Potter et al., 1989). By lowering DE intake, a decrease in heat production, and thus heat load might be expected.

GROWTH

Energy Requirements for Maintenance and Gain

The energy requirement of a growing horse is the sum of the energy needed for maintenance and the energy needed for gain. The daily DE requirement was previously estimated by the following equation (NRC, 1989):

$$DE (Mcal/d) = (1.4 + 0.03 \times BW) + (4.81 + 1.17X - 0.023X^2) \times ADG$$

where X = age in months; BW = body weight in kilograms; and ADG = average daily gain in kilograms. There is good agreement between actual energy intakes that have been reported in several studies and the energy intakes predicted by this equation (Figure 1-2). The studies that were reviewed for Figure 1-2 were Ott et al. (1979); Knight and Tyznik (1985); Ott and Asquith (1986); Gibbs et al. (1987); Schryver et al. (1987); Cymbaluk and Christison (1989); Cymbaluk et al. (1989); Davison et al. (1989); Scott et al.

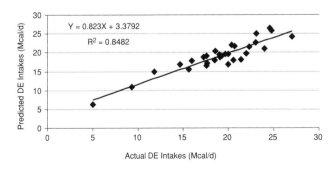

FIGURE 1-2 Comparison of digestible energy (DE) intakes of growing horses as predicted by NRC (1989) and actual intakes reported in the literature.

(1989); Buffington et al. (1992); Saastamoinen et al. (1993); Ott and Asquith (1995); Coleman et al. (1997); Ousey et al. (1997); Cooper et al., (1999); Ott and Kivipelto, (1999); Bell et al. (2001); and Ott et al. (2005).

In the equation developed in 1989 (NRC, 1989), the energy required for maintenance in growing horses was estimated using the same method as the energy required for maintenance in adult horses. This equation predicts that maintenance requirements on a body weight basis will be somewhat higher for a 200-kg weanling (37 kcal/kg BW) than for a 500-kg horse (32.8 kcal/kg BW). Coenen (2000) suggested the maintenance requirement of growing horses decreases from 210 kcal/kg $BW^{0.75}$ at 3 to 6 months of age to 151 kcal/kg $BW^{0.75}$ for horses between 13 and 18 months of age. Horses older than 18 months were estimated to have maintenance requirements similar to mature horses (Coenen, 2000). Using the estimates of Coenen (2000), the maintenance component for a 200-kg weanling would be about 56 kcal/kg BW. In addition, Arieli et al. (1995) determined that heat production in young calves ranged from 105 to 130 kcal/kg $BW^{0.75}$, which is much higher than estimated fasting heat production in mature cows (NRC, 2001). Ousey et al. (1997) estimated the daily net energy for maintenance (NE_m) of neonatal foals at about 67 kcal/kg BW. They also estimated that the conversion of DE to NE was greater than 95 percent in milk-fed foals. In limit-fed and ad libitum–fed growing horses (6–24 months of age), Cymbaluk et al. (1989) reported maintenance requirements to be 37.8 and 35.6 kcal DE/kg BW, respectively. The horses in that study were kept in a barn with 6 hours of daily turnout exercise. Mean daily temperature during the study was above freezing, but minimum and maximum temperatures ranged from −20.6 to 26.6°C. In that study, the maintenance component of the daily energy requirement may have been elevated due to environmental effects, but other factors such as increased voluntary activity and increased ratio of surface area to body weight could also result in an increased maintenance component in young horses. Figure 1-3 shows the effect of age on DE_m when the values from Ousey et al. (1997) and Cymbaluk et al. (1989) are combined with estimates for 24- and 36-month-old horses of 36.3 and 33.3 kcal/kg BW, respectively. These values for horses at 24 and 36 months are the same as the elevated and average maintenance requirements derived for mature horses.

Based on the values shown in Figure 1-3, DE_m for growing horses may be estimated using the following equation:

$$DE \text{ (kcal/kg BW/d)} = 56.5X^{-0.145} \ (R^2 = 0.99) \quad (1\text{-}1)$$

where X = age in months. This equation appears to fit the available data well, but it is based on very few data points, and therefore may under- or overestimate DE_m in growing horses. However, the estimates derived by Equation 1-1 for growing horses between the ages of 6 and 18 months are only slightly higher than estimates that would be derived from scaling the maintenance requirements of growing horses to metabolic body size. Therefore, the estimates of maintenance derived by Equation 1-1 are used in this document for growing horses. Additional research is needed to provide accurate estimates of the maintenance component for horses of different ages.

To obtain estimates of the amount of DE required for each kilogram of gain, data from several studies were summarized (Ott et al., 1979; Knight and Tyznik, 1985; Ott and

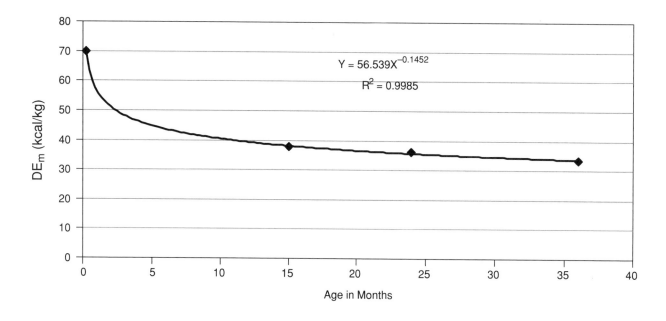

FIGURE 1-3 Effect of age on digestible energy for maintenance (DE_m) (kcal/kg BW) in growing horses.

Asquith, 1986; Gibbs et al., 1987; Schryver et al., 1987; Cymbaluk and Christison, 1989; Cymbaluk et al., 1989; Davison et al., 1989; Scott et al., 1989; Buffington et al., 1992; Saastamoinen et al., 1993; Ott and Asquith, 1995; Coleman et al., 1997; Ousey et al., 1997; Cooper et al., 1999; Ott and Kivipelto, 1999; Bell et al., 2001; Ott et al., 2005). For each study the maintenance requirement (determined using Equation 1-1) was subtracted from DE intake to obtain the DE available for gain. The amount of DE available for gain was then divided by ADG to arrive at the energy cost (DE) for 1 kg of gain. Figure 1-4 shows the relationship of age to the amount of DE required per kilogram of gain. It is apparent in Figure 1-4 that there is considerable variation in the amount of DE needed for a kilogram of gain at any age. There are several potential explanations for the observed variation in DE required per kilogram of gain. The DE required for each unit of body weight gain will be influenced by the composition of the gain (amount of fat and protein). Not all horses at a given age were growing at the same rate, and it is possible that rate of gain influenced composition of gain. In addition, gender may influence composition of gain. Most studies did not separate their results by gender. In addition, the composition of the diet may contribute to differences in the amount of DE required per kilogram of gain. The efficiency of DE use in high-forage diets may be lower than the efficiency of DE use when high-concentrate diets are fed. In the studies that were reviewed, the composition of the diets varied from milk replacer to predominantly concentrate to predominantly forage. Some diets contained added fat. Finally, the amount of DE utilized for gain for horses in each study was determined as the difference between the maintenance component and the DE intake. The maintenance component was related to age only and did not account for differences in activity or thermal challenges that might have occurred in the various studies. There was insufficient information to determine effects due to gender and there was only one value for horses older than 18 months. This equation may underestimate the DE required for gain in animals more than 18 months of age. Using the data in Figure 1-4, Equation 1-2 was obtained. Because Equation 1-2 was developed from mean values reported in the literature and not from observations on individual horses, it is likely that the R^2 is overestimated:

DE (Mcal) for gain = $(1.99 + 1.21X - (0.021X^2)) \times$ (1-2)
ADG ($R^2 = 0.65$)

where X = age in months and ADG = average daily gain in kilograms.

Using Equation 1-2, the amount of energy required for gain by growing horses of different ages may be estimated. The predicted amount of DE necessary for 1 kg of gain increases from 6 months to 24 months of age (Table 1-4). This equation is not appropriate for predicting the DE necessary for gain in mature horses. For young growing horses, the values for DE/kg gain in Table 1-4 are somewhat lower than the values suggested previously (NRC, 1989).

Growth Rate

The daily energy requirements for growing horses are greatly influenced by the rate of growth of the animal. Growth rate often varies among breeds or types in cattle and swine, and nutrient recommendations have been developed to account for some of these differences (NRC, 1998, 2001). Extensive, well-documented growth data are available for Thoroughbreds (Green, 1969; Hintz et al., 1979; Ruff et al., 1993; Thompson, 1995; Jelan et al., 1996; Pagan et al.,

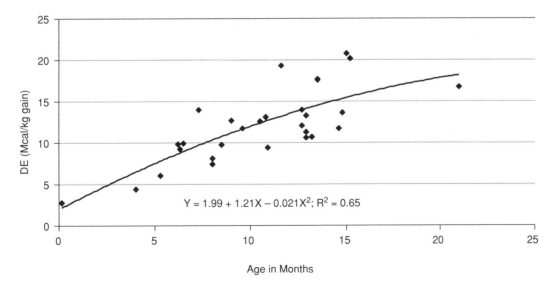

FIGURE 1-4 Relationship between age (in months) and the amount of digestible energy (DE) (Mcal) required above maintenance per kilogram of gain in growing horses.

TABLE 1-4 Effect of Age on the Amount of Digestible Energy (DE) Required per Kilogram of Gain (above maintenance) for Growing Horses

Age of Horse	DE for Gain (Mcal/kg gain)
6 months	8.5
12 months	13.5
18 months	17.0
24 months	18.9

1996; Kavazis and Ott, 2003), but the available data for other breeds are less comprehensive or entirely absent. Growth data were found for Hanovarians (Vervuert et al., 2003), Morgan horses (Lawrence et al., 2003), Swedish Standardbreds (Sandgren et al., 1993), Arabians (Reed and Dunn, 1977), and ponies (Jordan, 1977). No recent data sets containing sequential body weight measurements were found for Quarter horses, but numerous studies have reported body weights at different ages (Russell et al., 1986; Davison et al., 1989; Lawrence et al., 1987, 1991; Coleman et al., 1997). Some of the studies cited above separated growth information by gender, but others did not.

Because of the limited data available for most breeds, it was not possible to develop breed-specific growth curves at this time. However, it has been proposed that the body weight of a growing horse at any given age can be predicted from mature body weight (Coenen, 2000; Austbo, 2004), which would allow prediction of growth rate for horses of different breeds and mature body weights. This method would also allow prediction of differences between males and females based on expected differences in mature body weight.

Body weight data for growing horses were summarized by breed using previously cited growth studies and a few additional unpublished data sets on Quarter horses (Cooper, personal communication; Cymbaluk, personal communication) and Belgian foals (Cymbaluk, personal communication). Mature weights were estimated from the body weights of sires and dams cited in individual studies (Jordan, 1977) or from the mature weight given in the study (Reed and Dunn, 1977). When mature weights were not available for a specific study, the literature was searched for estimates of mature body weights in each breed. The mature body weight for Thoroughbreds was developed from body weights of broodmares and stallions (Siciliano et al., 1993; Pagan et al., 1996; Ordakowski et al., 2001; Williams et al., 2001). Mature body weight for Quarter horses was developed from body weights of mares (Webb et al., 1991; Lawrence et al., 1992a; Coleman et al., 1997; Cymbaluk, personal communication). Mature body weight for Swedish Standardbreds was estimated from data of Malinowski et al. (2002) and Palmgren Karlsson et al. (2002). No mature weights were found for Morgan or Hanovarian horses. Therefore, mature body weight for Morgan horses was obtained from the same farm that provided the growth measurements of the Morgan horses (Green, personal communication). Mature body weights for Swedish warmbloods (Johnston et al., 2002) were used to estimate the mature weight of Hanovarians. The following mature body weights (Kg) were used: Thoroughbred, 580; Hanovarian, 580; Swedish Standardbred, 500; Quarter horse, 555; Belgian, 863; Morgan, 454; Arabian, 455; pony, 195.

Once mean growth data for each breed were converted to a percentage of mature body weight, the data were fitted to a curve. The NLIN procedure of the Statistical Analysis System (SAS) (SAS/STAT, 1999) was used to calculate weighted least squares estimates of parameters a and c of the following non-linear model:

Percent mature body weight = a + ((100 − a) (1 − e^{-ct}))

where a = percent mature body weight at birth; c = rate constant; t = age in months; e = 2.7183. The resulting equation was derived:

$$Y = 9.7 + (100 - 9.7) \times (1 - (e^{(-0.0772 \times X)})) \ (R^2 = 0.99) \quad (1\text{-}3)$$

where Y = percent mature body weight and X = months of age. Equation 1-3 was derived from mean data that were pooled within a breed, and not from observations on individual horses. Therefore the R^2 given for Equation 1-3 is probably overestimated.

The percent of mature body weight predicted by Equation 1-3 is compared to the estimates of Austbo (2004) and Coenen (2000) in Table 1-5.

Equation 1-3 may be used to calculate expected body weight during growth if an estimate of mature body weight is available. Table 1-6 shows body weights predicted by Equation 1-3 for growing horses expected to mature at 200, 400, 500, 600, and 900 kg. Table 1-6 also shows the body weights previously suggested for horses of various ages (NRC, 1989). Equation 1-3 predicts slightly lower body weights at most ages for growing horses expected to mature at 500 kg or less than NRC (1989). However, Equation 1-3 tends to predict larger body weights during growth than NRC (1989) for horses 600 kg and greater. Body weights in NRC (1989) appear to have been scaled to assume a longer

TABLE 1-5 Summary of Estimates of the Relationship Between Age and Percentage of Mature Body Weight in Growing Horses

	Birth	6 mo	9 mo	12 mo	18 mo
Equation 1-3	9.7	43.2	54.9	64.2	77.5
Coenen, 2000[a]	9.95	46.2	56.4	64.2	75.9
Austbo, 2004	10.0	47.0	58.0	67.0	82.0

[a]500-kg horse.

TABLE 1-6 Body Weight Predicted by Equation 1-3 and Expected Mature Body Weight and Body Weight Estimated in the Previous NRC (1989) for Growing Horses (values in parentheses represent % of mature body weight)

Mature Wt/Age		NRC (1989)	Equation 1-3
200 kg	4 mo	75 (37.5%)	67.4 (33.7%)
	6 mo	95	86.4
	12 mo	140	128.5
	18 mo	170	155
	24 mo	185 (92.5%)	172 (86%)
	36 mo	No value	189
400 kg	4 mo	145 (36.3%)	134.8 (33.6%)
	6 mo	180	173
	12 mo	265	257
	18 mo	330	310
	24 mo	365 (91.2%)	343.4 (85.9%)
	36 mo	No value	379
500 kg	4 mo	175 (35%)	168.5 (33.7%)
	6 mo	215	215.9
	12 mo	325	321.2
	18 mo	400	387.5
	24 mo	450 (90%)	429.2 (86%)
	36 mo	No value	472
600 kg	4 mo	200 (33.3%)	202.1 (33.7%)
	6 mo	245	259
	12 mo	375	385.5
	18 mo	475	465
	24 mo	540 (90%)	515 (86%)
	36 mo	No value	566.4
900 kg	4 mo	275 (30.6%)	303.2 (33.7%)
	6 mo	335	388.6
	12 mo	500	578.2
	18 mo	665	697.5
	24 mo	760 (84.4%)	773 (85.9%)
	36 mo	No value	850

maturation curve for heavy-weight horses. For example, NRC (1989) estimated that a foal expected to mature at 200 kg would have reached 37.5 percent of mature weight at 4 months of age, whereas a foal expected to mature at 900 kg would have reached 30.6 percent of mature body weight at the same age. The data sets used to develop Equation 1-3 were insufficient to determine whether large breeds mature more rapidly than small breeds using statistical analyses. However, there were a few data points for ponies, Thoroughbreds, and draft horses at similar ages. The percentage of mature weight at 4 months of age was 33.3 percent, 33.7 percent, and 32.2 percent, for ponies, Thoroughbreds, and Belgians, respectively. At 6 months of age, percentage of mature weight was 42 percent for ponies and 42.4 percent for Thoroughbreds (data not available for draft horses). At 12 months of age, percentage of mature weight was 75 percent for ponies and 69 percent for Thoroughbreds (data not available for draft horses). The similarity of the available values, particularly in early growth, indicates that one curve may be used for a variety of breeds. However, it is likely that

Equation 1-3 is best suited to estimating weight of horses with an expected mature weight of 450 to 650 kg.

The ability of Equation 1-3 to predict body weight in growing horses was tested using three independent data sets that contained 550 measurements on horses between birth and 16 months of age. Expected mature weight was calculated from dam weight and sire weight, from dam weight and the average weight of sire's breed, or from the breed average, depending upon the information contained in each data set. Horses included in the data sets were of Thoroughbred or stock-type (Quarter horse, Appaloosa, or Paint) breeding. For these data sets, the body weights predicted from expected mature body weight and Equation 1-3 and the actual body weights were not different for horses less than 9 months of age, or older than 12 months of age ($P > 0.05$). However, between 9 and 12 months of age, the average predicted body weight was higher ($P < 0.05$) than the actual body weight. Equation 1-3 predicts that ADG will decrease with age. However, data collected on horses in commercial environments do not always reflect this trend. Pagan et al. (1996) reported that ADG of Thoroughbred yearlings in central Kentucky was lower in January and February than in April and May, possibly due to milder temperatures and increased pasture availability in April and May. Rates of gain for Thoroughbreds in Japan have been reported to be 0.40 to 0.50 kg/d at 11 months and 0.4 to 0.7 kg/d at 13 to 15 months, with the slower growth observed in winter and the faster growth observed in summer (Asai, 2000). Staniar et al (2004) also reported a lag in growth during the winter months followed by accelerated growth in the spring for pastured Thoroughbred horses. Therefore, Equation 1-3 overestimates percent of mature body weight and ADG during the winter for pastured horses kept in northern climates and underestimates ADG in the subsequent spring. However, for horses with an expected mature body weight of 580 kg, the body weight and ADG predicted at 6 months and 15 months of age (250 kg and 415 kg, respectively) are similar to body weights reported by Pagan et al. (1996) for Thoroughbreds. In addition, the predicted weight at 16.5 months of age for horses expected to mature at 580 kg is similar to the actual weight reported by Staniar et al. (2004) for Thoroughbreds. Independent data for horses older than 16 months of age were not available to test Equation 1-3. However the body weight predicted by Equation 1-3 for an 18-month-old horse with an expected mature body weight of 580 kg was similar to the body weight reported for 18-month-old Thoroughbreds at a commercial sale (Pagan et al., 2005b).

Segmental models have also been used to predict growth in horses (Kavazis and Ott, 2003; Delobel et al., 2005). Segmental models may provide a better estimate of growth in horses affected by seasonal factors; however, it was the consensus of the Committee on Nutrient Requirements of Horses that it was more desirable to use a continuous model to predict growth. Therefore, Equation 1-3 is used in this document to estimate body weight and ADG of growing horses.

Ideally, ADG and body weight will be known for individual horses. However, when it is not possible to weigh horses, body weight and ADG may be estimated using the equations above. Although this prediction equation may be used to predict body weight and average daily gain of horses beyond 18 months of age, users should recognize that the imposition of training can markedly affect the accrual of body weight. In addition, horses used for intense competitive purposes, such as racing, will typically weigh less than a similarly aged horse used for breeding or for recreation. Because many of the values used to generate these prediction equations were obtained from commercial horse enterprises, this prediction equation should represent the average of modern-day growth rates. However, it is recognized that it may be desirable to accelerate growth rate to produce horses suitable for specific purposes such as competition or sale (NRC, 1989; Martin-Rosset, 2000). In addition slower growth rates may be suitable for horses that will not be utilized or marketed until they reach a later stage of maturity. Therefore, users should modify dietary nutrient intakes to attain the desired growth rate necessary to meet management goals.

Daily DE Intakes for Growing Horses

Daily DE requirements for growing horses are determined as the sum of the requirement for maintenance and the requirement for gain. As noted previously, the maintenance requirement will vary with age of horse and body weight (Equation 1-1). The requirement for gain will vary with age of horse and rate of gain (Equation 1-2). The daily DE requirement of growing horses can be calculated by combining Equation 1-1 and Equation 1-2 to form Equation 1-4:

$$DE \text{ (Mcal/d)} = (56.5X^{-0.145}) \times BW + (1.99 + 1.21X - 0.021X^2) \times ADG \quad (1\text{-}4)$$

where X = the age in months; ADG = average daily gain in kilogram; and BW = body weight in kilograms.

The relationship between predicted daily DE intakes and reported daily DE intakes from published studies is shown in Figure 1-5. Although Equation 1-4 appears to predict daily DE intakes of growing horses more closely than the equation used previously (NRC, 1989), this may be because the studies used to generate Figure 1-5 included those that were used to generate Equation 1-2, which is a component of Equation 1-4 (Ott et al., 1979; Knight and Tyznik, 1985; Ott and Asquith, 1986; Gibbs et al., 1987; Schryver at al., 1987; Cymbaluk and Christison, 1989; Cymbaluk et al., 1989; Davison et al., 1989; Scott et al., 1989; Buffington et al., 1992; Saastamoinen et al., 1993; Ott and Asquith, 1995; Coleman et al., 1997; Ousey et al., 1997; Cooper et al., 1999; Ott and Kivipelto, 1999; Bell et al., 2001; Ott et al., 2005). In addition, the values shown in Figure 1-5 represent means for groups of horses, rather than observations on individual horses. Therefore it is likely that the variation associated with differences in predicted and actual DE intakes of individual horses will be much greater than is illustrated by Figure 1-5. Unfortunately, independent data sets were not available to test this equation for individual horses.

REPRODUCTION

Breeding Stallions

Stallions are generally considered to have higher maintenance requirements than mares or geldings (Cuddeford, 2004; Martin-Rosset and Vermorel, 2004). The amount of dietary energy required in the breeding season will likely be affected by breeding frequency. Horses that make a few

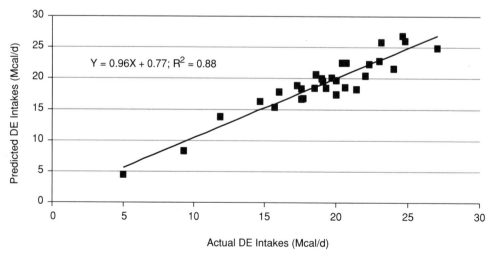

FIGURE 1-5 Digestible energy (DE) intakes of growing horses as predicted by Equation 1-4 and actual intakes reported in the literature.

mounts each week in live cover or artificial insemination programs would be expected to have lower energy requirements than horses that make more than a dozen mounts each week in intensively managed live cover programs. Limited data on DE intakes of breeding stallions are available. One field study estimated that Thoroughbred stallions (590 kg) covering 70 to 90 mares/month were receiving approximately 25 Mcal DE/d (42.4 kcal/kg BW) (Siciliano et al., 1993). This estimate is slightly higher than the recommendation of the previous edition of this publication (NRC, 1989), where the requirement for breeding stallions was considered to be equivalent to the requirement for light work. The DE requirement for breeding stallions in heavy use is estimated to be 20 percent higher than maintenance, and breeding stallions are considered to have an elevated maintenance requirement during the nonbreeding season (36.3 kcal/kg BW).

Pregnancy

During pregnancy, energy will be used for maintenance of the dam, deposition of fetal and placental tissue, hypertrophy of the uterus, mammary development, and maintenance of the fetus, placenta, mammary and additional uterine tissue. In studies with other livestock species, sacrifice of pregnant females has provided information about the amount of fetal, placental, and uterine tissue accumulated at various stages of gestation. In the pig, which also has a diffuse placenta, more than 50 percent of the final placental and uterine weight had accumulated by midgestation (Ji et al., 2005). At parturition, placental weight (without fluids) is about 4 kg for a 500-kg mare (Allen et al., 2002; Whitehead et al., 2004). The few measurements of uterine and placental tissue accretion in midgestation mares indicate that uterine and placental tissue accretion occurs during the second trimester (Ginther, 1992). If uterine development parallels placental development, then there would be an increase in uterine tissue of 4 kg during gestation. There are insufficient data to determine whether the rate of nonfetal tissue accretion during gestation follows a linear function in mares. However, Bell et al. (1995) reported that tissue accumulation in the gravid uterus of cows was a linear process. Therefore the rate of total nonfetal tissue accretion (uterus and placenta) in a 500 kg-horse is estimated at about 45 g/d (0.09 g/kg maternal BW/day) from day 150 through day 330 of gestation. Although the amount of nonfetal tissue accretion is not great, this tissue appears to be very active metabolically (Fowden et al., 2000a,b), and thus has a higher maintenance requirement per unit of weight.

The existing data on fetal development have been drawn from studies on foals that were aborted or stillborn between day 150 and term of gestation (Meyer and Ahlswede, 1978; Platt, 1978; Giussani et al., 2005). Using the data reported in these papers, the percent of birth weight accumulated during days 150 to 330 of gestation were calculated and are presented in Figure 1-6. Birth weight was estimated at 9.7 percent of dam weight.

Several equations were developed from the data in Figure 1-6. The resulting equations (where X = days of gestation) were:

Fetal weight as a percent of birth weight = (1-5a)
$0.5321X - 87.996$ ($R^2 = 0.855$)

Fetal weight as a percent of birth weight = (1-5b)
$2.456 + 0.0015X^2 - 0.2198X$ ($R^2 = 0.874$)

Fetal weight as a percent of birth weight = (1-5c)
$0.8875e^{0.0144X}$ ($R^2 = 0.903$)

Fetal weight as a percent of birth weight = (1-5d)
$1 \times 10^{-7}X^{3.5512}$ ($R^2 = 0.929$)

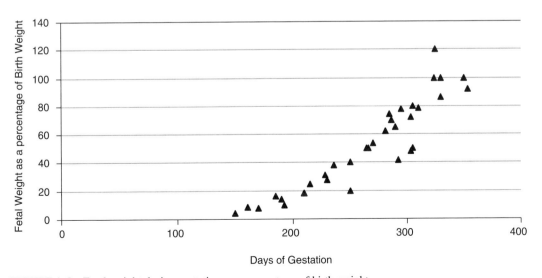

FIGURE 1-6 Fetal weight during gestation as a percentage of birth weight.

Although the coefficients of determination were relatively high for all equations, not all equations predicted the same gestation length. For example, using Equation 1-5a, the fetus would reach birth weight at 353 days, whereas with Equation 1-5c the fetus would reach birth weight at about 328 days of gestation. Equations 1-5b and 1-5d predict that the fetus would reach birth weight at 339 and 342 days, respectively. Equation 1-5d appears to provide a more biological approximation of the data than Equation 1-5b (Figure 1-7), and thus Equation 1-5d is used to predict the fetal weight as a percent of birth weight.

Fetal weight during gestation may be calculated from birth weight, which is estimated as 9.7 percent of the expected mature weight (Equation 1-3). Because the data used to develop Equation 1-5d were taken from non-normal foals, it is possible that the resulting estimates may underestimate development of normal foals. However, data on fetal development of normal foals at various stages of gestation were not found during a search of the literature.

Using information discussed above and Equation 1-5d, the total accretion of fetal and nonfetal tissue during gestation was calculated and the additional maintenance requirement of these tissues as well as the energy retained in these tissues estimated. The accumulated fetal and nonfetal tissues associated with pregnancy are more metabolically active than other maternal tissue and a higher maintenance cost (66.6 kcal/kg BW) was estimated. This estimate was based on studies by Fowden et al. (2000a) using horses and by Reynolds et al. (1986) using cattle. This rate was applied only to the accumulating tissues of conception. Therefore, the additional maintenance requirement was calculated as the product of weight of tissue accumulated and a maintenance DE cost for those tissues of 66.6 kcal/kg BW. The energy cost of tissue deposition was determined using the assumptions that the efficiency of DE use for tissue deposition during pregnancy is 60 percent (NRC, 1989) and that each unit of gain is 20 percent protein and 3 percent lipid.

The resulting estimates of DE intakes for mares with body weights between 400 and 600 kg are slightly higher than previous estimates (NRC, 1989) that were calculated at 11 percent, 13 percent, and 20 percent increments above maintenance in the 9th, 10th and 11th months of gestation, respectively. Mares in late gestation with DE intakes 10 percent above the previous recommendation have been reported to maintain fat mass (Filho et al., 2005). In another study, mares with estimated DE intakes slightly above the previous recommendation did not gain weight during the last 60 days of gestation but had apparently normal foals (Kowalski et al., 1990). Because fetal growth is greatest during the last 60 days of gestation, an increase in mare body weight would be expected if the energy requirements for maintenance and tissue deposition were met. The failure of mares to gain weight suggests that the amount of DE consumed was not adequate to meet the needs for maintenance and tissue deposition, and that mares were mobilizing body stores to meet the needs of fetal development. The current recommendations for 500-kg pregnant mares are approximately 5 to 8 percent above the 1989 recommendations; in addition, the current recommendations suggest increasing DE intakes above maintenance earlier in gestation.

The current estimates for DE intakes by draft-type mares are much higher than most previous estimates (NRC, 1989; Coenen, 2000; Martin-Rosset, 2000). However, one study utilizing pregnant draft-type mares (Doreau et al., 1991) fed diets providing DE intakes similar to those recommended here. The higher estimates of DE intakes by draft-type mares

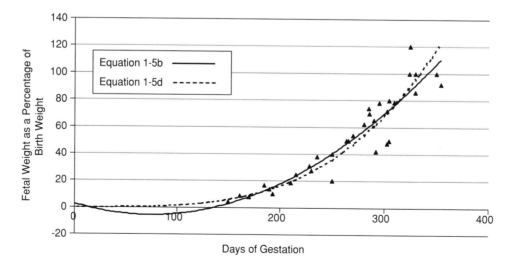

FIGURE 1-7 Comparison of two equations (1-5b and 1-5d) that predict fetal weight as a percentage of birth weight.

arise from the maintenance component associated with the dam, which is higher than in the previous edition of this publication (NRC, 1989). For mares with body weights above 700 kg, a maintenance requirement of 30.3 kcal DE/kg BW (minimal maintenance) may be more appropriate.

The current recommendations do not allow for accretion of maternal fat stores during gestation, and thus apply to mares that enter midgestation in at least moderate body condition (CS > 5). Mares that have inadequate body condition (CS < 5) in early or midgestation should be fed additional energy to reach a body condition score of at least 5 by the 9th month of gestation. Additional DE would also be necessary to meet the maintenance requirements of mares kept in environmentally stressful conditions during gestation.

Foal birth weight is estimated at 9.7 percent of nonpregnant mare weight. Additional weight accrues from the other products of conception, such as the placenta and associated fluids. Therefore, mares that conceive in a moderate body condition would be expected to increase in body weight by 12 to 15 percent during gestation. In the computer program that accompanies this document, the majority of the increase in mare weight coincides with the majority of the increase in weight of the fetus that occurs primarily in the last 3 months of gestation. However, it appears possible that an increase in mare body weight in the last 3 months of gestation is not necessary if mares gain weight earlier and are in adequate body condition. Kowalski et al. (1990) found that mares with an average condition score of 6 did not gain weight during the last 90 days of gestation but produced apparently normal foals. Even though the mares did not gain weight during the last 90 days, the difference in pre- and post-foaling weight was 14 percent of the post-foaling weight. In another study, mare body weight increased by 14 percent during gestation but the majority of weight gain occurred in the second trimester, rather than the last trimester (Lawrence et al., 1992a). Banach and Evans (1981) restricted the energy intake of pregnant mares during the last 90 days, causing the mares to lose weight. They reported that mares delivered normal weight foals (49 kg; 9.6 percent of postpartum dam weight). The mean gestation length for the mares was 350 days. Hines et al. (1987) also restricted energy intake by mares in late gestation, resulting in loss of weight and body condition. Mares fed the energy-restricted diet had longer gestation lengths than mares fed energy-adequate diets. These authors did not report foal weight. Henneke et al. (1984) also restricted energy of mares in late gestation, causing a reduction in body condition. Gestation length of restricted mares did not differ from the gestation length of mares fed to increase body condition during late gestation. Birth weight of foals from restricted mares was similar to the birth weight of foals from the mares fed to gain condition during late gestation. The results of these studies indicate that mares in moderate body condition can utilize body stores to support fetal development if energy is partially restricted in late gestation. Whether this situation affects the well-being of the equine fetus is unknown. In studies cited above, the amount of energy fed was less than amounts recommended for pregnant mares, but was close to or slightly above the maintenance requirements of the mares. The effects of long-term or more drastic energy restriction on gestating mares and the development of their foals has not been studied. Silver and Fowden (1982) reported that complete feed withdrawal for 12 to 30 hours during late gestation resulted in increased uterine prostaglandin production. These authors suggested that extended interruptions in feed intake should be avoided during late gestation.

Lactation

Studies with lactating mares have produced variable estimates of daily milk output. Estimates in early lactation have ranged from 2.3 kg milk/100 kg BW (Gibbs et al., 1982) to 3.8 kg milk/100 kg BW (Doreau et al., 1992; Martin et al., 1992). The differences in measurements may arise from variation in breeds, diets, or method of measurement. Using draft-type mares, Doreau et al. (1986) reported that daily milk output increased from 2.6 kg/100 kg BW in week 1 to 3.1 kg/100 kg BW in weeks 4 and 8. In a later study, milk output of draft mares was 2.7 kg/100 kg BW in week 1 and 3.8 kg/100 kg BW in week 8 (Doreau et al., 1992). Using Thoroughbred and Standardbred mares, Oftedal et al. (1983) reported that daily milk output was 3.1, 2.9, and 3.4 kg/100 kg BW at 11, 25, and 39 days postpartum, respectively. The daily amounts of milk (kg/d) estimated by Oftedal et al. (1983) were similar to amounts measured by Glade (1991) using Thoroughbred mares. In light horse mares (Anglo-Arab and Selle Francais), milk production at 4 weeks of lactation was 3.4 kg/100 kg BW. The lowest daily milk outputs were reported by Gibbs et al. (1982) in Quarter horse mares, which may suggest a breed effect on milk production. However, Martin et al. (1992) reported milk outputs above 3.8 kg/100 kg BW in Australian Stockhorses. Most of the previously mentioned studies used isotope dilution methods to estimate daily milk output, although Gibbs et al. (1982) and Glade (1991) utilized weigh-suckle-weigh techniques. In the study by Glade, foals were allowed to nurse every 2 hours, whereas in the study by Gibbs et al. foals were allowed to nurse every 3 hours. It is possible that less frequent nursing resulted in the somewhat lower milk output estimates of Gibbs et al. (1982).

A few studies have examined the effects of dietary energy and protein intake on milk output by mares. Doreau et al. (1992) found that mares fed a high-concentrate, high-energy diet produced about 10 percent more milk than mares fed a high-forage diet that was adequate in energy. However, the milk produced by mares receiving the high-energy, high-concentrate diet was slightly lower in fat and protein than milk produced by mares receiving the high-forage diet. As a result, even though the amount of milk produced was different between diets, the total milk energy output was similar and foal growth was not affected by the diet of the mares. Mares receiving the high-energy, high-concentrate diet gained more weight than mares receiving the high-forage diet. Pagan et al. (1984) studied the effect of energy restriction on lactating pony mares. Although milk production was not measured, average daily gain of the foals was not affected by either mild energy restriction or mild energy excess. Mares receiving restricted dietary energy lost weight, whereas mares receiving excess energy gained weight. Dietary protein has been reported to have a small effect on milk yield (Gibbs et al., 1982), but Martin et al. (1991) did not find any effect of a protein supplement on milk yield in pastured mares.

A review of studies on milk production suggested that mares will produce approximately 3 kg milk/100 kg BW in early lactation and 2 kg milk/100 kg BW in late lactation (NRC, 1989). More recently published studies have reported higher levels of milk production in early lactation, and Santos et al. (2005) reported that milk production in Lusitano mares was greater than 2 percent of body weight at day 120 of lactation. Therefore, it is possible that milk production is somewhat higher that previously estimated (NRC, 1989). Because the transition from early lactation to late lactation is probably gradual, data from available studies were summarized to estimate milk production by day of lactation. The equation to estimate milk production is:

$$Y = a \times (d^{0.0953}) \times e^{(-0.0043d)} \qquad (1\text{-}6)$$

where Y = daily milk yield in kilograms; a = 0.0274287 × mature weight in kilograms; and d = day of lactation.

The gross energy content of mare milk has previously been summarized as 580 kcal/kg, 530 kcal/kg, and 500 kcal/kg, in weeks 1 to 4, 5 to 8, and 9 to 21, respectively (NRC, 1989). Martin et al. (1992) reported the mean gross energy of milk to be 480, 470, and 450 kcal/kg, at 11, 41, and 71 days of lactation. Doreau et al. (1992) found that gross energy declined from 560 kcal/kg milk in week 1 of lactation to 450 kcal/kg milk in week 8. These data suggest that the concentration of gross energy in milk decreases during the lactation period. However, Hoffman et al. (1998) reported that the concentrations of fat and lactose were higher at 4 months of lactation than at 1 month of lactation in Thoroughbred mares. Hoffman et al. (1998) did not report gross energy concentration in their samples. If gross energy is estimated from the concentration of fat, protein, and lactose, then gross energy content was 580 kcal/kg milk at 1 and 2 months of lactation and 600 kcal/kg milk at 6 months of lactation. When all data were summarized, a significant relationship between milk energy concentration and stage of lactation was not obtained. Dietary energy amount or source appears to influence the energy composition of milk. Mares receiving an energy-adequate, high-forage diet had higher concentrations of fat and energy in milk than mares fed a high-energy, high-concentrate diet (Doreau et al., 1992). Pagan and Hintz (1986c) reported that increased energy intake decreased the concentration of fat and energy in milk from pony mares. Davison et al. (1991) found that adding fat to the diets of lactating mares increased the concentration of fat in the milk. However, Hoffman et al. (1998) did not report an increase in milk fat when pastured mares received a supplement containing 10 percent fat. It appears that the energy concentration may be influenced by several factors, including energy source and amount as well as stage of lactation.

The DE requirement for lactation was calculated as the sum of the DE utilized for milk production and the DE utilized for maintenance. The amount of energy secreted in milk each day was calculated as the product of daily milk output and the gross energy content of milk (estimated at 500 kcal/kg milk). To estimate daily milk production for each month of lactation, the total milk produced per month was calculated and a daily average was obtained. The amount of DE needed for milk production is calculated using an efficiency of DE use for lactation of 60 percent (NRC, 1978).

The maintenance requirement of lactating mares has previously been assumed to be the same as for other adult horses (NRC, 1989). However, several factors may contribute to an elevated maintenance requirement in lactating mares such as increased activity associated with maternal behavior and increased feed intake; therefore, the elevated maintenance estimate that was discussed in this chapter's maintenance section of 36.3 kcal/kg BW was used for lactating mares.

The recommendations for DE intakes by lactating mares assume that the mare enters lactation with a body condition score of at least 5 (moderate), and that she will not gain or lose weight during lactation. If a change in body condition of the mare is desirable, then either more or less energy should be fed. Small to moderate increases or decreases in energy intake of lactating mares in moderate body condition do not appear to alter milk production. Pony mares with DE intakes approximately 15 percent above or 15 percent below the estimated requirement gained or lost body weight, but their foals grew similarly to foals of mares consuming DE at the estimated requirement (Pagan et al., 1984). However, when energy restriction is more severe or extended, lactation may be affected (Banach and Evans, 1985).

For 200-kg mares, the current estimates for DE intakes are somewhat lower than previous estimates (NRC, 1989). Milk production for pony mares in early lactation was previously estimated at 4 percent of body weight (NRC, 1989). Pagan et al. (1984) estimated the DE requirements of 200-kg lactating mares at 12.9 Mcal/d, which is also lower than the previous estimate (NRC, 1989). For mares with mature weights of 400–600 kg, the current DE recommendations for early lactation are somewhat higher than previous rec-

ENERGY

ommendations (NRC, 1989). Lactating Thoroughbred mares weighing 460–475 kg maintained body weight when fed diets containing 28–31 Mcal DE/d (Glade, 1991). Similarly, Quarter horse mares (approximately 520 kg) maintained body weight when fed diets estimated to contain 29–31 Mcal DE/d (Gibbs et al., 1982). The current estimates for draft-type mares are markedly higher than the 1989 estimates due to the higher maintenance requirement used in the current recommendations. In a study by Doreau et al. (1992), draft-type mares (730 kg) consumed diets containing approximately 71 or 47 Mcal DE/d. Mares consuming 71 Mcal/day gained 1.18 kg/d, whereas mares consuming 47 Mcal DE gained 0.18 kg/d. These data suggest that the draft mares used approximately 24 Mcal of DE/kg of gain and that the mares fed the lower energy diet would have been in energy balance at a daily DE intake of 43 Mcal/day. Using the current set of assumptions (with a maintenance component of 36.3 kcal/kg BW) to determine DE, a 730-kg lactating mare would require approximately 46 Mcal of DE in early lactation. If a maintenance component of 33.3 kcal/kg BW is used, the daily DE intake is estimated at about 44 Mcal. Morrison (1961) suggested that lactating draft mares (730 kg) performing light work should be fed 10 to 12.5 kg TDN or 44 to 55 Mcal DE. The conversion of TDN to DE assumes 1 kg TDN = 4.4 Mcal DE (NRC, 1978). When daily DE intake recommendation is corrected for the additional work, the resulting DE intake is approximately 38–47 Mcal/d for a lactating 730-kg mare. Therefore, for lactating mares weighing more than 700 kg, a daily maintenance component of 33.3 kcal/kg BW is suggested.

Reproductive Efficiency

The energy status of broodmares can affect several components of reproductive efficiency, including conception rate, length of the anovulatory period, and number of cycles to conception. Henneke et al. (1984) found that mares entering the breeding season in a moderate body condition required fewer cycles for conception and had higher conception rates than mares entering the breeding season in thin condition. These researchers also reported that mares that foaled in a thin body condition and remained thin during lactation had a longer interval from parturition to the second postpartum estrus. The condition scoring system used by these researchers is shown in Table 1-7. Other condition scoring systems have been developed for horses, but this system has been the most widely applied in nutrition studies with horses. Where condition scores are noted in this chapter, they were determined using the system in Table 1-7.

Kubiak et al. (1987) reported that mares entering the breeding season with a mean condition score of 5.3 ovulated sooner than mares that entered the season at condition scores below 5. Mares with a condition score above 5 in that study also tended to have a shorter initial estrus period. Mares that entered the breeding season in a moderately fat or fat body condition did not have impaired reproductive efficiency compared to mares that entered the breeding season in moderate or thin condition (Henneke et al., 1984). Gentry et al. (2002) found that open mares maintained in moderately fat to fat body condition (condition score 6.5 to 8) during the fall and winter often continued to cycle throughout

TABLE 1-7 A Condition Scoring System for Horses[a]

Score		Description
1	Poor	Animal extremely emaciated; spinous processes, ribs, tailhead, tuber coxae, and ischii projecting prominently; bone structure of withers, shoulders, and neck easily noticeable, no fatty tissue can be felt
2	Very thin	Animal emaciated; slight fat covering over base of spinous processes; transverse processes of lumbar vertebrae feel rounded; spinous processes, ribs, tailhead, tuber coxae, and ischii prominent; withers, shoulders, and neck structure faintly discernible
3	Thin	Fat buildup about halfway on spinous processes; transverse processes cannot be felt; slight fat cover over ribs; spinous processes and ribs easily discernible; tailhead prominent, but individual vertebrae cannot be identified visually; tuber coxae appear rounded but easily discernible; tuber ischii not distinguishable; withers, shoulders, and neck accentuated
4	Moderately thin	Slight ridge along back; faint outline of ribs discernible; tailhead prominence depends on conformation, fat can be felt around it; tuber coxae not discernible; withers, shoulders, and neck not obviously thin
5	Moderate	Back is flat (no crease or ridge); ribs not visually distinguishable but easily felt; fat around tailhead beginning to feel spongy; withers appear rounded over spinous processes; shoulders and neck blend smoothly into body
6	Moderately fleshy	May have slight crease down back; fat over ribs spongy; fat around tailhead soft; fat beginning to be deposited along the side of withers, behind shoulders, and along the sides of neck
7	Fleshy	May have crease down back; individual ribs can be felt, but noticeable filling between ribs with fat; fat around tailhead soft; fat deposited along withers, behind shoulders, and along neck
8	Fat	Crease down back; difficult to feel ribs; fat around tailhead very soft; area along withers filled with fat; area behind shoulder filled with fat; noticeable thickening of neck; fat deposited along inner thighs
9	Extremely fat	Obvious crease down back; patchy fat appearing over ribs; bulging fat around tailhead, along withers, behind shoulders, and along neck; fat along inner thighs may rub together; flank filled with fat

[a]SOURCE: Adapted from Henneke et al. (1983).

the winter. Mares in fat body condition at parturition had foaling characteristics similar to mares in moderate body condition at parturition (Kubiak et al., 1988). In addition, mares in fat and moderate body condition had similar intervals from parturition to foal heat ovulation, and from parturition to the second postpartum ovulation (Cavinder et al., 2005).

Sudden or chronic energy restriction, as well as energy supplementation of broodmares, may also affect reproductive efficiency. When mares that entered the fall in a moderately fat or fat body condition were fed energy-restricted diets, all mares became anovulatory within 12 weeks of the onset of restriction and remained anovulatory for an extended period (Gentry et al., 2002). Similarly, Kubiak et al. (1987) found that mares that entered the breeding season in a thin body condition and remained thin had an extended anovulatory period. In some instances, the reproductive efficiency of mares that began the breeding season in a thin condition was improved when sufficient energy was supplied to increase body weight and condition (Henneke et al., 1984; Kubiak et al., 1987). However, in a field study conducted by Henneke et al. (1984), mares that entered the breeding season in thin condition and gained weight during the breeding season remained less reproductively efficient than mares that entered the breeding season at condition scores above 5.

Many studies have been conducted to investigate the mechanism that governs the interaction between energy status and reproductive efficiency in mares. Initial attention focused on the effects of energy restriction on luteinizing hormone (LH) responses in mares (Hines et al., 1987). Subsequent studies have examined the relationships among short-term feed deprivation or long-term feed restriction on growth hormone (GH), IGF-I (insulin-like growth factor I), thyroid hormones, prolactin, insulin, and leptin. Energy restriction appears to result in a rapid decrease in IGF-I concentrations in nonpregnant mares, but growth hormone and thyroid hormone responses were less affected (Sticker et al., 1995). McManus and Fitzgerald (2000) reported that leptin concentrations decreased in mares subjected to 24 hours of feed deprivation, while serum concentrations of follicle stimulating hormone (FSH), prolactin, and LH were not affected. Similarly, Buff et al. (2005) reported that 48 hours of feed deprivation resulted in decreased leptin concentrations. Gentry et al. (2002) compared the hormonal responses of mares receiving a nutritionally adequate diet and a restricted diet during the fall and winter. Mares in the adequately fed group maintained condition scores of 6.5 to 8, whereas mares in the restricted group began the study with condition scores of 6.5 to 8 but eventually reached condition scores of 3 to 3.5. Most of the mares in the adequately fed group continued to cycle during the fall and winter, but all mares in the restricted group entered an anovulatory state. Basal concentrations of LH, FSH, thyroid stimulating hormone (TSH), GH, or insulin that were measured at each week were not affected by feed restriction. However, restricted mares had a reduced LH response to gonadotropin releasing hormone (GnRH) and a reduced prolactin response to thyroid releasing hormone (TRH). Leptin concentrations decreased in both groups with time, but were lower in mares receiving the restricted diet. Although it is possible that changes in leptin are involved in the mechanism that allows diet to affect reproductive efficiency, a clear relationship has not been demonstrated at this time.

A number of studies have demonstrated that energy restriction or low body condition can negatively impact reproductive efficiency in mares. Therefore, it is recommended that mares used for breeding be maintained at a condition score of at least 5. Maintaining broodmares at a high condition score (condition scores of 7 or 8) does not impair or improve reproductive efficiency (Cavinder et al., 2005). Mares maintained in situations that elevate energy requirements (such as cold) should be fed sufficient energy to meet the increased needs for maintenance, or they should have sufficient body stores to meet energy needs without decreasing condition score below 5. Similarly, mares that have difficulty maintaining body condition during late gestation or lactation should be fed to accrete sufficient body stores to prevent a decline in body condition below 5 when energy needs increase.

EXERCISE

Oxygen Utilization During Exercise

The amount of energy utilized during exercise must be known in order to estimate the DE requirements of exercising horses. The amount of energy utilized during exercise depends upon the duration and the intensity of the exercise. The duration of an exercise bout is relatively easy to measure, but the intensity of exercise is much more difficult to characterize. Factors that influence intensity include the speed of travel, ground resistance (moving on sand versus a flat surface), and the incline of the terrain. Other factors germane to equine events include number and height of jumping efforts, performance of extended and collected gaits, and the amount of weight carried or pulled.

Oxygen consumption during exercise is often measured as a means of estimating energy expenditure during work. Several studies have investigated the relationship between oxygen consumption and speed of travel of horses. Hiraga et al. (1995) reported that oxygen utilization was linearly related to speed for horses running on a level treadmill. Eaton (1994) has also reported a linear relationship between speed and oxygen. Subsequently, Eaton et al. (1995b) reported a nonlinear relationship between speed and oxygen utilization for horses exercising on a level treadmill. Similarly Pagan and Hintz (1986b) found a nonlinear relationship between energy expended (calculated from oxygen consumption) and speed when horses exercised on a level track. The equations of Eaton et al. (1995b) and Pagan and Hintz (1986b) yield similar values for horses exercising at 300 meters/minute (m/min). However, at speeds above 400 m/min, the equations produce very different estimates of energy use. As the measurements made by Eaton et al. included a wider range of speeds, it is likely that their equation provides a better estimate of oxygen use than the equation of Pagan and Hintz (1986b) at speeds above 400 m/min. However, the equation from Eaton et al. (1995b) probably overestimates oxygen utilization at slow speeds (walking and slow trotting).

Although it seems reasonable that an equation relating speed of travel to oxygen use could be used to estimate the energy requirements of exercising horses, there are several complicating factors. The equation of Eaton et al. (1995b) was derived from horses running on a treadmill, rather than on a typical track or arena surface. When trotters were tested on a treadmill and on a track, heart rate at a given speed was lower on the treadmill, suggesting that exercise on a treadmill may not precisely replicate exercise on a track, even though speed is the same (Couroucé et al., 1999). Compared to horses on the track, horses on the treadmill did not pull a sulky, which probably accounted for most of the differences observed. Other differences between the treadmill and the track, such as ground reaction forces, wind resistance, and psychological factors, were also suggested. In addition, it is possible that biomechanical factors or conformational factors could alter the relationship between speed and oxygen utilization. In a study comparing oxygen utilization of small ponies (171 kg), medium ponies (319 kg), and Thoroughbreds (487 kg), ponies reached 40, 60, 80, and 100 percent of maximum oxygen consumption at slower speeds than the Thoroughbreds (Katz et al., 2000). Hoyt and Taylor (1981) demonstrated that the gait of the horse affected oxygen utilization at a given speed. Their data indicated that horses appear to select gaits to maximize energy efficiency, and that shortening or lengthening of a stride may be energetically quite expensive. Eaton et al. (1995b) concluded that the most efficient speed for Thoroughbred horses exercising on a level or an inclined treadmill was 3 to 6 meters/second (m/s), and horses generally changed from a trot to a canter at 5 to 6 m/s. Other factors influencing oxygen utilization at a given speed include level of warm-up (Tyler et al, 1996; McCutcheon et al., 1999), conditioning (Eaton et al., 1999; Katz et al., 2000), and possibly body composition (Kearns et al., 2002a). In summary, it is clear that it may be difficult to precisely predict oxygen utilization from speed of travel for a specific individual. Nonetheless, within an individual, oxygen utilization, and thus energy use, usually increases with speed.

Oxygen utilization is increased by 25–35 percent when horses exercise on a slight incline compared to a flat surface (Eaton et al., 1995b). At steeper inclines, the effect on oxygen use is much greater. At a slope of 6.25 percent, oxygen consumption increased 76 percent in Standardbreds at the trot (Thornton et al., 1987). Oxygen utilization of horses galloping on a 10 percent incline has been observed to be approximately 100–150 percent higher than when horses gallop on a flat surface (Eaton et al., 1995b; Hiraga et al., 1995). When horses walked or trotted on a dry treadmill or on a treadmill in water at the depth of the horse's fetlock or elbow, heart rate was increased (Voss et al., 2002). Although oxygen utilization was not measured, the increase in heart rate suggests that oxygen utilization is increased by other factors that increase resistance to movement. Changing the amount of weight carried will change the amount of oxygen utilized (Thornton et al., 1987). Therefore, if estimates of oxygen utilization are used to estimate energy requirements in horses they should take into account the amount of weight carried (i.e., the rider).

Measurements of oxygen utilization made during exercise probably account for most of the energy utilized. However, as exercise becomes more intense, the anaerobic component of energy expenditure will increase. Although the contribution of anaerobic metabolism to total energy utilization is relatively small at light to moderate workloads, it may be as high as 30 percent during maximal exercise (Eaton et al., 1995a).

Energy Requirements of Exercising Horses

The daily energy requirements of an equine athlete may be partitioned into at least two compartments, which include the amount of energy required for the daily exercise effort and the amount of energy required for maintenance. A third compartment may be the amount of energy required for all other activities associated with a performance horse's daily life (such as transportation to and from events). This compartment could be accounted for separately, or it could be added to the maintenance or exercise components, but it should be considered. Doherty et al. (1997) have suggested that energy use during transportation in a trailer may be similar to the amount of energy used during walking. Therefore, several hours of transportation a week could add significantly to total energy requirements.

As noted previously, the amount of energy utilized during any exercise bout will depend on factors such as incline, speed, and ground resistance. It is relatively simple to calculate the energy utilized by an unloaded horse trotting or cantering on a level treadmill, but it is much more difficult to calculate the energy utilized by a loaded (ridden) horse trotting and cantering up and down hills or jumping obstacles. Attempts to convert theoretical estimates of oxygen consumption to practical estimates of dietary energy need are fraught with pitfalls. Factors that can potentially affect the reliability of the process include differences among horses, level of training, type of exercise, rider weight and experience, climate, and ground conditions. An excellent review of the energy costs associated with a 3-day event has been published (Jones and Carlson, 1995), and models to estimate uphill and downhill running have also been published

(Schroter and Marlin, 2002). However, estimates of energy utilization during many equine events are not available. Perhaps more importantly, the average daily energy requirement of an individual horse is more closely related to the activities performed during training than the energy expended in a single event.

There is a strong relationship between heart rate and oxygen utilization (Eaton et al., 1995b; Coenen, 2005); therefore, it may be possible to estimate energy expenditure from heart rate (Coenen, 2005), particularly at submaximal exercise intensities. Oxygen utilization is related more closely to percentage of maximal heart rate than to actual heart rate. The maximum heart rate of an individual horse may vary with age and breed, and, therefore, to estimate the percentage of heart rate maximum achieved during a specific work bout, it is necessary to know the maximal heart rate of an individual horse. However, it is difficult for many equestrians to impose a workload sufficient to elicit maximum heart rate. It is more practical to use heart rate as a guide to oxygen consumption than percentage of heart rate maximum achieved during various exercise bouts. At the very least, heart rate can be used to assess the relative intensity of a work bout for a given horse. The availability of on-board heart rate monitors for horses makes it possible to determine heart rate during the various stages of an exercise bout and even calculate a mean heart rate that could be used to estimate mean energy expenditure. Eaton et al. (1995b) derived the following equation to relate oxygen utilization to heart rate:

Oxygen Utilization (ml O_2/kg BW/min) = $0.833 \times (HR) - 54.7$ ($R^2 = 0.865$)

where HR = heart rate in beats/min. This equation produces reasonable estimates of oxygen utilization at high heart rates but not at low heart rates. Coenen (2005) summarized oxygen consumption data from 87 studies and developed the following equation:

Oxygen Utilization (ml O_2/kg BW/min) = $0.0019 \times (HR)^{2.0653}$ ($R^2 = 0.9$)

where HR = heart rate in beats/min. (Note: this is not the equation published in the original reference, which had a typographical error). This equation (Coenen, 2005) provides a better estimate of oxygen utilization at lower heart rates than the equation of Eaton et al. (1995b).

Table 1-8 shows the estimated oxygen utilization and energy utilization at various heart rates for a 500-kg horse with a 50-kg rider. By using heart rate, rather than speed alone, a more comprehensive estimate of work intensity is provided. Also, heart rate can be used to estimate oxygen consumption for some activities where speed might be irrelevant (such as cutting), or where the relationship between speed and oxygen consumption might not be known, such as for horses performing specialized gaits. The values in Table 1-8 have not been corrected for resting oxygen utilization, and therefore slightly overestimate the energy cost of exercise above maintenance. This overestimation would be of minor importance to horses exercising for short periods of time, but could be of significant importance when calculating the energy requirements of horses exercising for extended periods. In addition, at high heart rates, the energy expenditure calculated from oxygen utilization will underestimate the true energy utilization because oxygen utilization does not account for the anaerobic energy component.

In order for heart rate measurements to be a useful indicator of exercise intensity, the heart rate must be determined during exercise and not after exercise or at a rest break. Heart rate decreases rapidly (within a few seconds) after most exercise, and thus post-exercise heart rate is not a good indicator of exercising heart rate. Heart rate measurements made when a horse is excited due to new surroundings or another situation may overestimate the effect of the actual work performed. As it is not always possible to measure heart rate under practical conditions, a brief review of selected studies that have measured heart rates in horses during various activities is provided. Conditioned Arabian horses trotting on a level treadmill at 3.6 m/s had heart rates of 90 to 100 beats/min (Bullimore et al., 2000), whereas conditioned Thoroughbred horses exercising at 6 and 8.5 m/sec on a level treadmill had heart rates of 115 and 145 beats/min, respectively (Danielsen et al., 1995). Older unfit mares had heart rates of 120 to 140 during free lunging in a round pen at a trot (Powell et al., 2002). (Ridgway) (1994) suggests that unfit horses ridden at a working trot (160 to 210 m/min) will have heart rates of 120 to 150 beats/min, whereas conditioned horses performing the same work will have heart rates of 70 to 110 beats/min. The heart rates of French trotters on a sand training track were approximately 180 and 190 beats/min at 490 and 560 m/min, respectively (Couroucé et al., 1999). Horses performing reining-type exercise have heart rates between 160 and 180 beats/min (Howard et al., 2003), and horses performing cutting-type exercise have been reported to have heart rates of 200 beats/min (Webb et al., 1987). Peak heart rates in 3-day eventing horses exercising on the beach at 450–500 m/min

TABLE 1-8 Estimated Oxygen Consumption and Net Energy Utilization of a 500-kg Horse Ridden by a 50-kg Rider at Various Heart Rates

Heart Rate (beats/min)	Oxygen Utilization[a] (ml O_2/kg BW/min)	Oxygen Utilization[b] (liters/min)	Energy Utilization[c] (kcal/min)
60	9	5.0	24
90	21	11.6	56
120	37	20.4	99
150	59	32.5	158
180	86	47.3	230

[a] Where oxygen utilization (ml/kg/min) = $0.0019 \times HR^{2.0653}$.
[b] For a 500-kg horse with a 50-kg rider (550-kg total weight).
[c] Where 1 liter of oxygen utilized is equivalent to 4.86 kcal.

have been reported to range from 126–151 beats/min, whereas heart rates in a "paddock canter" at 350–400 m/min were 127–141 beats/min, and the peak heart rate of one horse performing gallops on a hill was 205 beats/min (Serrano et al., 2002). The peak heart rates represented the most strenuous portion of a workout. Heart rate in elite show jumpers is elevated prior to entering the arena and may increase to 200 beats/min by the end of the round (Clayton, 1994). Racing (flat or harness) results in maximal heart rates (> 210 beats/min).

Although energy expenditure can be estimated on a daily basis, it is more practical to evaluate energy expenditure over a longer period in order to determine a mean daily energy expenditure. Table 1-9 shows a hypothetical example of the estimated weekly energy expenditure of a horse utilized for recreational riding.

The mean daily energy expenditure in Table 1-9 of 1.5 Mcal/day represents the NE used during exercise. In order to estimate daily DE requirements, the efficiency of conversion of DE to NE during exercise must be known. Pagan and Hintz (1986b) originally estimated the efficiency of DE use for exercise at 57 percent. However, much lower efficiencies have been suggested (Harris, 1997; Pagan et al., 2005a). A number of studies (Webb et al., 1987; Freeman et al., 1988; Bullimore et al., 2000; Graham-Thiers et al., 2000) that reported body weight, weekly exercise program, and either feed intake or DE intake were reviewed to examine the efficiency of DE use for exercise. When maintenance is estimated at 33.3 kcal/kg BW, the estimated efficiency of DE use for exercise ranged from approximately 20–50 percent. Based on estimates of feed intake and typical training programs, the efficiency of DE use for exercise by race horses would be 20 percent or lower. If the elevated maintenance estimate is used in the equations (36.3 kcal/kg BW), somewhat higher efficiencies of DE use for exercise can be calculated, but for most studies, the values would still be below 50 percent. Additional research is needed to determine the efficiency of DE use for exercise in horses performing different types of work. In addition, there are probably individual differences among horses, as well as differences due to feed intake and diet composition that should be characterized. However, in the absence of more specific data, it is estimated that the efficiency of DE use for exercise is 30 percent for horses engaged in strenuous activities and 40 percent or higher for horses engaged in moderate or mild exercise.

The cost of exercise must be added to the cost of maintenance to determine the daily DE requirement of performance horses. Maintenance estimates have usually been made using sedentary animals. It is possible that athletic horses have a somewhat higher maintenance requirement than a sedentary horse. One factor that could influence the maintenance requirement of a performance horse is total feed intake. Several studies have reported that the mean daily dry matter intake of race horses exceeds 2.2 percent of body weight (Zmija et al., 1991; Gallagher et al., 1992a,b). A horse's response to its stabling environment may also affect maintenance requirements. A survey of Thoroughbred, Standardbred, and pleasure horse stables found that approximately 12 percent of horses exhibited some type of compulsive behavior such as cribbing, weaving, or stall-kicking (Luescher et al., 1998). The performance of a compulsive behavior could increase the maintenance requirement. Other stabling factors that have not been assessed but could influence maintenance requirements include amount of turnout, activity in the stable, and even comfort associated with stall size, ventilation, temperature, or bedding.

Most researchers who have measured oxygen utilization during work have not accounted for the energy costs of an elevated post-exercise metabolic rate (or of walking during a recovery period) in their calculations of energy use. For 1 hour after a short-term, moderately intense exercise bout, oxygen utilization was elevated by about 11 percent above the pre-exercise value (Dunn et al., 1991). Body temperature, heart rate, and respiration will remain elevated after exercise in horses for various lengths of time, depending upon the fitness of the horse, the type of exercise performed, envi-

TABLE 1-9 Hypothetical Weekly Net Energy Expenditure (above maintenance) of a 500-kg Horse Used for Recreational Riding

Day of Week	Type of Exercise	Average HR during Exercise	Energy Utilization[a] for Exercise (Mcal/d)
Monday	45 min riding in arena[b]	100	3.1
Tuesday	45 min on trail (mostly walking)	60	1.1
Wednesday	No exercise	0	0
Thursday	45 min riding in arena	100	3.1
Friday	No exercise	0	0
Saturday	2 hours trail riding (mostly walking)	60	2.9
Sunday	No exercise	0	0
		Mean daily energy expenditure above maintenance	1.5 Mcal/d

[a]For calculations see Table 1-8.
[b]Includes walk, trot, and canter.

ronmental conditions, and other factors. A post-exercise elevation in metabolic rate could increase the maintenance requirement. It is possible that the average maintenance component of 33.3 kcal/kg BW/d is appropriate for some performance horses, but that the elevated maintenance requirement discussed in the maintenance section (36.3 kcal/kg BW/d) is appropriate for others, particularly if horses are transported long distances to competitions.

Given the discussion and equations reported above, it is possible to calculate an estimate of DE requirements for an individual horse, based on body weight, weight of rider, and individual work program. However, as this approach is not practical for every situation, general categories of exercising horses have been devised. The previous edition of this document used three categories of work (light, moderate, and intense). Other publications have listed as many as seven categories (Lewis, 1995). Four categories of work are suggested here: light, moderate, heavy, and very heavy. The DE requirements for horses in these categories are calculated using the following equations:

Light work:
$$DE (Mcal/d) = (0.0333 \times BW) \times 1.20 \quad (1\text{-}7a)$$

Moderate work:
$$DE (Mcal/d) = (0.0333 \times BW) \times 1.40 \quad (1\text{-}7b)$$

Heavy work:
$$DE (Mcal/d) = (0.0333 \times BW) \times 1.60 \quad (1\text{-}7c)$$

Very heavy work:
$$DE (Mcal/d) = (0.0363 \times BW) \times 1.9 \quad (1\text{-}7d)$$

The assignment of the DE increments above maintenance (20, 40, 60, and 90 percent) to the words "light," "moderate," "heavy," and "very heavy" are arbitrary. Other categories and descriptors could be used instead. Table 1-10 provides estimates of weekly workloads for each category. The estimated workloads should be used only as a guide, as there are many combinations of work intensity and work duration that could not be included in a single table. In addition, the heart rates that are associated with each category in the table should not be used to define that category. The heart rates given in each category are consistent with the amount of work performed over the duration specified.

These suggested DE intakes (Table 1-10) appear to be consistent with estimates from several studies. Several studies have reported that horses in race training (450–500 kg) have DE intakes above 30 Mcal/day (Zmija et al., 1991; Gallagher et al., 1992a,b; Southwood et al., 1993). McGowan et al. (2002) reported that polo ponies were fed approximately 11 kg of hay and 2 kg of concentrate per day, which would result in a DE intake of about 26 Mcal/day,

TABLE 1-10 Example Weekly Workloads of Horses in the Light, Moderate, Heavy, and Very Heavy Exercise Categories

Exercise Category	Mean Heart Rate[a]	Description[b]	Types of Events[c]
Light	80 beats/min	1–3 hours per week; 40% walk, 50% trot, 10% canter	Recreational riding Beginning of training programs Show horses (occasional)
Moderate	90 beats/min	3–5 hours per week; 30% walk, 55% trot, 10% canter, 5% low jumping, cutting, other skill work	School horses Recreational riding Beginning of training/breaking Show horses (frequent) Polo Ranch work
Heavy	110 beats/min	4–5 hours per week; 20% walk, 50% trot, 15% canter, 15% gallop, jumping, other skill work	Ranch work Polo Show horses (frequent, strenuous events) Low-medium level eventing Race training (middle stages)
Very Heavy	110–150 beats/min	Various; ranges from 1 hour per week speed work to 6–12 hours per week slow work	Racing (Quarter horse, Thoroughbred, Standardbred, Endurance) Elite 3-day event

[a] Mean heart rate over the entire exercise bout.
[b] These are general descriptions based on weekly totals of work and do not include all combinations of work intensities and duration. The hours of work performed per week in any particular category could be much more than the estimate given, if the work intensity was much lower. For example, horses in the light category could be exercised for more than 3 hours per week if the work intensity was much lower (see Table 1-9); and horses in the moderate category could be exercised for more than 5 hours per week if the work intensity were lower than the mean heart rate given.
[c] For additional discussion of the sources of variation in energy requirements, see explanation in the text.

which is similar to a previous estimate for 475-kg polo ponies (Hintz et al., 1971). Crandell (2002) reported that endurance horses are fed approximately 24 Mcal DE/day, but noted that many horses receive pasture that could not be quantified. For a 425-kg endurance horse, 24 Mcal/day would exceed maintenance requirements by 57–73 percent (using a maintenance requirement of 36.3 or 33.3 kcal/kg BW, respectively). The DE requirements for equitation horses were estimated at about 140 percent of maintenance (Hintz et al., 1971). Webb et al. (1987) reported that cutting horses (470 kg) in a lean body condition consumed about 19 Mcal/day, which would be about 25 percent above maintenance and much lower than the estimate suggested here. However, it was not clear whether these horses were actively engaged in competition; therefore, cutting horses should probably be included in the moderate category.

Although the guidelines above should be helpful in determining whether an individual horse should be classified in the light, moderate, heavy, or very heavy work category, it is likely these categories will not apply to all horses. There are numerous factors that could potentially affect the energy needed by a performance horse including level of fitness, skill, and weight of the rider, climate conditions, breed, and housing conditions. Therefore, these recommendations should be applied in combination with other criteria such as body condition, performance, and maintenance of body weight.

EFFECTS OF ENERGY DEFICIENCY AND EXCESS

In most cases, energy deficiencies and excesses are easily identified by weight loss or weight gain. Because it is difficult for many horse owners to regularly weigh horses, use of a body condition scoring system may help determine whether a horse is gaining or losing weight. A number of condition scoring systems have been developed for horses and even for donkeys (see Chapter 13). Some systems have used a 9- or 10-point scale, whereas others have used a 5-point scale. Regardless of the details of any one method, to be most useful the system must be applied consistently over time. A body condition scoring system for horses that has been widely used for many years (Henneke et al., 1983) is shown in Table 1-7. This system scores horses on fat cover at several locations on the body, with a low score of 1 being applied to an extremely thin horse and a high score of 9 being applied to a very fat horse. A condition score of 5 is considered moderate. Condition scoring has been used to assess the condition of horses in various physiological states. As mentioned previously, reproductive efficiency is optimized with a body condition score of at least 5. Similarly, the body condition score of select Thoroughbred yearlings at public auction was between 5 and 6. For performance horses, lower body condition scores may be appropriate. Body condition scores for endurance horses completing a race have been reported to range from 3 to 5.5 (Garlinghouse and Burrill, 1998). In that study, condition scores of 4, 4.5, or 5 were most frequent, and no horses with a body condition score below 3 completed the race. Mean condition score for endurance horses had previously been reported to be 4.67 (Lawrence et al., 1992b). Some studies have shown no disadvantages to very high condition scores in broodmares (Henneke et al., 1983; Kubiak et al., 1989; Cavinder et al., 2005). However, Hoffman et al. (2003) suggested that very fat horses may have disturbed metabolic and endocrine regulation, although specific consequences to animal health were not reported. Therefore, at this time the optimal body condition for a horse is not known.

When horses have body condition scores outside the desired range, energy balance may be manipulated to produce weight loss or weight gain. Although condition score is often reported in equine nutrition studies, the amount of weight loss or gain necessary to achieve a change in body condition score has not been well studied. Heusner (1993) found that weight gains of 33 to 45 kg were associated with an increase in condition score of approximately two units (from 4 to 6) in mature horses (approximately 480–580 kg). Consequently, it appears that each unit of condition score increase requires about 16–20 kg of weight gain. The amount of weight needed to change condition score by one unit will vary with the mature weight of the horse.

To alter energy balance, either energy expenditure or energy intake can be manipulated. The most common means of increasing energy expenditure is to increase activity, usually by imposing a regular exercise program. Energy expenditure may be decreased by reducing the amount of regular exercise. For horses that are not receiving forced exercise, energy expenditure may be reduced by limiting activity or by reducing environmental stresses impacting the horse (i.e., providing shelter during cold wet weather).

When it is not desirable or practical to alter energy expenditure, energy intake may be manipulated. The relationships among energy intake, change in body weight, and change in body condition score have not been well described in horses. One recommendation suggested that a change in condition score could be achieved if DE intake were increased or decreased 10–15 percent above or below maintenance (NRC, 1989). Recent information suggests that this recommendation may not be realistic for many situations in which weight gain is desired. The amount of DE required per kilogram of gain will depend on several factors including composition of gain and composition of diet. The amount of DE required per kilogram of gain typically increases with maturity. In a study by Heusner (1993), mature horses required approximately 24 Mcal of DE (above maintenance) per kilogram of gain. Martin-Rosset and Vermorel (1991) estimated that 0.99 Mcal ME/d was required above maintenance for mature Standardbred geldings consuming a mixed diet to gain 5.6 kg over a 3-month period. This amount of ME is approximately equivalent to 18 Mcal DE/kg gain. Using two different methods of determining

DE intake in Belgian and Percheron horses, Potter et al. (1987) suggested that 16–20.7 Mcal of DE were needed per kg (gain).

It seems reasonable to estimate that 16–24 Mcal of DE are required per kilogram of gain for mature horses, based on the results of the previously mentioned studies. The amount of energy needed per unit of gain will be influenced by the composition of gain. The composition of gain could be influenced by the body composition of the animal as well as other factors. The efficiency of DE conversion to NE varies among energy sources; therefore, less DE may be needed per unit of gain when a high-fat diet is offered than when a high-fiber diet is fed. Using the observations discussed above, it is possible to develop an approximate estimate of the amount of DE required above maintenance to increase the condition score of a horse one unit. Table 1-11 shows the estimated amount of DE above maintenance that would be needed to change the condition score of a 500-kg horse from a score of 4 to a score of 5 over different periods of time. These estimates have been derived from limited data and have not been tested under controlled conditions. Therefore, the estimates in Table 1-11 may under- or overestimate the amount of DE needed to change the condition score of a horse, particularly when applied to animals at the extreme ranges of the condition scoring range.

As noted above, deprivation of calories will result in weight loss. The composition of weight loss in horses has not been investigated, although it is likely that thin individuals lose lean body mass as well as fat mass when calories are restricted. Chronic calorie restriction resulting in severe weight loss can result in starvation. Horses that have been starved require careful management (see Chapter 12).

Short-term calorie restriction results in adaptive metabolic changes in horses. When food is withheld for an extended period (~ 12 hours), hepatic glycogenolysis and gluconeogenesis will maintain blood glucose levels and the mobilization of free fatty acids from adipose tissue will provide fuel for many tissues. In most cases, these responses do not have negative consequences for horses. However, in some equids, particularly ponies and donkeys, prolonged periods of negative energy balance may result in severe hyperlipidemina that may progress to the clinical syndrome of equine hyperlipemia. In horses, hyperlipidemia is generally defined as serum triglyceride concentration in excess of 500 mg/dl, whereas hyperlipemia is characterized by lipemia (a milky discoloration of the plasma), as well as hypertriglyceridemia. In the clinical syndrome of equine hyperlipemia, affected animals have hyperlipemia as well as signs of hepatic and/or renal failure. Severe liver and kidney damage occurs due to excessive accumulation of lipid, and death rate is high (Watson and Love, 1994). The onset of hyperlipemia usually follows a period of negative energy balance that can arise from feed restriction, decreased feed intake due to disease, or increased energy demand due to pregnancy or lactation. Watson (1998) has proposed that hyperlipemia results from abnormal regulation of hormone sensitive lipase (HSL), the enzyme responsible for stimulating lipolysis in adipose. When HSL is stimulated during negative energy balance or a stressful event in susceptible animals, excessive amounts of free fatty acids are released from adipose. These free fatty acids are taken up by the liver, re-esterified into triglycerides, and then released into the circulation or retained in the liver, eventually causing liver and kidney damage (Watson, 1998). Mares (particularly late in gestation or early in lactation) appear to be more susceptible to equine hyperlipemia than geldings or stallions, and obesity may also increase risk (Jeffcott and Field, 1985; Watson et al., 1992). As noted above, ponies and donkeys are more likely to be affected than horses. For animals in high-risk categories, it may be prudent to avoid periods of extended or severe energy restriction. Unfortunately, there do not appear to be any quantitative data available at this time to describe the severity or duration of restriction necessary to precipitate the onset of this syndrome.

REFERENCES

Allen, W. R., S. Wilsher, C. Turnbull, F. Stewart, J. Ousey, P. D. Rossdale, and A.L. Fowden. 2002. Influence of maternal size on placental, fetal and postnatal growth in the horse. I. Development in utero. Reproduction 123:445–453.

Anderson, C. E., G. D. Potter, J. L. Krieder, and C. C. Courtney. 1983. Digestible energy requirements for exercising horses. J. Anim. Sci. 56:91–95.

Argenzio, R. A., and H. F. Hintz. 1970. Glucose tolerance and effect of volatile fatty acid on plasma glucose concentration in ponies. J. Anim. Sci. 30:514–519.

Arieli, A., J. W. Schrama, W. van der Hel, and M. W. Verstegen. 1995. Development of metabolic partitioning in young calves. J. Dairy Sci. 78:1154–1162.

Asai, Y. 2000. Japanese feeding standards. Pp. 145–158 in Proc., 2000 Equine Nutr. Conf. for Feed Manufacturers, Kentucky Equine Research, Inc. Versailles KY.

Austbo, D. 2004. The Scandinavian adaptation of the French UFC System. Pp. 69–78 in Nutrition of the Performance Horse, V. Julliand and W. Martin-Rosset, eds. EAAP Publication No. 111. Netherlands: Wageningen Academic Publishers.

Austbo, D. 2005. Rations for intensive growth in young horses. Pp. 137–146 in The Growing Horse: Nutrition and Prevention on Growth

TABLE 1-11 Estimated Increase in Digestible Energy (DE) Intake Necessary to Change the Condition Score of a 500-kg horse from 4 to 5[a]

Time Period to Accomplish Gain	DE above Maintenance (Mcal/d)	Percent Increase in DE above Maintenance
60 days	5.3 – 6.7	32 – 41 percent
90 days	3.6 – 4.4	22 – 27 percent
120 days	2.7 – 3.3	16 – 21 percent
150 days	2.1 – 2.7	13 – 16 percent
180 days	1.8 – 2.2	11 – 14 percent

[a]Assumptions: 1 unit of change of condition score requires 16 to 20 kg of gain and 1 kg gain requires 20 Mcal DE above maintenance.

Disorders, V. Julliand and W. Martin-Rosset, eds. EAAP Publication No. 114. Netherlands: Wageningen Academic Publishers.

Banach, M. A., and J. W. Evans. 1981. Effects of inadequate energy during gestation and lactation on the estrous cycle and conception rates of mares and on their foal weights. Pp. 97–100 in Proc. 7th Equine Nutr. Physiol. Soc. Symp., Warrenton, VA.

Barth, K. M., J. W. Williams, and D. G. Brown. 1977. Digestible energy requirements of working and non-working ponies. J. Anim. Sci. 44:585–589.

Bell, A. W., R. Slepetis, and R. A. Ehrhardt. 1995. Growth and accretion of energy and protein in the gravid uterus during late pregnancy in Holstein cows. J. Dairy Sci. 78:1954–1961.

Bell, R. A., B. D. Nielsen, K. Waite, D. Rosenstein, and M. Orth. 2001. Daily access to pasture turnout prevents loss of mineral in the third metacarpus of Arabian weanlings. J. Anim. Sci. 79:1142–1150.

Birnie, J. W., R. E. Agnew, and F. J. Gordon. 2000. The influence of body condition on the fasting energy metabolism of nonpregnant, nonlactating dairy cows. J. Dairy Sci. 83:1217–1223.

Blaxter, K. L. 1989. Energy Metabolism in Animals and Man. Cambridge, UK: Cambridge University Press.

Booth, M. E. 1998. Factors influencing energy requirements of native ponies living outdoors in the United Kingdom. Ph.D. Thesis. University of Edinburgh.

Buff, P. R., C. D. Morrison, V. K. Ganjam, and D. H. Keisler. 2005. Effects of short-term feed deprivation and melatonin implants on circadian patterns of leptin in the horse. J. Anim. Sci. 83:1023–1032.

Buffington, C. A., D. A. Knight, C. W. Kohn, J. E. Madigan, and P. A. Scaman. 1992. Effect of protein source in liquid formula diets on food intake, physiologic values and growth of equine neonates. Am. J. Vet. Res. 53:1941–1946.

Bullimore, S. R., J. D. Pagan, P. A. Harris, K. E. Hoekstra, K. A. Roose, S. C. Gardner, and R. J. Geor. 2000. Carbohydrate supplementation of horses during endurance exercise: comparison of fructose and glucose. J. Nutr. 130:1760–1765.

Bush, J. A., D. E. Freeman, K. H. Kline, N. R. Merchen, and G. C. Fahey, Jr. 2001. Dietary fat supplementation effects on in vitro nutrient disappearance and in vivo nutrient intake and total digestibility by horses. J. Anim. Sci. 79:232–239.

Cavinder, C. A., M. M. Vogelsang, D. W. Forrest, P. G. Gibbs, and T. L. Blanchard. 2005. Reproductive parameters of fat vs moderately conditioned mares following parturition. Pp. 65–70 in Proc. 19th Equine Science Soc., Tucson, AZ.

Clayton, H. M. 1994. Training show jumpers. Pp. 429–438 in The Athletic Horse, D. R. Hodgson and R. J. Rose, eds. Philadelphia, PA: W. B. Saunders.

Coenen, M. 2000. German feeding standards. Pp. 159–173 in Proc., 2000 Equine Nutr. Conf. for Feed Manufacturers, Kentucky Equine Research, Inc., Versailles, KY.

Coenen, M. 2005. About the predictability of oxygen consumption and energy expenditure in the exercising horse. Pp. 123 in Proc. 19th Equine Science Soc., Tucson, AZ.

Coleman, R. J., G. W. Mathison, L. Burwash, and J. D. Milligan. 1997. The effect of protein supplementation of alfalfa diets on the growth of weanling horses. Pp. 59–64 in Proc. 15th Equine Nutr. Physiol. Soc. Symp., Ft. Worth, TX.

Cooper, S. R., D. R. Topliff, D. W. Freeman, J. E. Breazile, and R. D. Geisert. 1999. Effect of dietary cation anion difference on growth and serum osteocalcin levels in weanling horses. Pp. 110–120 in Proc. 16th Equine Nutr. Physiol. Soc. Symp., Raleigh, NC.

Couroucé, A., O. Geffroy, E. Barrey, B. Auvinet, and R. J. Rose. 1999. Comparison of exercise tests in French trotters under training track, racetrack and treadmill conditions. Equine Vet. J. Suppl. 30:528–532.

Crandell, K. 2002. Trends in feeding the American endurance horse. Pp. 135–138 in Proc. 2002 Equine Nutr. Conf., Kentucky Equine Research, Inc., Versailles, KY.

Cuddeford, D. 2004. A comparison of energy feeding systems for horses. Pp. 79–88 in Nutrition of the Performance Horse, V. Julliand and W. Martin-Rosset, eds. EAAP Publication No. 111.

Cymbaluk, N. F. 1990. Cold housing effects on growth and nutrient demand of young horses. J. Anim. Sci. 68:3152–3162.

Cymbaluk, N. F. 1994. Thermoregulation of horses in cold winter weather: a review. Livest. Prod. Sci. 40:65–71.

Cymbaluk, N. F., and G. I. Christison. 1989. Effects of diet and climate on growing horses. J. Anim. Sci. 67:48–59.

Cymbaluk, N., and G. Christison. 1990. Environmental effect on thermoregulation and nutrition of horses. Vet. Clin. North Am. Equine Pract. 6(2):355–372.

Cymbaluk, N. F., and G. I. Christison. 1993. Cold weather—does it affect foal growth. P. 7 in 4th Internat. Env. Symp., Am. Soc. Agr. Eng., St. Joseph, MI.

Cymbaluk, N. F., G. I. Christison, and D. H. Leach. 1989. Energy uptake and utilization by limit and ad libitum fed growing horses. J. Anim. Sci. 67:403–413.

Cymbaluk, N. F., M. E. Smart, F. Bristol, and V. A. Ponteaux. 1993. Importance of milk replacer intake and composition in rearing orphan foals. Can. Vet. J. 34:479–486.

Danielsen, K., L. M. Lawrence, P. Siciliano, D. Powell, and K. Thompson. 1995. Effect of diet on weight and plasma variables in endurance exercised horses. Equine Vet. J. Suppl. 18:372–377.

Davison, K. E., G. D. Potter, J. W. Evans, L. W. Greene, P. S. Hargis, C. D. Corn, and S. P. Webb. 1989. Growth and nutrient utilization in weanling horses fed added dietary fat. Pp. 95–100 in Proc. 11th Equine Nutr. Physiol. Soc. Symp., Stillwater, OK.

Davison, K. E., G. D. Potter, L. W. Greene, J. W. Evans, and W. C. MacMullan. 1991. Lactation and reproductive performance of mares fed added dietary fat during late gestation and early lactation. J. Equine Vet. Sci. 11:111–115.

Delobel, A., B. Vandervorst, J. P. Lejeune, V. De Behr, D. Serteyn, I. Durfrasne, and L. Istasse. 2005. First results from a morphological approach to draught foal and filly growth in the Ardennes: 2. Calculating growth curves. Pp. 77–78 in The Growing Horse: Nutrition and Prevention of Growth Disorders, V. Julliand and W. Martin-Rosset, eds. EAAP Publication No. 114. Netherlands: Wageningen Academic Publishers.

Doherty, O., M. Booth, N. Waran, C. Salthouse, and D. Cuddeford. 1997. Study of the heart rate and energy expenditure of ponies during transport. Vet. Rec. 141:589–592.

Doreau M., S. Boulot, W. Martin-Rosset, and J. Robelin. 1986. Relationship between nutrient intake, growth and body composition of the nursing foal. Reprod. Nutr. Develop. 26(2 B):683–690.

Doreau, M., S. Boulot and W. Martin-Rosset. 1991. Effect of parity and physiological state on intake, milk production and blood parameters in lactating mares differing in body size. Anim. Prod. 53:111–118.

Doreau, M., S. Boulot, D. Bauchart, J. P. Barlet, and W. Martin-Rosset. 1992. Voluntary intake, milk production and plasma metabolites in nursing mares fed two different diets. J. Nutr. 122:992.

Dunn, E. L., H. F. Hintz, and H. F. Schryver. 1991. Magnitude and duration of the elevation in oxygen consumption after exercise. Pp. 267–268 in Proc. 12th Equine Nutr. Physiol. Soc. Symp., Calgary, Alberta.

Eaton, M. D. 1994. Energetics and performance. Pp. 49–61 in The Athletic Horse, D. R. Hodgson and R. J. Rose, eds. Philadelphia, PA: W. B. Saunders.

Eaton, M. D., D. L. Evans, D. R. Hodgson, and R. J. Rose. 1995a. Maximal accumulated oxygen deficit in Thoroughbred horses. J. Appl. Physiol. 78:1564–1568.

Eaton, M. D., D. L. Evans, D. R. Hodgson, and R. J. Rose. 1995b. Effect of treadmill incline and speed on metabolic rate during exercise in Thoroughbred horses. J. Appl. Physiol. 79:951–957.

Eaton, M. D., D. R. Hodgson, D. L. Evans, and R. J. Rose. 1999. Effects of low and moderate intensity training on metabolic responses to exercise in Thoroughbreds. Equine Vet. J. Suppl. 30:521–527.

Ferrell, C. L. 1988. Energy metabolism. Pp 250–268 in The Ruminant Animal. Digestive physiology and nutrition, D. C. Church, ed. Englewood Cliffs, NJ: Prentice Hall.

Filho, H., C. Manso, M. Watford, and K. H. Mckeever. 2005. Body composition in transition mares and suckling foals. Pp. 303–304 in The Growing Horse: Nutrition and Prevention of Growth Disorders, V. Julliand and W. Martin-Rosset, eds. EAAP Publication No. 114. Netherlands: Wageningen Academic Publishers.

Fonnesbeck, P. V. 1981. Estimating digestible energy and TDN for horses with chemical analysis of feeds. J. Anim. Sci. 53 (Supplement 1):241 (Abstr.).

Fowden, A. L., A. J. Forehead, K. White, and P. M. Taylor. 2000a. Equine uteroplacental metabolism at mid- and late gestation. Exp. Physiol. 85:539–545.

Fowden, A. L., P. M. Taylor, K. L. White, and A. J. Forehead. 2000b. Ontogenic and nutritionally induced changes in fetal metabolism in the horse. J. Physiol. 528:209–219.

Freeman, D. W., G. D. Potter, G. T. Schelling, and J. L. Kreider. 1988. Nitrogen metabolism in mature horses at varying levels of work. J. Anim. Sci. 66:407–412.

Gallagher, K., J. Leech, and H. Stowe. 1992a. Protein, energy and dry matter consumption by racing Thoroughbreds: a field survey. J. Equine Vet. Sci. 12:43–48.

Gallagher, K., J. Leech, and H. Stowe. 1992b. Protein, energy and dry matter consumption by racing Standardbreds: a field survey. J. Equine Vet. Sci. 12:382–388.

Garlinghouse, S. E., and M. J. Burrill. 1998. Relationship of body condition score to completion rate during 160 mile endurance races. Equine Vet. J. Suppl. 30:591–595.

Gentry, L. R., D. L. Thompson, G. T. Gentry, Jr., K. A. Davis, R. A. Godke, and J. A. Cartmill. 2002. The relationship between body condition, leptin, and reproductive and hormonal characteristics of mares during the seasonal anovulatory period. J. Anim. Sci. 80:2695–2703.

Geor, R. J., L. J. McCutcheon, and M. I. Lindinger. 1996. Adaptations to daily exercise in hot and humid ambient conditions in trained Thoroughbred horses. Equine Vet. J. Suppl. 22:63–68.

Geor, R. J., L. J. McCutcheon, G. L. Exker, and M. I. Lindinger. 2000. Heat storage in horses during submaximal exercise before and after humid heat acclimation. J. Appl. Physiol. 89:2283–2293.

Gibbs, P. G., G. D. Potter, R. W. Blake, and W. C. McMullan. 1982. Milk production of Quarter Horse mares during 150 days of lactation. J. Anim. Sci. 54:496–499.

Gibbs, P. G., D. H. Sigler, and T. B. Goehring. 1987. Influence of diet on growth and development of yearling horses. Pp. 37–42 in Proc. 10th Equine Nutr. Physiol. Soc. Symp., Ft. Collins, CO.

Ginther, O. 1992. Reproductive Biology of the Mare. 2nd ed. Madison: University of Wisconsin.

Giussani, D. A., A. J. Forehead, and A. L. Fowden. 2005. Development of cardiovascular function in the horse fetus. J. Physiol. 565:1019–1030.

Glade, M. J. 1991. Dietary yeast culture supplementation of mares during late gestation and early lactation. J. Equine Vet. Sci. 11:10–16.

Glinsky, M. J., R. M. Smith, H. R. Spires, and C. L. Davis. 1976. Measurement of volatile fatty acid production rates in the cecum of the pony. J. Anim. Sci. 42:1465–1470.

Graham-Thiers, P., D. S. Kronfeld, K. A. Kline, D. J. Sklan, and P. A. Harris. 2000. Protein status of exercising Arabian horses fed diets containing 14 percent or 7.5 percent protein fortified with lysine and threonine. J. Equine Vet. Sci. 20:516–521.

Green, D. A. 1969. A study of growth rate in Thoroughbred foals. Br. Vet. J. 124:539–546.

Harris, P. 1997. Energy sources and requirements of the exercising horse. Annu. Rev. Nutr. 17:185–210.

Henneke, D., G. Potter, J. Kreider, and B. Yates. 1983. Relationship between condition score, physical measurements and body fat percentage in mares. Equine Vet. J. 15:371–372.

Henneke, D. G., G. D. Potter, and J. L. Kreider. 1984. Body condition during pregnancy and lactation and reproductive efficiency in mares. Theriogenology 21:897–909.

Heusner, G. 1993. Ad libitum feeding of mature horses to achieve rapid weight gain. P. 86 in Proc. 13th Equine Nutr. Physiol. Soc. Symp., Gainesville, FL.

Hines, K. K., S. L. Hodge, J. L. Kreider, G. D. Potter, and P. G. Harms. 1987. Relationship between body condition and levels of serum luteinizing hormone in postpartum mares. Theriogenology 28:815–825.

Hintz, H. F., and N. F. Cymbaluk. 1994. Nutrition of the horse. Annu. Rev. Nutr. 14:243–267.

Hintz, H. F., S. J. Roberts, S. W. Sabin, and H. F. Schryver. 1971. Energy requirements of light horses for various activities. J. Anim. Sci. 32:100–102.

Hintz, H. F., R. L. Hintz, and L. D. Van Vleck. 1979. Growth rate of Thoroughbreds. Effect of age of dam, year and month of birth and sex of foal. J. Anim. Sci. 48:480–487.

Hintz, H. F., J. Scott, L. V. Soderholm, and J. Williams. 1985. Extruded feeds for horses. Pp. 174–176 in Proc. 9th Equine Nutr. Physiol. Symp., East Lansing, MI.

Hiraga, A., M. Kai, K. Kubo, Y. Yamaya, and B. Kipp. 1995. The effects of incline on cardiopulmonary function during exercise in the horse. J. Equine Sci. 6:55–60.

Hoffman, R. M., D. S. Kronfeld, H. S. Herblein, W. S. Swecker, W. L. Cooper, and P. A. Harris. 1998. Dietary carbohydrates and fat influence milk composition and fatty acid profile of mare's milk. J. Nutr. 128:2708S–2711S.

Hoffman, R. M., R. C. Boston, D. Stefanovski, D. S. Kronfeld, and P. A. Harris. 2003. Obesity and diet affect glucose dynamics and insulin sensitivity in Thoroughbred geldings. J. Anim. Sci. 81:2333–2342.

Howard, A. D., G. D. Potter, E. M. Michael, P. G. Gibbs, D. M. Hood, and B. D. Scott. 2003. Heart rates, cortisol and serum cholesterol in exercising horses fed diets supplemented with omega-3 fatty acids. Pp. 41–46 in Proc. 18th Equine Nutr. Physiol. Soc. Symp., East Lansing, MI.

Hoyt, D. F., and C. R. Taylor. 1981. Gait and the energetics locomotion in horses. Nature 292:239–240

Jansen, W. L., J. van der Kuilen, S. N. J. Geelen, and A. C. Beynen. 2000. The effect of replacing nonstructural carbohydrates with soybean oil on the digestibility of fibre in trotting horses. Equine Vet. J. 32:27–30.

Jansen, W. L., S. N. J. Geelen, J. van der Kuilen, and A. C. Beynen. 2002. Dietary soyabean oil depressed the apparent digestibility of fibre in trotters when substituted for an iso-energetic amount of corn starch or glucose. Equine Vet. J. 34:302–305.

Jeffcott, L. B., and J. R. Field. 1985. Epidemiological aspects of hyperlipaemia in ponies in southeastern Australia. Austral. Vet. J. 62:140–141.

Jelan, Z., L. Jeffcott, N. Lundeheim, and M. Osborne. 1996. Growth rates in Thoroughbred foals. Pferdeheilkunde 12:291–295.

Ji, F., G. Wu, J. R. Blanton, Jr., and S.W. Kim. 2005. Changes in weight and composition in various tissues of pregnant gilts and their nutritional implications. J. Anim. Sci. 83:366–375.

Johnston, C., H. Holm, M. Faber, C. Erichsen, P. Eksell, and S. Drevemo. 2002. Effect of conformational aspects on the movement of the equine back. Equine Vet. J. Suppl. 34:314–318.

Jones, J. H., and G. P. Carlson. 1995. Estimation of metabolic energy cost and heat production during a 3-day event. Equine Vet. J. Suppl. 20:23–30.

Jordan, R. M. 1977. Growth pattern of ponies. Pp. 63–70 in Proc. 5th Equine Nutr. Soc. Symp., St. Louis, MO.

Kane, E. J., J. P. Baker, and L. S. Bull. 1979. Utilization of a corn oil supplemented diet by the pony. J. Anim. Sci. 48:1379–1383.

Kane, R. A., M. Fisher, D. Parrett, and L. M. Lawrence. 1987. Estimating fatness in horses. Pp. 127–131 in Proc. 10th Equine Nutr. Physiol. Soc. Symp., Ft. Collins, CO.

Katz, L. M., W. M. Bayly, M. J. Roeder, J. K. Kingston, and M. T. Hines. 2000. Effects of training on maximum oxygen consumption of ponies. Am. J. Vet. Res. 81:986–991.

Kavazis A. N., and E. A. Ott. 2003. Growth rates of Thoroughbred horses raised in Florida. J. Equine Vet. Sci. 23:353–357.

Kearns, C. F., K. H. McKeever, H. John-Alder, T. Abe, and W. F. Brechue. 2002a. Relationship between body composition, blood volume and maximal oxygen uptake. Equine Vet. J. Suppl. 34:485–490.

Kearns, C. F., K. H. McKeever, K. H. Kumagi, and T. Abe. 2002b. Fat-free mass is related to one mile race performance in elite Standardbred horses. Vet. J. 163:260–266.

Kienzle, E., S. Fehrle, and B. Opitz. 2002. Interactions between the apparent energy and nutrient digestibilities of a concentrate mixture and roughages and horses. J. Nutr. 132:1778S–1780S.

Knight, D., and W. Tyznik. 1985. Effect of artificial rearing on the growth of foals. J. Anim. Sci. 60:1–5.

Kowalski, J., J. Williams, and H. Hintz. 1990. Weight gains of mares during the last trimester of gestation. Equine Pract. 12:6–8.

Kronfeld, D. S. 1996. Dietary fat affects heat production and other variables of equine performance under hot and humid conditions. Equine Vet. J. (Supplement 22):24–34.

Kubiak, J. R., B. H. Crawford, E. L. Squires, R. H. Wrigley, and G. M. Ward. 1987. The influence of energy intake and percentage of body fat on the reproductive performance of nonpregnant mares. Theriogenology 28:587–598.

Kubiak, J. R., J. W. Evans, G. D. Potter, P. G. Harms, and W. L. Jenkins. 1988. Parturition in the multiparous mare fed to obesity. J. Equine Vet. Sci. 8:233–238.

Lawrence, L., M. Murphy, K. Bump, D. Weston, and J. Key. 1991. Growth responses in hand-reared and naturally reared Quarter Horse Foals. Equine Pract. 13:19–23.

Lawrence, L., J. DiPietro, K. Ewert, D. Parrett, L. Moser, and D. Powell. 1992a. Changes in body weight and condition in gestating mares. J. Equine Vet. Sci. 12:355–358.

Lawrence, L., S. Jackson, K. Kline, L. Moser, D. Powell, and M. Biel. 1992b. Observations on body weight and condition of horses in a 150-mile endurance ride. J. Equine Vet. Sci. 12:320–324.

Lawrence, L. A., H. R. Hearne, S. P. Davis, J. D. Pagan, A. Fitzgerald, and E. A. Greene. 2003. Characteristics of growth in Morgan horses. Pp. 317–322 in Proc. 18th Equine Nutr. Physiol. Soc. Symp., East Lansing, MI.

Lawrence, L. M., R. A. Kane, P. A. Miller, S. R. Reece, and C. Hartman. 1986. Urea space determination and body composition in horses. J. Anim. Sci. 63(Supplement 1):233.

Lawrence, L. M., K. J. Moore, H. F. Hintz, E. H. Jaster, and L. Wischover. 1987. Acceptability of alfalfa hay treated with an organic acid preservative for horses. Can. J. Anim. Sci. 67:217–220.

Lewis, L. D. 1995. Equine Clinical Nutrition. Philadelphia: Lea & Febiger.

Lieb, S. 1971. Cecal absorption and hepatic utilization of glucose and VFA in portal-carotid catheterized equine. M.S. Thesis. University of Kentucky, Lexington KY.

Luescher, U. A., D. B. McKeown, and H. Dean. 1998. A cross-sectional study on compulsive behaviour (stable vices) in horses. Equine Vet. J. Suppl. 27:14–18.

Malinowski, K., C. L. Betros, L. Flora, C. F. Kearns, and K. H. McKeever. 2002. Effect of training on age-related change in plasma insulin and glucose. Equine Vet. J. Suppl. 34:147–153.

Marlin, D. J., C. M. Scott, R. C. Schroter, R. C. Harris, P. A. Harris, C. A. Roberts, and P. C. Mills. 1999. Physiological responses of horses to a treadmill simulated speed and endurance test in high heat and humidity before and after humid heat acclimation. Equine Vet. J. 31:31–42.

Marlin, D. J., R. C. Shroter, S. L. White, P. Maykuth, G. Matthesen, P. C. Mills, N. Waran, and P. Harris. 2001. Recover from transport and acclimatisation of competition horses in a hot humid environment. Equine Vet. J. 33:371–379.

Martin, R. G., N. P. McMeniman, and K. F. Dowsett. 1991. Effects of a protein deficient diet and urea supplementation on lactating mares. J. Reprod. Fert. Suppl. 44:543–550.

Martin, R. G., N. P. McMeniman, and K. F. Dowsett. 1992. Milk and water intakes of foals sucking grazing mares. Equine Vet. J. 24:295–299.

Martin-Rosset, W. 2000. Feeding standards for energy and protein for horses in France. Pp. 31–94 in Proc., 2000 Equine Nutr. Conf. for Feed Manufacturers, Kentucky Equine Research Inc., Versailles, KY.

Martin-Rosset, W., and M. Vermorel. 1991. Maintenance energy requirement variations determined by indirect calorimetry and feeding trials in light horses. J. Equine Vet. Sci. 11:42–45.

Martin-Rosset, W., and M. Vermorel. 2004. Evaluation and expression of energy allowances and energy value of feeds in the UFC system for the performance horse. Pp. 29–60 in Nutrition of the Performance Horse, V. Julliand and W. Martin-Rosset, eds. EAAP Publication No. 111. Netherlands: Wageningen Academic Publishers.

Martin-Rosset, W., M. Vermorel, M. Doreau, J. L. Tisserand, and J. Andieu. 1994. The French horse feed evaluation systems and recommended allowances for energy and protein. Livest. Prod. Sci. 40:37–56.

McBride, G. E., R. J. Christopherson, and W. Sauer. 1985. Metabolic rate and plasma thyroid concentrations of mature horses in response to changes in ambient temperatures. Can. J. Anim. Sci. 65:375–382.

McLeod, K. R. and R. L. Baldwin, IV. 2000. Effects of diet forage:concentrate ratio and metabolizable energy intake on visceral organ growth and in vitro oxidative capacity of gut tissues in sheep. J. Anim. Sci 78:760–770.

McCutcheon, L. J., R. J. Geor, and K. W. Hinchcliff. 1999. Effects of prior exercise on muscle metabolism during sprint exercise in horses. J. Appl. Physiol. 87:1914–1922.

McGowan, C. M., R. E. Posner, and R. M. Christly. 2002. Incidence of exertional rhabdomyolysis in polo horses in the USA and the United Kingdom in the 1999/2000 season. Vet. Rec. 150:535–537.

McManus, C. J., and B. P. Fitzgerald. 2000. Effects of a single day of feed restriction on changes in serum leptin, gonadotropins, prolactin, and metabolites in ages and young mares. Domestic Animal Endocrinology 19:1–13.

McMiken, D. F. 1983. An energetic basis of equine performance. Equine Vet. J. 15:123–133.

Meyer, H., and L. Ahlswede. 1978. The intra-uterine growth and body composition of foals and the nutrient requirements of pregnant mares. Anim. Res. Dev. 8:86–111.

Morgan, K. 1997. Effects of short-term changes in ambient air temperature or altered insulation in horses. J. Thermal Biol. 22:187–194.

Morgan, K. 1998. Thermoneutral zone and critical temperatures of horses. J. Thermal Biol. 23:59–61.

Morgan, K., A. Ehrlemark, and K. Sallvik. 1997. Dissipation of heat from standing horses exposed to ambient temperatures between –3°C and 37°C. J. Thermal Biol. 22:177–186.

Morrison, F.B. 1961. Feeds and Feeding, Abridged. Claremont, Ontario: Morrison Pub. Co.

Mostert, H. J., R. J. Lund, A. J. Guthrie, and P. J. Cilliers. 1996. Integrative model for predicting thermal balance in exercising horses. Equine Vet. J. Suppl. 22:7–15.

NRC (National Research Council). 1978. Nutrient Requirements of Horses, 4th rev. ed. Washington, DC: National Academy Press.

NRC. 1981. Effect of Environment on Nutrient Requirements of Domestic Animals. Washington, DC: National Academy Press.

NRC. 1989. Nutrient Requirements of Horses, 5th rev. ed. Washington, DC: National Academy Press.

NRC. 1998. Nutrient Requirements of Swine. Washington, DC.: National Academy Press.

NRC. 2000. Nutrient Requirements of Beef Cattle. Washington, DC: National Academy Press.

NRC. 2001. Nutrient Requirements of Dairy Cattle. Washington, DC: National Academy Press.

Oftedal, O. T., H. F. Hintz, and H. F. Schryver. 1983. Lactation in the horse: milk composition and intake by foals. J. Nutr. 113:2196–2206.

Ordakowski, A. L., D. S. Kronfeld, C. A. Williams, and L. S. Gay. 2001. Folate status during lactation and growth in the Thoroughbred. Pp. 134–135 in Proc. 17th Equine Nutr. Physiol. Soc. Symp., Lexington, KY.

Ott, E. A. 2005. Influence of temperature stress on the energy and protein metabolism and requirements of the working horse. Livestock Prod. Sci. 92:123–130.

Ott, E. A., and R. L. Asquith. 1986. Influence of level of feeding and nutrient content of the concentrate on the growth and development of yearling horses. J. Anim. Sci. 62:290–299.

Ott, E. A., and R. L. Asquith. 1995. Trace mineral supplementation of yearling horses. J. Anim. Sci. 73:466–471.

Ott, E., and J. Kivipelto. 1999. Influence of chromium tripicolinate on growth and glucose metabolism in yearling horses. J. Anim. Sci. 77:3022–3030.

Ott, E. A., R. L. Asquith, J. P. Feaster, and F. G. Martin. 1979. Influence of protein level and quality on the growth and development of yearling foals. J. Anim. Sci. 49:620–628.

Ott, E. A., M. P. Brown, G. D. Roberts, and J. Kivipelto. 2005. Influence of starch intake on growth and skeletal development of weanling horses. J. Anim. Sci. 83:1033–1043.

Ousey, J. C., 1997. Thermoregulation and the energy requirement of the newborn foal, with reference to prematurity. Equine Vet. J. 24:104–108.

Ousey, J. C., A. J. McArthur, P. R. Murgatroyd, J. H. Stewart, and P. D. Rossdale. 1992. Thermoregulation and total body insulation in the neonatal foal. J. Thermal Biol. 17:1–10.

Ousey, J. C., S. Prandi, J. Zimmer, N. Holdstock, and P. D. Rossdale. 1997. Effects of various feeding regimens on the energy balance of equine neonates. Am. J. Vet. Res. 58:1243–1251.

Pagan, J. D. 1998. Measuring the digestible energy content of horse feeds. Pp. 71–76 in Advances in Equine Nutrition, J. D. Pagan, ed. Nottingham, UK: Nottingham University Press.

Pagan, J. D., and H. F. Hintz. 1986a. Equine Energetics I. J. Anim. Sci. 63:816–822.

Pagan, J. D., and H. F. Hintz. 1986b. Equine Energetics II. Energy expenditure in horses during submaximal exercise. J. Anim. Sci. 63:822–830.

Pagan, J. D., and H. F. Hintz. 1986c. Composition of milk from pony mares fed various levels of digestible energy. Cornell Vet. 76:139–148.

Pagan, J. D., H. F. Hintz, and T. R. Rounsaville. 1984. The digestible energy requirements of lactating pony mares. J. Anim. Sci. 58:1382–1387.

Pagan, J., S. Jackson, and S. Caddel. 1996. A summary of growth rates in Thoroughbreds in Kentucky. Pferdeheilkunde 12:285–289.

Pagan, J. D., P. Harris, T. Brewster-Barnes, S. E. Duren, and S. G. Jackson. 1998. Exercise affects digestibility and rate of passage of an all forage and mixed diets in Thoroughbred horses. J. Nutr. 128:2704s–2707s.

Pagan, J., G. Cowley, D. Nash, A. Fitzgerald, L. White, and M. Mohr. 2005a. The efficiency of utilization of digestible energy during submaximal exercise. Pp.199–204 in Proc. 19th Equine Science Symp., Tucson, AZ.

Pagan, J. D., A. Koch, S. Caddel, and D. Nash. 2005b. Size of Thoroughbred yearlings presented for auction at Keeneland Sales affects selling price. Pp. 224–225 in Proc. 19th Equine Science Symp., Tucson, AZ.

Palmgren Karlsson, C. A. Jansson, B. Essen-Gustavsson, and J. E. Lindberg. 2002. Effect of molassed sugar beet pulp on nutrient utilisation and metabolic parameters during exercise. Equine Vet. J. Suppl. 34: 44–49.

Pethick, D. W., R. J. Rose, W. L. Bryden, and J. M. Gooden. 1993. Nutrient utilization by the hindlimb of Thoroughbred horses at rest. Equine Vet. J. 25:41–44.

Platt, H. 1978. Growth and maturity in the equine fetus. J. Royal Soc. Med. 71:658–661.

Potter, G. D., J. W. Evans, G. W. Webb, and S. P. Webb. 1987. Digestible energy requirements of Belgian and Percheron horses. Pp. 133–138 in Proc. 10th Equine Nutr. Physiol. Soc. Symp., Ft. Collins, CO.

Potter, G. D., S. P. Webb, J. W. Evans, and G. W. Webb. 1989. Digestible energy requirements for work and maintenance of horses fed conventional and fat-supplemented diets. Pp. 145–150 in Proc. 11th Equine Nutr. Physiol. Soc. Symp., Stillwater, OK,

Powell, D., S. E. Reedy, D. R. Sessions and B. P. Fitzgerald. 2002. Effect of short term exercise training on insulin sensitivity in obese and lean mares. Equine Vet. J. Suppl. 34:81–84.

Reed, K. R., and N. K. Dunn. 1977. Growth and development of the Arabian horse. Pp. 76–90 in Proc. 5th Equine Nutr. Soc. Symp., St. Louis, MO.

Reynolds, L. P., C. L. Ferrell, D. A. Robertson, and S. P. Ford. 1986. Metabolism of the gravid uterus, foetus and utero-placenta at several stages of gestation in cows. J. Agric. Sci. 106:437–442.

Rich, V. B., J. P. Fontenot, and T. N. Meacham. 1981. Digestibility of animal, vegetable and blended fats by equine. Pp. 30–34 in Proc. 7th Equine Nutr. Physiol. Soc. Symp., Warrenton, WV.

Ridgway, K. J. 1994. Training endurance horses. Pp. 409–418 in The Athletic Horse, D. R. Hodgson and R. J. Rose, eds. Philadelphia: W. B. Saunders.

Robb, J., R. B. Harper, H. F. Hintz, J. T. Reid, J. E. Lowe, H. F. Schryver, and M. S. Rhee. 1972. Chemical composition and energy value of the body, fatty acid composition of adipose tissue and liver and kidney size in the horse. Anim. Prod. 14:25–34.

Ruff, S. J., C. H. Wood, D. K. Aaron, and L. M. Lawrence. 1993. A comparison of growth rates of normal Thoroughbred foals and foals diagnosed with cervical vertebral malformation. J. Equine Vet. Sci. 13:596–599.

Russell, M. A., A. V. Rodiek, and L. M. Lawrence. 1986. Effect of meal schedules and fasting on selected plasma free amino acids in horses. J. Anim. Sci 63:1428–1431.

Saastamoinen, M. T., S. Hyppa, and K. Huovinen. 1993. Effect of dietary fat supplementation and energy to protein ratio on growth and blood metabolites of weanling foals. J. Anim. Physiol Anim. Nutr. 71:179–188.

Sandgren B., G. Dalin, J. Carlsten, and N. Lundheim. 1993. Development of osteochondrosis in the tarsocrural joint and osteochondral fragments in the fetlock joints of Standardbred trotters. II. Body measurements and clinical findings. Equine Vet. J. Suppl. 16:48–53.

Santos, A. S., B. C. Sousa, L. C. Leitão, V. C. Alves. 2005. Yield and composition of milk from Lusitano lactating mares. Pferdeheilkunde 21(Supplement):115–116.

SAS/STAT. 1999. Statistical Analysis System. Cary, NC: SAS Institute.

Schroter, R. C., and D. J. Marlin. 2002. Modelling the cost of transport in competitions over ground of variable slope. Equine Vet. J. Suppl. 34: 397–401.

Schryver, H. F., H. F. Hintz, J. E. Lowe, R. L. Hintz, R. B. Harper, and J. T. Reid. 1974. Mineral composition of the whole body, liver and bone of young horses. J. Nutr. 104:126–132.

Schryver, H. F., D. W. Meakim, J. E. Lowe, J. Williams, L. V. Soderholm, and H. F. Hintz. 1987. Growth and calcium metabolism in horses fed varying levels of protein. Equine Vet. J. 19:280–287.

Scott, B. D., G. D. Potter, J. W. Evans, J. C. Reagor, G. W. Webb, and S. P. Webb. 1989. Growth and feed utilization by yearling horses fed added dietary fat. J. Equine Vet. Sci. 9:210–214.

Senft, R. L., and L. R. Rittenhouse. 1985. Effects of day-to-day weather fluctuations on grazing behavior of horses. Proc. Western Section Am. Soc. Anim. Sci. 36:298–300.

Serrano, M. G., D. L Evans, and J. L. Hodgson. 2002. Heart rate and blood lactate responses during exercise in preparation for eventing competition. Equine Vet. J. Suppl. 34:135–139.

Siciliano, P. D., C. H. Wood, L. M. Lawrence, and S. E. Duren. 1993. Utilization of a field study to evaluate digestible energy requirements of breeding stallions. Pp. 293–298 in Proc. 13th Equine Nutr. Physiol. Soc. Symp., Gainesville, FL.

Silver, M., and A. L. Fowden. 1982. Uterine prostaglandin F metabolite production in relation to glucose availability in late pregnancy and in a possible influence of diet on time of delivery in the mare. J. Reprod. Fert. Suppl. 32:511–519.

Simmons, H. A., and E. J. H. Ford. 1991. Gluconeogenesis from propionate produced in the colon of the horse. Br. Vet. J. 147:340–345.

Southwood, L. L., D. L. Evans, W. L. Bryden, and R. J. Rose. 1993. Nutrient intake of horses in Thoroughbred and Standardbred stables. Austral. Vet. J. 70:164–168.

Staniar, W. B., D. S. Kronfeld, K. H. Treiber, R. K. Splan, and P. A. Harris. 2004. Growth rate consists of baseline and systematic deviation components in Thoroughbreds. J. Anim. Sci. 82:1007–1015.

Sticker, L. S., D. L. Thompson, Jr., J. M. Fernandez, L. D. Bunting, and C. L. Depew. 1995. Dietary protein and(or) energy restriction in mares: plasma growth hormone, IGF-I, prolactin, cortisol, and thyroid hormone responses to feeding, glucose, and epinephrine. J. Anim. Sci. 73:1424–1432.

Stillions, M. C., and W. E. Nelson. 1972. Digestible energy during maintenance of the light horse. J. Anim. Sci. 34:981–982.

Thompson, K. N. 1995. Skeletal growth rates of weanling and yearling Thoroughbred horses. J. Anim Sci. 73:2513–2517.

Thornton, J., J. Pagan, and S. Persson. 1987. The oxygen cost of weight loading and inclined treadmill exercise in the horse. Pp 206–215 in Equine Exercise Physiology 2, J. R. Gillespie and N. E. Robinson, eds. Davis, CA: ICEEP Publ.

Tyler, C. M., D. R. Hodgson, and R. J. Rose. 1996. Effect of warm-up on energy supply during high intensity exercise in horses. Equine Vet. J. 28:117–120.

Vermorel, M., and W. Martin-Rosset. 1997. Concepts, scientific bases, structure and validation of the French horse net energy system (UFC). Livest. Prod. Sci. 47:261–275.

Vermorel, M., W. Martin-Rosset, and J. Vernet. 1991. Energy utilization of two diets for maintenance by horses; agreement with the new French net energy system. J. Equine Vet. Sci. 11:33–35.

Vermorel, M., W. Martin-Rosset, and J. Vernet. 1997a. Energy utilisation of twelve forage or mixed diets for maintenance by sport horses. Livest. Prod. Sci. 47:157–167.

Vermorel, M., J. Vernet, and W. Martin-Rosset. 1997b. Digestive and energy utilisation of two diets by ponies and horses. Livest. Prod. Sci. 51:13–19.

Vernet, J., M. Vermorel, and W. Martin-Rosset. 1995. Energy cost of eating long hay, straw and pelleted food in sport horses. Anim. Sci. 61:581–588.

Vervuert, I., M. Coenen, A. Borchers, M. Granel, S.Winkelsett, L. Christmann, O. Distl, E. Bruns, and B. Hertsch. 2003. Growth rates and the incidence of osteochondrotic lesions in Hanovarian warmblood foals. Pp. 107–112 in Proc. 18th Equine Nutr. Physiol. Soc. Symp., East Lansing, MI.

Voss, B., E. Mohr, and H. Krzywanek. 2002. Effects of aqua-treadmill exercise on selected blood parameters and on heart rate variability of horses. J. Vet. Med. 49A:137–143.

Watson, T. 1998. Equine hyperlipaemia. Pp. 23–40 in Metabolic and Endocrine Problems of the Horse, T. Watson, ed. London: Harcourt Brace and Co.

Watson, T. D. G., and S. Love. 1994. Equine hyperlipidemia. Compend. Continuing Education 16:89–98.

Watson, T., D. Murphy, and S. Love. 1992. Equine hyperlipaemia in the United Kingdom. Vet. Rec. 131:48–51.

Webb, S. P., G. D. Potter, and J. W. Evans. 1987. Physiologic and metabolic response of race and cutting horses to added dietary fat. P. 115 in Proc. 10th Equine Nutr. Physiol. Soc. Symp., Fort Collins, CO.

Webb, G. W., S. P. Webb, and D. K. Hansen. 1991. Digestibility of wheat straw or ammoniated wheat straw in equine diets. Pp. 261–262 in Proc. 12th Equine Nutr. Physiol. Soc. Symp., Calgary, Alberta.

Westervelt, R. G., J. R. Stouffer, and H. F. Hintz. 1976. Estimating fatness in horses and ponies. J. Anim. Sci. 43:781–785.

Whitehead, A. E., R. Foster, and T. Chenier. 2004. Placental characteristics of Standardbred mares. Pp. 71–75 in Proceedings of the Workshop on the Equine Placenta, University of Kentucky, Lexington, KY.

Williams, C. A., D. S. Kronfeld, W. B. Staniar, and P. A. Harris. 2001. Plasma glucose and insulin responses of Thoroughbred mares fed a meal high in starch and sugar or fat and fiber. J. Anim. Sci. 79:2196–2200.

Wooden G. R., K. L. Knox, and C. L. Wild. 1970. Energy metabolism in light horses. J. Anim. Sci. 30:544–548.

Zeyner, A., and E. Kienzle. 2002. A method to estimate digestible energy in horse feed. J. Nutr. 132:1771S–1773S.

Zmija, G., H. Meyer, and E. Kienzle. 1991. Feeds and feeding in German training stables of race horses. Pp. 85–90 in Proc. 12th Equine Nutr. Physiol. Soc. Symp., Calgary, Alberta.

2

Carbohydrates

CARBOHYDRATES IN FEEDS

Carbohydrates are the principal sources of energy in horse diets. Most of the carbohydrates in equine diets originate from forages, grains, and grain byproducts. Carbohydrates may be categorized by degree of polymerization (DP), and are often referred to as mono-, di-, oligo-, or polysaccharides. Monosaccharides of nutritional importance include glucose, fructose, galactose, mannose, arabinose, and xylose. Free monosaccharides occur in low concentrations in plants, but they are important constituents of the oligosaccharides and polysaccharides found in horse feeds. There are a few disaccharides of nutritional importance for horses. Lactose, a disaccharide composed of glucose and galactose, is an important nutrient source to the nursing foal. Maltose, a disaccharide consisting of two glucose units, is produced in the gastrointestinal tract by the action of amylase on starch, and may then be further digested to glucose. Oligosaccharides are compounds composed of short chains of monosaccharides (DP of 3-10). Oligosaccharides occurring in animal feeds include raffinose, stachyose, and fructooligosaccharides (FOS). The term "fructan" is often used to describe carbohydrates containing multiple fructose units. Therefore, fructooligogoasaccharides and inulin are types of fructans. Some fructans may be considered polysaccharides by the strict definition that polysaccharides contain more than 10 monosaccharide units. However, compared to many other polysaccharides, fructan polysaccharides have a lower degree of polymerization (Tungland and Meyer, 2002). Polysaccharides are the largest and most complex category of carbohydrates in horse feeds. Starch and cellulose are the most common polysaccharides in horse diets. Pectin and hemicellulose are also polysaccharides.

All carbohydrates contain similar amounts of gross energy. However, when utilized by the horse, they provide variable amounts of digestible energy (DE), metabolizable energy (ME), or net energy (NE). Carbohydrates digested and absorbed as monosaccharides in the small intestine yield more energy than carbohydrates digested by microbial action. The type of linkage between the monosaccharide residues in the oligosaccharides and polysaccharides has a great influence on the site of digestion of these compounds, and thus their nutritional value to the horse. Hydrolysis of the α1-6 and the α1-4 linkages of starch and maltose can occur in the equine small intestine, but horses do not produce the enzymes necessary to digest the β1-4 linkages found in cellulose or the mixed linkages found in hemicellulose. Therefore, digestion of cellulose and hemicellulose must occur as a result of microbial fermentation. Stachyose, raffinose, β-glucans, and pectin are also resistant to enzymatic hydrolysis.

A variety of systems have been developed to classify plant carbohydrates. Some methods have classified carbohydrates according to their role in the plant, whereas other systems have attempted to classify carbohydrates in ways that have significance to animal or human nutrition. The analytical methods used to determine the carbohydrate composition of feeds are discussed in Chapter 10. There are readily available methods for measuring some, but not all carbohydrate components in animal feeds. Because some components have traditionally been difficult to measure, many carbohydrate partitioning systems have used collective terms such as nonstarch polysaccharides or total dietary fiber (Figure 10-1). The most common system of analysis for feeds is the system initially developed by Van Soest in the late 1960s. This system separates the feed into neutral detergent solubles and neutral detergent fiber (NDF). The NDF fraction contains cellulose, most hemicellulose, and lignin. For many years, the amount of nonstructural carbohydrate (NSC) in a feed was determined by subtracting the amount of NDF, protein, ether extract, and ash from total dry matter (DM). More recently, the term "nonfibrous" (or nonfiber) carbohydrates (NFC) has been used to represent this difference, whereas "nonstructural carbohydrate" has been used to describe a chemically analyzed fraction of a feed (NRC, 2001). The NFC fraction is comprised of all carbohydrates not found in the NDF component of a feed. The NSC fraction includes mono- and disaccharides, oligosaccharides (including fructan) and starch (Hall, 2003). Few commercial feed analysis laboratories completely fractionate the carbohydrates that make up NSC, but in most feeds, the amount of NSC can be approximated by summing the amount of starch and the amount of water-soluble carbohydrates (WSC). The extent to which the sum of starch and WSC accounts for all NSC depends on the analytical procedures used to measure these fractions. The quantitative difference between NSC and NFC is relatively small for some feeds such as cereal grains, but can be quite large for many other feeds (Table 2-1). Marked differences between NSC and NFC occur in feeds that contain significant amounts of pectin.

The system of partitioning carbohydrates into NDF and NFC fractions was developed for use in ruminant nutrition. This system is also useful for partitioning carbohydrates in horse feeds, particularly if additional analyses for other carbohydrate fractions, such as starch, are also available. Table 2-2 shows representative values for the NDF, NFC, and starch content of a number of common horse feeds. These values were obtained from a commercial feed library (Dairy One, 2005). It should be noted that the carbohydrate composition of a feed can vary greatly, especially for forages and byproducts; therefore, analysis of individual feed ingredients is the best method of estimating carbohydrate composition. Because NDF and NFC are heterogeneous mixtures of carbohydrates that vary in digestibility, additional partitioning of carbohydrate fractions may be useful. In 2001, Hoffman et al. proposed that a relevant system for partitioning carbohydrates in equine feeds would include at least three fractions. The three fractions are: (1) hydrolyzable carbohydrates (CHO-H), which can be digested in the small intestine; (2) rapidly fermented carbohydrates (CHO-F_R), which are readily available for microbial fermentation; and (3) slowly fermentable carbohydrates (CHO-F_S). They suggested the hydrolyzable fraction included hexoses, disaccharides, some oligosaccharides, and the nonresistant starches. Although some fermentation of these compounds may occur in the stomach, the primary products of digestion of these compounds are monosaccharides, and thus the energy yield is relatively high. The rapidly fermentable fraction included pectin, fructan, and some oligosaccharides not digested in the small intestine. Resistant starch and neutral detergent hemicellulose could also be included in the rapidly fermented fraction. In human nutrition, starch that is not easily digested in the small intestine is categorized as resistant starch (Englyst and Englyst, 2005). Hoffman et al. (2001) suggested that lactate and propionate are the primary products of the rapidly fermented carbohydrates in horses. However, lactate production from pectin fermentation by rumen bacteria is low and acetate production is high (Strobel and Russell, 1986). Also, Moore-Colyer et al. (2000) did not report increased lactate concentrations in the cecum of ponies fed sugar beet feed as compared to ponies fed hay cubes. The slowly fermented carbohydrate fraction includes cellulose, hemicellulose, and ligno-cellulose that result primarily in the production of acetate in the large intestine. The system proposed by Hoffman et al. (2001) may allow better understanding of the energy value of the carbohydrate portion of the feed as it separates the components that are absorbed as glucose from those that are fermented to volatile fatty acids (VFAs). Unfortunately, methods for analyzing all of these fractions are not readily available. A comparison of the various analytical and nutritional methods of classifying carbohydrates is shown in Figure 10-1.

CARBOHYDRATE DIGESTION

Structural carbohydrates are important sources of energy in horse diets. The microbial production of VFAs in the cecum may be sufficient to meet up to 30 percent of a horse's energy needs at maintenance (Glinsky et al., 1976). Additional VFAs are produced in the colon. Therefore, the contribution of VFAs to total daily energy utilization must be great, particularly for horses consuming all-forage diets. Acetate is the principal VFA produced, but propionate and butyrate production may also be significant (Hintz et al., 1971; Moore-Colyer et al., 2000). Acetate may be used directly for energy. Pethick et al. (1993) studied acetate uptake by the hind limb of resting horses and estimated that acetate oxidation was responsible for about 30 percent of the energy utilized by the limb. In addition, Pratt et al. (1999) reported that the clearance rate of infused acetate was increased during exercise. Acetate that is not used immediately is probably used for the synthesis of long-chain fatty acids, which may be stored or, in the lactating mare, secreted into the milk. Doreau et al. (1992) reported that mares consuming high-forage rations produced milk with a higher concentration of fat than mares fed a high-concentrate ration. The

TABLE 2-1 Neutral Detergent Fiber (NDF), Nonfiber Carbohydrate (NFC), and Nonstructural Carbohydrate (NSC) Composition of Selected Feedstuffs[a] on a Dry Matter Basis (NRC, 2001)

Feedstuff	%NDF	%NFC[b]	%NSC[c]
Alfalfa hay	43.1	22.0	12.5
Beet pulp	47.3	36.2	19.5
Corn gluten meal	7.0	17.3	12.0
Mixed, mostly grass hay	60.9	16.6	13.6
Soybean meal (48% CP)	9.6	34.4	17.2
Soy hulls	66.6	14.1	5.3

[a]The values shown here may vary from those shown elsewhere in this document. The values are provided to illustrate differences among feeds and carbohydrate categories. Actual values for individual feeds may vary by stage of maturity, variety, source, etc.
[b]%NFC = 100 − (%CP + %NDF + %EE + %Ash).
[c]%NSC determined by measurement using the methods described by Smith (1981).

TABLE 2-2 Carbohydrate Composition (dry matter basis) of Selected Feed Ingredients[a]

Feed	%NDF	%ADF	%NFC[b]	%Starch
Grass pasture				
Mean (SD)	58.8 (11.9)	35.6 (7.8)	19.6 (6.7)	3.5 (2.9)
Range	46.9–70.6	27.6–43.5	12.9–26.2	0.6–6.4
Observations	4,229	4,135	3,469	1,186
Mixed, mostly grass pasture				
Mean (SD)	51.9 (10.0)	30.8 (6.1)	20.6 (6.8)	3.1 (2.3)
Range	41.9–61.9	24.7–36.9	13.8–27.3	0.8–5.4
Observations	3,649	3,455	2,395	1,536
Fresh Bermuda grass				
Mean (SD)	66.7 (6.1)	38.4 (4.2)	14.0 (4.5)	2.6 (2.3)
Range	60.6–72.8	34.3–42.6	9.5–18.5	0.3–4.9
Observations	304	304	285	46
Alfalfa cubes				
Mean (SD)	43.3 (7.0)	33.6 (5.0)	26.6 (4.5)	2.0 (1.2)
Range	36.4–50.3	28.6–38.6	22.1–31.1	0.8–3.2
Observations	319	319	224	144
Legume hay				
Mean (SD)	38.5 (5.4)	30.0 (4.1)	30.8 (3.7)	2.4 (1.2)
Range	33.1–43.9	26.0–34.1	27.1–34.5	1.3–3.6
Observations	64,704	64,673	46,133	23,738
Grass hay				
Mean (SD)	63.8 (6.4)	39.2 (4.6)	19.5 (6.7)	2.8 (1.5)
Range	57.4–70.2	34.6–43.7	14.8–24.2	1.3–4.2
Observations	19,935	19,716	15,951	9,682
Mixed, mostly grass hay				
Mean (SD)	60.8 (7.2)	38.8 (4.6)	20.9 (4.6)	2.7 (1.4)
Range	53.7–68.0	34.2–43.5	16.3–25.5	1.4–4.1
Observations	15,666	15,661	11,319	6,721
Bermuda grass hay				
Mean (SD)	67.7 (5.3)	35.6 (4.1)	16.5 (4.5)	6.1 (3.0)
Range	62.4–73.0	31.6–39.7	12.0–21.0	3.1–9.0
Observations	4,874	4,874	3,529	1,989
Barley				
Mean (SD)	19.6 (6.8)	7.7 (3.9)	63.9 (8.3)	53.9 (9.4)
Range	12.8–26.4	3.7–11.6	55.6–72.3	44.5–63.2
Observations	523	511	346	218
Steam flaked corn				
Mean (SD)	9.1 (1.9)	3.5 (1.0)	78.4 (3.5)	72.3 (4.8)
Range	7.2–11.0	2.6–4.5	74.9–81.9	67.5–77.1
Observations	139	136	135	98
Oats				
Mean (SD)	27.9 (9.8)	13.5 (5.4)	50.9 (9.1)	44.3 (10.3)
Range	18.0–37.7	8.1–18.9	41.9–60.0	34.0–54.5
Observations	263	260	201	125
Wheat midds				
Mean (SD)	37.1 (6.5)	12.9 (2.8)	37.9 (7.7)	26.0 (9.1)
Range	30.7–43.6	10.1–15.7	30.1–45.6	16.9–35.1
Observations	420	414	303	116
Molasses				
Mean (SD)	0.7 (0.7)	0.3 (0.4)	76.7 (13.9)	1.1 (1.6)
Range	0–1.4	0–0.7	62.8–90.6	0–2.8
Observations	114	114	65	41
Beet pulp				
Mean (SD)	41.9 (5.8)	25.6 (4.0)	44.4 (6.3)	1.3 (1.0)
Range	36.1–47.7	21.6–29.5	38.1–50.6	0.3–2.4
Observations	359	380	284	141
Corn gluten feed				
Mean (SD)	36.0 (7.3)	11.1 (3.2)	33.4 (6.7)	16.8 (8.0)
Range	28.6–43.3	7.9–14.3	26.7–40.1	8.7–24.8
Observations	330	342	260	50

TABLE 2-2 continued

Feed	%NDF	%ADF	%NFC[b]	%Starch
Distillers dried grains				
Mean (SD)	33.9 (4.2)	17.1 (3.9)	24.9 (5.0)	5.7 (3.0)
Range	29.7–38.1	13.3–21.0	19.9–29.9	2.7–8.7
Observations	1,427	1,453	1,134	795
Oat hulls				
Mean (SD)	69.9 (14.4)	39.7 (8.9)	[c]	[c]
Range	55.6–84.3	30.7–48.7		
Observations	19	18		
Rice bran				
Mean (SD)	30.2 (11.8)	18.1 (13.0)	14.3 (10.5)	18.4 (9.8)
Range	18.6–42.0	5.1–31.1	0–31.1	8.6–28.1
Observations	110	110	86	51
Extruded soybeans				
Mean (SD)	17.8 (4.5)	11.4 (3.1)	20.3 (4.2)	2.4 (1.5)
Range	13.4–22.3	8.3–14.5	16.1–24.6	1.0–3.9
Observations	60	59	39	15
Soybean meal				
Mean (SD)	13.1 (5.4)	8.4 (3.0)	28.3 (4.6)	2.0 (1.1)
Range	7.7–18.5	5.5–11.4	23.7–32.9	0.8–3.1
Observations	1,273	1,253	1,044	188
Soy hulls				
Mean (SD)	61.7 (3.3)	44.0 (8.3)	19.7 (4.0)	1.7 (1.2)
Range	53.4–70.1	37.5–50.6	15.7–23.8	0.5–2.8
Observations	297	357	218	75

[a]Data taken from Dairy One website, September 2005. The values listed here may vary from those in feed composition tables elsewhere in this document. The values shown here were drawn from a commercial website and reflect the diversity of feeds submitted for analysis.
[b]NFC as determined by difference: %NFC = 100 – (%CP + %NDF + %EE + %Ash).
[c]Fewer than 10 observations available.

propionate produced by microbial fermentation may be used for hepatic glucose synthesis. This gluconeogenic mechanism is probably very important in maintaining glucose homeostasis in forage-fed horses (Argenzio and Hintz, 1970; Simmons and Ford, 1991). The role of butyrate in equine gastrointestinal health has not been well studied, but it is generally accepted as important in other species. Although cellulose is the most abundant carbohydrate in most forages, other carbohydrates contribute to the energy produced from the microbial fermentation in the gastrointestinal tract, including hemicellulose, pectin, fructan, and the β-glucans. As noted above, not all carbohydrates are fermented at the same rate or produce the same proportions of VFAs. Differences in the amounts of various carbohydrates found in forages are discussed in depth in Chapter 8.

Diet composition, particularly carbohydrate composition, may affect the microbial population of the large intestine as well as the proportions of VFAs that are produced. Feeding a high-starch diet (30% starch; 3.4 g starch/kg body weight [BW]/meal) has been reported to decrease the concentration of celluloytic bacteria but increase the concentration of total anaerobic bacteria, lactic-acid utilizing bacteria, lactobacilli, and streptococci in the cecum (Medina et al., 2002). The concentrations of lactobaccilli and streptococci in the colon were also increased in response to the high-starch diet (Medina et al. 2002). Moore and Dehority (1993) reported minimal differences in cecal cellulolytic bacterial concentrations in ponies receiving diets consisting of 90 percent hay and 10 percent concentrate compared to ponies receiving 60 percent hay and 40 percent concentrate. However, the higher concentrate diet was associated with increased total bacterial and protozoal concentrations in the colon. The composition of the carbohydrates in the diet may also affect VFA production in the large intestine. The molar percentage of acetate in the cecum decreased, and the molar percentage of propionate increased, when ponies were fed diets with increasing amounts of corn (Hintz et al., 1971). In that study, diet did not alter the proportion of acetate and propionate in the colon, but the total VFA concentrations were reduced in response to the diet containing 63 percent ground corn. Medina et al. (2002) found lower cecal acetate concentrations and increased cecal propionate concentrations in horses fed a high-starch diet. The effect of diet on acetate and propionate in the colon was less pronounced; however, the high-starch diet increased lactic acid concentrations and decreased pH in the cecum and colon (Medina et al., 2002).

In ruminants, adequate consumption of structural carbohydrates is believed to be important for gastrointestinal health (NRC, 2001). Minimum NDF recommendations for the total diet of dairy cattle vary with source of NDF in the diet and other factors such as particle size. Chewing activity, and thus saliva production, has been suggested as an important consideration for gastrointestinal health and productivity in dairy cows. Ruminant nutritionists have attempted to assess the amount and form of fiber in a diet that allows for adequate chewing and saliva production. Concepts such as "effective fiber," "physically effective fiber," and "effective NDF" have been developed to assess the ability of various diets to maintain production and gastrointestinal health in dairy cattle (Mertens, 1997). Similar concepts have not been developed in horses, but research on the effect of fiber amount and type on digestion and gastrointestinal health is needed. The amount of fiber in the diet may also affect the weight of the gastrointestinal tract. High-fiber diets tend to hold more water, thus increasing total weight of the gastrointestinal tract (Coenen and Meyer, 1987). However, the mass of the gastrointestinal tissue may also be increased. McLeod and Baldwin (2000) reported that lambs fed a high forage diet at 2-times maintenance had heavier gut tissues than lambs fed an isocaloric high-concentrate diet. The gastrointestinal tract has a high metabolic rate; thus, an increase in gut size could account for elevated maintenance requirements in forage-fed animals.

The digestion and metabolism of structural carbohydrates in the large intestine may be able to meet the energy needs of many horses at maintenance, but this source of energy alone is unable to meet the needs of horses with higher requirements. Traditionally, dietary energy density has been increased by adding grains (oats, barley, corn, or others) or grain byproducts to the horse's diet. Most of the energy in grains is found as starch.

Total tract starch disappearance in the horse is very high (> 90 percent), but the extent of prececal starch digestion is variable. Starch is often viewed as a homogenous entity, but there is structural variation in the starch found in different foods. There are two main components of starch: amylose and amylopectin. Amylose is a straight chain structure of glucose units. Amylopectin is a branched chain of glucose units. The proportions of amylose and amylopectin in starch vary by cereal grain and with other factors, including maturity and variety (Van Soest, 1994). Interrupting the crystalline structure of starch may increase digestibility. A common method of altering the crystalline structure is gelatinization, which occurs with moist heating. However, under some conditions, amylose that has been heated and allowed to recrystalize can be less susceptible to enzymatic digestion than the original starch. The starch that reaches the large intestine is categorized as resistant starch in human nutrition (Englyst et al., 1996; Englyst and Englyst, 2005). Resistant starch includes starch that is not accessible to digestive enzymes due to its structure or encapsulation in plant cell structures and starch that has been modified by certain types of processing (Cummings et al., 1996; Tharanathan, 2002). A system for characterizing the availability of the starch found in various horse feeds has not been developed, but could be a useful tool. Enzymatic digestion of starch occurs in the small intestine, but starch is also susceptible to microbial fermentation. The equine stomach contains microbes capable of fermenting carbohydrates (Kern et al., 1974). Healy et al. (1995) reported increased lactate concentrations in gastric fluid obtained from ponies fed a large concentrate meal, and other researchers have reported significant dry matter and starch disappearance to occur in the stomach (de Fombelle et al., 2003; Varloud et al., 2003). It is also possible that fructan can be hydrolyzed to some extent by gastric acid (Van Soest, 1994) or fermented in the stomach.

Most glucose absorption appears to occur in the proximal small intestine (Dyer et al., 2002), so factors that decrease retention time in the proximal small intestine may decrease small intestinal glucose absorption. The type and amount of forage in the diet may alter small intestinal starch digestibility (Meyer et al., 1993), possibly by affecting digesta flow in the small intestine. The abundance of amylase in the digestive secretions, as well as the opportunity for amylase to associate with dietary starch, may also influence the variability in starch disappearance from the small intestine. Relatively little is known about the factors that affect the quantity of digestive enzymes secreted into the equine gastrointestinal tract. The ability of horses to produce the enzymes associated with lactose digestion decrease with age (Roberts et al., 1973). In other species of animals, diet composition has been shown to have variable effects on the secretion and activity of enzymes associated with carbohydrate digestion (Zebrowska and Low, 1987; Flores et al., 1988; Swanson et al., 2000). The amount of amylase measured in the pancreatic tissue of horses fed either hay or hay and concentrate for at least 8 weeks was not affected by diet (Kienzle et al., 1994). However, in another experiment, the amylase activity (on a wet weight basis) of jejunal chyme was higher when horses received a diet with added corn, oats, or barley than when they received only hay (Kienzle, et al., 1994). These authors noted that amylase activity in jejunal chyme was subject to variation among individuals. Further research is needed to define the factors that influence the amount and activity of carbohydrate-digesting enzymes in the horse.

Grain processing may influence the extent of prececal starch disappearance by decreasing particle size and increasing surface area. Gelatinization of starch may also occur with some processing methods. The ability of various processing methods to enhance small intestinal starch disappearance is discussed in Chapter 8. There are differences in prececal starch disappearance among different types of grains (Radicke et al., 1991; Kienzle et al., 1992; Meyer et al., 1993; de Fombelle et al., 2004), with oat starch generally being more digestible in the small intestine than corn starch or barley starch. The amount of starch consumed at one time may also affect the percentage of starch that disappears before reaching the large intestine. When a small amount of oats was fed to horses, approximately 80 percent of the starch was digested and absorbed prior to reaching the terminal ileum, but when a larger amount of oats was fed, starch disappearance before reaching the ileum was only 58 percent (Potter et al., 1992).

Starch that is not digested in the small intestine enters the large intestine, where it will be fermented. When starch is fermented, its net energy value is lower than when it is absorbed as glucose. Also, starch flow to the large intestine may alter the microbial environment. In certain cases, this may be beneficial to the horse. Kienzle et al. (2002) suggested that addition of concentrate to a straw diet improved the utilization of the straw, possibly by providing additional nutrients that enhanced the activity of the microbial population. However, negative effects of starch bypass to the large intestine may also occur. Feeding a high-starch diet (30% starch; 3.4 g starch/kg BW/meal) has been reported to decrease the concentration of celluloytic bacteria in the cecum (Medina et al., 2002). In addition, several studies have reported decreased colon and/or cecal pH in horses or ponies fed high concentrate/starch diets (Willard et al., 1977; Radicke et al., 1991; Medina et al., 2002). To avoid a decrease in large intestinal pH, high-starch feeds should not be offered in amounts that result in significant starch overflow to the large intestine. One researcher has suggested that the capacity of the small intestine for starch digestion is reached at a starch intake of 3.5 to 4 g/kg BW (Potter et al., 1992). However, Radicke et al. (1991) found that cecal pH was suppressed with starch intakes between 2 and 3 g/kg BW.

CARBOHYDRATE METABOLISM AND STORAGE

Blood glucose concentrations rise when a meal high in starch is consumed. Insulin levels also increase, which enhances glucose uptake by many tissues, including muscle and adipose. The increase in blood glucose is generally related to the amount and availability of starch consumed (or glucose when a source of free glucose is fed). In humans, the term "glycemic index" (GI) has been used to characterize the magnitude of the blood glucose increase to various foods. The primary purpose of the GI in human nutrition was to provide a means of comparing carbohydrate sources in order to manage hyperglycemia. The GI has been defined as the incremental area under the blood glucose response curve of a 50-g carbohydrate portion of a test food, expressed as a percentage of the blood glucose response curve to the same amount of carbohydrate from a standard food consumed by the same person (FAO/WHO, 1998). The 50-g carbohydrate portion should contain 50 g of glycemic or "available" carbohydrate, and the standard food may be either white bread or glucose (FAO/WHO, 1998). The FAO/WHO guideline suggested testing the standard food at least three times in each subject in order to obtain a representative mean response. The guideline also discussed the method of determining available carbohydrate in the test food. Application of the GI in human nutrition has some limitations (Monro, 2003). A GI that compares an equivalent amount of the test food to the standard has been suggested (Monro, 2003). This system would place food substitutions on an equal-weight basis rather than an equal-carbohydrate basis. Monro (2003) also suggested that a GI determined with a specific amount of carbohydrate (50 g) may not represent responses to other levels of intake.

Recently, several studies have attempted to apply the GI concept to horse feeds. The methods that have been used in horses have been extremely variable, making it difficult to interpret the results across studies. The glucose response to the carbohydrate in test feeds has been compared to the response to an equivalent amount of glucose administered by nasogastric tube (Jose-Cunilleras et al., 2004) or to oats or corn (Pagan et al., 1999; Vervuert et al., 2003, 2004, 2005; Rodiek and Stull, 2005). Using a readily consumed grain as the standard removes any effect associated with the administration of glucose by nasogastric tube, but the chemical composition of a grain may vary from one study to another. Another source of variation among studies with horses has been the amount of feed or carbohydrate offered. Among studies that have determined GI for horse feeds, there has been little consistency in the amount of carbohydrate offered to horses. In one study, the amount of hydrolyzable carbohydrate was approximately 900 g/484-kg horse (Jose-Cunilleras et al., 2004). In other studies, smaller amounts of hydrolyzable carbohydrates have been fed (Vervuert et al., 2003, 2004). When the glycemic responses to several feeds were compared to oats, the relative GI values were affected by the amount of the test feeds and the oats that were offered (0.75, 1.5, or 2.5 kg) (Pagan et al., 1999). Feeds have not always been offered in equicarbohydrate amounts or equal food amounts. One study compared feeds that provided similar amounts of calories that resulted in large differences in both total hydrolyzable carbohydrate intake and total feed intake among feeds (Rodiek and Stull, 2005). An advantage of this method would be that feed substitutions in horse diets are often made on a caloric basis. However, a disadvantage relates to the time required to consume the feed provided and the effects this may have on the glucose response curve. With appropriate standardization, there may be some application of the GI to horse nutrition; however, many factors will have to be considered, including the age, breed, and physiological state of the horse, as well as the physical form of the feed. In addition, a GI system must account not only for differences among feeds when they are fed separately, but also when they are mixed with other ingredients as is common in the horse industry. For example, Pagan et al. (1999) reported that the glycemic response of horses consuming sweet feed was reduced when vegetable oil was added to the feed.

Absorbed glucose may be used for immediate energy or it may be stored for later use. The storage carbohydrate in animals is glycogen, and the main storage sites are muscle and liver. Glucose that is not utilized for immediate energy or for glycogen synthesis may also be used for fat synthesis. Glycogen stored in the muscle is available only to the muscle as a fuel source. However, glycogen stored in the liver may be broken down to augment glucose availability to other tissues. Maintaining adequate blood glucose concentration is important for the central nervous system. The developing fetus is also an important consumer of glucose (Fowden et al., 2000a,b). Carbohydrates are an important source of energy to the exercising horse. The contribution of carbohydrate to energy production increases with increasing work intensity, partly due to increasing recruitment of fast-twitch muscle fibers. Muscle fibers in the horse are usually grouped into three categories: Type I, Type IIA, and Type IIX. The Type I fibers are highly oxidative and are well equipped to use fat as a substrate. Type I fibers are recruited for activities that do not require great force generation. Type II fibers, particularly the Type IIX fibers, are more suited to rapid contraction and high force generation and thus must be used during speed or strength work. Type IIX fibers are highly glycolytic and, thus, prefer carbohydrate as an energy source over fat.

The carbohydrate utilized during exercise may arise from muscle glycogen stores or from blood glucose derived from the diet or from hepatic glycogenolysis or hepatic gluconeogenesis. Muscle and liver glycogen stores can decrease dramatically when strenuous exercise continues for an extended period. When horses exercised for 1 hour at 500 m/min or for 4 hours at 300 m/min, muscle glycogen stores were depleted by approximately 60 percent (Lindholm et al., 1974). In that study, liver glycogen was depleted by approximately 40 percent in the 1-hour exercise bout and 90 percent in the 4-hour exercise bout. The extent of muscle glycogen depletion is affected by exercise intensity and duration. Muscle glycogen depletion increased from approximately 13 percent during a 506-m sprint, to approximately 35 percent during a 1,025-m sprint (Nimmo and Snow, 1983). When exercise distance was increased to 3,620 m and average speed was decreased, glycogen depletion decreased to about 20 percent. Although the amount of muscle glycogen utilized during short-term, high-intensity exercise is lower than the amount used during long-term, moderate exercise, the rate of utilization is much higher.

Maintaining adequate carbohydrate availability is important for performance. When human athletes initiate exercise with reduced muscle glycogen stores, fatigue resistance during long-term exercise is decreased. The effect of diminished glycogen stores on performance of short-term, high-intensity exercise is less well understood. There was no difference in the physical performance of horses that started high-intensity exercise with normal muscle glycogen stores or with slightly depleted (~ 22 percent below normal) muscle glycogen stores (Davie et al., 1996). However, when muscle glycogen stores were severely depleted (~ 55 percent) prior to high-intensity exercise, run time to fatigue was decreased (Lacombe et al., 1999). Topliff et al. (1983, 1985) also reported decreased performance when exercise was initiated with reduced muscle glycogen stores.

A number of strategies have been explored to either enhance initial muscle glycogen stores or enhance repletion of glycogen stores after exercise. It has been demonstrated that muscle glycogen levels in human athletes can be elevated above normal if an individual exercises and consumes a low-carbohydrate diet for a few days and then consumes a high-carbohydrate diet and limits exercise just prior to an event. This practice of "carbohydrate loading" appears to be most beneficial prior to the performance of long-term, moderate exercise. Carbohydrate loading has gained limited acceptance for horses, possibly because many performance horses already receive diets high in hydrolyzable carbohydrates. Also, traditional horse feeding recommendations have warned against sudden changes in diet in order to minimize digestive disturbances (Lewis, 1995), and recent research has linked the consumption of diets high in hydrolyzable carbohydrates to increased incidence of some muscular disorders such as equine polysaccharide storage myopathy (see Chapter 12). Finally, there is no clear evidence that carbohydrate loading has significant benefits to equine athletes. Topliff et al. (1983, 1985) did not find a positive effect on performance when muscle glycogen levels were elevated above normal after using a carbohydrate-loading feeding program in horses.

The ability to rapidly replete muscle glycogen stores following exercise may be important to subsequent performance for some activities. An initial study on glycogen repletion in exercised horses suggested that the rate of repletion was fastest in the first few hours after exercise (Snow et al., 1987). Repletion appeared to be faster in horses fed hay and grain after exercise than in horses fed only hay. At 28 hours post-exercise, muscle glycogen concentrations were 90 percent of pre-exercise values when horses were fed hay and grain, but only 71.7 percent of pre-exercise values when they received hay only. Interestingly, at 68 hours post-exercise, muscle glycogen concentrations were 84 and 76 percent of initial concentrations in horses fed the hay-and-concentrate diet or the hay diet, respectively. Recent studies have demonstrated that relatively extreme procedures are necessary to significantly enhance the rate of muscle glycogen repletion in horses after exercise. Continuous intravenous administration of dextrose/glucose at a rate of 6 g/kg BW (3 kg/500-kg horse) during the first several hours after glycogen-depleting exercise enhances the rate of glycogen resynthesis in horses (Davie et al., 1995; Lacombe et al., 2001). When glucose was administered at a lower rate (2 g/kg BW) by nasogastric tube, glycogen resynthesis was not increased above the control (Nout et al., 2003). In a subsequent study, horses were given a low soluble carbohydrate diet (hay), a mixed soluble carbohydrate diet (hay and grain), or a high soluble carbohydrate diet (grain only) for 72 hours after glycogen-depleting exercise (Lacombe et al., 2004). There was no difference in rate of glycogen resynthesis when horses were fed the hay diet or the hay/grain diet. Glycogen resynthesis was greater in horses fed only grain, compared to the other treatments. However, the authors noted that water consumption and the restoration of body weight were also less in horses fed only the concentrate, and they cautioned that the feeding of large amounts of soluble carbohydrates in the post-exercise period could predispose horses to gastrointestinal disorders A few studies have examined the effects of exercise, training, and post-exercise carbohydrate administration on glucose transporters (GLUT) in equine skeletal muscle in order to develop a better understanding of post-exercise glycogen repletion. After a single bout of moderate exercise, skeletal muscle content of glucose transporter-4 (GLUT-4) protein was not increased (Nout et al., 2003). However, GLUT-4 protein content and/or GLUT-4 mRNA were increased in equine skeletal muscle after a 3-day regimen of strenuous, glycogen-depleting exercise (Lacombe et al., 2003; Jose-Cunilleras et al., 2005). The GLUT-4 protein content was also increased after 6 weeks of training (McCutcheon et al., 2002). These studies suggest that some types of exercise can modify the amount of glucose transporters present in skeletal muscle in horses. It has also been hypothesized that post-exercise administration of carbohydrate would increase GLUT-4 protein or GLUT-4 mRNA in equine skeletal muscle after glycogen-depleting exercise (Lacombe et al., 2003; Jose-Cunilleras et al., 2005). However, intravenous administration of glucose after exercise did not elevate GLUT-4 protein content, even though glycogen repletion was increased. Similarly, feeding corn in the post-exercise period (as compared to no food or only hay) did not affect GLUT-4 protein content or GLUT-4 mRNA in skeletal muscle. These initial studies did not provide evidence that the GLUT-4 transporter in equine skeletal muscle was sensitive to carbohydrate administration after exercise. It was suggested that methods that examine plasma membrane isolates might be more revealing than methods that measured total GLUT-4 (Lacombe et al., 2003). It was also suggested that variables such as muscle glycogen content and insulin response may be involved in regulating post-exercise carbohydrate metabolism (Jose-Cunilleras et al., 2005; Pratt et al., 2005). Clearly, further research is needed to elucidate the mechanisms that control glycogen in repletion in horses.

The effect of providing additional carbohydrate to exercising horses before or during exercise has received considerable attention. Consumption of grain a few hours prior to exercise results in increased plasma glucose, increased serum insulin, and decreased plasma free fatty acid concentrations when exercise begins (Lawrence et al., 1993). However, after several minutes of exercise, a decrease in plasma glucose concentration has been observed in horses consuming a grain meal a few hours prior to exercise (Lawrence et al., 1993, 1995; Stull and Rodiek, 1995). This decrease in plasma glucose may result from enhanced glucose uptake by exercising muscle under the influence of elevated insulin concentrations. Providing a grain meal 2 to 3 hours prior to exercise (compared to hay or no food) resulted in increased carbohydrate and decreased lipid oxidation during exercise (Jose-Cunilleras et al., 2002). Insulin is a potent inhibitor of lipolysis and lipid oxidation may have been reduced due to decreased free fatty acid availability. Providing a grain meal a few hours prior to exercise did not reduce muscle glycogen utilization (Lawrence et al., 1993, 1995; Jose-Cunilleras et al., 2002), although liver glycogen may have been spared in one study (Lawrence et al., 1993). The response to a pre-exercise meal of grain may be affected by the timing of the meal and whether forage is also fed (Pagan and Harris, 1999). In addition, the effects of a pre-exercise meal may be attenuated during long-term exercise or when horses perform repeated bouts of exercise (Lawrence et al., 1995).

In humans, fatigue can be delayed if carbohydrate is consumed during long-term, moderate exercise, possibly by offsetting the decline in carbohydrate available from endogenous sources. Intravenous infusion of glucose during 90 minutes of exercise in horses increased total carbohydrate oxidation, reduced endogenous glucose production, and did not alter glycogen utilization in horses (Geor et al., 2000). Intravenous administration of glucose has been shown to increase time to fatigue in horses (Farris et al., 1995, 1999). However, in these studies, signs of reduced carbohydrate availability, such as hypoglycemia, did not occur in control horses. Nonetheless, the increased performance of horses given additional carbohydrate is in agreement with findings in human athletes. The authors of these studies noted that the intermittent feeding of horses during long-term exercise might not duplicate the effects of intravenous glucose infusion. Bullimore et al. (2000) administered glucose, fructose, or a glucose-fructose combination to horses in the middle of an exercise bout, but did not compare their results to a control condition. Because carbohydrate stores are limited, but fat stores are not, practices that enhance fat utilization and spare glycogen use are considered desirable. Factors affecting lipid metabolism in exercising horses are discussed in Chapter 3.

REFERENCES

Argenzio, R., and H. F. Hintz. 1970. Glucose tolerance and effect of volatile fatty acid on plasma glucose concentration in ponies. J. Anim. Sci. 30:514–519.

Bullimore, S. R., J. D. Pagan, P. A. Harris, K. E. Hoekstra, K. A. Roose, S. C. Gardner, and R. J. Geor. 2000. Carbohydrate supplementation of horses during endurance exercise: comparison of fructose and glucose. J. Nutr. 130:1760–1765.

Coenen, M., and H. Meyer. 1987. Water and electrolyte content of the equine gastrointestinal tract in dependence on ration type. Pp. 531–536 in Proc. 10th Equine Nutr. Physiol. Soc. Symp., Ft. Collins, CO.

Cummings, J. H., E. R. Beatty, S. M. Kingman, S. A. Bingham, and H. N. Englyst. 1996. Digestion and physiological properties of resistant starch in the human large bowel. Br. J. Nutr. 75:733–747.

Dairy One. 2005. Feed Composition Library. Available at http://www.dairyone.com/Forage/FeedComp/default.asp. Accessed September 1, 2005.

Davie, A., D. L. Evans, and D. R. Hodgson. 1995. Effects of intravenous dextrose infusion on muscle glycogen resynthesis after intense exercise. Equine Vet. J. 18S:195–198.

Davie, A. J., D. L. Evans, D. R. Hodgson, and R. J. Rose. 1996. Effects of glycogen depletion on high intensity exercise performance and glycogen utilisation. Pferdeheilkunde 12:482–484.

de Fombelle, A., A. G. Goachet, M. Varloud, P. Boisot, and V. Julliand. 2003. Effects of diet on prececal digestion of different starches in the horse measured with the nylon bag technique. Pp. 115–116. Proc. 18th Equine Nutr. Physiol. Soc. Symp., East Lansing, MI.

de Fombelle, A., L. Veiga, C. Drogoul, and V. Julliand. 2004. Effect of diet composition and feeding pattern on the prececal digestibility of starches from diverse botanical origins measured with the mobile nylon bag technique. J. Anim. Sci. 82:3625–3634.

Doreau, M., S. Boulot, D. Bauchart, J. P. Barlet, and W. Martin-Rosset. 1992. Voluntary intake, milk production and plasma metabolites in nursing mares fed two different diets. J. Nutr. 122:992–999.

Dyer, J., E. Fernandez-Castano-Merediz, K. S. Salmon, C. J. Proudman, G. B. Edwards, and S. P. Shirazi-Beechey. 2002. Molecular characterisation of carbohydrate digestion and absorption in equine small intestine. Equine Vet. J. 34:349–358.

Englyst, H. N., S. M. Kingman, G. J. Hudson, and J. H. Cummings. 1996. Measurement of resistant starch in vitro and in vivo. Br. J. Nutr. 75:749–755.

Englyst, K. N., and H. N. Englyst. 2005. Carbohydrate availability. Br. J. Nutr. 94:1–11.

FAO/WHO (Food and Agriculture Organization/World Health Organization). 1998. Carbohydrates in human nutrition (FAO Food and Nutrition Paper 66). Available at http://www.fao.org/docrep/W8079E/w8079e00.htm. Accessed on March 23, 2006.

Farris, J. W., K. W. Hinchcliff, K. H. McKeever, and D. R. Lamb. 1995. Glucose infusion increases maximal duration of prolonged treadmill exercise in Standardbred horses. Equine Vet. J. Suppl. 18:357–361.

Farris, J. W., K. W. Hinchcliff, K. H. McKeever, D. R. Lamb, and D. L. Thompson. 1998. Effect of tryptophan and of glucose on exercise capacity of horses. J. Appl. Physiol. 85:807–816.

Flores, C. A., P. M. Brannon, S. A. Bustamante, J. Bezerra, K. T. Butler, T. Goda, and O. Koldovsky. 1988. Effect of diet on intestinal and pancreatic enzyme activities in the pig. J. Pediatr. Gastroenterol. Nutr. 7:914–921.

Fowden, A. L., A. J. Forehead, K. White, and P. M. Taylor. 2000a. Equine uteroplacental metabolism at mid- and late gestation. Exp. Physiol. 85:539–45.

Fowden, A. L., P. M. Taylor, K. L. White, and A. J. Forehead. 2000b. Ontogenic and nutritionally induced changes in fetal metabolism in the horse. J. Physiol. 528:209–219.

Geor, R. J., K. W. Hinchcliff, and R. A. Sams. 2000. Glucose infusion attenuates endogenous glucose production and enhances glucose use of horses during exercise. J. Appl. Physiol. 88:1765–1776.

Glinsky, M. J., R. M. Smith, H. R. Spires, and C. L. Davis. 1976. Measurement of volatile fatty acid production rates in the cecum of the pony. J. Anim. Sci. 42:1465–1470.

Hall, M. B. 2003. Challenges with nonfiber carbohydrate methods. J. Anim. Sci. 81:3226–3232.

Healy, H. P., P. D. Siciliano and L. M. Lawrence, 1995. Effect of concentrate form on blood and gastric fluid variables in ponies. J. Equine Vet. Sci. 15:423–428.

Hintz, H. F., R. A. Argenzio, and H. F. Schryver. 1971. Digestion coefficients, blood glucose levels, and molar percentage of volatile fatty acids in intestinal fluid of ponies fed varying forage-grain ratios. J. Anim. Sci. 33:992–995.

Hoffman, R. M., J. A. Wilson, D. S. Kronfeld, W. L. Cooper, L. A. Lawrence, D. Sklan, and P. A. Harris. 2001. Hydrolyzable carbohydrates in pasture, hay and horse feeds: direct assay and seasonal variation. J. Anim. Sci. 79:500–506.

Jose-Cunilleras, E., K. W. Hinchcliff, R. A. Sams, S. T. Devor, and J. K. Linderman. 2002. Glycemic index of a meal fed before exercise alters substrate use and glucose flux in exercising horses. J. Appl. Physiol. 92:117–128.

Jose-Cunilleras, E., L. E. Taylor, and K. W. Hinchcliff. 2004. Glycemic index of cracked corn, oat groats and rolled barley in horses. J. Anim. Sci. 82:2623–2629.

Jose-Cunilleras, E., H. A. Hayes, R. E. Toribio, L. E. Mathes, and K. W. Hinchcliff. 2005. Expression of equine glucose transporter type 4 in skeletal muscle after glycogen depleting exercise. Am. J. Vet. Res. 66:379–385.

Kern, D. L., L. L. Slyter, J. M. Weaver, E. C. Leffel, and G. Samuelson. 1973. Pony cecum vs steer rumen: Effect of oat and hay on the microbial ecosystem. J. Anim. Sci. 37:463–469.

Kern, D. L., L. L. Slyter, E. C. Leffel, J. M. Weaver, R. R. Oltjen. 1974. Ponies vs. Steers: microbial and chemical characteristics of intestinal ingesta. J. Anim. Sci. 38:559–564.

Kienzle, E., S. Radicke, W. Wilke, E. Landes, and H. Meyer. 1992. Pre-ilieal starch digestion in relation to source and preparation of starch. Pferdeheilkunde (1. European Conference on Horse Nutrition):103–106.

Kienzle, E., S. Radicke, E. Landes, D. Kleffken, M. Illenseer, and H. Meyer. 1994. Activity of amylase in the gastrointestinal tract of the horse. J. Anim. Physiol. Anim Nutr. 72:234–241.

Kienzle, E., S. Fehrle, and B. Optiz. 2002. Interactions between the apparent energy and nutrient digestibilities of a concentrate mixture and roughages in horses. J. Nutr. 132:1778S–1780S.

Lacombe, V. A., K. W. Hinchcliff, R. J. Geor, and M. A. Lauderdale. 1999. Exercise that induces substantial muscle glycogen depletion impairs subsequent aerobic capacity. Equine Vet. J. Suppl. 30:293–297.

Lacombe, V. A., K. W. Hinchcliff, R. J. Geor, and C. R. Baskin. 2001. Muscle glycogen depletion and subsequent replenishment affect anaerobic capacity of horses. J. Appl. Physiol. 91:1782–1790.

Lacombe, V. A., K. W. Hinchcliff, and S. T. Devor. 2003. Effects of exercise and glucose administration on content of insulin-sensitive glucose transporter in equine skeletal muscle. Am. J. Vet. Res. 64: 1500–1506.

Lacombe, V. A., K. W. Hinchcliff, C. W. Kohn, S. T. Devor, and L. E. Taylor. 2004. Effects of feeding meals with various soluble-carbohydrate content on muscle glycogen synthesis after exercise in horses. Am. J. Vet. Res. 65:916–923.

Lawrence, L. M., L. V. Soderholm, A. Roberts, J. Williams, and H. F. Hintz. 1993. Feeding status affects glucose metabolism in exercising horses. J. Nutr. 123:2152–2157.

Lawrence, L. M., J. Williams, L. V. Soderholm, A. M. Roberts, and H. F. Hintz. 1995. Effect of feeding state on the response of horses to repeated bouts of intense exercise. Equine Vet. J. 27S:27–30.

Lewis, L. D. 1995. Equine Clinical Nutrition. Media, PA: Williams and Wilkens.

Lindholm, A., H. Bjerneld, and B. Saltin. 1974. Glycogen depletion pattern in muscle fibers of trotting horses. Acta. Physiol. Scand. 90:475–484.

McCutcheon, L. J., R. J. Geor and K. W. Hinchcliff. 2002. Changes in skeletal muscle GLUT4 content and muscle membrane glucose transport following 6 weeks of exercise training. Equine Vet. J. Suppl. 34:199–204.

McLeod, K. R., and R. L. Baldwin, VI. 2000. Effects of diet forage:concentrate ratio and metabolizable energy intake on visceral organ growth and in vitro oxidative capacity of gut tissues in sheep. J. Anim. Sci. 78:760–770.

Medina, B., I. D. Girard, E. Jacotot, and V. Julliand. 2002. Effect of a preparation of Sacchromyces cervisiae on microbial profiles and fermentation patterns in the large intestine of horses fed a high fiber or a high starch diet. J. Anim. Sci. 80:2600–2609.

Mertens, D. R. 1997. Creating a system for meeting the fiber requirements of dairy cows. J. Dairy Sci. 80:1463–1481.

Meyer, H., S. Radicke, E. Kienzle, S. Wilke, and D. Kleffen. 1993. Investigations on preileal digestion of oats, corn and barley starch in relation to grain processing. Pp. 92–97 in Proc. 13th Equine Nutr. Physiol. Soc. Symp., Gainesville, FL.

Monro, J. 2003. Redefining the glycemic index for dietary management of postprandial glycemia. J. Nutr. 133:4256–4258.

Moore, B. E., and B. A. Dehority. 1993. Effects of diet and hindgut defaunation on diet digestibility and microbial concentrations in the cecum and colon of the horse. J. Anim. Sci. 71:3350–3358.

Moore-Colyer, M. J. S., J. J. Hyslop, A. C. Longland, and D. Cuddeford. 2000. Intra-cecal fermentation parameters in ponies fed botanically diverse fibre-based diets. Anim. Feed Sci. Tech. 84:183–197.

Nimmo, M. A., and D. H. Snow. 1983. Changes in muscle glycogen, lactate and pyruvate concentrations in the Thoroughbred horse following maximal exercise. Pp. 237–243 in Equine Exercise Physiology, D. H. Snow, S. G. B. Persson, and R. J. Rose, eds. Cambridge: Granta Editions.

Nout, Y. S., K. W. Hinchcliff, E. Jose-Cunilleras, L. R. Dearth, G. S. Sivko, and J. W. DeWille. 2003. Effect of moderate exercise immediately followed by induced hyperglycemia on gene expression and content of the glucose transporter-4 protein in skeletal muscles of horses. Am. J. Vet. Res. 64:1401–1408.

NRC (National Research Council). 2001. Nutrient Requirements of Dairy Cattle. Washington, DC: National Academy Press.

Pagan, J. D., and P. A. Harris. 1999. The effects of timing and amount of forage and grain on exercise response in Thoroughbred horses. Equine Vet. J. 30:451–458.

Pagan, J. D., P. A. Harris, M. A. P. Kennedy, N. Davidson, and K. E. Hoekstra. 1999. Feed type and intake affect glycemic response in Thoroughbred horses. Pp.147–149 in Proc. 1999 Equine Nutr. Conf. Feed Manufact., Lexington, KY.

Pethick, D. W., R. J. Rose, W. L. Bryden, and J. M. Gooden. 1993. Nutrient utilization by the hindlimb of Thoroughbred horses at rest. Equine Vet. J. 25:41–44.

Potter, G., F. Arnold, D. Householder, D. Hansen, and K. Bowen. 1992. Digestion of starch in the small or large intestine of the equine. Pferdeheilkunde (1. European Conference on Horse Nutrition):109–111.

Pratt, S., R. Geor, and J. McCutcheon. 2005. Insulin sensitivity after exercise in the horse. P. 120 in Proc. Equine Science Soc., Tucson AZ.

Pratt, S. E., L. M. Lawrence, L. K. Warren, and D. Powell. 1999. P. 7 in Effect of sodium acetate infusion on the exercising horse. Proc. 16th Equine Nutr. Physiol. Soc. Symp., Raleigh, NC.

Radicke, S., E. Kienzle, and H. Meyer. 1991. Preileal apparent digestibility of oats and cornstarch and consequences for cecal metabolism. Pp. 43–48 in Proc. 12th Equine Nutr. Physiol. Soc. Symp., Calgary, Alberta.

Roberts, M. C., D. E. Kidder and F. W. G. Hill. 1973. Small intestinal beta-galactosidatse activity in the horse. Gut 14:535–540.

Rodiek A.V., and C. Stull. 2005. Glycemic index of common horse feeds. Pp. 154–155 in Proc. 19th Equine Science Symp., Tucson, AZ.

Simmons, H. A., and E. J. H. Ford. 1991. Gluconeogenesis from propionate produced in the colon of the horse. Br. Vet. J. 147:340–345.

Smith, D. 1981. Removing and analyzing total non-structural carbohydrates from plant tissues. Wisconsin Ag. Exp. Stn. Rep. No R2107, Madison.

Snow, D. H., R. C. Harris, J. C. Harman, and D. J. Marlin. 1987. Glycogen repletion patterns following different diets. Pp. 701–710 in Equine Exercise Physiology 2, J. R. Gillespie and N. E. Robinson, eds. Davis, CA: ICEEP Publications.

Strobel, H. J., and J. B. Russell. 1986. Effect of pH and energy spilling on bacterial protein synthesis by carbohydrate limited cultures of mixed rumen bacteria. J. Dairy Sci. 69:2941–2947.

Stull, C., and A. V. Rodiek. 1995. Effects of post prandial interval and feed type on substrate availability during exercise. Equine Vet. J. Suppl. 18:362–366.

Swanson, K. C., J. C. Matthews, A. D. Matthews, J. A. Howell, C. J. Richards, and D. L. Harmon. 2000. Dietary carbohydrate source and energy intake influence the expression of pancreatic amylase in lambs. J. Nutr. 130:2157–2165.

Tharanathan, R. N. 2002. Food-derived carbohydrates—Structural complexity and functional diversity. Critical Rev. Biotech. 22:65–84.

Topliff, D. R., G. D. Potter, T. R. Dutson, J. L. Kreider, and G. T. Jessup. 1983. Diet manipulation and muscle glycogen in the equine. Pp. 119–124 in Proc. 8th Equine Nutr. Physiol. Soc. Symp., Lexington, KY.

Topliff, D. R., G. D. Potter, J. L. Kreider, T. R. Dutson, and G. T. Jessup. 1985. Diet manipulation, muscle glycogen metabolism and anaerobic work performance in the equine. Pp. 224–229 in Proc. 9th Equine Nutr. Physiol. Soc. Symp., East Lansing, MI.

Tungland, B. C. and D. Meyer. 2002, Nondigestible oligo- and polysaccharides (dietary fiber): their physiology and role in human health and food. Comprehensive Reviews in Food Science and Food Safety 1:73–80.

Van Soest, P. J. 1994. Carbohydrates. Pp. 156–176 in Nutritional Ecology of the Ruminant 2nd ed: Ithaca, NY: Cornell University Press.

Varloud, M., A. G. Goachet, A. de Fombelle, A. Guyonvarch and V. Julliand. 2003. Effect of the diet on prececal digestibility of the dietary starch measured in horses with acid insoluble ash as an internal marker. Pp. 117–118 in Proc. 18th Equine Nutr. Physiol. Soc. Symp., East Lansing MI.

Vervuert, I., M. Coenen, and C. Bothe. 2003. Effects of oat processing on the glycaemic and insulin responses in horses. J. Anim. Physiol. Anim Nutr. 87:96–104.

Vervuert, I., M. Coenen, and C. Bothe. 2004. Effects of corn processing on the glycaemic and insulinaemic responses in horses. J. Anim. Physiol. Anim. Nutr. 88:348–355.

Vervuert, I., M. Coenen, and C. Bothe. 2005. Glycaemic and insulinaemic indexes of different mechanical and thermal processes grains for horses. Pp. 154–155 in Proc. 19th Equine Science Symp., Tucson, AZ.

Willard, J. G., J. C. Willard, S. A. Wolfram and J. P. Baker. 1977. Effect of diet on cecal pH and feeding behavior of horses. J. Anim. Sci. 45:87–93.

Zebrowska, T., and A. G. Low. 1987. The influence of diets based on whole wheat, wheat flour and wheat bran on the exocrine pancreatic secretion in pigs. J. Nutr. 117:1212–1216.

3

Fats and Fatty Acids

INTRODUCTION

Fats or oils are generally used in equine diets to increase energy density and/or substitute for hydrolyzable and rapidly fermentable carbohydrates in the form of cereal grains. However, fat supplementation has other potential benefits, including improved energetic efficiency (Kronfeld, 1996), enhanced body condition, diminished excitability (Holland et al., 1996a), and metabolic adaptations that increase fat oxidation during exercise (Dunnett et al., 2002). Dietary fats also serve as carriers for fat-soluble vitamins and supply the essential fatty acids (EFAs) linoleic acid and α-linolenic acid that are not synthesized by the body, although an EFA requirement for horses has not been determined. All fatty acids serve structural functions, and several of the polyunsaturated fatty acids (PUFAs) are precursors of the prostaglandins and other eicosanoids, which are important for a host of cellular functions.

From a biochemical viewpoint, fats belong to a broad group of compounds known as lipids that can be glycerol or nonglycerol based. Glycerol-based lipids include the glycolipids, phospholipids, and triglycerides (also termed triacylglycerols). Triglycerides consist of three fatty acid molecules linked to a glycerol backbone. Cholesterol and its fatty acid esters are nonglycerol-based lipids. Included in this category of lipids are waxes, terpenes, cerebrosides, and various sterols.

Fatty acids may be designated on the basis of the number of carbon atoms they contain and the number of double bonds. Long-chain fatty acids contain 16 to 20 carbon atoms, medium-chain fatty acids contain 6 to 10 carbons, and short-chain or volatile fatty acids (VFAs), produced in the intestinal tract by bacterial fermentation, contain only 2 to 5 carbons. Saturated fatty acids (SFAs) contain no double bonds, monounsaturated (MUFAs) a single double bond, and PUFAs two or more double bonds. Fatty acids are also described by the position of the first double bond relative to the methyl end of the molecule (the omega [ω] end), in the form of A:Bω-C (or A:Bn-C), where A is the number of carbon atoms in the chain, B is the number of double bonds, and C is the position of the first double bond from the methyl terminus. For example, linoleic acid is referred to as 18:2n-6 because it contains 18 carbon atoms and 2 double bonds, the first between carbons 6 and 7 counted from the methyl terminus. Fatty acids with the first double bond in this position are commonly referred to as omega-6 fatty acids, whereas fatty acids with the first double bond between carbons 3 and 4 (e.g., α-linolenic, 18:3ω-3) are in the omega-3 series.

Triglycerides exist as fats or oils at room temperature according to their physical properties of the component fatty acids. Triglycerides with a high proportion of relatively short-chain fatty acids or unsaturated fatty acids tend to be liquid (oils) at room temperature. Saturated fatty acids have a higher melting point and exist as solids (fats) at room temperature.

SOURCES OF DIETARY FATS AND FATTY ACIDS

Both animal fats and vegetable fats or oils have been fed to horses, although use of vegetable sources is more prevalent in part due to superior palatability. In one study that examined the palatability of several animal and vegetable fats and oils, corn oil was the most palatable (Holland et al., 1998). In this study, diets containing up to 15 percent added fat as corn oil were readily accepted by horses. Several other vegetable sources, including seed and fruit oils (e.g., soy, canola, linseed [or flax], sunflower, safflower, coconut, and peanut) and other feed byproducts with relatively high fat content (e.g., lecithin, stabilized rice bran, wheat germ, and copra), appear to have acceptable palatability and are widely used in horse diets. Fish oil (menhaden) and medium-chain triglycerides (MCTs) also have been fed to horses. Use of these different fat and oil sources can be dictated by cost and availability. Table 8-5 provides the fatty acid composition of some of the fats and oils added to horse diets.

DIGESTIBILITY AND ENERGY VALUE OF FATS

In general, there is an increase in the digestibility of fat when fats or oils are added to forages or grains (Potter et al., 1992). Mean estimates of apparent digestibilities of fats in horses and ponies are 42–49 percent for forages (Fonnesbeck et al., 1967; Bowman et al., 1979; Sturgeon et al., 2000), 55–76 percent for grains (Hintz and Schryver, 1989), and 88–94 percent for added fats and oils (Kane et al., 1979; McCann et al., 1987). Kronfeld et al. (2004) compiled published data from digestibility studies in which five basal (hay and grain mixes without added fats; 23–37 g fat/kg dry matter [DM]) and 18 test feeds with added fats (76–233 g fat/kg DM) were evaluated (Rich, 1980; Custalow, 1992; Holland, 1994; Bowman et al., 1979). This analysis demonstrated mean apparent digestibilities (D_a) of 55, 81, and 95 percent for fat in, respectively, forages, mixed feeds with added fat, and added fats. Encapsulation of fat within cereal grains or oilseeds may decrease the availability of these fats for digestion in the small intestine. The low true digestibility (D_t) of forage fat may be explained by the poor digestibility of waxes, pigments, and other non-triglyceride lipid components. Kronfeld et al. (2004) also reported that the true digestibility of added fats approached 100 percent with an endogenous fecal fat of 0.22 g/kg body weight (BW)/d. Maximal fat digestibility occurred between 100 and 150 g/kg DM and was sustained to 230 g/kg DM, suggesting high capacity for fat digestion in horses adapted to fat-supplemented rations. However, the results of other studies have suggested a lower upper limit in fat digestibility in horses. In an analysis of data from 225 digestion trials evaluating rations with varying amounts of partially hydrogenated soy oil, Zeyner (2002) reported a strong positive relationship between the D_a of fat and the amount of fat in the diet, but only up to approximately 7 percent DM. Assuming a gross energy value of 9.5 Mcal/kg for fat, caloric values for fat in forages, mixed feeds, and added vegetable fats have been estimated at 5.2, 7.7, and 9 Mcal/kg, respectively (Kronfeld et al., 2004). More precise digestible energy (DE) values can be calculated from measured fat content (g/kg) using the equation developed by Kronfeld et al. (2004): Energy value (Mcal/kg) = $0.095(92 - 92e^{(-\text{ether extract}/342)})$.

In other species, there is evidence that degree of saturation, melting point, and possibly fatty acid (FA) chain length affect the digestibility of added fats. Saturated fats are less digestible than unsaturated fats, while the digestibility is inversely related to the melting point of the FA. These factors are of minor importance in horse nutrition given the widespread use of vegetable oils containing predominantly unsaturated FAs. In two studies (McCann et al., 1987; Kronfeld et al., 2004), an effect of chain length or saturation of FAs on digestibility was not detected when comparing vegetable oils (corn, soy, soy lecithin, peanut), tallow, and vegetable-tallow blends.

In ruminants, the addition of oils to rations decreases ruminal fermentation of fiber (Coppock and Wilks, 1991), an effect not observed when encapsulated or protected fat is fed. There is conflicting evidence regarding the effects of added fat on the utilization of other nutrients in equine rations. The addition of corn oil at up to 15 percent of the total diet (DM basis) had no effect on fiber digestibility in three studies (Bowman et al., 1979; Kane et al., 1979; Bush et al., 2001). The digestibility of calcium, phosphorus, and magnesium also were largely unchanged in horses fed fat-supplemented diets (Bowman et al., 1979; Rich, 1980; McCann et al., 1987). The preileal digestibility of protein was slightly lower in horses fed coconut or soybean oils at 0.5 or 1 g/kg BW/d (Meyer et al., 1997). Kronfeld et al. (2004) reported that the addition of corn oil (up to 233 g/kg DM), tallow (up to 190 g/kg DM), or 50:50 soy lecithin and soy oil (100 g/kg DM) had no effect on DM, crude protein (CP), or acid detergent fiber (ADF) digestibility. Zeyner (2002) reported increased fiber digestibility of a mixed hay and concentrate ration with isoenergetic exchange of micronized corn (3 g starch/kg BW) by soy oil (up to 14 percent of DM). However, a further increase in the fat content of the ration (22 and 32 percent of DM) resulted in a statistically significant depression of gut microbial fermentative activity and decreased fiber digestibility. Jansen and co-workers reported a negative associative effect of soy oil on crude fiber (CF), neutral detergent fiber (NDF), ADF, and nitrogen-free extract (NFE) digestibility when horses were fed hay and isocaloric concentrates with different amounts of cornstarch, glucose, and soy oil (Jansen et al., 2000, 2001, 2002). In one of these studies (Jansen et al., 2001), CF digestibility was 71 percent and 55 percent in the control and fat-supplemented feeds (soybean oil 158 g/kg DM), respectively. Regression analysis of ether extract (EE) intake (as soybean oil) on CF digestibility showed that an increase of 10 g/kg DM of soybean oil resulted in a 0.9 percent decrease in apparent total tract digestibility (Jansen et al., 2001). The reason(s) for this apparent adverse effect of soy oil on fiber digestibility have not been elucidated. However, one possible explanation could be inadequate accommodation to the oil-supplemented ration. Zeyner (2002) reported decreased fiber digestibility with rapid substitution of cereal starch by soy oil (0.33 g soy oil/kg BW/d). This adverse effect was not evident after a 3-week accommodation period. Another explanation may be a specific negative effect of soybean oil at high levels of inclusion. Zeyner (2002) demonstrated no adverse effects in horses accommodated to soy oil-supplemented rations containing up to 0.7 g oil/kg BW/d. However, decreased fiber digestibility was observed in horses fed 1 g soy oil/kg/d. Therefore, at least for soy oil, 0.7 g/kg BW/d is suggested as an upper limit of fat inclusion.

Kronfeld et al. (2004) reported that rapid introduction of fat-supplemented diets is associated with greasy feces (steatorrhea) and increased fecal output, an indication that some fat has escaped digestion. These adverse effects are apparently avoided if fat is gradually introduced to the ration, with an accommodation period of 4 to 14 days depending on the level of fat supplementation.

PHYSIOLOGIC EFFECTS OF DIETARY FAT

Effects on Lipid and Carbohydrate Metabolism

Studies in humans and in rodent species have shown that high-fat diets result in enhanced capacity for fatty acid oxidation in skeletal muscle. Enhanced expression and activity of proteins and enzymes associated with the transport of free fatty acids (FFA) into muscle and β-oxidation underlie this increase in fat oxidation. There is some evidence that dietary fat supplementation results in similar adaptations in fat metabolism of horses, although some reports are conflicting and few studies quantitatively assessed fat oxidation. Fat supplementation has been demonstrated to increase postheparin plasma hepatic and lipoprotein lipase (LPL) activities, decrease plasma triglyceride (TAG) concentrations by as much as 55 percent, and increase plasma cholesterol and phospholipid concentrations (Orme et al., 1997; Geelen et al., 1999). In Warmblood horses fed soy oil at 0, 0.33, 0.67, 1, and 1.33 g/kg BW/d, there were dose-dependent increases in serum VFA, phospholipids, and total cholesterol concentrations, as well as the proportion of α-lipoproteins (Zeyner, 2002). Serum TAG concentrations were decreased relative to the control diet at the 0.33 and 0.67 g/kg soy oil dosages, but significantly increased at the 1 and 1.33 g/kg dosages (Zeyner, 2002). In one study a dose-response relationship was detected between fat intake (3 to 10.8 percent fat, as soybean oil) and heparin-released plasma lipoprotein lipase activity (Geelen et al., 2001a). Specifically, an increase in fat intake by 1 g/kg DM was associated with an increase in LPL activity by 0.98 micromoles of fatty acid released per hour. As LPL is involved in the removal of FFA and glycerol from triglyceride-rich lipoprotein particles in tissue capillaries of skeletal muscle and adipose tissues, the increase in LPL activity with fat-supplementation indicates increased availability of FFA in these tissue beds. Geelen et al. (2001b) demonstrated decreases in the activities of acetyl-CoA carboxylase and fatty acid synthase in the liver of Shetland ponies on a high-fat diet (118 g/kg DM). Thus, the fat-induced decrease in plasma TAG concentrations may be due to a decrease in de novo fatty acid synthesis.

There is conflicting evidence regarding the effects of fat supplementation on the skeletal muscle activities of enzymes involved in oxidative metabolism. In Thoroughbred horses, 10 weeks of fat supplementation (soybean oil, 80 g/kg DM; control and fat-supplemented diets supplied 0.22 and 1 g/kg BW, respectively) resulted in increases in the activities of citrate synthase (CS) and β-hydroxyacyl CoA dehydrogenase (HAD) in skeletal (middle gluteal) muscle (Orme et al., 1997). On the other hand, the feeding of a high-fat diet (118 g/kg DM vs. control diet 15 g/kg DM) to Shetland ponies for 45 days was without effect on the activities of CS and HAD in gluteus and semitendinosus muscle, although an increase in CS activity was detected in the masseter muscle (Geelen et al., 2001b). Similarly, the activities of CS, HAD, hexokinase, and phosphofructokinase in middle gluteal muscle were unchanged in Standardbred horses fed a high-fat diet (Geelen et al., 2000).

The replacement of starch by fat or oils in concentrate feeds resulted in decreased blood glycemic and insulinemic responses to meal feeding (Williams et al., 2001; Zeyner et al., 2005). In mature Thoroughbred horses, the consumption of a fat and fiber supplement (approximately 10 percent nonstructural carbohydrates [NSC]; where NSC was determined by difference), when compared to a sweet feed supplement (approximately 50 percent NSC), resulted in a 65 percent and 85 percent decrease in, respectively, glycemic and insulinemic response (Williams et al., 2001). The feeding of a sweet feed (50 percent NSC, as determined by direct analysis) to mature Thoroughbred geldings maintained at pasture resulted in decreased insulin sensitivity when compared to the feeding of a high-fat, low-NSC (10 percent fat, 10 percent NSC in DM) feed or pasture alone (Hoffman et al., 2003).

Substrate Storage

There is conflicting information on the effects of dietary fat supplementation on muscle glycogen storage. In several studies, muscle glycogen content was increased after oil or fat supplementation, while other studies reported no change or a moderate decrease in muscle glycogen content. Five different studies from a single laboratory examined the effects of feeding a fat-supplemented concentrate (100 g tallow/kg DM in a grain-based concentrate) for 3–4 weeks (Meyers et al., 1987; Oldham et al., 1990; Jones et al., 1991; Scott et al., 1992; Julen et al., 1995). In these studies, (the concentrates were fed) with hay in a ratio of 65:35 to 75:25 such that the concentration of fat in the total diet was approximately 6–7 percent. A consistent finding was increased glycogen storage, with muscle glycogen content increasing by as much as 50 percent. In another study, Harkins et al. (1992) measured muscle glycogen in Thoroughbred horses fed a control diet of hay and a pelleted concentrate for 3 weeks followed by a fat-supplemented diet (corn oil, 3 percent DM) for a further 3 weeks, and mean muscle glycogen was 15.8 percent higher after oil supplementation. However, as hay was not fed with the fat-supplemented diet, absolute starch intake was higher for the fat-supplemented diet when compared to the control diet. These differences in fiber and starch intake confounded interpretation of the apparent change in muscle glycogen content. Hambleton et al. (1980)

measured muscle (quadriceps femoris m.) glycogen in horses conditioned for 3 weeks and fed diets containing 4 percent, 8 percent, 12 percent, or 16 percent soybean oil. Muscle glycogen content was measured before and after 6 hours of exercise (trotting interspersed with walking). Although mean values for muscle glycogen were higher in the 8 percent and 12 percent diets when compared to the other diets, statistically significant differences were not detected. This study has been consistently misquoted in the literature as demonstrating an effect of dietary fat on muscle glycogen content.

Other investigators have reported either no change (Essen-Gustavsson et al., 1991; Eaton et al., 1995; Orme et al., 1997; Hyyppa et al., 1999; MacLeay et al., 1999) or a moderate decrease (Pagan et al., 1987; Geelen et al., 2001b) in muscle glycogen storage following 3–10 weeks of fat supplementation. In two studies, liver glycogen content also decreased after oil supplementation (Pagan et al., 1987; Geelen et al., 2001b). A fat-supplemented diet (5 percent DM) slowed the rate of muscle glycogen replenishment in horses not accommodated to fat feeding (Hyyppa et al., 1999). However, the rate of post-exercise muscle glycogen resynthesis was not different from the control diet after an adaptation period of 3 weeks. In summary, there is no consensus on the effects of dietary fat supplementation on muscle glycogen storage in horses. The variability in results between the different studies could be due to differences in diet composition, duration of fat supplementation, muscle sampling and analysis techniques, and breed, age, and training state of the horses studied.

There is also conflicting information regarding the effects of a fat-supplemented diet on muscle triglyceride content. Essen-Gustavsson et al. (1991) demonstrated no change in the triglyceride content of middle gluteal muscle from Standardbred horses fed a fat-supplemented diet (60 g/kg DM) for 5 weeks. Orme et al. (1997) also reported no change in middle gluteal muscle triglyceride content of Thoroughbred horses provided oil supplementation (80 g soybean oil/kg DM) for 10 weeks. On the other hand, Geelen et al. (2001b) found an 80 percent increase in the semimembranosus triglyceride content of ponies fed a diet that provided 118 g soybean oil/kg DM.

Metabolic Responses to Exercise

Several studies have assessed the effects of fat supplementation on metabolic responses to exercise. The focus of earlier studies was the effects of fat supplementation on the concentrations of various plasma substrates or metabolites (e.g., glucose, FFA, TAG, and lactate) during exercise (Slade et al., 1975; Hintz et al., 1978; Hambleton et al., 1980; Hintz et al., 1982; Duren et al., 1987; Ferrante et al., 1994). More recent studies sought to obtain quantitative measures of substrate oxidation (Pagan et al., 1987, 2002; Dunnett et al., 2002). In general, fat supplementation (animal or vegetable fat at 8 percent or more of total DM) has been associated with mitigation of exercise-associated decreases in plasma glucose concentrations and increased TAG and FFA during prolonged, low-intensity exercise (Slade et al., 1975; Hintz et al., 1978; Hambleton et al., 1980; Hintz et al., 1982; Duren et al., 1987). Maintenance of higher plasma glucose concentrations has been taken as evidence of a glucose-sparing effect of fat supplementation. This hypothesis was supported by a recent study in which tracer-determined blood glucose utilization during 90 minutes of exercise at 30 percent of maximum aerobic capacity (Vo_2max) was lower after 5 weeks adaptation to a diet providing 29 percent DE from fat (corn oil) (Pagan et al., 2002).

In a small group (n = 4) of conditioned Thoroughbred horses, supplementation with soybean oil (20 percent of DE from oil) resulted in a decrease in respiratory exchange ratio (RER) during low- (trot at 3.2 m/s) and medium- (canter at 7 m/s) intensity treadmill (0° incline) exercise (Dunnett et al., 2002). This metabolic response during low-intensity exercise was apparent after 3 weeks of oil supplementation, but was not evident at higher workloads (canter at 10 m/s), perhaps reflecting greater dependence on carbohydrate metabolism during intense exercise. Two other studies have also reported a fat supplementation-induced decrease in the RER of horses during low-intensity exercise (Pagan et al., 1987, 2002). Overall, these findings suggest an increase in the utilization of fat, with a concomitant decrease in carbohydrate utilization, during low- and moderate-intensity exercise following oil supplementation. However, oil supplementation does not appear to alter substrate oxidation at high exercise intensities (> 50–60 percent Vo_2max). The increase in fat oxidation during low-intensity exercise may be related to changes in plasma lipase activity and mechanisms for fat utilization in skeletal muscle. In the study by Dunnett et al. (2002), parallel increases in plasma total lipase activity, circulating FFA during exercise, and activity of CS in skeletal muscle were detected. However, whereas the fat-supplementation–induced decrease in RER was correlated to the increase in muscle CS activity ($r^2 = 0.95$), there was no relationship to changes in FFA concentrations or to total lipase or β-hydroxyacyl CoA dehydrogenase activities.

The length of time required for expression of these metabolic adaptations to dietary oil has been debated. Some nutritionists have advocated that a minimum of 10–12 weeks is required for full adaptation (Kronfeld and Harris, 2003). However, metabolic adaptations to oil supplementation have been observed as early as 3–5 weeks after the start of supplementation (Pagan et al., 1987, 1995; Orme et al., 1997; Pagan et al., 2002). Thus, whereas a 2–3 month period may be required for complete adaptation to an oil-supplemented diet, some of the metabolic responses are evident much earlier. Importantly, the metabolic response to oil supplementation is apparently transient and dependent on its continued use. In one study, the effects on RER were abolished within

5 weeks of withdrawal of the oil-supplemented diet (Dunnett et al., 2002).

Whereas the aforementioned adaptations in lipid metabolism (e.g., decreased RER during low-intensity exercise) might imply a sparing of muscle glycogen, the available data do not support this view. Essen-Gustavsson et al. (1991) and Pagan et al. (1987) reported no effect of fat supplementation (approximately 7 percent of total DM intake) on muscle glycogen utilization of Standardbred horses during 60–100 minutes of submaximal exercise. Similarly, Harkins et al. (1992) and Eaton et al. (1995) reported no change in net muscle glycogen utilization in fat-supplemented Thoroughbred horses undertaking exercise that simulated race performance. Other researchers (Oldham et al., 1990; Jones et al., 1991; Scott et al., 1992; Hughes et al., 1995) have reported higher net muscle glycogen utilization and plasma lactate concentrations and improved performance during exercise tests consisting of multiple sprints (e.g., 4 × 600 m). The improved performance was attributed to the higher glycogen stores and maintenance of anaerobic energy transduction during sprint exercise.

A single study has examined the effects of dietary fish (menhaden) oil supplementation on metabolic response to incremental treadmill exercise in horses (O'Connor et al., 2004). Horses were assigned to either a fish oil (n = 6) or corn oil (n = 4) treatment in which the oil (324 mg/kg BW) was supplemented to a hay and concentrate ration for 63 days. The horses underwent moderate physical conditioning 5 days/week and completed an incremental exercise test after 63 days. During the test, horses that received fish oil had significantly lower heart rate and serum free fatty acid, glycerol, and cholesterol concentrations when compared to the corn oil treatment. The physiological importance of these findings remains to be determined.

Acid-Base Responses

Adaptation to a fat-supplemented diet influences blood acid-base responses to exercise. During a treadmill exercise test, venous pH was higher (~ 7.44–7.46) in Arabian horses fed a diet supplemented with corn oil (100 g/kg DM) when compared to the control diet (~ 7.40–7.42) at speeds between 3 and 6 m/s (Taylor et al., 1995; Kronfeld et al., 1998). There also was a decrease in venous blood pCO_2 during repeated sprints, which was attributed to a lower RER associated with enhanced fat oxidation, although RER was not measured (Kronfeld et al., 1998). Graham-Thiers et al. (2001) showed that dietary protein restriction (crude protein 7.5 g/100 g with supplemental L-lysine [0.5 percent] and L-threonine [0.3 percent]) had an additive effect with fat supplementation (corn oil, 100 g/kg DM) in the mitigation of the acidogenic effects of exercise. The biological significance of these small alterations in acid-base response to exercise is unclear.

This research group (Ferrante et al., 1994; Taylor et al., 1995) also reported higher plasma lactate concentrations during repeated sprints or incremental exercise in horses fed an oil-supplemented diet. The mechanism of this response is unclear. One hypothesis is that "fat adaptation" confers improved metabolic regulation of glucose utilization in muscle, with glycogen sparing at work of low intensity but enhanced glycolysis and lactate production during exercise requiring higher power output (Kronfeld et al., 1998). An alternative explanation is down regulation in the activity of skeletal muscle pyruvate dehydrogenase in response to oil feeding, as has been observed in humans (Spriet and Watt, 2003). It should also be noted that other researchers have reported lower plasma lactate accumulation during submaximal incremental exercise when horses are fed an oil-supplemented (11.8 percent fat, DM basis) diet (Sloet van Oldruitenborgh-Oosterbaan et al., 2002).

Athletic Performance

A number of researchers have attempted to determine the effects of fat supplementation on athletic performance. It has been hypothesized that adaptation to fat supplementation results in an improvement in the athletic performance of horses. Several theoretical explanations have been put forth as explanations for enhanced athletic performance with the feeding of higher-fat diets, including: (1) an improved power-to-weight ratio due to a reduction in DM intake and bowel ballast; (2) decreased metabolic heat production associated with feeding and exercise (Kronfeld, 1996); (3) enhanced stamina as a result of muscle glycogen sparing (Kronfeld et al., 1998); (4) improved sprint performance due to increased energy transduction from anaerobic glycolysis (Oldham et al., 1990; Kronfeld et al., 1998); and (5) mitigation of acidemia during high-intensity exercise (Kronfeld et al., 1998). However, the results of studies examining the effects of fat supplementation in horses on athletic performance are equivocal. Some authors have reported improved performance (Oldham et al., 1990; Harkins et al., 1992; Eaton et al., 1995), while others have found no change (Topliff et al., 1983; Pagan et al., 1987; Essen-Gustavsson et al., 1991; Hyyppa et al., 1999). Harkins et al. (1992) reported that 14 of 15 horses ran a 1,600-m simulated race faster when fed a fat-supplemented diet (corn oil, 3 percent DM for 3 weeks) compared to the control ration. Mean race time improved 2.5 s (2.1 percent) after consuming the fat-added diet. However, as discussed above, this experiment was inappropriately designed. A longitudinal design was used with all horses completing the control-diet race first, with the fat-diet race undertaken after a further 3 weeks of training. It is possible, therefore, that the observed decrease in simulated race time was due to training rather than oil supplementation. Furthermore, as the horses were not fed hay during the second diet period, it is possible the faster race time was associated with a reduction in gut weight.

Four weeks of fat supplementation (12 percent DE from corn oil) was associated with a small but statistically significant increase in run time to fatigue in Thoroughbred horses undertaking treadmill exercise at an intensity equivalent to 120 percent of $\text{V}o_2\text{max}$ (Eaton et al., 1995). Earlier studies of the effects of fat supplementation found enhanced performance during exercise protocols consisting of repeated sprints (Meyers et al., 1987; Oldham et al., 1990; Scott et al., 1992) or efforts during protocols that simulated exercise undertaken by cutting horses (Webb et al., 1987). Improved work performance during high-intensity exercise was attributed to increases in resting muscle glycogen content and the rate of glycogen utilization. However, in the study by Eaton et al. (1995), there was no effect of diet on glycogen utilization rate during exercise.

Several factors could account for the variability in results between studies, including the type and amount of fat supplemented, duration of fat feeding, variation in the intensity and duration of exercise tests, small number of horses per treatment (most often fewer than six), and differences in the conditioning status of the horses.

Behavior

There are limited published data on the effects of fat supplementation on behavior of horses. Holland et al. (1996a) evaluated the effects of fat supplementation on spontaneous activity (distance moved per day, measured by use of a pedometer) and reactivity (responses to pressure, loud noise, and sudden visual stimuli) in eight horses. The control diet (CON) contained chopped hay, corn, oats, beet pulp, and molasses, while the three test diets contained an additional 10 percent (by weight) corn oil (CO), soy lecithin-corn oil (SL-CO), or soy lecithin-soy oil (SL-SO), with small decreases in hay, grains, and molasses. Horses were fed each diet in random order for four 3-week periods. When compared to CON, spontaneous activity was less in horses fed SL-CO (~ 4 km/day vs. ~ 5 km/day in CON) but unaffected by the CO or SL-SO diets. Similarly, there was no consistent effect of fat supplementation on measures of reactivity, although startle response to the sudden opening of an umbrella was decreased in all three diets. In studies examining the effect of dietary energy source on the clinical expression of recurrent exertional rhabdomyolysis in Thoroughbreds, researchers have reported decreased excitability, nervousness, and resting heart rate when the horses were consuming a fat-supplemented ration when compared to a high-grain ration (MacLeay et al., 2000; McKenzie et al., 2003). These authors suggested that the effect of fat supplementation on the behavior of RER-affected horses was due to the exclusion of dietary starch rather than a specific effect of dietary fat. Other researchers have reported a reduction in the exercise-associated increase in plasma cortisol concentration in horses fed a fat-supplemented ration (Crandell et al., 1999; Graham-Thiers et al., 2001).

Holland et al. (1996b) found lower plasma cortisol concentrations in 4- to 5-month-old foals fed a fat-and-fiber supplement when compared to a starch and sugar (sweet feed) supplement. Subjectively, the foals fed the fat-and-fiber supplement were less stressed after weaning. In a longitudinal study of growing horses, supplementation with a fat and fiber concentrate was associated with lower apparent distress at weaning and diminished responses to standardized temperament tests when compared to a starch-and-sugar concentrate (Nicol et al., 2005).

Lactation, Reproductive Performance, and Growth

Davison et al. (1987, 1991) added 5 percent animal fat to concentrates fed to pregnant and lactating Quarter horse mares. Feed consumption was lower during gestation, while growth rate tended to be higher in foals of mares fed the supplemented diet compared to mares and foals fed the unsupplemented diet (Davison et al., 1987, 1991). Fat supplementation increased milk fat concentration at days 10 and 60 of lactation, but protein and total solids content were unaffected. The feeding of fat to mares during late gestation and early lactation did not affect reproductive performance (Davison et al., 1991). Growth of Thoroughbred weanlings kept at pasture and fed a 10-percent fat supplement was not different when compared to weanlings fed an isocaloric supplement rich in starch and sugar (Hoffman et al., 1999).

Health Effects of Dietary (n-3) vs. (n-6) Fatty Acids

In other species, the two recognized EFAs are linoleic acid (18:2, n-6) and α-linolenic acid (18:3, n-3), both of which are PUFAs. Mammals lack the desaturase enzymes necessary to introduce double bonds into fatty acid chains that are more than nine carbons from the carboxyl terminus. Therefore, mammals are unable to synthesize n-3 and n-6 fatty acids, and they must be supplied in the diet (Dunbar and Bauer, 2002).

Soy, corn, sunflower, and safflower oils are rich in linoleic acid, while α-linolenic acid is the major fatty acid in linseed and flaxseed oils. Soy and canola oils also contain α-linolenic acid. The fatty acids in oils obtained from coldwater fish (e.g., menhaden oil) are rich in the n-3 fatty acids eicosapentaenoic acid (EPA) and docosahexaenoic acid (DHA). When supplied in the diet, EFAs can be converted to long-chain PUFAs by desaturase and chain-elongation enzymes located in the cellular endoplasmic reticulum. Linoleic acid is desaturated and elongated to yield arachidonic acid (20:4, n-6) and other long-chain PUFAs that are incorporated into cell membrane phospholipids, while metabolism of α-linolenic acid yields eicosapentaenoic acid (EPA; 20:5, n-3) and docosapentaenoic acid (22:5, n-3). Docosapentaenoic acid may be retroconverted to EPA (20:5, n-3) or further metabolized to DHA (22:6, n-3).

In human and animal nutrition there is interest in the potential health benefits of n-3 fatty acid supplementation (or alterations in the dietary n-6:n-3 ratio). The dietary n-6 vs. n-3 PUFA ratio affects the fatty acid composition of cell membranes (Simopoulos, 1999). When the diet of humans is supplemented with fish oil, the ingested EPA and DHA partially replace n-6 fatty acids (especially arachidonic acid) in cell membranes, particularly those of platelets, erythrocytes, neutrophils, and monocytes. This alteration in membrane fatty acid composition reduces the quantity of arachidonic acid available for eicosanoid synthesis, alters the spectrum of eicosanoids synthesized, and lessens the inflammatory and prothrombotic responses to physical or chemical stimuli (Hulbert et al., 2005). In addition, EPA competitively inhibits the activity of the enzyme cyclooxygenase, which is necessary for eicosanoid synthesis (Weber et al., 1986).

Several studies in horses have examined the effects of n-3 fatty acid supplementation on plasma fatty acid composition and various physiologic responses. Henry et al. (1990) fed horses a complete pelleted ration containing 8 percent (by weight) raw linseed oil vs. a control ration without added linseed oil. After 8 weeks on the ration, the mean procoagulant activity and thromboxane B_2 production by endotoxin-stimulated monocytes from horses consuming the linseed oil ration decreased by 51 percent and 71 percent, respectively, compared with cells from horses consuming the control ration. Fatty acid analysis of membrane phospholipids demonstrated a decrease in the n-6:n-3 ratio in monocytes from horses fed the linseed oil ration (Henry et al., 1990). In a companion study (Morris et al., 1991), it was shown that endotoxin-induced synthesis of tumor necrosis factor by peritoneal macrophages was lower in horses fed the linseed oil ration when compared to cells from horses fed the control ration. This research group also demonstrated that intravenous administration of a single dose of a 20 percent lipid emulsion enriched with n-3 fatty acids to healthy horses resulted in decreased inflammatory mediator synthesis (thromboxane, TNF-alpha) by monocytes and a lower n-6:n-3 fatty acid ratio in cell membranes when compared to the infusion of a lipid emulsion enriched with n-6 fatty acids (McCann et al., 2000). However, the feeding of an 8 percent linseed oil ration for 8 weeks did not alter the in vivo response of horses to the infusion of *Escherichia coli* 055:B5 endotoxin (0.03 mg/kg BW, infused over 30 minutes) (Henry et al., 1991). In another study, there were statistically significant increases in the plasma concentrations of α-linolenic acid (18:3, n-3) and EPA, but not DHA, in horses fed a 10 percent flaxseed oil-enriched complete pellet (80 percent of the ration) and hay (20 percent) for 16 weeks. However, in vitro measures of platelet aggregation were not altered by the supplementation of flaxseed oil (Hansen et al., 2002). More marked increases in plasma concentrations of EPA and DHA were observed when healthy horses were fed ration supplemented with fish (menhaden) oil. Hall et al. (2004a) fed horses diets supplemented with either 3 percent (by weight) corn oil or fish oil for 14 weeks. At 12 weeks, horses fed fish oil had increased plasma concentrations of EPA (27-fold; 8.5 vs. 0.3 g/100g fatty acids), DHA (34-fold; 5.1 vs. 0.1 g/100 g fatty acids), and arachidonic acid (8.3-fold; 4.1 vs. 0.5 g/100 g fatty acids). Neutrophils from horses fed fish oil produced 17.6-fold more leukotriene B_5 (LTB_5) compared with horses fed corn oil, and the ratio of LTB_5 to leukotriene B_4 was 4-fold high in horses fed fish oil. In addition, the quantity of prostaglandin E_2 by endotoxin-stimulated bronchoalveolar fluid (BALF) cells was lower in fish oil-fed when compared to corn oil-fed horses. However, the production of TNF-alpha by BALF cells did not differ between diets and cell-mediated immunity, assessed by the skin response to injection of the keyhole limpet hemocyanin, was similar in the corn oil- and fish oil-fed horses (Hall et al., 2004b).

Supplementation of horses with recurrent seasonal pruritis ("sweet itch") with large amounts of flaxseed (454 g flaxseed/450 kg BW) was associated with a significant decrease in the allergic skin response to *Culicoides* extract, suggesting a possible benefit of flaxseed in the management of horses with this condition. However, in another study, supplementation with flax oil did not alter clinical signs in horses with *Culicoides* hypersensitivity (Friberg and Logas, 1999).

In summary, the data from studies in which horses were fed diets enriched with omega-3 (n-3) fatty acids (linseed, flaxseed, or fish oils) have demonstrated modulation of inflammatory mediator synthesis by cells harvested from blood, peritoneal fluid, or respiratory secretions. However, physiological importance of these findings is unclear, and further research is needed to determine the effects of n-3 fatty acid supplementation in the treatment and prevention of inflammatory diseases in horses (e.g., recurrent airway obstruction) (McCann and Carrick, 1998).

REQUIREMENTS, DEFICIENCIES, AND EXCESSES

Dietary fats or oils are required to facilitate absorption of the fat-soluble vitamins A, D, E, and K, and as a source of the EFAs, linoleic and α-linolenic. There have been no reports of EFA deficiency in horses. In other species, an EFA deficiency causes dry coat, scaly skin, hair loss, and, with prolonged deficiency, development of exudative dermatitis (Connor, 2000). Decreased reproductive efficiency and fetal abnormalities are other potential consequences of an EFA deficiency. No clinical abnormalities were observed in ponies fed extremely low-fat diets (0.05 percent and 0.22 percent total fat containing, respectively, 0.03 and 0.14 percent linoleic acid) for 7 months (Sallmann et al., 1991). However, a substantial decrease in plasma and tissue vitamin E concentration was observed in ponies fed the 0.05 percent fat diet, suggesting that there was inadequate intestinal absorption of this fat-soluble vitamin.

A suggested dietary minimum for linoleic acid is 0.5 percent of DM. This minimum is easily achieved when supplemental fat is fed, as fats and oils added to equine rations are high in linoleic acid (see Table 8-5). Because fat is energy dense, one concern with the feeding of fat-supplemented diets is weight gain associated with the provision of DE in excess of needs. The promotion of weight gain in hard keeper horses is a common rationale for the addition of fat to equine diets. For less active or easy keeper horses, however, use of fat-supplemented energy concentrates may lead to undesirable weight gain. Metabolic utilization of absorbed fat is highly efficient. In ponies fed supplemental corn oil, the DE to net energy (NE) conversion efficiency was about 85 percent (Kane et al., 1979). The comparative efficiency for a hay/grain diet is less than 60 percent. Accordingly, the NE of fat-supplemented feeds is higher than is predicted by estimation of the DE content.

In Shetland ponies, there is evidence that fat supplementation (soybean oil, 10 percent DM) results in glucose intolerance (Schmidt et al., 2001). When ponies were fed to meet DE requirement (15.5 MJ DE/100 kg BW), mean plasma glucose concentrations during an oral glucose tolerance test (1 g/kg BW) were approximately 40 percent higher in the fat-supplemented diet when compared to the control diet. Furthermore, the feeding of a hypercaloric (18.5 MJ DE/100 kg BW) fat-enriched diet resulted in a 25-fold increase in plasma insulin concentrations after oral glucose loading. Thus, glucose intolerance and insulin resistance may occur in ponies fed fat-supplemented diets, particularly when energy intake exceeds requirements. As insulin resistance is considered a risk factor for laminitis in ponies, some caution in the feeding of fat-supplemented diets is warranted.

Most of the studies evaluating the effects of fat supplementation in horses have been of short duration (less than 3 months). However, Pagan et al. (1995) observed no adverse effects in 2-year-old Thoroughbreds fed supplemental fat (soybean oil, 12 percent DE) for 7 months. Harris et al. (1999) reported no apparent adverse effects of feeding a diet supplemented with either an unsaturated or saturated vegetable oil for 6 months at 20 percent DE after 10 months at 12 percent DE. In Warmblood-type horses, no detrimental effects on blood biochemical variables were observed after feeding a mixed diet containing 14 percent and 16.3 percent partially hydrogenated soy oil for, respectively, 168 (Zeyner and Dittrich, 2003) and 390 (Zeyner et al., 2002) days.

REFERENCES

Bowman, V. A., J. P. Fontenot, T. N. Meacham, and K. E. Webb. 1979. Acceptability and digestibility of animal, vegetable and blended fats by equine. Pp. 74–75 in Proc. 6th Equine Nutr. Physiol. Soc. Symp., College Station, TX.

Bush, J. A., D. E. Freeman, K. H. Kline, N. R. Merchen, and G. C. Fahey, Jr. 2001. Dietary fat supplementation effects on in vitro nutrient disappearance and in vivo nutrient intake and total digestibility by horses. J. Anim. Sci. 79:232–239.

Connor, W. E. 2000. Importance of n-3 fatty acids in health and disease. Am. J. Clin. Nutr. 71(suppl):171S–175S.

Coppock, C.E., and D. L. Wilks. 1991. Supplemental fat in high energy rations for lactating cows: effects on intake, digestion, milk yield and composition. J. Anim. Sci. 69:3826–3837.

Crandell, K. G., J. D. Pagan, P. Harris, and S. E. Duren. 1999. A comparison of grain, oil and beet pulp as energy sources for the exercised horse. Equine Vet. J. Suppl. 30:485–489.

Custalow, S. E. 1992. Lactate and Glucose Responses to Exercise in the Horse: Influence of Interval Training and Dietary Fat. M.S. Thesis. Virginia Polytechnic Institute and State University, Blacksburg.

Davison, K. E., G. D. Potter, J. W. Evans, L. W. Greene, P. S. Hargis, C. D. Corn, and S. P. Webb. 1987. Growth and nutrient utilization in weanling horses fed added dietary fat. Pp. 95–100 in Proc. 11th Equine Nutr. Physiol. Soc. Symp., Stillwater, OK.

Davison, K. E., G. D. Potter, L. W. Greene, J. W. Evans, and W. C. MacMullan. 1991. Lactation and reproductive performance of mares fed added dietary fat during late gestation and early lactation. J. Equine Vet. Sci. 11:111–115.

Dunbar, B. L., and J. E. Bauer. 2002. Metabolism of dietary essential fatty acids and their conversion to long-chain polyunsaturated metabolites. J. Am. Vet. Med. Assoc. 220:1621–1626.

Dunnett, C. E., D. J. Marlin, and R. C. Harris. 2002. Effect of dietary lipid on response to exercise: relationship to metabolic adaptation. Equine Vet. J. Suppl. 34:75–80.

Duren, S. E., S. G. Jackson, J. P. Baker, and D. K. Aaron. 1987. Effect of dietary fat on blood parameters in exercised Thoroughbred horses. Pp. 674–685 in Equine Exercise Physiology 2, J. R. Gillespie and N. E. Robinson, eds. Davis, CA: ICEEP Publications.

Eaton, M. D., D. R. Hodgson, and D. L. Evans. 1995. Effect of diet containing supplementary fat on the effectiveness for high intensity exercise. Equine Vet. J. Suppl 18:353–356.

Essen-Gustavsson, B., E. Blomstrand, K. Karlstrom, A. Lindholm, and S. G. B. Persson. 1991. Influence of diet on substrate metabolism during exercise. Pp. 288–298 in Equine Exercise Physiology 3, S. G. B. Persson, A. Lindholm, and L. B. Jeffcott, eds. Upsala: ICEEP Publications.

Ferrante, P. L., D. S. Kronfeld, L. E. Taylor, and T. N. Meacham. 1994. Blood lactate concentration during exercise in horses fed a high-fat diet and administered sodium bicarbonate. J. Nutr. 124:2738S–2739S.

Fonnesbeck, P. V., R. K. Lydman, G. W. Vander Noot, and L. D. Symons. 1967. Digestibility of the proximate nutrients of forage by horses. J. Anim. Sci. 26:1039–1045.

Friberg, C. A., and D. Logas. 1999. Treatment of culicoides hypersensitive horses with high-dose n-3 fatty acids: a double-blinded crossover study. Vet. Dermatol. 10:117–122.

Geelen, S. N. J., M. M. Sloet van Oldruitenborgh-Oosterbaan, and A. C. Beynen. 1999. Dietary fat supplementation and equine plasma lipid metabolism. Equine Vet. J. Suppl. 30:475–478.

Geelen, S. N. J., W. L. Jansen, M. J. H. Geelen, M. M. Sloet van Oldruitenborgh-Oosterbaan, and A. C. Beynen. 2000. Lipid metabolism in equines fed a fat-rich diet. Int. J. Vitam. Nutr. Res. 70:148–152.

Geelen, S. N. J., W. L. Jansen, M. M. Sloet van Oldruitenborgh-Oosterbaan, H. J. Breukink, and A. C. Beynen. 2001a. Fat feeding increases equine heparin-released lipoprotein lipase activity. J. Vet. Int. Med. 15:478–481.

Geelen, S. N. J., C. Blazquez, M. J. H. Geelen, M. M. Sloet van Oldruitenborgh-Oosterbaan, and A. C. Beynen. 2001b. High fat intake lowers fatty acid synthesis and raises fatty acid oxidation in aerobic muscle in Shetland ponies. Br. J. Nutr. 86:31–36.

Graham-Thiers, P., D. S. Kronfeld, and D. J. Sklan. 2001. Dietary protein restriction and fat supplementation diminish the acidogenic effect of exercise during repeated sprints in horses. J. Nutr. 131:1959–1964.

Hall, J. A., R. J. Van Saun, and R. C. Wander. 2004a. Dietary (n-3) fatty acids from menhaden fish oil alter plasma fatty acids and leukotriene B synthesis in healthy horses. J. Vet. Int. Med. 18:871–879.

Hall, J. A., R. J. Van Saun, S. J. Tournquist, J. L. Grandin, E. C. Pearson, and R. C. Wander. 2004b. Effect of type of dietary polyunsaturated fatty acid supplement (corn oil or fish oil) on immune responses in healthy horses. J. Vet. Int. Med. 18:880–886.

Hambleton, P. L., L. M. Slade, D. W. Hamar, E. W. Kienholz, and L. D. Lewis. 1980. Dietary fat and exercise conditioning effect on metabolic parameters in the horse. J. Anim. Sci. 51:1330–1339.

Hansen, R. A., C. J. Savage, K. Reidlinger, J. L. Traub-Dargatz, G. K. Ogilvie, D. Mitchell, and M. J. Fettman. 2002. Effects of dietary flaxseed oil supplementation on equine plasma fatty acid concentrations and whole blood platelet aggregation. J. Vet. Int. Med. 16:457–463.

Harkins, J. D., G. S. Morris, R. T. Tulley, A. G. Nelson, and S. G. Kamerling. 1992. Effect of added dietary fat on racing performance in Thoroughbred horses. J. Equine Vet. Sci. 12:123–129.

Harris, P. A., J. D. Pagan, K. G. Crandell, and N. P. Davidson. 1999. Effect of feeding Thoroughbred horses a high unsaturated or saturated vegetable oil supplemented diet for 6 months following a 10 month fat acclimation. Equine Vet. J. Suppl. 30:468–474.

Henry, M. M., J. N. Moore, E. B. Feldman, J. K. Fischer, and B. Russell. 1990. Effect of dietary alpha-linolenic acid on equine monocyte procoagulant activity and eicosanoid synthesis. Circ. Shock 32:173–188.

Henry, M. M., J. N. Moore, and J. K. Fischer. 1991. Influence of an omega-3 fatty acid-enriched ration on in vivo responses of horses to endotoxin. Am. J. Vet. Res. 52:523–527.

Hintz, H. F., and F. F. Schryver. 1989. Digestibility of various sources of fat by horses. Pp. 44–48 in Cornell Nutr. Conf. for Feed Manuf., Syracuse, NY.

Hintz, H. F., M. W. Ross, F. R. Lesser, P. F. Leids, K. K. White, J. E. Lowe, C. E. Short, and H. F. Schryver. 1978. The value of dietary fat for working horses. 1. Biochemical and hematological evaluations. J. Equine Med. Surg. 2:483.

Hintz, H. F., J. E. Lowe, K. K. White, C. E. Short, and M. Ross. 1982. Nutritional value of fat for exercising horses. Unpublished data, Cornell University.

Hoffman, R. M., L. A. Lawrence, D. S. Kronfeld, W. L. Cooper, D. J. Sklan, J. J. Dascanio, and P. A. Harris. 1999. Dietary carbohydrates and fat influence radiographic bone mineral content of growing foals. J. Anim. Sci. 77:3330–3338.

Hoffman, R. M., R. C. Boston, D. Stefanovski, D. S. Kronfeld, and P. A. Harris. 2003. Obesity and diet affect glucose dynamics and insulin sensitivity in Thoroughbred geldings. J. Anim. Sci. 81:2333–2342.

Holland, J. L. 1994. Lecithin Containing Diets for the Horse: Acceptance, Digestibility and Effects on Behavior. M.S. Thesis. Virginia Polytechnic Institute and State Univ., Blacksburg.

Holland, J. L., D. S. Kronfeld, and T. N. Meacham. 1996a. Behavior of horses is affected by soy lecithin and corn oil in the diet. J. Anim. Sci. 74:1252–1255.

Holland, J. L., D. S. Kronfeld, R. M. Hoffman, and K. M. Griewe-Crandell. 1996b. Weaning stress is affected by nutrition and weaning methods. Pferdeheilkunde 12:257–260.

Holland, J. L., D. S. Kronfeld, G. A. Rich, K. A. Kline, J. P. Fontenot, T. N. Meacham, and P. A. Harris. 1998. Acceptance of fat and lecithin containing diets by horses. Appl. Anim. Behav. Sci. 56:91–96.

Hughes, S. F., G. D. Potter, L. W. Greene, T. W. Odom, and M. Murray-Gerzik. 1995. Adaptation of Thoroughbred horses in training to a fat supplemented diet. Equine Vet. J. Suppl. 18:349–352.

Hulbert, A. J., N. Turner, L. H. Storlein, and P. L. Else. 2005. Dietary fats and membrane function: implications for metabolism and disease. Biol. Rev. 80:155–159.

Hyyppa, S., M. Saastamoinen, and A. R. Poso. 1999. Effect of a post exercise fat-supplemented diet on muscle glycogen repletion. Equine Vet. J. Suppl. 30:493–498.

Jansen, W. L., J. van der Kuilen, S. N. J. Geelen, and A. C. Beynen. 2000. The effect of replacing nonstructural carbohydrates with soybean oil on the digestibility of fiber in trotting horses. Equine Vet. J. 32:27–30.

Jansen, W. L., J. van der Kuilen, S. N. Geelen, and A. C. Beynen. 2001. The apparent digestibility of fiber when dietary soybean oil is substituted for an iso-energetic amount of glucose. Arch. Tierernahr. 54:297–304.

Jansen, W. L., S. N. J. Geelen, J. van der Kuilen, and A. C. Beynen. 2002. Dietary soyabean oil depressed the apparent digestibility of fibre in trotters when substituted for an iso-energetic amount of corn starch or glucose. Equine Vet. J. 34:302–305.

Jones, D. L., G. D. Potter, L. W. Greene, and T. W. Odom. 1991. Muscle glycogen concentrations in exercised miniature horses at various body conditions and fed a control or fat-supplemented diet. P. 109 in Proc. 12th Equine Nutr. Phys. Soc. Symp., Calgary, Alberta.

Julen, T. R., G. D. Potter, L. W. Greene, and G. G. Stott. 1995. Adaptation to a fat-supplemented diet by cutting horses. Pp. 56–61 in Proc. 14th Equine Nutr. Physiol. Soc. Symp., Ontario, CA.

Kane, E. J., J. P. Baker, and L. S. Bull. 1979. Utilization of a corn oil supplemented diet by the pony. J. Anim. Sci. 48:1379–1383.

Kronfeld, D. S. 1996. Dietary fat affects heat production and other variables of equine performance under hot and humid conditions. Equine Vet. J. Suppl. 22:24–34.

Kronfeld, D. S., and P. A. Harris. 2003. Equine grain-associated disorders. Comp. Contin. Educ. Pract. Vet. 25:974–983.

Kronfeld, D. S., S. E. Custalow, P. L. Ferrante, L. E. Taylor, J. A. Wilson, and W. Tiegs. 1998. Acid-base responses of fat-adapted horses: relevance to hard work in the heat. Appl. Anim. Behav. 59:61–72.

Kronfeld, D. S., J. L. Holland, G. A. Rich, S. E. Custalow, J. P. Fontenot, T. N. Meacham, D. J. Sklan, and P. A. Harris. 2004. Fat digestibility in Equus caballus follows increasing first-order kinetics. J. Anim. Sci. 82:1773–1780.

MacLeay, J. M., S. J. Valberg, J. D. Pagan, F. de laCorte, J. Roberts, J. Billstrom, J. McGinnity, and H. Kaese. 1999. Effect of diet on thoroughbred horses with recurrent exertional rhabdomyolysis performing a standardised exercise test. Equine Vet. J. Suppl. 30:458–462.

MacLeay, J. M., S. J. Valberg, J. Pagan, J. A. Billstrom, and J. Roberts. 2000. Effect of diet and exercise intensity on serum CK activity in Thoroughbreds with recurrent exertional rhabdomyolysis. Am. J. Vet. Res. 61:1390–1395.

McCann, J. S., T. N. Meacham, and J. P. Fontenot. 1987. Energy utilization and blood traits of ponies fed fat-supplemented diets. J. Anim. Sci. 65:1019–1026.

McCann, M. E., and J. B. Carrick. 1998. Potential uses of ω-3 fatty acids in equine diseases. Comp. Cont. Educ. Pract. Vet. 20:637–641.

McCann, M. E., J. N. Moore, J. B. Carrick, and M. H. Barton. 2000. Effect of intravenous infusion of omega-3 and omega-6 lipid emulsions on equine monocytes fatty acid composition and inflammatory mediator production in vitro. Shock 14:222–228.

McKenzie, E. C., S. J. Valberg, S. Godden, J. D. Pagan, J. M. MacLeay, R. J. Geor, and G. P. Carlson. 2003. Effect of dietary starch, fat and bicarbonate content on exercise responses and serum creatine kinase activity in equine recurrent exertional rhabdomyolysis. J. Vet. Int. Med. 17:693–701.

Meyer, H., C. Flothow, and S. Radicke. 1997. Preileal digestibility of coconut and soybean oil in horses and their influence on metabolites of microbial origin of the proximal digestive tract. Arch. Anim. Nutr. 50:63–74.

Meyers, M. C., G. D. Potter, L. W. Greene, S. F. Crouse, and J. W. Evans. 1987. Physiological and metabolic response of exercising horses to added dietary fat. Pp. 107–113 in Proc. 10th Equine Nutr. Physiol. Soc. Symp., Fort Collins, CO.

Morris, D. D., M. M. Henry, J. N. Moore, and J. K. Fisher. 1991. Effect of dietary alpha-linolenic acid on endotoxin-induced production of tumor necrosis factor by peritoneal macrophages in horses. Am. J. Vet. Res. 52:528–532.

Nicol, C. J., A. J. Badwell-Waters, R. Rice, A. Kelland, A. D. Wilson, and P. A. Harris. 2005. The effects of diet and weaning method on the behavior of young horses. Appl. Anim. Behav. Sci. 95:205–221.

O'Connor, C. I., L. M. Lawrence, A. C. St. Lawrence, K. M. Janicki, L. K. Warren, and S. Hayes. 2004. The effect of dietary fish oil supplementation on exercising horses. J. Anim. Sci. 82:2978–2984.

Oldham, S. L., G. D. Potter, J. W. Evans, S. B. Smith, T. S. Taylor, and W. S. Barnes. 1990. Storage and mobilization of muscle glycogen in exercising horses fed a fat-supplemented diet. J. Equine Vet. Sci. 10:353–359.

Orme, C. E., R. C. Harris, D. J. Marlin, and J. Hurley. 1997. Metabolic adaptation to a fat-supplemented diet by the Thoroughbred horse. Br. J. Nutr. 78:443–458.

Pagan, J. D., B. Essen-Gustavsson, A. Lindholm, and J. Thornton. 1987. The effect of dietary energy source on exercise performance in Standardbred horses. Pp. 686–799 in Equine Exercise Physiology 2, J. R. Gillespie and N. E. Robinson, eds. Davis, CA: ICEEP Publications.

Pagan, J. D., I. Burger, and S. G. Jackson. 1995. The long term effects of feeding fat to 2-year-old Thoroughbreds in training. Equine Vet. J. Suppl. 18:343–348.

Pagan, J. D., R. J. Geor, P. A. Harris, K. Hoekstra, S. Gardner, C. Hudson, and A. Prince. 2002. Effects of fat adaptation on glucose kinetics and substrate oxidation during low-intensity exercise. Equine Vet. J. Suppl. 34:33–38.

Potter, G. D., S. L. Hughes, T. R. Julen, and S. L. Swinney. 1992. A review of research on digestion and utilization of fat by the equine. Pferdeheilkunde Sonderheft 1:119–123.

Rich, V. A. B. 1980. Digestibility and Palatability of Animal, Vegetable and Animal-Vegetable Blended Fats by the Equine. Ph.D. Diss., Virginia Polytechnic Institute and State Univ., Blacksburg.

Sallmann H. P., E. Kienzle, H. Fuhrmann, D. Grunwald, I. Eilmans, and H. Meyer. 1991. Metabolic consequences of feeding ponies with marginal amounts of fat. Pp. 81–82 in Proc. 12th Equine Nutr. Physiol. Soc. Symp., Calgary, Alberta.

Schmidt, O., E. Deegen, H. Fuhrmann, R. Duhlmeier, and H. P. Sallmann. 2001. Effects of fat feeding and energy level on plasma metabolites and hormones in Shetland ponies. J. Vet. Med. 48A:39–49.

Scott, B. D., G. D. Potter, L. W. Greene, P. S. Hargis and J. G. Anderson. 1992. Efficacy of a fat-supplemented diet on muscle glycogen concentrations in exercising Thoroughbred horses maintained in varying body conditions. J. Equine Vet. Sci. 12:105–109.

Simopoulos, A. P. 1999. Essential fatty acids in health and chronic disease. Am. J. Clin. Nutr. 70 (Suppl):560S–569S.

Slade, L. M., L. D. Lewis, C. R. Quinn, and M. L. Chandler. 1975. Nutritional adaptations of horses for endurance performance. Pp. 114–128 in Proc. 4th Equine Nutr. Physiol. Soc. Symp., Pomona, Calif.

Sloet van Oldruitenborgh-Oosterbaan, M. M., M. P. Annee, E. J. M. M. Verdegaal, A. G. Lemens, and A. C. Beynen. 2002. Exercise and metabolism-associated blood variables in Standardbreds fed either a low- or a high-fat diet. Equine Vet. J. Suppl. 34:29–32.

Spriet, L. L., and M. J. Watt. 2003. Regulatory mechanisms in the interaction between carbohydrate and lipid oxidation during exercise. Acta. Physiol. Scand. 178:443–452.

Sturgeon, L. S., L. A. Baker, J. L. Pipkin, J. C. Haliburton, and N. K. Chirase. 2000. The digestibility and mineral availability of matua, bermuda grass, and alfalfa hay in mature horses. J. Equine Vet. Sci. 20:45–48.

Taylor, L. E., P. L. Ferrante, D. S. Kronfeld, and T. N. Meacham. 1995. Acid-base variables during incremental exercise in sprint-trained horses fed a high-fat diet. J. Anim. Sci. 73:2009–2018.

Topliff, D. R., G. D. Potter, T. R. Dutson, J. L. Kreider, and G. T. Jessup. 1983. Diet manipulation and muscle glycogen in the equine. Pp. 224–229 in Proc. 8th Equine Nutr. Physiol. Soc. Symp., Lexington, KY.

Webb, S. P., G. D. Potter, and J. W. Evans. 1987. Physiologic and metabolic response of race and cutting horses to added dietary fat. P. 115 in Proc. 10th Equine Nutr. Physiol. Soc. Symp., Fort Collins, CO.

Weber, P. C., S. Fischer, C. von Schacky, R. Lorenz, and T. Strasser. 1986. Dietary omega-3 polyunsaturated fatty acids and eicosanoid formation in man. Pp. 49–60 in Health Effects of Polyunsaturated Fatty Acids in Seafoods, A. P. Simipoulos, R. R. Kifer, and R. E. Martin, eds. Orlando, FL: Academic Press.

Williams, C. A., D. S. Kronfeld, W. B. Staniar, and P. A. Harris. 2001. Plasma glucose and insulin responses of Thoroughbred mares fed a meal high in starch and sugar or fat and fiber. J. Anim. Sci. 79:2196–2200.

Zeyner, A. 2002. Ernährungsphysiologische Wirkungen eines Austusches von starker-eichen Konponenten durch Sojaöl in der Reitpferdeernährung. Göttingen: Georg-August-University, Habilitation thesis.

Zeyner, A., and A. Dittrich. 2003. Digestibility of energy, proximate nutrients and minerals and indicators of gut microbial activity in horses fed a moderate amount of soybean oil over 168 days. Proc. Soc. Nutr. Physiol. 12:98.

Zeyner, A., J. Bessert, and J. M. Gropp. 2002. Effect of feeding exercised horses on high starch or high fat diets for 390 days. Equine Vet. J. Suppl. 34:50–57.

Zeyner, A., C. Hoffmeister, A. Einspanier, and O. Lengwenat. 2005. Glycemic and insulinemic response of Quarter horses to concentrates high in fat and low in soluble carbohydrates. P. 312 in Proc. 19th Equine Sci. Soc., Tucson, AZ.

4

Proteins and Amino Acids

INTRODUCTION

Protein is a major component of most tissues in the body, second only to water. All tissues in the body are made of protein along with enzymes, hormones, and antibodies. Protein is made of chains of amino acids. Twenty so-called "primary" amino acids make up most proteins. The types of amino acids incorporated into a protein chain as well as the length of the protein chain differentiate one protein from another. Therefore, the horse's requirement is actually for amino acids. Individual amino acid requirements (with the exception of lysine) have not been established for the horse. As a nonruminant species, there are 10 presumed essential amino acids for the horse: arginine, histidine, isoleucine, leucine, lysine, methionine, phenylalanine, threonine, tryptophan, and valine (NRC, 1998). These are amino acids that cannot be synthesized by the body in sufficient quantities to meet the demand for them. All the necessary amino acids required for a protein to be made must be present at the same time. One that is present in less than adequate amounts is referred to as a limiting amino acid because it will limit protein synthesis. The challenge in feeding horses is to provide adequate quantities of protein that will allow for sufficient concentrations of circulating amino acids in the blood that the body can draw on to synthesize tissues, enzymes, and hormones, as well as repair tissues.

PROTEIN DIGESTION AND UTILIZATION

Dietary protein is digested mainly in the foregut of the horse through enzymatic digestion in the stomach and small intestine. Enzymatic digestion of protein in the stomach occurs via pepsin, which has specificity for peptide bonds involving aromatic L-amino acids such as phenylalanine and tryptophan. Pancreatic proteases secreted into the small intestine continue protein breakdown and enable absorption of amino acids and dipeptides in the small intestine. Dipeptides are hydrolyzed to amino acids in the gut wall and add to the circulating pool of amino acids in the blood. Nonprotein nitrogen (NPN) sources, such as free amino acids and urea, are also absorbed in the small intestine. Protein and NPN escaping digestion in the foregut enter the hindgut where they are available for degradation and the synthesis of microbial protein. Studies have reported an increase in plasma ammonia concentrations when protein sources were infused directly into the cecum (Reitnour and Salsbury, 1975), suggesting that ammonia is the main nitrogen product absorbed from the hindgut. There is no evidence that amino acids from microbial protein synthesis are absorbed in sufficient quantities to significantly contribute to the amino acid pool for the horse. Cecal administration of 75 g of lysine did not increase plasma lysine in horses, in contrast to a dramatic increase in plasma lysine with a gastric dose of lysine (Wysocki and Baker, 1975). If the hindgut were of significant importance in protein digestion, it would be expected that cecal infusion of protein sources would result in improved nitrogen balance, but this has proven not to be the case (Reitnour and Salsbury, 1972). Another study showed a high correlation between blood amino acids and dietary amino acids, but no correlation between cecal amino acid concentrations and blood amino acids (Reitnour et al., 1970). These observations suggest that the horse is sensitive to the quality of protein in the diet (amino acid profile), and despite evidence that there is microbial synthesis of amino acids in the hindgut, these amino acids are not absorbed for the horse's benefit. It seems evident that the quality of the protein source should be considered carefully in the horse's diet.

Feeding NPN sources, such as urea, is not useful to the horse in most circumstances. Hintz et al. (1970) reported ammonia toxicity and death of ponies (125 to 136 kg) when 450 g of urea was fed orally. Inclusion of urea in the diet has been reported to improve nitrogen retention in cases where dietary protein appeared to be deficient, but not in cases where other protein sources have been used such as soybean meal (Slade et al., 1970). Inclusion of urea in the diet has consistently increased blood and urine urea concentrations, suggesting that the dietary urea contributed to excess nitrogen in the body, resulting in the increase in blood urea and excretion of urea in urine (Slade et al., 1970; Hintz and Schryver, 1972; Martin et al., 1991, 1996). Urea intake of as little as 0.9 percent of the diet (0.14 g urea/kg BW/d) was reported to increase plasma urea nitrogen (PUN) over the control ration (Hintz and Schryver, 1972), while the other studies fed urea at a rate of 2 to 3 percent of the diet and reported similar increases in PUN over control rations (Slade et al., 1970; Martin et al., 1991, 1996). These studies support the conclusion that urea and other sources of NPN in the form of urea are of little to no nutritional benefit to the horse.

Protein Digestibility

The quality of the dietary protein should be considered when selecting a protein source for the horse's diet. Protein quality is a function of the amino acid profile and the digestibility of the protein source. The higher the digestibility (especially the foregut digestibility) of the protein source, the higher the absorption of amino acids to contribute to the amino acid pool for tissue synthesis and repair.

Digestibility of nitrogen (N) or crude protein (CP) is correlated to dry matter (DM) intake as well as CP concentration in the diet. As DM intake and CP concentration increase, so does CP digestibility (Slade et al., 1970). Combining means of nitrogen digestibility from several studies (N = 16) provided evidence of this across a range of nitrogen intakes between 0.035 g N/kg BW/d to 0.57 g N/kg BW/d. Total tract apparent digestibility of CP varies based on protein source (e.g., fishmeal vs. corn gluten meal) and components of the diet (e.g., forage vs. concentrate), as well as with the ratio of forage to concentrate in the daily ration. Within forages, apparent total tract CP digestibility varies from 73-83 percent for alfalfa, 57-64 percent for Coastal Bermudagrass, and 67-74 percent for other grasses such as fescue and bromegrass. Gibbs et al. (1988) examined the difference in foregut and hindgut digestibility of forages. Apparent prececal digestibility was 28.5 percent for alfalfa and 16.8 percent for Coastal Bermudagrass. Endogenous fecal nitrogen in the study was estimated to be 5.8 mg N/g DM intake resulting in true prececal digestibility of protein from the forages of 37 percent.

Other digestibility studies have fed concentrates in high proportion to forage when determining nitrogen digestibility. Feeding corn, oats, or sorghum in combination with Coastal Bermudagrass hay (3:1 concentrate to forage ratio) resulted in apparent total tract protein digestibility of 88, 82.8, and 84.6 percent respectively. Apparent prececal protein digestion was 38.5, 45.8, and 56.1 percent for corn-, oat-, and sorghum-based diets. This study determined the apparent protein digestibility of the grain portion of the diet by difference (by subtracting the predetermined apparent digestibility of the hay from a previous study), resulting in apparent prececal protein digestibility of 48.1, 53.9, and 70.7 percent for the three diets (corn, oats, and sorghum) and apparent overall tract protein digestion of 98.1, 88.5, and 93.1 percent, respectively (Gibbs et al., 1996). A similar trial was conducted to evaluate protein digestibility of protein supplements. Soybean meal (SBM) and cottonseed meal (CSM) were evaluated. Upper tract apparent protein digestibility was 50.9 and 42.4 percent for SBM and CSM, respectively. Endogenous nitrogen in the upper tract was estimated at 3.5 mg N/g DM intake. True protein digestibility was calculated to be 90.9 and 87.1 percent for SBM and CSM, respectively. Calculating the apparent digestibility of the protein supplement by difference results in prececal digestibility of 52.5 and 81.2 percent for SBM and CSM, respectively, and total tract digestibility of 92.2 and 85 percent for SBM and CSM, respectively. Apparent prececal digestibilities increased from 48 to 59.6 percent as SBM increased in the diet from 0.85 percent of DM intake to 2.85 percent of DM intake and total tract digestibility varied from 77.9 to 87.2 percent with the same increasing amounts of SBM. This study also calculated the true prececal digestibility of SBM to be 72.2 percent (Farley et al., 1995). Potter et al. (1992) fed forage and concentrate with a higher percentage of forage in the ration when compared to other studies evaluating digestibility (50:50 concentrate to forage) and reported apparent prececal digestibilities of 67.3, 70.3, and 75.9 percent for oats, SBM, and CSM, respectively, when fed in combination with Coastal Bermudagrass hay. Relative prececal digestion of protein appears to be 25–30 percent of the dietary protein when diets contain only forage and approaches 70–75 percent when diets contain protein supplements such as SBM or CSM in combination with forage. Compiling means from studies that have reported nitrogen intake as well as fecal nitrogen (N = 16) resulted in an estimate of apparent nitrogen digestibility of 79 percent for the total tract when linear regression was applied to the data ($r^2 = 0.94$) (Figure 4-1). Comparing digestibility between diets that were a mix of concentrate and forage to those containing only forage did not result in a significant difference in digestibility (77 percent for forage-only diets). The same approach of compiling means from studies (N = 4) that reported nitrogen intake as well as foregut N disappearance was used to evaluate apparent prececal nitrogen digestibility. It determined digestibility to be 51 percent when including all diets ($r^2 = 0.83$) (Figure 4-2). Only one study (Gibbs et al., 1988) estimated apparent prececal nitrogen digestibility with all forage diets and reported a slightly lower prececal digestibility (42 percent).

The studies reviewed to determine these estimates of protein digestibility in the total tract, as well as prececal digestibility, utilized sources of protein such as SBM, CSM, linseed meal, brewer's dried grains, fishmeal, milk byproducts, and corn gluten meal. If other sources of protein are utilized that have not been included in this review, this may affect overall protein digestibility and thus protein requirements when using that particular source of protein.

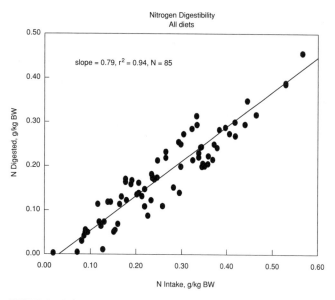

FIGURE 4-1 Regression of means from nitrogen digestibility studies for sedentary horses. The slope of the fitted line represents a 79 percent digestibility for dietary protein (Slade et al., 1970; Hintz et al., 1971; Hintz and Schryver, 1972; Harper and Vander Noot, 1974; Reitnour and Salsbury, 1976; Meyer, 1985; Freeman et al., 1986, 1988; Gibbs et al., 1988, 1996; Potter et al., 1992; Farley et al., 1995; Martin et al., 1996; van Niekerk and van Nierkerk, 1997a; de Almeida et al., 1998a; Olsman et al., 2003).

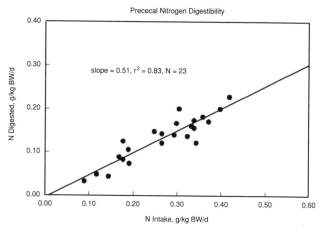

FIGURE 4-2 Regression of means from nitrogen digestibility studies evaluating foregut vs. total tract digestibility of nitrogen. The slope of the fitted line indicates a 51 percent digestibility for dietary protein (Gibbs et al., 1988, 1996; Potter et al., 1992; Farley et al., 1995).

A study by de Almeida et al. (1998b) determined individual amino acid digestibilities using foals and reported increasing apparent digestibility of amino acids as the concentrations increased in the diet. An increase in amino acid digestibility with increasing amino acid intake is consistent with the increase in protein digestibility with increasing protein intake. Apparent digestibilities ranged from a low of 52.8 percent for glycine to a high of 86.3 percent for isoleucine. Apparent lysine digestibility was 63.8 percent in this study. Slightly higher digestibilities were reported by van Niekerk and van Niekerk (1997a) for lysine (79 percent), threonine (79 percent), isoleucine (80 percent), leucine (82 percent), methionine (81 percent), and arginine (90 percent) in pregnant mares.

Nitrogen balance studies have resulted in various estimates of the amounts of nitrogen needed to maintain zero nitrogen balance. The differences in estimates may be explained by variation in nitrogen digestibility. Therefore, 100 g of CP from SBM may be different from 100 g of CP from fishmeal nutritionally to the horse, because of differences in the amino acid profile and digestibility of the protein source. Understanding protein digestibility in the horse enables protein requirements to be expressed in terms of digestible protein (DP) instead of CP. When protein requirements are expressed in terms of DP, diets can be balanced in terms of DP, provided data are available regarding the DP concentration of feedstuffs. In France, protein requirements and protein content of feeds are expressed in terms of MADC (Matières Azotées Digestibles Cheval). This system was developed to account for differences in digestibility of various sources of protein and availability of protein digestion products in the small vs. large intestine. Estimates of true ileal digestibility of protein have been made for hays, concentrates, and mixed diets. Adjustments for total tract digestibility have been made in this system due to the fact that nitrogen of endogenous origin and nitrogen of microbial origin cannot be differentiated in the feces (Martin-Rosset et al., 1994). This system provides insight into considering available protein for the horse rather than CP. Improvement of this system and more research can assist in expressing the protein requirements for the horse in the future in terms of DP rather than CP. The lack of information regarding DP and amino acid availabilities in feedstuffs prevents doing this at this time. More information about estimating DP in feedstuffs for horses is given in Chapter 8.

Protein Bioavailability

Proteins that are digested in the foregut are potentially available to the horse to contribute to the amino acid pool in the body, whereas those that pass to the hindgut are not. Thus, proteins that are largely digested in the equine foregut are of higher quality than those that are mainly degraded in the cecum and colon. In addition to its foregut digestibility, the quality of a protein supplement is further determined by its amino acid profile rather than its crude protein content. As a consequence, nitrogen balance studies found that different amounts of protein were required for zero nitrogen retention when different protein sources were fed. Thus zero nitrogen balances were observed for fishmeal, SBM, and corn gluten meal at intakes of 0.57, 0.8, and 1.18 g N/kg BW/d, respectively. Such results suggest that different protein sources have varying foregut digestibilities and/or amino acid profiles, and thus differ in their biological value to the horse.

A number of studies have determined DP values for a limited number of feeds in horses, but as yet insufficient data are available for the horse in order for DP to be the standard expression for describing either the protein requirements of horses or the protein quality of the wide range of feedstuffs given to them. Crude protein is simply nitrogen × 6.25. Not all CP is available to the animal and adjusting CP content for protein that is not available to the horse could allow estimation of digestible or "available protein" (AP). Available protein can be estimated by subtracting NPN and acid detergent insoluble nitrogen (ADIN), which represents "bound" protein, from CP values for the feeds. Thus, AP is a calculated estimate of protein that may be available to the horse, while DP is based on whole tract digestibility studies that measured the amount of protein apparently digested in vivo. For more information on protein analysis in feeds, see Chapter 10. Studies that evaluated protein digestibility in the horse were used to evaluate the concept of AP. Digestible protein intake was calculated using the digestibility for protein observed in the respective study. The AP of the diet in each study and the respective AP intake was then calculated using the diet and intake data provided in the study. The intake of AP was compared to the DP intake. There was a high correlation between the two variables ($r^2 = 0.91$) (Figure 4-3). Additional research is required to evaluate this concept in vivo, but it could be the next step in progressing from CP to DP in terms of expressing protein requirements for horses.

Data from appropriate studies were subjected to linear and/or nonlinear regression to obtain estimates of requirements in the following sections. This approach is different from the previous edition and results in changes in the calculation of protein requirements for horses in various physiological states.

MAINTENANCE

Nitrogen balance studies in mature horses and ponies have concluded that between 400 and 800 mg DP/kg BW/d is necessary to achieve nitrogen balance in the sedentary horse. However, different protein sources have been used in the various studies. Taking into account true digestibility may reduce the variation. Linear regression of means from studies (providing adequate data to calculate nitrogen balance) using fishmeal, SBM, and corn gluten meal resulted in zero nitrogen balance at intakes of 0.57, 0.80, and 1.18 g N/kg BW/d respectively.

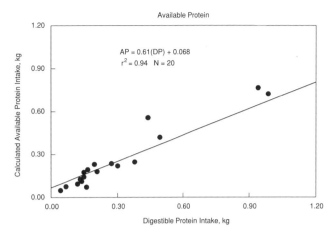

FIGURE 4-3 Relationship between calculated available protein (AP) intake and digestible protein (DP) intake (AP = CP − (NPN + ADIN)) (Hintz and Schryver, 1972; Reitnour and Salsbury, 1972; Reitnour and Salsbury, 1975; Glade et al., 1985; Gibbs et al., 1988, 1996; Farley et al., 1995; Crozier et al., 1997; LaCasha et al., 1999).

When protein needs are evaluated, energy intake must be adequate. Horses fed only 700 mg CP/kg BW/d (350 g/d for a 500-kg horse) lost weight even when energy intake was adequate. These horses continued to lose weight when energy intake was deficient despite CP intakes of 1,300 mg/kg BW/d (650 g CP for a 500-kg horse) (Sticker et al., 1995). Therefore, when CP is deficient, weight loss results; however, when energy is deficient despite CP being adequate, weight loss still results.

Endogenous urinary and fecal nitrogen have been evaluated in several studies in an attempt to estimate the minimal protein needs of the horse. Based on these evaluations, 400 mg DP/kg BW/d has been determined to be the minimum protein need (Reitnour and Salsbury, 1976; Patterson et al., 1985). Higher estimates have been reported by others: 440 mg DP/kg BW/d by Harper and Vander Noot (1974), 545 mg DP/kg BW/d by Olsman et al. (2003), 580 mg DP/kg BW/d by Slade et al. (1970), and 631 mg DP/kg BW/d by Hintz and Schryver (1972). Meyer (1985) estimated endogenous losses (fecal, urine, and cutaneous) to be approximately 57 g N/kg BW/day, suggesting a minimum of 500 mg DP/kg BW/d, but also recommended 714 mg DP/kg BW/d to allow for some reserves of nitrogen in the body. The recommendation was based on a 20 percent increase in DP over the minimal nitrogen need to build up nitrogen reserves and assumed 50 percent efficiency of use for the nitrogen. Intakes of < 400 mg DP/kg BW/d are inadequate. Horses being fed 264 and 310 mg DP/kg BW/d were in negative nitrogen balance (Martin et al., 1996; Olsman et al., 2003). The NRC (1989) CP requirement for maintenance (656 g CP/d for 500-kg horse) assumes a 46 percent digestibility and an all-forage diet. This equates to approximately 600 mg DP/kg BW/d.

Applying linear regression to means from studies (N = 12) that measured nitrogen intake and nitrogen retention resulted in 619 mg DP/kg BW/d (813 mg CP/kg BW/d) for zero nitrogen retention ($r^2 = 0.76$). Thus, based on these data, the minimum digestible protein intake for horses in maintenance should be > 620 mg DP/kg BW/d. Because nitrogen balance can underestimate true nitrogen loss from the body due to measuring error as well as nitrogen losses from hair, skin, and sweat, some allowances for nitrogen retention greater than zero should be made when determining the minimum requirement. This would help compensate for errors in nitrogen balance data as well as allow for some nitrogen reserves in the body. Fitting the same data to a broken-line model estimates the requirement to be 0.202 g N/kg BW/d, resulting in a CP equivalent of 1.26 g/kg BW/d (Figure 4-3). Thus, the equation for determining the CP for the horse in average maintenance would be BW × 1.26 g/kg BW/d. For a 500-kg horse this would equate to 630 g CP/d. Using the 95 percent confidence interval for the data determines the requirement to be between 1.08 g CP/kg BW/d to 1.44 g CP/kg BW/d, which would provide three levels of maintenance similar to those described for energy requirements (Chapter 1), based on the assumption that horses that are more active without forced exercise would have more lean tissue to support. Therefore, minimum CP needs for the maintenance horse can be calculated using the equation: BW × 1.08 g CP/kg BW/d and the need for horses determined to be in elevated maintenance can be calculated by the equation: BW × 1.44 g CP/kg BW/d.

Crude protein requirements for the horse can be calculated using the following equations:

Minimum: BW × 1.08 g CP/kg BW/d

Average: BW × 1.26 g CP/kg BW/d

Elevated: BW × 1.44 g CP/kg BW/d

Studies evaluating lysine requirements of sedentary adult horses have not been conducted. The lysine requirement for maintenance has, in the past, been based on the average lysine content in most protein sources fed to horses. Using means from studies (N = 7) that reported diet composition, intake, and N retention, linear regression was applied and resulted in an intake of 0.036 g lysine/kg BW/d for zero N retention, representing the minimum need for lysine at maintenance. Broken-line analysis (Figure 4-4) identified a plateau in N retention for maintenance horses at an intake of 0.054 g lysine/kg BW/d. The equation to calculate the minimum lysine requirement for maintenance would be BW × 0.036 g/kg BW/d, while the optimum could be calculated with the equation: BW × 0.054 g/kg BW/d. This equates to a minimum of 18 g lysine per day and an optimum of 27 g lysine per day for the 500-kg horse. With a CP requirement of 630 g for the 500-kg horse, the lysine requirement of 27 g/d is equal to 4.3 percent of the CP requirement. Therefore, the requirement for lysine for horses in minimal and elevated maintenance can be calculated by multiplying the CP requirement by 4.3 percent. It is important to emphasize that the relationship between CP and lysine should result in lysine being 4.3 percent of the CP requirement. If the protein sources utilized in the ration do not provide this amount of lysine, this could alter the CP requirement as well.

The lysine requirement for horses in maintenance can be calculated as follows:

Lysine (g/d) = CP requirement × 4.3 percent

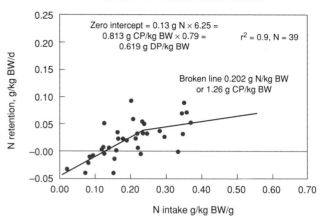

FIGURE 4-4 Linear and nonlinear regression for nitrogen balance for horses at maintenance. Linear regression determined zero N retention to be 0.126 g N/kg BW and broken-line analysis estimated the requirement to be 0.202 g N/kg BW (Slade et al., 1970; Hintz and Schryver, 1972; Reitnour and Salsbury, 1972, 1976; Harper and Vander Noot, 1974; Meyer, 1983a, 1985; Freeman et al., 1986, 1988; Gibbs et al., 1988; Martin et al., 1996; Olsman et al., 2003).

GROWTH

Hintz et al. (1971) studied 4-month-old growing horses and reported maximal nitrogen retention and average daily gain (ADG) when horses consumed 4.25 g CP/kg BW/d from a diet in which the supplemental protein was provided by "milk product blend" (2.77 g DP/kg BW/d). These young horses had greater ADG when fed milk protein compared to linseed meal (Hintz et al., 1971). Other studies have reported greater ADG for young horses (< 8 months of age) fed milk protein over SBM (Borton et al., 1973) or barley (Saastamoinen and Koskinen, 1993), while SBM proved superior for ADG compared to brewer's dried grains (BDG) (Ott et al., 1979). However, when canola meal was fed as the protein source to horses 6 months of age, ADG was equal to that produced by SBM (Cymbaluk, 1990). Urea as a dietary source of nitrogen did not improve ADG in growing horses younger than 8 months of age (Dubose, 1983; Godbee and Slade, 1981). This reinforces the idea that the horse is sensitive to protein quality. This is especially true in the growing horse where lysine has been found to be the first limiting amino acid.

Average daily gain was maximized for weanlings (6 months of age) when 5.05 g CP/kg BW/d was consumed SBM, and a reduction in ADG was reported when intake reached 5.45 g CP/kg BW/d (Yoakam et al., 1978). If a 79 percent protein digestibility is assumed, this equates to maximal growth at 3.95 g DP/kg BW/d. Other studies have reported improved ADG when weanlings (4 to 6 months of age) consumed at least 4.1 g CP/kg BW/d (Pulse et al., 1973), 4.57 g CP/kg BW/d (Jordan and Myers, 1972), and 3.37 g CP/kg BW/d from SBM (Schryver et al., 1987). Combining data from several studies, fitting it to a broken-line model estimate, and extrapolating to different mature body weights, the requirement becomes 4 g CP/kg BW/d for weanlings between 4 and 10 months of age with an expected mature body weight of 500 kg. This equals 672 g CP/d for the 4-month-old (168-kg) weanling. Subtracting the maintenance requirement (1.44 g CP/kg BW/d) from the total CP results in a 50 percent efficiency of use of the remaining CP for gain (0.84 kg/d), assuming the gain is 20 percent protein. This efficiency of use of CP for gain can be used to calculate the CP requirement for gain with an adjustment for digestibility and adding this amount of CP to the daily maintenance requirement.

De Almeida et al. (1998b) estimated total endogenous nitrogen losses in yearling horses to be 588.8 mg CP/kg BW/d and found nitrogen retention was maximized at a protein intake of 3.2 g CP/kg BW/d (2.4 g DP/kg BW/d). This study also compared prececal and postileal digestibility and determined that the majority of protein digestion took place in the foregut. Yearlings (315–333 days of age) have had greater ADGs when fed at least 3.3 g CP/kg BW/d when fed SBM and alfalfa (Ott and Kivipelto, 2002), and 3 g CP/kg BW/d when fed SBM and Bermudagrass hay (Ott and Asquith, 1986). Analysis of means from studies providing intake data as well as ADG reported improved ADG with increasing CP intake up to 3.3 g CP/kg BW/d for yearlings between 11 and 17 months of age. Calculating the efficiency of use of CP for gain (after subtracting the CP needed for maintenance) in studies reporting CP intake, BW and ADG resulted in average efficiency of only 30 percent for horses over 11 months of age. A 321-kg yearling (12 months old) gaining 0.45 kg/d would require 462 g CP/d for maintenance needs (1.44 g CP/kg BW/d) and 380 g CP/d for gain after adjusting for efficiency of use and digestibility assuming gain is 20 percent protein.

Young horses (< 10 months of age) have also responded to amino acid supplementation of diets. Improvement of the amino acid profile of the diet has resulted in improved ADG as well as an ability to lower the overall quantity of CP in the diet. Ott and Kivipelto (2002) concluded through regression analysis that lysine was the most important factor affecting growth, and Ott et al. (1981) earlier concluded that CP could be reduced in the diet if lysine intake was adequate. Studies have concluded that lysine intake for weanlings (4 to 10 months of age) should be 33 to 42 g/d (151 to 179 mg lysine/kg BW/d) to improve ADGs (Breuer and Golden, 1971; Ott et al., 1979; Ott and Kivipelto, 2002). Lysine supplementation of linseed meal (Hintz et al., 1971) and brewer's dried grains (Ott et al., 1979) yielded ADG similar to those reported with milk protein and SBM respectively. Using the data (means) from studies that reported ADG as well as diet, body weight, and feed intake, estimates of amino acid intake can be made. The broken-line model estimated the lysine requirement to be 168 mg/kg BW/d. For the 4-month-old 168-kg weanling, this would be 28 g lysine/d. This amount of lysine is equivalent to 4.3 percent of the horse's CP requirement. Therefore, the lysine requirement for weanling horses between 4–10 months of age is 4.3 percent of the CP requirement.

Yearlings (11–17 months of age) have also responded to lysine supplementation. Studies have concluded that between 48–50 g lysine/d (154–175 mg lysine/kg BW/d) for improved growth was necessary. In yearlings, lysine supplementation has improved ADG reported from CSM- and BDG-based rations (Potter and Hutchon, 1975; Ott et al., 1981). Graham et al. (1994) evaluated threonine as a potentially limiting amino acid for yearling horses. Improved growth and reduced serum urea nitrogen concentrations were reported in yearlings fed 45 g of lysine (127 mg/kg BW/d) and 39 g of threonine (110 mg/kg BW/d) per day compared to yearlings receiving no amino acid supplementation or supplemental lysine of 42 g/d (116 mg/kg BW/d). A reduction in serum urea nitrogen would provide evidence of a reduction in excess amino acids presumably from an improvement in amino acid balance and utilization for tissue synthesis. This study also supported the idea that improvement of protein quality can allow reduction of the overall concentration of CP in the diet.

Most studies have only utilized sedentary growing horses to evaluate CP requirements. Orton et al. (1985) compared groups of 2-year-olds fed low and high amounts of dietary protein as well as combinations of exercise and control groups. Exercise improved the utilization of the dietary protein in the low-protein group (1.45 g CP/kg BW/d). Average daily gain was equal to that of the group consuming 3 g CP/kg BW/d with or without exercise. This increase in dietary protein utilization was also reported in 9-month-old weanlings (1.76 g CP/kg BW/d with exercise yielded similar ADG as 3.1 g CP/kg BW/d with or without exercise) and yearlings (2 g CP/kg BW/d with exercise had ADG similar to consumption of 3.4 g CP/kg BW/d with or without exercise) (Orton et al., 1985). Certainly it seems that exercise improved digestibility in the low-protein exercise group allowing for improved efficiency of use of the dietary protein. The decrease in activity observed with stabled horses as well as horses with minimal exercise may be at a disadvantage for optimal protein utilization.

Nutrient requirements for growing horses less than 4 months of age and greater than 18 months of age have received very little attention in published research. Studies involving horses less than 4 months of age have reported ADG between 0.86 and 1.57 kg/d feeding between 300 and 700 g CP/d (Lawrence et al., 1991; Cymbaluk et al., 1993; Breuer et al., 1996). These ADG fall into the normal growth curve reported in Chapter 1 for horses with an expected mature weight of 500 kg. Body weights were not always reported in the studies so it is not possible to express CP on a BW basis. Rations also varied from nursing foals receiving only milk for a period of time, foals nursing and receiving creep feed, and foals receiving milk replacer and creep feed, making it difficult to make comparisons. This is an area of research that needs to be addressed.

It is important that lysine amount to 4.3 percent of the CP requirement for growing horses. If protein sources in the ration do not provide this relationship between lysine and CP, the overall CP requirement of the animal may need to be increased compared to recommendations made here.

The protein requirements for growing horses can be calculated as follows:

CP requirement = (BW × 1.44 g CP/kg BW) plus ((ADG × 0.20)/E)/0.79

where E = efficiency of use of dietary protein, which is estimated to be 50 percent for horses 4–6 months of age, 45 percent for horses 7 and 8 months of age, 40 percent for horses 9 and 10 months of age, 35 percent for horses 11 months of age, and 30 percent for horses 12 months of age or older.

Lysine requirements can be calculated by multiplying the CP requirement by 4.3 percent.

PREGNANCY

Protein requirements for pregnant mares have received little attention. Pregnant mares fed 1.86 g CP/kg BW/d had no apparent ill effects (Boyer et al., 1999); however, pregnant mares that were fed < 2.0 g CP/kg BW/d (1,000 g CP/d for the 500-kg horse) lost weight and had a higher incidence of early fetal loss than mares fed ≥ 2.8 g CP/kg BW/d (1,400 g CP/d for the 500-kg horse). Digestibility of CP in van Nierkerk and van Nierkerk's 1997a study was approximately 80 percent, resulting in DP intakes of 1.6 and 2.2 g/kg BW/d for the apparently deficient and adequate groups mentioned previously. Mares fed the apparently deficient amount of dietary protein were slower to begin ovulating after the anovulatory period than mares fed higher amounts of dietary protein (van Niekerk and van Niekerk, 1997c).

The slow return to cycling in these mares is possibly due to low progesterone concentrations that were reported in all of the mares in the protein-deficient group. Progesterone is produced by the corpus luteum, which is critical to the maintenance of early pregnancy (van Niekerk and van Niekerk, 1998). Holtan and Hunt (1983) reported a positive linear relationship between dietary protein and progesterone concentrations. This study did not report intakes but fed CP concentrations of 8.6, 11.4, and 17.2 percent CP and found 6.5, 7.9, and 10.3 ng/ml progesterone, respectively. Pregnant mares generally have circulating progesterone concentrations of 7 to 10 ng/ml after day 60 of gestation (Terblanche and Maree, 1981). A study evaluating nitrogen balance in mares in early pregnancy reported mares in positive nitrogen balance with 1.86 g CP/kg BW/d (930 g CP/d for the 500-kg horse) (Boyer et al., 1999). This study also evaluated CP digestibility and determined it to be only 51.7 percent for the all-forage diet, which equates to a DP amount of only 950 mg DP/kg BW/d for these mares in early to mid-gestation (4.5–9 months of pregnancy). Boyer et al. (1999) concluded that approximately 1,100 g CP/d for mares in early pregnancy to be appropriate. However, an amount of protein intake that created negative nitrogen balance was not evaluated. The lower amount of acceptable protein intake for mares in early to mid-gestation has not been investigated thoroughly. In the study by van Niekerk and van Niekerk (1997a) the CP:DE ratio was < 35 in mares that lost weight and had higher incidence of fetal loss compared to the other groups with (CP:DE) ratios ≥ 38. The study by Boyer et al. (1999) had a CP:DE ratio of 40. It can be concluded that feeding mares in early to mid-gestation at an average maintenance level of protein intake (1.26 g CP/kg BW/d) is adequate, but more research needs to be done to determine more precisely the needs of the mare in early to mid-pregnancy. Therefore, the equation to determine CP requirements for pregnant mares from conception through the 4th month of gestation is:

CP = BW × 1.26 g CP/kg BW/d

Studies utilizing in utero measurements as well as aborted fetuses have reported fetal weight gain in the third trimester to be related to gestational age (Y = –20.7 + 0.00067X^2, r^2 = 0.84, where Y = fetal body weight in kg and X = gestational age in days; Platt, 1984). Therefore, at the start of the last trimester (day 240), the fetus would be 17.9 kg, 28.1 kg at day 270, 39.6 kg at day 300, and 52.3 kg at day 330. Fetal birth weight is estimated to be approximately 9.7 percent of the mare's body weight. Therefore, this equation appears to work well for the 500-kg mare. The rates of growth estimated from the equation equate to approximately 0.38 kg of weight gain/d for the fetus. Fowden et al. (2000) used ponies in studies that reported fetal weights. Plotting linear regression of mean weights of fetuses of known gestational age results in a fetal growth equation of Y = 0.13x –

24.8 where Y = fetal weight in kg and x = gestational age in days ($r^2 = 0.98$). From this equation, at the start of the last trimester (day 240), the fetus would be 7.2 kg, 10.3 kg at day 270, 14.2 kg at day 300, and 18.1 kg at day 330. This equation would presumably work well for the 200-kg pony. The rate of gain in the fetus from these data is 0.13 kg of weight gain/d. Meyer (1983a) reported that newborn foals were 17.1 percent CP. If the neonatal foal is also similar in composition in utero, this would equate into 65 g CP deposited per day in the horse mare and 22.5 g CP deposited per day in the pony mare. This does not take into account other protein needs of the uterus. Using only fetal protein deposition and the 50 percent efficiency of use of protein in pregnancy for fetal growth estimated by Meyer (1983a) results in an additional need of 130 g CP/d and 45 g CP/d over maintenance for fetal growth in the horse and pony, respectively. Using a digestibility of 79 percent, in order to provide 130 g and 45 g of protein for fetal growth, an additional 165 g and 57 g of CP must be provided in the diet for horses (500kg) and ponies (200kg), respectively. Bell et al. (1995) determined body composition of calves of known gestational age. Nonlinear regression was applied, and an equation estimated total fetal and uterine protein deposition. Fetal protein deposition was much higher for calves than that estimated by Platt's (1984) equation and Meyer's (1983a) estimation of fetal protein composition for horses. The difference between fetal protein deposition and total uterine protein deposition (assumed to be placental protein need), however, was approximately 20 g CP/d. Using 50 percent efficiency, this adds 40 g CP/d to the mare's need during mid- to late pregnancy. Therefore, the 500-kg mare would need 802, 845, and 863 g CP for the 9th, 10th, and 11th month of pregnancy, respectively. Using the available data, a growth curve for the fetus was derived for the 5th through 11th months of gestation. Based on estimated protein composition of the fetus, as well as the rate of fetal gain, estimates of protein needs above maintenance were made with an allowance for placental and uterine protein needs included.

The difficulty in determining dietary protein needs of the pregnant mare is that the mare readily utilizes body reserves to support the fetus. Meyer (1996) speculated that the pregnant mare adjusts for marginal energy, protein, and mineral deficiencies by mobilizing body reserves and prolonging gestation time. Kowalski et al. (1990) weighed 10 pregnant Thoroughbred mares every 14 days for the last 3 months of gestation. The diets provided 23 Mcal DE/d and the mares averaged a body condition score of 6. There were no significant weight gains in the last 3 months of pregnancy, leading the authors to conclude that the mares used body reserves to support the pregnancy. Lawrence et al. (1992) also found no significant weight gains for mares in the last trimester. In this study, mares were evaluated throughout pregnancy, and it was determined that the significant increase in weight gain actually occurred in the second trimester of pregnancy rather than the third. All mares delivered normal size foals, adding support to the hypothesis that mares may store reserves during the earlier stages of pregnancy and mobilize reserves in the last trimester.

The amino acid requirements of the pregnant mare have not been addressed. Van Niekerk and van Niekerk (1997b) reported lower fetal loss during pregnancy in mares fed ≥ 110 mg lysine/kg BW/d. No other information regarding lysine needs of the pregnant mare is available at this time to the best of the available knowledge. Without any available data regarding the amino acid needs of the pregnant mare, the lysine requirement for pregnancy will be estimated to be 4.3 percent of the CP requirement. Therefore, the lysine requirement for pregnancy can be calculated by multiplying the CP requirement by 4.3 percent. Protein sources should be of high quality and allow the CP relationship with lysine to have lysine at 4.3 percent of the CP. If this is not achieved because of lower-quality protein sources, the CP requirement may need to be increased.

The protein requirements for pregnancy can be estimated as follows:

Early pregnancy (conception through the 4th month):
Protein requirements = BW × 1.26 g CP/kg BW/d

Pregnancy from the 5th month through parturition:
Protein requirements = BW × 1.26 g CP/kg BW/d
plus ((fetal gain in kg/0.5)/0.79

where 0.5 represents the efficiency factor and 0.79 represents the digestibility of the protein. The lysine requirement can be calculated by multiplying the CP requirement by 4.3 percent.

LACTATION

Lactating mares fed < 2.8 g CP/kg BW/d lost weight and produced less milk than mares fed at least 3.2 g CP/kg BW/d. Foals also gained more weight in this study when mares were fed at least 3.2 g CP/kg BW/d (van Niekerk and van Niekerk, 1997b). In Martin et al. (1991) mares fed only 1.26 g CP/kg BW/d lost weight. Despite increasing the CP via urea supplementation to an amount of 2 g CP/kg BW/d, the mares still lost weight. Milk production in this study was reduced; foals had slower growth and higher plasma urea nitrogen concentrations. Mares in the study had higher plasma urea nitrogen concentrations as well when fed urea. This suggests that urea is not appropriate for lactating mares and only high-quality protein should be fed (Martin et al., 1991). Jordan (1983) reported that lactating mares fed < 3 g CP/kg BW lost weight. Inclusion of SBM as the protein source in the diet reduced the daily weight loss compared to diets without SBM, but did not prevent weight loss until CP intake reached an amount of 3 g /kg BW/d. Foal ADG did not differ among any of the groups, suggesting milk production and composition were not affected by the apparent lack of dietary protein. This suggests the mare readily utilizes body reserves during lactation.

The amount of milk production by mares has been documented in several studies and reported to vary between 1.9–3.9 percent of the mare's body weight throughout lactation (up to 6 months). The same studies reported a very consistent protein content of milk: from 3.1 to 3.3 percent in early lactation (generally colostrums) and gradually declining to 1.6 to 1.9 percent in later lactation (Doreau et al., 1986, 1990; Smolders et al., 1990; Martin et al., 1992; Mariani et al., 2001). Broken-line analysis of means from these studies produced a linear decline in CP content of milk from day 1 to day 22 of lactation and then the concentration of crude protein in milk reached a plateau at 1.96 percent. Dietary protein intake in these studies was not determined to affect milk production or crude protein composition of milk. One exception reported that mares fed supplemental SBM (diet provided 1,674 g CP/d) compared to mares fed a diet without supplemental SBM (diet provided 1,568 g CP/d) had higher concentrations of amino acids in milk, with the exception of cysteine. The amino acid profile as expressed as a percent of milk protein was not different, however. The foals nursing these mares had higher withers height consistently throughout the study, suggesting the protein quantity and/or quality was better for their growth (Glade and Luba, 1990).

Lactating mares fed diets containing 129 g CP/kg DM or 142 g CP/kg DM (from SBM) produced between 2.6 to 3.9 percent BW in milk/d between weeks 1 and 8 of lactation. Based on the overall intake of CP, between 126 to 150 g CP was needed per kg milk produced in the first week of lactation. This declined to 110 to 120 g CP/kg milk in week 8 of lactation (Doreau et al., 1992). Using these values, a 500-kg mare producing 3.2 percent of her BW (16 kg/d) would need 2,400 g CP/d in early lactation and 1,920 g CP/d in late lactation to support this amount of production. This is much higher than other estimates. Doreau et al. (1992) calculated the daily output of CP from this study to be an average of 590 g, based on milk production at 3.2 percent of the mare's body weight. Adding this amount of protein, adjusting for 50 percent efficiency of use, to the assumed maintenance need of the mare would result in a requirement of 1,587 g CP/d. Average milk production, from the previous studies mentioned, was 3, 2.9, 2.8, 2, and 1.9 percent of the mare's BW between 1 and 5 months of lactation, respectively. Linear regression of means from studies reporting milk CP concentrations prior to day 22 of lactation determined that the percent of CP in milk can be calculated from the equation Y = 3.43 − 0.066x where Y = CP percent of milk and x = days in milk (r^2 = 0.7). After day 22, milk protein concentration seems to plateau at approximately 1.96 percent CP. In general, the mare requires between 20 and 34 g CP/kg milk/d in the first month of lactation and approximately 20 g CP/kg milk produced/d for the remainder of lactation. Adjusting for efficiency of utilization (assumed to be 50 percent), an additional 40 to 68 g DP/kg milk must be provided above maintenance during the first month of lactation and approximately 40 additional g of DP/kg milk must be provided above maintenance in later lactation. Using a digestibility of 79 percent results in 51 to 86 g CP/kg milk during the first month of lactation, and 51 g CP/kg milk thereafter above maintenance needs of the mare (presumably elevated maintenance). The equation to determine the CP requirements for lactation is BW × 1.44 g CP/kg BW/d plus milk production (kg/d) × 50 g CP/kg milk.

Wickens et al. (2002) estimated requirements for amino acids during lactation based on the ratios of amino acids to lysine in milk. Assuming an average lysine content of 1.7 g/kg milk and 65 percent utilization efficiency, a dietary lysine requirement was estimated to be 2.62 g digestible lysine/kg milk. If a 500-kg mare produces an average of 3.2 percent of her body weight in milk/d, she will require 41.9 g of digestible lysine per day above maintenance. The estimated amino acid requirements based on the amino acid profile of milk and the lysine requirement are as follows (grams of digestible amino acids/kg milk): arginine, 1.81; histidine, 0.86; isoleucine, 2.04; leucine, 3.85; lysine, 2.62; methionine, 0.84; phenylalanine, 1.39; threonine, 1.88; valine, 2.54.

Lysine requirements for lactation are estimated by the equation: kg milk/d × 3.3 g lysine per kg milk plus the maintenance requirement for lysine. Based on the amount of lysine needed during lactation, it is important that high-quality protein sources be fed to lactating mares. If poor-quality protein sources are utilized and the same CP:lysine relationship is not achieved as recommended here, CP requirements may need to be increased.

The protein requirements for lactation can be calculated as follows:

CP requirement = BW × 1.44 g CP/kg BW/d
plus milk production (kg/d) × 50 g CP/kg milk

Lysine needs can be calculated by multiplying milk production (kg/d) by 3.3 g lysine per kg milk in addition to the maintenance requirement for lysine.

EXERCISE

There is some evidence that the exercising horse requires additional protein per kilogram of body weight for developing muscle and repair of damaged muscle. The increased protein need is typically achieved by an increase in DM intake to increase energy intake. However, with an increase in use of higher fat feeds, the increase in energy intake will not always result in a concurrent increase in protein intake. Therefore, attention needs to be paid to amounts of protein consumed.

Freeman et al. (1988) reported an increase in nitrogen retention for exercising horses as exercise load increased. The increase in nitrogen retention was still evident after exercise had ceased during a deconditioning period, which suggests additional protein was needed for developing muscle mass and repairing tissues. Horses retained an additional 0.37 g CP/kg BW/d during exercise compared to rest periods. Working backwards using a 50 percent efficiency of use of the available protein equates into a predicted additional need of 0.74 g CP/kg BW for exercising horses over maintenance. For the 500-kg horse, this would be 370 g CP in addition to maintenance; however, this study did not account for nitrogen lost in sweat. Estimating the amount of protein lost in sweat in this study accounts for 0.23 g of CP/kg BW out of the additional 0.37 g CP/kg that was apparently retained. This leaves 0.14 g CP/kg BW unaccounted for in nitrogen losses and may represent the additional protein need over maintenance for exercising horses. Freeman et al. (1986) reported an increase in RNA concentration in biceps fermoris muscle biopsies for horses in a conditioning program. An increase in RNA concentration has been reported in hypertrophied muscle in other species. This evidence in combination with a decrease in body fat without a decrease in BW suggests a gain in muscle and likely an increase in protein needs to support the muscle gain.

Wickens et al. (2003) fed exercising horses (moderate intensity) various amounts of dietary protein (677 g/d, 790 g/d, 903 g/d, 1,016 g/d, and 1,129 g/d). Nitrogen retention was maximized when horses were fed the diet providing 1,016 g CP/d compared to the diet providing 903 g CP/d and the diet providing 1,129 g CP/d. The data from these studies result in a recommendation of 1.9 to 2.1 g CP/kg BW/d for moderately exercised horses. If 79 percent digestibility is assumed, this equates to 1.5 to 1.66 g DP/kg BW/d. For the 500-kg horse, this would result in a requirement of 950 to 1,050 g CP/d or a digestible protein need of 750 to 830 g DP/d. Wickens et al. (2005) used 3-methylhistidine (3MH) to estimate protein requirements for exercising horses by evaluating the breakpoint at which 3MH concentrations were minimized for horses fed various amounts of dietary protein. Muscle protein turnover can be estimated using 3MH. The 3MH method has limitations, particularly the fact that it measures muscle protein turnover and not whole body protein turnover. However, the amount of muscle protein in the body far exceeds that of other proteins in the body. These data predicted a crude protein requirement of 954 g/d (95 percent confidence interval: 823 to 1,085 g CP/d), which would equate to 1.9 g CP/kg BW/d or a range of 1.65 to 2.2 g CP/kg BW/d. These three studies (Freeman et al., 1986; Wickens et al., 2003; Wickens et al., 2005) are in close agreement with each other.

Other researchers have reported much lower CP needs for exercising horses. Patterson et al. (1985) determined mature horses at three different work intensities required about 410 mg DP/kg BW/d (260 g CP for a 500-kg horse). Orton et al. (1985) reported improved utilization of dietary protein when horses were exercised. Two-year-olds fed 1.2 g DP/kg BW/d had similar ADG to those fed 2.4 g DP/kg BW/d provided they were exercised. Those 2-year-olds fed similar amounts of protein (but did not receive exercise) did not achieve similar ADGs compared to those fed higher protein amounts. Interestingly, linear regression of means from studies (N = 5) utilizing exercising horses that provided information to calculate nitrogen balance finds zero nitrogen balance to be at 0.813 g CP/kg BW/d, which is exactly the same as zero nitrogen balance for horses at maintenance.

One source of nitrogen loss for the exercising horse, which has rarely been quantified, is nitrogen lost in sweat. Freeman et al. (1986) reported that water turnover rate increased in conditioning horses but urine output did not account for the losses, inferring that sweat losses increase greatly with intense exercise. Hodgson et al. (1993) estimated sweat loss at 10–12 L per hour. McCutcheon and Geor (1996) reported losses of approximately 1 percent of pre-exercise BW in training (50–60 percent of maximum volume of oxygen [VO_2max]) up to a loss of 2.6 percent of pre-exercise BW during a standard exercise test (SET) that approached 100 percent VO_2max. Sweat contains between 1–1.5 g of N/kg sweat (Meyer, 1987). Sweat loss is generally correlated to increases in activity, and losses have been estimated to be as high as 5 kg/100 kg BW during intense exercise (Meyer, 1987). This equates to approximately 38 g of N or 238 g CP for the 500-kg horse.

The protein requirement for the exercising horse is therefore based on the fact that additional muscle appears to be gained during conditioning and that nitrogen is lost in sweat. An additional need above maintenance is assumed with an adjustment for sweat loss added based on intensity of exercise. The additional protein needed for muscle can be calculated by:

Light exercise: BW × 0.089 g CP/kg BW/d

Moderate exercise: BW × 0.177 g CP/kg BW/d

Heavy exercise: BW × 0.266 g CP/kg BW/d

Very heavy exercise: BW × 0.354 g CP/kg BW/d

If sweat loss is estimated to be 0.25, 0.5, 1, and 2 percent of pre-exercise BW for light, moderate, heavy, and very heavy exercise, nitrogen loss would be 1.56, 3.13, 6.25, and 12.5 g, respectively, and equate to 9.75, 19.6, 39.1, and 78.1 g CP for the 500-kg horse. If a 50 percent efficiency of use is assumed for dietary CP to replace these losses (and assuming 79 percent digestibility of the dietary protein), the 500-kg exercising horse would need 24.7, 49.6, 99, and 197.7 g CP to replace nitrogen lost in sweat during light, moderate, heavy, and very heavy exercise, respectively. The adjustment for CP needed to replace nitrogen lost in sweat should be added to the additional need for CP for muscle development and the horse's maintenance requirement.

Plasma concentrations of branched-chain amino acids (BCAA; valine, leucine, and isoleucine) increase during exercise (Miller-Graber et al., 1990; Pösö et al., 1991; Assenza et al., 2004). These amino acids are oxidized for energy during exercise in the muscle. Trottier et al. (2002) reported decreases in plasma BCAA following exercise and during recovery. Reports on muscle BCAA are contradictory: Trottier et al. (2002) reported no change in muscle BCAA after exercise, whereas Essén-Gustavsson and Jensen-Waern (2002) reported an increase in BCAA following exercise. There have been a few studies trying to demonstrate a benefit (such as decreased lactate) with BCAA supplementation for exercise, but results have been inconclusive or flawed in their design (Glade, 1991; Casini et al., 2000).

Several studies at the University of Illinois determined that there was no detrimental effect of high protein intakes (18.5 percent CP, > 1,700 g CP/d, 3.3 g CP/kg BW/d) on exercise performance, but did speculate that high protein intakes may reduce glycogen (and thus available fuel for exercise) and exceed the capacity of the urea cycle (Miller and Lawrence, 1988; Miller-Graber et al., 1991). Graham-Thiers et al. (1999, 2001) reported improved acid-base balance (higher blood pH and bicarbonate) during repeated sprints for horses fed lower CP (725 g/d, 1.45 g CP/kg BW/d) fortified with amino acids (lysine and threonine) compared to higher protein intakes (> 1,400 g CP/d, 2.8 g CP/kg BW/d). Combining this information with the fact that excess amino acids increase urea formation and water loss through urination (Meyer, 1987) may suggest that careful attention to dietary protein intake for exercising horses is needed. The concept of lowering the overall CP concentration with fortification (adding limiting amino acids) has been demonstrated to be successful with growing horses (Graham et al., 1994; Stanier et al., 2001) and with exercising horses (Graham-Thiers et al., 1999, 2001).

Concentrations of certain plasma amino acids were reported by McKeever et al. (1986) to decrease with horses in a conditioning program, suggesting that amino acid intake was inadequate for the demands from the body. These horses were fed > 1,500 g CP/d (alfalfa hay and milo). The amino acid profile and the digestibility of the diet apparently influenced the available amino acids (which seemed to be inadequate), despite presumably more than adequate amounts of CP (McKeever et al., 1986). In a study utilizing young and aged exercising horses (Graham-Thiers et al., 2005), dietary protein amounts were fed either to provide current recommendations of dietary CP or supplementary lysine and threonine at an amount recommended for growth in an effort to evaluate the horse's ability to build and maintain muscle mass. The study reported lower plasma urea nitrogen and 3MH concentrations, as well as greater plasma creatinine and subjective muscle mass scores for horses fed the amino acid fortified diets. The lysine intake of the control group was above the current recommendation for lysine for exercising horses (Graham-Thiers et al., 2005). This study suggests that the balance of amino acids was improved with supplementation and the requirements of amino acids for mature exercising horses are not well defined and require further research.

Using means from studies (N = 3) that reported diet and intake, lysine intake was calculated. Broken-line analysis of the means for lysine intake and nitrogen retention in exercising horses resulted in a recommendation of 0.068 g lysine/kg BW/d for the exercising horse. This would result in a recommended lysine intake of 34 g/d for the 500-kg horse. The horses in these studies participated in moderate to heavy exercise. Therefore, the requirement for lysine for the exercising horse in moderate to heavy exercise can be calculated from the equation: BW × 0.068 g/kg BW/d. With a CP requirement of 768 g CP/d for the 500-kg horse in moderate exercise, the lysine requirement of 34 g/d represents 4.3 percent of the CP requirement. Thus the lysine requirement for exercising horses can be calculated by multiplying the CP requirement by 4.3 percent. In order for lysine to be 4.3 percent of the CP in a ration, good-quality sources of protein must be used. If poor-quality sources of protein are incorporated in the horse's ration, lysine needs may not be met and CP requirements may need to be increased compared to those recommended in this discussion.

Protein requirements for exercising horses can be calculated by the following equation:

$$BW \times MG \text{ plus } ((BW \times SL \times 7.8 \text{ g/kg})/0.50)/0.79,$$
plus the maintenance requirement for protein

where MG = muscle gain and SL = sweat loss. Muscle gain is estimated to be 0.089 g CP/kg BW for light exercise, 0.177 g CP/kg BW for moderate exercise, 0.266 g CP/kg BW for heavy exercise, and 0.354 g CP/kg BW for very heavy exercise. Sweat loss is estimated to be 0.25, 0.50, 1, and 2 percent of BW for light, moderate, heavy, and very heavy exercise respectively. Lysine needs can be calculated by multiplying the CP requirement by 4.3 percent.

IDEAL PROTEIN

Protein quality has been mentioned in this discussion several times and should be of concern with the horse's sensitivity to amino acid profiles in the diet. The concept of ideal protein is used in feeding swine and poultry. Ideal protein is based on formulating a diet with amino acids, not just in the correct amounts, but also in the proper ratios to one another. Ideal protein is defined as a protein that includes the minimum quantity of each essential amino acid compatible with maximum utilization of the protein as a whole. The estimation of ideal protein in swine is based on results from experiments involving the removal of a single amino acid at a time from a casein diet and measuring nitrogen balance. The assumption is that the removal of the most limiting amino acid results in the greatest reduction in nitrogen balance. There is also the assumption that ideal protein would closely resemble the amino acid profile of the likely end product of amino acid use in the body—largely muscle tissue. The ratios for ideal protein for growth in swine are in close agreement with the ratios of amino acids in swine muscle tissue. Ideal protein ratios are normally established by comparing all other essential amino acids to lysine. In this approach, lysine is assigned a value of 100.

Specific studies in horses have not been done to evaluate ideal protein by removal of amino acids from the diet; however, ideal protein for horses may be able to be estimated from the ratios of amino acids in muscle of the horse. With that in mind, the ratios of amino acids in muscle of the horse are: lysine, 100; methionine, 27; threonine, 61; isoleucine, 55; leucine, 107; histidine, 58; phenylalanine, 60; valine, 62; and arginine, 76; with no information available for tryptophan (Bryden, 1991). With this information and the assumption that ideal protein in the diet should reflect muscle tissue amino acid profiles, the formulation of the diet can attempt to achieve these ratios. Also, since the ratios are based on lysine and the lysine requirement has been determined for the growing horse, estimates of the requirements for the other amino acids can be made.

It would also seem logical that the amino acid profile and corresponding ratios to lysine found in milk would correspond reasonably well to the dietary amino acid needs of growth in the foal. Several studies have evaluated amino acid composition of a mare's milk. The ratios of the amino acids in milk relative to lysine (set to 100) are as follows: arginine, 70 to 82; histidine, 29 to 37; isoleucine, 53 to 79; leucine, 127 to 147 methionine, 29 to 35; phenylalanine, 53 to 59; threonine, 53 to 68; and valine, 64 to 97. These ratios are in close agreement with the ratios in muscle with the exceptions of histidine, leucine, and valine (Davis et al., 1994; Doreau et al., 1990; Wickens et al., 2002; Stamper et al., 2005). Stamper et al. (2005) used these ratios to evaluate foal milk replacer and reported arginine, isoleucine, and leucine lower in relation to lysine than in mare's milk. This information may help to improve formulation of milk replacers in the future.

Synthetic amino acids such as lysine and threonine have been utilized in rations of growing horses (Ott et al., 1979; Graham et al., 1994; Stanier et al., 2001) and exercising horses (Graham-Thiers et al., 2001, 2003, 2005) as a means to improve protein quality in the ration. It should be noted that the addition of synthetic amino acids to rations alters the balance of amino acids. The balance created by supplementation may or may not lend itself to the concept of ideal protein.

PROTEIN DEFICIENCY

Reduced intake of protein results in decreased growth in horses despite adequate energy; however, energy is normally the first limiter for growth (Ott and Asquith, 1986; Stanier et al., 2001). As discussed earlier, a protein deficiency results in weight loss in adult horses, fetal loss in pregnant mares, and decreases in milk production in lactating mares. In exercising horses, a lack of protein will result in a loss of muscle as would also be seen in sedentary adult horses. Other indicators of protein deficiency include reduced feed intake, poor hair growth, and reduced hoof growth (NRC, 1989).

PROTEIN EXCESS

Not much evidence exists concerning the effect of excess protein consumption. Meyer (1987) pointed out that excess protein is degraded and results in an increase in urea, which will be excreted in the urine. This will increase water loss from the body and may increase the water need of the horse. One study reported a growth reduction when protein was fed at 5.45 g CP/kg BW/d (Yoakam et al., 1978). More recently, higher protein intakes in exercising horses resulted in lower blood pH at rest and during sprinting exercise. Therefore, protein in excess may interfere with acid-base balance during exercise (Graham-Thiers et al., 1999, 2001). An increase in calcium loss with high protein intakes has been reported in other species. Glade et al. (1985) reported an increased calcium and phosphorus loss when weanling horses were fed > 1,000 g CP/d. Other studies have not supported these conclusions. The effect of high protein intakes on calcium balance needs further investigation. This, along with other reasons to avoid excess protein, should be considered. Unlike many other species, longevity is a concern for horses and skeletal development in the young horse (which is affected by calcium balance) is crucial to its usefulness.

Concern for the environment has grown in recent years and led to regulations regarding waste management in cattle and swine. One of the concerns is nitrogen excretion from the animal due to excess protein in the diet. Lawrence et al. (2003) reviewed studies reporting nitrogen excretion in sedentary and exercising horses. Regression analysis determined, on average, horses excreted (via manure and urine) 89 g N/d at rest and 99 g N/d if the horses were exercising.

SUMMARY—FEEDING PROTEIN

Total tract and precaecal digestibility vary with protein source and protein concentration in the diet. It is important to consider the amino acid profile and precaecal digestibility of feedstuffs in addition to total crude protein, especially in rations fed to growing horses and those in high states of production.

Several factors can affect amino acid digestion in horses. As summarized by Gibbs and Potter (2002), these include site of digestion, feedstuff variation, biological value of protein, protein intake, amount consumed, and transit time through the digestive tract. In addition to emphasizing the need to evaluate amino acid content and availability in growing horse rations, Gibbs and Potter (2002), using results from several trials, provided supportive evidence of the need to supply amino acids in smaller, more frequent meals per day as compared to twice-daily feedings of rapidly growing horses.

Rations should be evaluated for amino acid content and availability, especially for those fed to growing horses and those in states of production. If using low-quality protein roughages, growing horses and lactating mare diets should be formulated so that 60 percent or more of the total protein is supplied by a high-quality protein supplement. Splitting high-protein rations meal fed to growing horses into three or more feedings per day may enhance amino acid absorption in the small intestine, although more research is necessary to more accurately define influences of diet, individual horses, and feeding schedules.

REFERENCES

Assenza, A., D. Bergero, M. Tarantola, G. Piccione, and G. Caola. 2004. Blood serum branched chain amino acids and tryptophan modifications in horses competing in long distance rides of different length. J. Anim. Physiol. Anim. Nutr. 88:172–177.

Bell, A. W., R. Slepetis, and R. A. Ehrhardt. 1995. Growth and accretion of energy and protein in the gravid uterus during late pregnancy in Holstein cows. J. Dairy Sci. 78:1954–1961.

Borton, A., D. R. Anderson, and S. Lyford. 1973. Studies of protein quality and quantity in the early weaned foal. P. 19 in Proc. 3rd Equine Nutr. Physiol. Soc. Symp., Gainesville, FL.

Boyer, J., N. Cymbaluk, B. Kyle, D. Brown, and H. Hintz. 1999. Nitrogen metabolism in pregnant mares fed grass hays containing different concentrations of protein. J. Anim. Sci. 77(Suppl. 1):202.

Breuer, L. H., and D. L. Golden. 1971. Lysine requirement of the immature equine. J. Anim. Sci. 33:227.

Breuer, L. H., R. A. Zimmerman, and J. D. Pagan. 1996. Effect of supplemental energy intake on growth of suckling quarter horse foals. Pferdeheilkunde 12:249–250.

Bryden, W. L. 1991. Amino acid requirements of horses estimated from tissue composition. P. 53 in Proc. Nutr. Soc. Aust. Kent Town, S. Australia.

Casini, L., D. Gatta, L. Magni, and B. Colombani. 2000. Effect of prolonged branched-chain amino acid supplementation on metabolic response to anaerobic exercise in Standardbreds. J. Equine Vet. Sci. 20:1–7.

Crozier, J. A., V. G. Allen, N. E. Jack, J. P. Fontenot, and M. A. Cochran. 1997. Digestibility, apparent mineral absorption, and voluntary intake by horses fed alfalfa, tall fescue, and Caucasian bluestem. J. Anim. Sci. 75:1651–1658.

Cymbaluk, N. F. 1990. Using canola meal in growing horse diets. Equine Pract. 12:13–19.

Cymbaluk, N. F., M. E. Smart, F. M. Bristol, and V. A. Pouteaux. 1993. Importance of milk replacer intake and composition in rearing orphan foals. Can. Vet. J. 34:479–486.

Davis, T. A., H. V. Nguyen, R. Garcia-Bravo, M. L. Fiorotto, E. M. Jackson, and P. J. Reeds. 1994. Amino acid composition of the milk of some mammalian species changes with stage of lactation. Br. J. Nutr. 72:845–853.

de Almeida, F. Q., S. de Campos Valdares Filo, J. L. Donzele, J. F. C. da Silva, M. I. Leao, P. R. Cecon, and C. de Queiroz. 1998a. Apparent and true prececal and total digestibility of protein in diets with different protein levels in equines. R. Bras. Zootec. 27:521–529.

de Almeida, F. Q., S. de Campos Valdares Filo, J. L. Donzele, J. F. C. da Silva, M. I. Leao, P. R. Cecon, and C. de Queiroz. 1998b. Endogenous amino acid composition and true prececal apparent and true digestibility of amino acids in diets for equines. R. Bras. Zootec. 27:546–555.

Doreau, M., S. Boulot, W. Martin-Rosset, and J. Robelin. 1986. Relationship between nutrient intake, growth and body composition of the nursing foal. Reprod. Nutr. Dev. 26:683–690.

Doreau, M., S. Boulot, J. P. Barlet, and P. Patureau-Mirand. 1990. Yield and composition of milk from lactating mares: effect of lactation stage and individual differences. J. Dairy Res. 57:449–454.

Doreau, M., S. Boulot, D. Bauchart, J. P. Barlet, and W. Martin-Rosset. 1992. Voluntary intake, milk production and plasma metabolites in nursing mares fed two different diets. J. Nutr. 122:992–999.

Dubose, E. 1983. Utilization of urea and lysine diets for growth by young equines. P. 107 in Proc. 8th Equine Nutr. Physiol. Soc. Symp., Lexington, KY.

Essén-Gustavsson, B., and M. Jensen-Waern. 2002. Effect of an endurance race on muscle amino acids, pro- and macroglycogen and triglycerides. Equine Vet. J. Suppl. 34:209–213.

Farley, E. B., G. D. Potter, P. G. Gibbs, J. Schumacher, and M. Murray-Gerzik. 1995. Digestion of soybean meal protein in the equine small and large intestine at varying levels of intake. J. Equine Vet. Sci. 15:391–397.

Fowden, A. L., P. M. Taylor, K. L. White, and A. J. Forhead. 2000. Ontogenic and nutritionally induced changes in fetal metabolism in the horse. J. Physiol. 528:209–219.

Freeman, D. W., G. D. Potter, G. T. Schelling, and J. L. Kreider. 1986. Nitrogen metabolism in the mature physically conditioned horse I. Response to conditioning. Equine Pract. 8(5):6–9.

Freeman, D. W., G. D. Potter, G. T. Schelling, and J. L. Kreider. 1988. Nitrogen metabolism in mature horses at varying levels of work. J. Anim. Sci. 66:407–412.

Gibbs, P. G., and G. D. Potter. 2002. Concepts in protein digestion and amino acid requirements of young horses. Prof. Anim. Scientist 18:295–301.

Gibbs, P. G., G. D. Potter, G. T. Schelling, and C. J. Boyd. 1988. Digestion of hay protein in different segments of the equine digestive tract. J. Anim. Sci. 66:400–406.

Gibbs, P. G., G. D. Potter, G. T. Schelling, J. L. Kreider, and C. J. Boyd. 1996. The significance of small vs large intestinal digestion of cereal grain and oilseed protein in the equine. J. Equine Vet. Sci. 16:60–65.

Glade, M. J. 1991. Timed administration of leucine, isoleucine, valine, glutamine and carnitine to enhance athletic performance. Equine Athlete 4:7–10.

Glade, M. J., and N. K. Luba. 1990. Benefits to foals of feeding soybean meal to lactating broodmares. J. Equine Vet. Sci. 10:422–428.

Glade, M. J., D. Beller, J. Bergen, D. Berry, E. Blonder, J. Bradley, M. Cupelo, and J. Dallas. 1985. Dietary protein in excess of requirements inhibits renal calcium and phosphorus reabsorption in young horses. Nutr. Rep. Int. 31:649–659.

Godbee, R. G., and L. M. Slade. 1981. The effect of urea or soybean meal on the growth and protein status of young horses. J. Anim. Sci. 53:670–676.

Graham, P. M., E. A. Ott, J. H. Brendemuhl, and S. H. TenBroeck. 1994. The effect of supplemental lysine and threonine on growth and development of yearling horses. J. Anim. Sci. 72:380–386.

Graham-Thiers, P. M., D. S. Kronfeld, and K. A. Kline. 1999. Dietary protein moderates acid-base responses to repeated sprints. Equine Vet. J. Suppl. 30:463–467.

Graham-Thiers, P. M., D. S. Kronfeld, K. A. Kline, and D. J. Sklan. 2001. Dietary protein restriction and fat supplementation diminish the acidogenic effect of exercise during repeated sprints in horses. J. Nutr. 131:1959–1964.

Graham-Thiers, P. M., D. S. Kronfeld, C. Hatsell, K. Stevens, and K. McCreight. 2003. Amino acid supplementation improves muscle mass in aged horses. P. 134 in Proc. 18th Equine Nutr. Physiol. Soc. Symp., East Lansing, MI.

Graham-Thiers, P. M., D. S. Kronfeld, C. Hatsell, K. Stevens, and K. McCreight. 2005. Amino acid supplementation improves muscle mass in aged and young horses. J. Anim. Sci. 83:2783–2788.

Harper, O. F., and G. W. Vander Noot. 1974. Protein requirements of mature maintenance horses. J. Anim. Sci. 62:183 (abstr.).

Hintz, H. F., and H. F. Schryver. 1972. Nitrogen utilization in ponies. J. Anim. Sci. 34:592–595.

Hintz, H. F., J. E. Lowe, A. J. Clifford, and W. J. Visek. 1970. Ammonia intoxication resulting from urea ingestion by ponies. J. Am. Vet. Med. Assoc. 157:963–966.

Hintz, H. F., H. F. Schryver, and J. E. Lowe. 1971. Comparison of a blend of milk products and linseed meal as protein supplements for young growing horses. J. Anim. Sci. 33:1274–1276.

Hodgson, D. R., L. J. McCutcheon, S. K. Byrd, W. S. Brown, W. M. Bayly, G. L. Brengelmann, and P. D. Gollnick. 1993. Dissipation of metabolic heat in the horse during exercise. J. Appl. Physiol. 74:1161–1170.

Holtan, D.W., and J. D. Hunt. 1983. Effect of dietary protein on reproduction in mares. Pp.107–112 in Proc. 8th Equine Nutr. Physiol. Soc. Symp., Lexington, KY.

Jordan, R. M. 1983. Effect of energy and crude protein intake on lactating pony mares. Pp. 90–94 in Proc. 8th Equine Nutr. Physiol. Soc. Symp., Lexington, KY.

Jordan, R. M., and V. Myers. 1972. Effects of protein levels on the growth of weanling and yearling ponies. J. Anim. Sci. 34:578–581.

Kowalski, J., J. Williams, and H. Hintz. 1990. Weight gains of mares during the last trimester of gestation. Equine Pract. 12:6–10.

LaCasha, P. A., H. A. Brady, V. G. Allen, C. R. Richardson, and K. R. Pond. 1999. Voluntary intake, digestibility, and subsequent selection of Matua bromegrass, coastal bermudagrass, and alfalfa hays by yearling horses. J. Anim. Sci. 77:2766–2773.

Lawrence, L. M., M. Murphy, K. Bump, D. Weston, and J. Key. 1991. Growth responses in hand-reared and naturally reared Quarter Horse foals. Equine Pract. 13:19–26.

Lawrence, L. M., J. DiPietro, K. Ewert, D. Parrett, L. Moser, and D. Powell. 1992. Changes in body weight and condition of gestating mares. J. Equine Vet. Sci. 12:355–358.

Lawrence, L., J. Bicudo, and E. Wheeler. 2003. Relationships between intake and excretion for nitrogen and phosphorus in horses. Pp. 306–307 in Proc. 18th Equine Nutr. Physiol. Soc. Symp., East Lansing, MI.

Mariani, P., A. Summer, F. Martuzzi, P. Formaggioni, A. Sabbioni, and A. L. Catalano. 2001. Physiochemical properties, gross composition, energy value and nitrogen fractions of Haflinger nursing mare milk throughout 6 lactation months. Anim. Res. 50:415–425.

Martin, R. G., N. P. McMeniman, and K. F. Dowsett. 1991. Effects of protein deficient diet and urea supplementation on lactating mares. J. Reprod. Fert. Suppl. 44:543–550.

Martin, R. G., N. P. McMeniman, and K. F. Dowsett. 1992. Milk and water intakes of foals sucking grazing mares. Equine Vet. J. 24(4):295–299.

Martin, R. G., N. P. McMeniman, B. W. Norton, and K. F. Dowsett. 1996. Utilization of endogenous and dietary urea in the large intestine of the mature horse. Br. J. Nutr. 76:373–386.

Martin-Rosset, W., M. Vermorel, M. Doreau, J. L. Tisserand, and J. Andrieu. 1994. French horse feed evaluation systems and recommended allowances for energy and protein. Livest. Prod. Sci. 40:37–56.

McCutcheon, L. J., and R. J. Geor. 1996. Sweat fluid and ion losses in horses during training and competition in cool vs. hot ambient conditions: implications for ion supplementation. Equine Vet. J. 22 (Suppl.):54–62.

McKeever, K. H., W. A. Schurg, S. H. Jarrett, and V. A. Convertino. 1986. Resting concentrations of the plasma free amino acids in horses following chronic submaximal exercise training. J. Equine Vet. Sci. 6:87–92.

Meyer, H. 1983a. Protein metabolism and protein requirement in horses. Pp. 343–364 in Proc. IVth Int. Sym. Protein Metabolism Nutr., Clermont-Ferrand, France.

Meyer, H. 1983b. Intestinal protein and N metabolism in the horse. Pp. 113–116 in Proc. Horse Nutr. Symp., Uppsala, Sweden.

Meyer, H. 1985. Investigations to determine endogenous faecal and renal N losses in horses. P. 68 in Proc. 9th Equine Nutr. Physiol. Soc. Symp., East Lansing, MI.

Meyer, H. 1987. Nutrition of the equine athlete. Pp. 644–673 in Equine Exercise Physiology 2, J. R. Gillespie and N. E. Robinson, eds. Davis, CA: ICEEP Publications.

Meyer, H. 1996. Influence of feed intake and composition, feed and water restriction, and exercise on gastrointestinal fill in horses. Equine Pract. 18:20–23.

Miller, P. A., and L. A. Lawrence. 1988. The effect of dietary protein level on exercising horses. J. Anim. Sci. 66:2185–2192.

Miller-Graber, P. A., L. M. Lawrence, E. V. Kurcz, R. Kane, K. D. Bump, M. G. Fisher, and J. Smith. 1990. The free amino acid profile in the middle gluteal muscle before and after fatiguing exercise in the horse. Equine Vet. J. 22:209–210.

Miller-Graber, P. A., L. A. Lawrence, J. H. Foreman, K. D. Bump, M. G. Fisher, and E. V. Kurcz. 1991. Dietary protein level and energy metabolism during treadmill exercise in horses. J. Nutr. 121:1462–1469.

NRC (National Research Council). 1989. Nutrient Requirements of Horses. 5th ed. Washington, DC: National Academy Press.

NRC. 1998. Nutrient Requirements of Swine, 10th ed. Washington, DC: National Academy Press.

Olsman, A. F. S., W. L. Jansen, M. M. Sloet van Oldruttenborgh-Oosterbaan, and A. C. Beynen. 2003. Assessment of the minimum protein requirement of adult ponies. J. Anim. Physiol. Anim. Nutr. 87:205–212.

Orton, R. K., I. D. Hume, and R. A. Leng. 1985. Effects of level of dietary protein and exercise on growth rates of horses. Equine Vet. J. 17:381–385.

Ott, E. A., and R. L. Asquith. 1986. Influence of level of feeding and nutrient content of the concentrate on growth and development of yearling horses. J. Anim. Sci. 62:290–299.

Ott, E. A., and J. Kivipelto. 2002. Growth and development of yearling horses fed either alfalfa or coastal bermudagrass: hay and a concentrate formulated for bermudagrass hay. J. Equine Vet. Sci. 22:311–319.

Ott, E. A., R. L. Asquith, J. P. Feaster, and F. G. Martin. 1979. Influence of protein level and quality on growth and development of yearling foals. J. Anim. Sci. 49:620–626.

Ott, E. A., R. L. Asquith, and J. P. Feaster. 1981. Lysine supplementation of diets for yearling horses. J. Anim. Sci. 53:1496–1503.

Patterson, P. H., C. N. Coon, and I. M. Hughes. 1985. Protein requirements of mature working horses. J. Anim. Sci. 61:187–196.

Platt, H. 1984. Growth of the equine foetus. Equine Vet. J. 16:247–252.

Pösö, A. R., B. Essén-Gustavsson, A. Lindholm, and S. G. Persson. 1991. Exercise-induced changes in muscle and plasma amino acid levels in the Standardbred horse. Equine Ex. Physiol. 3:202–208.

Potter, G. D., and J. D. Huchton. 1975. Growth of yearling horses fed different sources of protein with supplemental lysine. P. 19 in Proc. 4th Equine Nutr. Physiol. Soc. Symp., Pomona, CA.

Potter, G. D., P. G. Gibbs, R. G. Haley, and C. Klendshoj. 1992. Digestion of protein in the small and large intestines of equines fed mixed diets. Pferdeheikunde 1:140–143.

Pulse, J., P. Baker, G. D. Potter, and J. Williard. 1973. Dietary protein level and growth of immature horses. J. Anim. Sci. 37:289–290.

Reitnour, C. M., and R. L. Salsbury. 1972. Digestion and utilization of cecally infused protein by the equine. J. Anim. Sci. 35(6):1190–1193.

Reitnour, C. M., and R. L. Salsbury. 1975. Effect of oral or cecal administration of protein supplements on equine plasma amino acids. Br. Vet. J. 131:466–472.

Reitnour, C. M., and R. L. Salsbury. 1976. Utilization of proteins by the equine species. Am. J. Vet. Res. 37:1065–1067.

Reitnour, C. M., J. P. Baker, G. E. Mitchell, Jr., C. O. Little, and D. D. Kratzer. 1970. Amino acids in equine cecal contents, cecal bacteria and serum. J. Nutr. 100:349–354.

Saastamoinen, M. T., and E. Koskinen. 1993. Influence of quality of dietary protein supplement and anabolic steroids on muscular and skeletal growth of foals. Anim. Prod. 56:135–144.

Schryver, H. F., D. W. Meakim, J. E. Lowe, J. Williams, L. V. Solderholm, and H. F. Hintz. 1987. Growth and calcium metabolism in horses fed varying levels of protein. Equine Vet. J. 19:280–287.

Slade, L. M., D. W. Robinson, and K. E. Casey. 1970. Nitrogen metabolism in nonruminant herbivores. I. The influence of nonprotein nitrogen and protein quality on the nitrogen retention of adult mares. J. Anim. Sci. 30:753–760.

Smolders, E. A., N. G. Van Der Veen, and A. Polanen. 1990. Composition of horse milk during the suckling period. Livest. Prod. Sci. 25:163–171.

Stamper, T., J. Moore, T. Tier, B. Nielsen, and N. Trottier. 2005. An ideal protein for the Arabian foal: insight into protein formulation of foal milk replacer. P. 182 in Proc. 19th Equine Sci. Soc., Tucson, AZ.

Stanier, W. B., D. S. Kronfeld, J. A. Wilson, L. A. Lawrence, W. L. Cooper, and P. A. Harris. 2001. Growth of Thoroughbreds fed a low-protein supplement fortified with lysine and threonine. J. Anim. Sci. 79:2143–2151.

Sticker, L. S., D. L. Thompson, Jr., J. M. Fernandez, L. D. Bunting, and C. L. DePew. 1995. Dietary protein and(or) energy restriction in mares: plasma glucose, insulin, nonesterfied fatty acid, and urea nitrogen responses to feeding, glucose, and epinephrine. J. Anim. Sci. 73:136–144.

Terblanche, H. M., and L. Maree. 1981. Plasma progesterone levels in the mare during the oestrous cycle and pregnancy. J. S. Afr. Vet. Assoc. 52:181–185.

Trottier, N. L., B. D. Nielsen, K. J. Lang, P. K. Ku, and H. C. Schott. 2002. Equine endurance exercise alters serum branched-chain amino acid and alanine concentrations. Equine Vet. J. Suppl. 34:168–172.

van Niekerk, F. E., and C. H. van Niekerk. 1997a. The effect of dietary protein on reproduction in the mare: I. The composition and evaluation of digestibility of dietary protein from different sources. J. S. Afr. Vet. Assoc. 68:78–80.

van Niekerk, F. E., and C. H. van Niekerk. 1997b. The effect of dietary protein on reproduction in the mare: II. Growth of foals, body mass of mares and serum protein concentration of mares during the anovulatory, transitional and pregnant periods. J. S. Afr. Vet. Assoc. 68:81–85.

van Niekerk, F. E., and C. H. van Niekerk. 1997c. The effect of dietary protein on reproduction in the mare: III. Ovarian and uterine changes during the anovulatory, transitional and ovulatory periods in the nonpregnant mare. J. S. Afr. Vet. Assoc. 68:86–92.

van Niekerk, F. E., and C. H. van Niekerk 1998. The effect of dietary protein on reproduction in the mare: VII. Embryonic development, early embryonic death, foetal losses and their relationship with serum progestagen. J. S. Afr. Vet. Assoc. 69:150–155.

Wickens, C. L., P. K. Ku, and N. L. Trottier. 2002. An ideal protein for the lactating mare. J. Anim. Sci. (Suppl. 1):155.

Wickens, C. L., J. Moore, J. Shelle, C. Skelly, H. M. Clayton, and N. L. Trottier. 2003. Effect of exercise on dietary protein requirement of the Arabian horse. P. 128 in Proc. 18th Equine Nutr. Physiol. Soc. Symp., East Lansing, MI.

Wickens, C. L., J. Moore, C. Wolf, C. Skelly, and N. Trottier. 2005. 3-methylhistidine as a response criterium to estimate dietary protein requirement of the exercising horse. P. 205 in Proc. 19th Equine Sci. Soc., Tucson, AZ.

Wysocki, A. A., and J. P. Baker. 1975. Utilization of bacterial protein from the lower gut of the equine. P. 21 in Proc. 4th Equine Nutr. Physiol. Soc. Symp., Pomona, CA.

Yoakam, S. C., W. W. Kirkham, and W. M. Beeson. 1978. Effect of protein level on growth in young ponies. J. Anim. Sci. 46:983–991.

5

Minerals

INTRODUCTION

While constituting only a minor part of the equine diet by weight, minerals play a critical role in the health of horses. Minerals are involved in a number of functions in the body, including physiological roles such as in acid-base balance, formation of structural components, enzymatic cofactors, and energy transfer. Some minerals are integral parts of vitamins, hormones, and amino acids. The horse obtains most of the necessary minerals from forages and concentrates. The mineral content of feeds and the availability of minerals vary with soil mineral concentrations, plant species, stage of maturity, and conditions of harvesting. The resulting variations in feed mineral content should be considered in assessing an animal's mineral status and formulating appropriate diets, as minerals are elements that cannot be created or destroyed under normal circumstances and must be provided in the ration. Minerals are typically classified as macrominerals—those typically found and needed in concentrations in the diet measured in g/kg or percentage—and microminerals—those measured in ppm or mg/kg. While the amounts of individual minerals in the ration are important, the ratios of all minerals should be taken into consideration, as minerals often influence the absorption, metabolism, and/or excretion of other nutrients. Therefore, excesses or deficiencies of certain minerals can alter the requirements of others. When appropriate, the maximum tolerable concentration of a mineral is provided from the publication *Mineral Tolerance of Animals* (NRC, 2005). This concentration is defined as the dietary amount that, when fed for an extended period of time, will not impair animal health and performance. This differs from a toxic amount. Also, this tolerable concentration is based upon all other nutrients in the diet being at or near the animal's requirement. When other minerals are provided at higher or lower concentrations, absorption of the mineral in question can be altered, thus influencing the maximum tolerable concentration. To determine mineral requirements of horses, balance studies need to be conducted that compare the amount of mineral consumed by the animal to the amount of mineral lost in the feces and urine and determined via total collections of both feces and urine. Collecting the total amount of urine voided in a 24-hour period can be labor intensive. The use of a urinary fractional electrolyte excretion test (FE test) has been used, which requires collecting only a single urine sample. Unfortunately, fractional excretion values of minerals do not always agree with results obtained through total volumetric urinary collection, suggesting less accuracy (McKeever et al., 2002; McKenzie et al., 2003). Some minerals are present in such minute concentrations that determining requirements through balance studies is extremely difficult. Furthermore, mineral balance studies have not been done in all ages and classes of horses. In such cases, requirements are estimated by examining what amounts have been fed without negative effects being observed and, as a result, might be more appropriately termed "recommendations." Sulfur and many of the microminerals would fit this description. For minerals such as these, the research has tended to examine concentrations in the diet. Besides still being provided as a concentration, the committee has made a transformation, based on expected daily intakes, in an attempt to determine what would be a reasonable recommendation for a daily allotment on a body weight basis. The committee encourages researchers to report data from future studies on a body weight basis instead of simply as a dietary concentration to aid in determining actual requirements. The committee also encourages more studies aimed at determining mineral requirements for growth, exercise, and pregnancy, as these are areas in which data seemed to be insufficient to adequately determine mineral requirements. For instance, in pregnancy, it is recognized that additional minerals are needed for embryonic and fetal growth, including those needed in the uterine fluid and for growth of the uterus. Though the additional amount needed might be small, it is likely important, but not enough data are available to make strong conclusions.

When sufficient data are available, the apparent digestibility of a given mineral can be calculated by subtracting the amount of a mineral in the feces from the amount fed to the horse, then dividing that difference by the total amount ingested. While easier to determine than the true digestibility, the apparent digestibility often is lower as some of the nutrient found in the feces can come from endogenous losses instead of a mineral that was not absorbed. To determine the true digestibility of a mineral, endogenous losses need to be determined and, to do so, various concentrations of a mineral are fed. The regression line obtained by plotting the amount of a mineral apparently absorbed (Y-axis) against the amount of a mineral fed (X-axis) can be used to estimate endogenous mineral losses, or the point where the mineral intake is at zero. In this procedure, various assumptions have to be made. One assumption is that absorption of the mineral follows a linear function. Another assumption is that endogenous secretions are constant. True digestibility is then represented as the amount absorbed (which is the amount of mineral fed minus the amount of mineral in feces and in the endogenous secretions) divided by the amount fed. Alternatively, true digestibility of the nutrient can be represented by the slope of the regression of the amount of mineral absorbed on dietary mineral intake (Pagan, 1994). By plotting retention (Y-axis) against intake (X-axis), a prediction can be made as to what dietary intake would result in no mineral being retained and the mineral balance would be zero, thus representing minimal requirements (Hintz and Schryver, 1972). Limitations to these methods include improper mineral recovery from the urine or feces due to improper laboratory procedures (O'Connor and Nielsen, 2006) or not accounting for minerals lost through avenues other than the urine or feces. Concentrations of minerals such as sodium and chloride need to be examined in other body secretions such as sweat, particularly in the exercising animal (Coenen, 2005). Animals retaining more mineral than they are losing are considered to be in a positive mineral balance. This is expected when an animal is growing and accreting minerals in various tissues. Once an animal is mature and in a homeostatic state, it is more likely that an animal should be in a near zero balance, though a slight positive balance may exist due to unaccounted-for mineral losses in tissues, such as hair or hoof growth. While analyzing substances, such as the hair of horses, has been performed by some investigators in an attempt to determine mineral status of horses (Asano et al., 2002), such techniques are of questionable use as they can be influenced by factors, such as coat color, that are independent of nutrition (Cape and Hintz, 1982; Asano et al., 2005). In contrast, mineral concentrations in the blood can sometimes be useful in determining whether a dietary deficiency or excess is present. Blood samples are more likely to provide information about phosphorus, magnesium, potassium, sodium, chloride, copper, manganese, selenium, and zinc status of a horse than they are the calcium, iodine, and cobalt status (Lewis, 1995).

Serum ferritin status is believed to be a better indicator of iron status than is blood or plasma iron concentration. With most minerals, ration evaluation and case history are still often needed to confirm problems. Additionally, proper sampling techniques and analysis need to be performed to ensure the greatest likelihood of meaningful results.

In some studies on mineral requirements of horses, the daily intake of the mineral of interest is reported on a body weight basis. However, in other studies, intake is reported as a concentration of the diet. Whenever possible, daily intake was converted to a body weight basis using feed intake and body weight information presented in individual studies. When feed intake was not reported, assumptions were made as to the average intake of each class of horse so that it was possible to provide an estimate of the amount of a given mineral needed per kg of body weight (BW). Obviously these estimates of feed intakes are not constant among horses but are needed to provide estimates of daily nutrient intakes. Horses at maintenance were assumed to eat 2 percent of their BW/d in dry matter feed, while growing horses were assumed to eat 2.5 percent, pregnant mares were assumed to eat 2 percent of their nonpregnant body weight, and lactating mares were assumed to eat 2.5 percent feed on a dry matter basis. With increasing intensities and durations of exercise, dry matter intake typically increases, though this does not necessarily occur—particularly if fat is substituted for carbohydrates in the diet. For light exercise, a dry matter intake of 2 percent was assumed, while 2.25 percent and 2.5 percent of BW/d were assumed to be the intake of moderate and heavily working horses, respectively. As noted previously, these assumptions were only used when there was insufficient information reported in an individual study to calculate mineral intake on a body weight basis. These estimates of intake are somewhat liberal and thus may overestimate the actual feed intake of study animals. However, by using a liberal estimate of intake, it seemed less likely that a requirement expressed on a body weight basis would be underestimated. As there is an apparent lack of research in determining mineral requirements of breeding stallions, they can be considered to be similar to maintenance values, though it is possible some differences do exist.

MACROMINERALS

Calcium

Function

About 99 percent of the calcium (Ca) in the body is found in the bones and teeth, with calcium constituting about 35 percent of equine bone (El Shorafa et al., 1979). Calcium also plays an important role in various functions within the body such as muscle contraction, the function of cell membranes, blood coagulation, and the regulation of many enzymes. Calcium homeostasis within the blood is critical. The skeleton, besides serving as structural support for the body, can serve as a readily available storage location for calcium.

Sources and Factors Influencing Absorption

Calcium carbonate, sulfate, and oxide are common inorganic forms of calcium (Highfill et al., 2005). A calcium-amino acid proteinate did not differ from calcium carbonate in absorption rate though more calcium was absorbed in the two supplemented groups than in a nonsupplemented diet (Highfill et al., 2005). Free-choice feeding of calcium supplements is not an effective means of ensuring adequate intake (Hintz, 1987a). Calcium supplements should be mixed with grain or other palatable materials to help ensure consumption.

The portion of dietary calcium that is absorbed varies in order to maintain normal calcium homeostasis (Jones and Rasmusson, 1980). In response to lowered ionized serum calcium concentrations, parathyroid hormone (PTH) secretion is stimulated in order to reestablish normal concentrations through stimulation of bone resorption and renal tubular calcium reabsorption (Bushinsky and Monk, 1998). Vitamin D mediates intestinal absorption of calcium and adaptation to dietary intake in most species, though Breidenbach et al. (1998) suggest that it does not play a key role in regulating calcium and inorganic phosphate homeostasis in the horse. Horses have a moderate or lacking increase of plasma calcium and at the same time a pronounced increase in plasma inorganic phosphate during vitamin D intoxification, potentially suggesting a different regulatory role of vitamin D in horses than in other species (Harmeyer and Schlumbohm, 2004). More research would need to be done to confirm this theory.

An absorption efficiency of 50 percent is used for all ages of horses. The true absorption efficiency can be as high as 70 percent with young horses but appears to decline as a horse matures. Throughout a horse's life, calcium absorption can vary depending upon many factors, so determining a specific absorption rate in an individual animal is difficult. Additionally, many mineral balance studies last 10 days or less, and horses likely are able to modulate the absorption efficiency of calcium to account for lowered dietary intakes (Hintz, 2000). Thus, a 50 percent absorption efficiency may be low, especially when calcium concentrations in the diet are low. However, Hintz (2000) contended making a liberal estimate is better than making a conservative estimate, as it will decrease the likelihood of developing a calcium deficiency. Pagan (1994) reported true calcium digestibility established over the course of many trials to be around 75 percent in mature horses. Other factors affecting calcium absorption include concentrations of calcium, phosphorus, phytate, and oxalate in the diet. As calcium concentrations increase, the absorption efficiency typically decreases; however, apparent calcium absorption was higher in horses fed alfalfa than grass hays (Cuddeford et al., 1990; Crozier et al., 1997). Sturgeon et al. (2000) reported an apparent calcium digestibility of 72 percent for alfalfa compared to only 40 percent for Bermudagrass. When mature ponies were fed 316 and 535 mg Ca/kg BW/d, van Doorn et al. (2004b) reported the apparent digestibility of calcium was around 28 percent as compared to 42 percent when the ponies were fed 148 mg Ca/kg of BW/d (dietary concentration equal to 0.78 percent calcium, which is still excessive for a maintenance diet). All ponies were in positive calcium balance, though calcium retention was greatest at the highest concentration of calcium fed. As mature animals would be expected to maintain a balance close to zero by adapting the digestibility or urinary excretion, van Doorn et al. (2004b) suggested that when the amount of absorbed calcium exceeds the amount that can be excreted with urine, the additional calcium is retained, resulting in a positive balance. In what tissue(s) the extra calcium is retained is unclear, though it is expected that the animals would need to eventually return to a homeostatic state if they were examined long enough, unless calcium is lost from hair, hoof, or sweat and not accounted for. While Hintz and Schryver (1973) reported that increasing the dietary concentration of magnesium increased calcium absorption, the absorption efficiency of calcium decreases as phosphorus increases in the diet due to the competitive nature of calcium and phosphorus absorption in the small intestine. This likely varies somewhat depending upon mineral source. Schryver et al. (1987b) reported true calcium digestibility increasing from 51 to 69 percent as the percentage of sodium chloride in the diet increased. Dietary oxalate decreases absorption of calcium quite dramatically and can play a role in a deficiency of absorbed calcium when not taken into consideration when balancing diets. Swartzmann et al. (1978) reported a reduction of calcium absorption by about 66 percent by the inclusion of 1 percent oxalic acid in equine diets. McKenzie et al. (1981) reported total dietary oxalate concentrations of 2.6 to 4.3 percent decreased calcium absorption as evidenced by a negative calcium balance resulting from a doubling of fecal calcium and decreased urinary calcium in comparison to control horses. Similar negative balances for calcium were observed by Blaney et al. (1981) in horses fed various tropical grass hays containing more than 0.5 percent total oxalate. When the calcium:oxalate ratio on a weight-to-weight basis was less than 0.5, it was concluded that horses could be at risk for nutritional secondary hyperparathyroidism. No difference in calcium absorption was reported by Hintz et al. (1984) from alfalfas containing 0.5 and 0.87 percent oxalic acid in which the calcium:oxalate ratios were 3 and 1.7, respectively. By contrast, there have been a few reports of calcinosis in horses due to the consumption of calcinogenic plants (Mello, 2003). The plants that have been documented to affect horses are *Cestrum diurnum* (in Florida) and *Tricetum flavescens* (in Austria). These plants increase release of $1,25(OH)_2D_3$, and can greatly increase calcium absorption, thereby resulting in hypercalcemia. Fortunately, such situations are rare.

Both intake and type of diet influence renal calcium excretion (Meyer, 1990). Calcium is not absorbed from the large intestine, emphasizing the need to have sufficient amounts to ensure adequate absorption from the small intestine (Stadermann et al., 1992). Dietary constituents can influence digestibility as prececal apparent digestibility of calcium is higher with alfalfa hay than with concentrate (Stadermann et al., 1992). Hoffman et al. (2000) reported lowered bone mineral content of the third metacarpus when feeding a fat- and fiber-based diet compared to a sugar- and starch-based diet, and thus expressed concerns over the potential binding of calcium by fat and fiber. A follow-up study showed that supplementing more than 0.9 percent calcium in a sweet feed had no effect on mineral content of the third metacarpus in fat- and fiber-fed foals, thus leading the authors to conclude that the transient lower bone mineral content observed in the prior study may be better attributed to nutrient-endocrine interactions than to calcium insufficiency (Hoffman et al., 2001). Grace et al. (2003) reported no change in apparent absorption of calcium when weanlings were fed diets ranging in concentration from 3.5 to 12 g Ca/kg DM. Additionally, no changes in bone strength were related to dietary calcium concentration. Though hypothesized that diets high in protein increase urinary calcium excretion with potential detriment to bone, no influence on bone density was reported due to varying protein intakes (Schryver et al., 1987a; Spooner et al., 2005) or protein quality (Smith et al., 2005). Besides diet, other factors can influence absorption. Cymbaluk et al. (1989) reported true calcium digestibilities decreased substantially from 6 to 24 months of age (though this was confounded with a change in calcium source), and the efficiency of calcium absorption was influenced by varying requirements during different stages of training (Stephens et al., 2001). At times when mineral deposition is occurring in bone, requirements would be expected to increase. Bone serves as a reservoir for calcium, and more calcium is needed from the diet when calcium is being placed into bone as compared to when calcium is being removed from bone during periods of disuse (Bronner, 1993). During initial periods of disuse, the calcium goes into the plasma, from which excess is secreted from the body. This appears to decrease calcium requirements (Nielsen et al., 1998a). Likewise, when mineral is being deposited into bone at times when exercise intensity is increasing, requirements are likely higher than when intensity of training is relatively constant. Exercise in mature horses did not alter apparent calcium digestibility (about 54 percent: Pagan et al., 1998).

Signs of Deficiency or Excess

Removing calcium from the skeleton to meet metabolic demands when dietary calcium intake is inadequate can result in a weakened skeleton if done in excess. The need to maintain blood calcium concentration within such a tight range renders total serum calcium a poor indicator of calcium status (Krook and Lowe, 1964) so even when an unbalanced diet is fed, calcium concentrations in the blood can remain relatively constant (de Behr et al., 2003). When fractionated out using a micropartition system, Lopez et al. (2006) reported total calcium in the serum of healthy horses to be composed of ionized calcium (48.5 ± 0.7 percent), protein-bound calcium (47.4 ± 0.9 percent), and calcium complexed with weak acids (4.1 ± 0.9 percent). The ionized fraction is thought to be the only physiologically active form and thus is the form that should be evaluated for clinical work. A normal reference range for total serum calcium has been given as 10.8 to 13.5 mg/dl serum and for ionized serum calcium as 6.44 to 6.74 mg/dl serum (Garcia-Lopez et al., 2001). An ionized serum calcium concentration of less than 6 mg/dl serum has also been used to define horses as hypocalcemic by Toribio et al. (2001). Calcium deficiencies often have a dramatic impact on skeletal integrity. A deficiency of calcium in the developing foal can lead to osteopenia. This condition is characterized by poor mineralization of the osteoid tissue and the probability of enlarged joints and crooked long bones. A survey of the severity of metabolic bone disease in yearlings and diet analysis on 19 Ohio and Kentucky horse farms revealed a negative linear relationship between dietary calcium intake and perceived severity of metabolic bone disease in young horses (Knight et al., 1985). Farms with yearlings having the lowest incidence of metabolic bone disease were fed diets containing 1.2 percent calcium, whereas yearlings with the most severe metabolic bone disease were on farms that fed diets with 0.2 percent calcium. It should be noted that this report did not have data on what the horses were consuming prior to the survey and it did not report differences in exercise afforded to the young horses—both of which likely could have influenced results. In the mature horse, inadequate dietary calcium can result in weakening of the bones and an insidious shifting lameness (Krook and Lowe, 1964).

Whitlock et al. (1970) fed diets with calcium:phosphorus ratios of 1.16:1 (0.43 percent calcium) and 4.12:1 (1.96 percent calcium) and observed a greater proportion of lamellar bone than osteonic bone in high-calcium horses; however, no clinically deleterious effects or gross morphological differences were detected. Krook and Maylin (1988) proposed that osteochondrosis may be associated with excess dietary calcium (e.g., from alfalfa hay) by producing hypercalcitoninism. However, calcium has been fed at more than five times the required concentration without detrimental effects, provided the phosphorus concentration is adequate (Jordan et al., 1975). When provided adequate, but not excessive, amounts of phosphorus, the maximum tolerable concentration of calcium in horse feed has been given as 2 percent of the diet (NRC, 2005). Recent work in other species has shown that calcium influences gastrin secretion

(Cheng et al., 1999; Dufner et al., 2005), indicating unnecessarily high dietary calcium may be implicated in gastric ulcers and should be avoided. More details on the calcium:phosphorus ratio are given in the phosphorus section and in Chapter 12.

Some work has been done in utilizing dietary cation-anion difference (DCAD) to influence calcium utilization. A low DCAD (defined as mEq (sodium + potassium) − chloride/kg dry matter) has been shown to increase urinary calcium loss in exercising horses (Wall et al., 1992) and perhaps leads to a calcium deficiency in growing horses (Wall et al., 1997). However, Cooper et al. (2000) reported that when fed a lower DCAD (defined as mEq (sodium + potassium) − (chloride + sulfur)/kg of diet DM), horses increased intestinal calcium absorption to compensate for increased urinary excretion of calcium. Using that same definition, Baker et al. (1998) indicated a low DCAD diet formulated with ammonium chloride resulted in a decrease in apparent calcium balance. Cooper et al. (2000) suggested the horse is able to maintain metabolic equilibrium despite the ratio of cations to anions in the diet and that horses can tolerate a wide variation in DCAD without experiencing adverse effects on skeletal growth. Likewise, McKenzie et al. (2002) found that varying DCAD did not alter daily balance of calcium and phosphorus. Data from Cooper et al. (1998) obtained after a 21-day diet adaptation period suggested horses are able to maintain normal acid-base status regardless of the dietary cation-anion balance of the diet. Whether this would be true in a longer duration study is not known.

Recommendations

Endogenous losses of calcium have been estimated to be 20 mg Ca/kg BW/d (Schryver et al., 1970, 1971a). Using that estimate and the absorption efficiency of 50 percent, the 1989 NRC proposed a 500-kg horse would require 20 g (500 kg × 20 mg/0.5) of dietary calcium (0.04 g of Ca/kg BW) or 1.22 g Ca/Mcal DE (digestible energy)/d for maintenance. Using data compiled from many studies, Pagan (1994) estimated endogenous calcium loss to be 17.4 g/d ($R^2 = 0.94$) for a 550-kg horse (about 31.6 mg/kg BW), which is higher than the 1989 NRC values. The true digestibility of calcium was estimated at 74.7 percent, which is also higher than 1989 NRC values. However, the resulting requirement for a 500-kg horse (21.2 g Ca/d) is similar to the 1989 NRC requirement (20 g/d). Regression analyses on the calcium data of Buchholz-Bryant et al. (2001) using 12 sedentary geldings of three different age groups at four time periods gives a calculated requirement of 0.043 g Ca/kg of BW. This would represent 21 g Ca/d for a 500-kg horse, which is similar to the recommendation of the 1989 NRC. Thus, the subcommittee saw no reason to change the maintenance calcium requirements. As noted in the section on exercise, after extended periods of stall rest, calcium requirements likely go up, even if horses are just returned to a pasture setting to compensate for bone loss associated with disuse.

Using the estimate of Schryver et al. (1974) that growing foals deposit approximately 16 g Ca/kg of gain, a 215-kg foal gaining 0.85 kg/d and having a calcium absorption efficiency of 50 percent would require 27.2 g/d (16 g × 0.85 kg of gain/0.5) of dietary calcium for skeletal growth plus 8.6 g/d (215 kg × 20 mg/0.5) to meet endogenous losses. However, a study by Cymbaluk et al. (1989) estimated endogenous fecal calcium to be 36 mg/kg BW in growing Quarter horses. While Hintz (1996) suggested there is little evidence for the calcium requirements of growing horses to be greatly changed from the 1989 NRC's recommendations, the apparent greater endogenous losses in growing horses compared to mature horses would increase the requirements of a 215-kg foal by an additional 6.9 g/d over what the 1989 NRC suggested—up to 42.7 g. While these horses were on a relatively high-forage diet during the study (about 50 to 90 percent), it is reasonable to believe growing horses have greater endogenous losses than a mature horse. In addition, Moffett et al. (2001) reported increased daily gains, as well as increased calcium retention, when yearlings were fed 0.48 percent calcium compared to 0.32 percent. Thus, the calcium requirement for growing horses not in training was increased to meet endogenous losses of 36 mg Ca/kg BW with a 50 percent absorption rate and to meet growth requirements of 16 g Ca/kg BW gain with a 50 percent absorption rate. The resultant requirement for calcium is (0.072 g × kg BW) + (32 g × ADG in kg).

In late gestation, calcium requirements for the mare are increased to meet the needs of fetal growth and tissue development. Approximately 11.1, 25.3, and 11.4 mg of Ca/kg of mare body weight are deposited daily in the fetus and membranes of mares in months 9, 10, and 11, respectively (Meyer and Ahlswede, 1978; Drepper et al., 1982). Though the substantial increase at 10 months of gestation is suspect, their findings may be supported by a study by House and Bell (1993) that examined fetal calves from slaughtered cows. At the end of gestation, calcium accretion in the fetus was 10.3 g/d at 280 days of gestation. Using the average cow weight of 714 kg, 14.4 mg of calcium were being deposited per kg of BW, which is comparable to the 11.4 mg Ca/kg of BW reported in horses at the end of gestation. Given that fetal calf growth increased from 329 g/d at 200 days post-mating to 456 g/d at 242 days post-mating and then declined to 296 g/d at 280 days of gestation, it seems plausible that the increased deposition of calcium in the 10th month of gestation in horses also represents the greatest period of fetal foal growth and the greatest need for calcium. Using an absorption efficiency of 50 percent, the calcium requirement during months 9, 10, and 11 of gestation for a 500-kg mare would be 11, 25, and 11 g/d, respectively, for fetal development. As data on the deposition rate of minerals in the fetus are very limited, a mean deposition rate (15.9 mg Ca/kg BW) was used for the last 3 months (NRC, 1989). Using the 50-percent absorption rate, 0.032 g Ca/kg BW is needed in addition to maintenance requirements during the last 3 months of gestation. Martin et al. (1996) evaluated prepartum mares fed either 0.55 percent calcium (0.076 g Ca/kg BW; above the 1989 NRC suggested minimum of 0.45 percent) or 0.35 percent calcium (0.045 g Ca/kg BW; below the suggested minimum) and concluded that the optimal dietary calcium concentration for prepartum mares was closer to 0.55 percent than 0.35 percent. The dietary concentration of 0.45 percent calcium recommended by the 1989 NRC for pregnant mares was not evaluated in this study, which appeared to confirm that 0.35 percent dietary calcium was not adequate for prepartum mares. However, in the study by Martin et al. (1996), the two treatment groups were maintained on separate farms and the treatment groups were not balanced for breed. In addition, the dietary calcium concentration was determined from estimated pasture intake (which was very different for the two groups), so the results may have been influenced by factors other than dietary calcium concentration. However, Glade (1993) confirmed that the dietary amount of calcium recommended for broodmares is a minimum and should not be reduced. Foals of mares fed calcium lower than the 1989 NRC requirements had mechanically weaker bones at birth compared to foals of mares fed the 1989 NRC recommended amounts. While the 1989 NRC based its recommendation on DE, the current method of determination results in a similar requirement and, at this time, there is no strong evidence to suggest a revision of that requirement. However, considering there is substantial fetal growth during months 7 and 8 of gestation, the requirement for those months is suggested as being an average of maintenance and late gestation. In summary, to meet endogenous losses of 20 mg Ca/kg BW with an absorption rate of 50 percent and to meet fetal deposition rate of 15.9 mg Ca/kg BW with a 50 percent absorption rate, the calcium requirement during months 9, 10, and 11 of pregnancy is calculated as (0.04 g Ca × kg BW) + (0.032 g Ca × kg BW) or simply (0.072 g Ca × kg BW). To meet endogenous losses of 20 mg Ca/kg BW with an absorption rate of 50 percent and to meet fetal deposition rate of 8 mg Ca/kg BW with a 50 percent absorption rate, the requirement for pregnancy during months 7 and 8 of gestation is calculated as (0.04 g × kg BW) + (0.016 g × kg BW) or simply (0.056 g × kg BW).

Though commonly recognized, additional demand for calcium during lactation was reconfirmed by Martin et al. (1996), who reported an increase in serum parathyroid hormone concentrations with a lactation-induced decrease in serum total and ionized calcium beginning 3 days prepartum and continuing until 2 days postpartum. Schryver et al. (1986b) reported that the daily calcium requirements for lactation range from 1.2 g/kg of fluid milk during the first postpartum week to 0.8 g/kg of fluid milk during weeks 15 to 17 postpartum. This is consistent with the data of Baucus et al. (1987). For a 500-kg mare producing 16 kg milk/d in early lactation and with a calcium absorption efficiency of 50 percent, the daily dietary calcium requirement would be 38.4 g (16 kg × 1.2 g/0.5) for milk production, in addition to 20 g for maintenance. This estimate of calcium requirement for milk production is consistent with that of Jarrige and Martin-Rosset (1981). When fed at the 1989 NRC recommended concentration, mares still lost bone density from the third metacarpal bone during the first 12 weeks of lactation but density was restored by 24 weeks postpartum (Glade, 1993). Mares fed 20 percent less calcium had not fully recovered third metacarpal bone density by 20 weeks after milk production had ceased (40 weeks after parturition). This suggests that rebred mares not fed sufficient calcium during lactation would have a greater demand for calcium throughout gestation as they attempt to restore the mineral lost from the skeleton during lactation. This work reaffirms that the dietary calcium recommendation of the 1989 NRC for lactation should not be reduced, though it is uncertain if the recommendation should be increased. Thus, the recommendations remain unchanged, although new estimates of milk production are used. Milk production is estimated at 0.032 kg milk per kg BW from foaling to 3 months, 0.026 kg milk per kg BW from 4 to 5 months, and 0.020 kg milk per kg BW after 5 months. The resultant equations for calcium requirements during lactation are:

Foaling to 3 months = (0.04 g × kg BW) + (0.032 × kg BW × 2.4 g)

4–5 months = (0.04 g × kg BW) + (0.026 × kg BW × 1.6 g)

> 5 months = (0.04 g × kg BW) + (0.020 × kg BW × 1.6 g)

Previously, it had been assumed that any additional calcium required for exercise would be met through the additional feed consumed to meet energy demands (NRC, 1989). The need for calcium is greatly influenced by bone development. Bone formation is impacted by exercise, or the lack thereof. When net bone deposition is increased, so is the need for calcium. When bone loss is occurring, requirements for calcium are lower as calcium is removed from the skeleton, goes into the plasma, and is lost through the urine and feces with an accompanying decreased need for calcium absorption (Nielsen et al., 1998a). Unfortunately, plasma calcium concentrations are of little use in assessing net calcium balance as horses in a negative calcium balance commonly have normal plasma or serum values (Rose, 1990) despite measurable changes in bone mineral content. Estimates of mineral content of the lower leg are reduced in young horses that are stalled without sufficient access to exercise as compared to horses kept on pasture (Hoekstra et al., 1999; Bell et al., 2001; Brama et al., 2002). Porr et al. (1998) reported stall rest for 12 weeks in mature Arabians similarly decreased third metacarpal bone mineral content estimates, which was not prevented by dietary calcium intake at twice the 1989 NRC recommended concentration (an excess of about 20 g of calcium). To compensate for mineral loss from the skeleton, Meyer (1987) suggested feeding 20 percent above the recommended amounts of calcium and phosphorus if horses have a prolonged period without activity once normal activity has returned. Short sprints are sufficient to stimulate bone formation, while exercising for longer distances, but at slower speeds, is less efficient. Vervuert et al. (2005a) reported draught load exercise with low velocities had no effect on calcium metabolism. In contrast, despite receiving the exact same diet, a single 82-m sprint five days per week increased indirect measures of third metacarpal bone mineral content and improved third metacarpus architecture in stalled weanlings compared to stalled weanlings afforded no exercise (Hiney et al., 2004). These studies demonstrate the importance of exercise in stimulating calcium deposition in the skeleton. Interestingly, a 10-year study in humans showed that calcium intake over that period was not associated with bone gain or bone strength (Lloyd et al., 2004). Instead, only exercise during adolescence, as determined by a sports exercise questionnaire, was significantly associated with increased bone mineral density and bone bending strength ($P < 0.01$). Similarly, Nielsen (2005) reported a much greater role in influencing markers of bone turnover in studies related to differences in exercise as compared to nutrition. Hence, the importance of exercise in young horses to maximize bone strength is underscored. If sufficient exercise is provided, extra dietary calcium can likely be utilized to improve bone strength. Exercise, particularly in the young horse, appears to increase calcium requirements above maintenance requirements. Gray et al. (1988) found horses in training had lower urinary calcium excretion, despite receiving more calcium, than horses not working, suggesting exercise increases the need for calcium. Exercised horses had a higher calcium balance than horses that were sedentary for 2 months and then exercised for 2 months (Elmore-Smith et al., 1999). In response to previously measured declines in mineral content of the third metacarpal bone (Nielsen et al., 1997, 1998a), calcium balance and retention were determined in 2-year-old racehorses placed into training receiving a total diet containing either 0.31 percent calcium (0.063 g × kg BW) or 0.38 percent calcium (0.074 g × kg BW) on an as-fed basis and consuming about 2 percent of their body weight daily (Nielsen et al., 1998b). Calcium retention was greater, as was mineral content of the third metacarpal bone, in horses fed 0.38 percent calcium (0.074 g × kg BW). Other studies also support the need for additional calcium for horses in training. Nolan et al. (2001) reported increased mineralization of the third metacarpal bone when 151 percent and 169 percent of the 1989 NRC recommended calcium amount were fed compared to 97 percent and 136 percent. Likewise, Michael et al. (2001) reported increased markers of bone formation and decreased markers of bone resorption in horses fed the two higher percentages of calcium compared to the two lower percentages. Unfortunately, neither Nolan et al. (2001) nor Michael et al. (2001) reported weight of the horses or feed intake, so calculating absolute intake on a body weight basis is not possible. If the feed intake of the horses was relatively low, the absolute amount taken in may have been closer to the amount recommended by the 1989 NRC than the concentrations would make it appear. Stephens et al. (2004) reported calcium retention to be maximal when calcium intake was 123 mg Ca/kg BW/d, which represents a 36 percent increase over the 1989 NRC recommendations for exercise. However, variation was great ($R^2 = 0.23$) for calcium retention vs. intake. Total concentrate and hay intake averaged 18 g/kg BW. Calcium intake was 135 ± 6 mg/kg BW/d at the start of the study and was 123 ± 4 mg/kg BW/d at the completion of the study at day 128. In these studies, the effects of additional calcium are often confounded with varying amounts of phosphorus and magnesium but demonstrate potential improvements in bone mineral content, and potentially strength, by feeding additional calcium over what was recommended by the 1989 NRC. When only the calcium concentration was altered, Schryver et al. (1978) suggested that 0.6 percent dietary calcium was not needed, compared to 0.4 percent calcium, when fed to yearling Standardbreds entering training. For horses consuming 2 percent of their body weight per day, as was the case in many of these studies, this would equate to 0.08 g Ca/kg BW. This is also supported by the data of Buchholz-Bryant et al. (2001). When their data for calcium intake for young horses in training are plotted against the amount retained, the linear regression response shows a requirement of 0.079 g Ca/kg BW. For horses that are rapidly growing (typically under 24 months of age), these requirements would usually be met by the requirements for growth (((0.072 g Ca × kg BW) + (32 g Ca × ADG in kg)) that have been increased from the 1989 NRC. As a result, the requirement for growing horses that are exercising is the same as the requirement for growth. Typically, this is equal or greater than the apparent recommendation for heavy exercise (0.08 g Ca × kg BW) only when average daily gain drops to 0.1 kg. It is likely the calcium requirement associated with exercise is less for mature horses. Mansell et al. (1999) found little difference in the response of bone to varying concentrations of dietary calcium but found bigger differences depending upon the age of horses. When calcium intake data of Buchholz-Bryant et al. (2001) for mature horses are plotted against retention, linear regression reveals a requirement of 0.04 g Ca/kg BW/d—the same as is required for maintenance. While it is likely the calcium requirement for mature horses is less than that of the younger horse, an insufficient number of studies have been performed to warrant lowering the requirement for heavy exercise in mature horses at this time. Because forces applied to the skeleton primarily regulate bone mineral deposition, which is one of the major needs for additional calcium, establishing calcium requirements for exercise is difficult and will vary depending upon the intensity of training and the influence upon the skeleton. The requirement will likely be closer to maintenance for horses not experiencing any high-speed work and for horses that are not increasing their intensity of training. Thus, the calcium recommendations for light and moderate exercise can be expected to be lower than that of heavy exercise and have been set at 0.06 g Ca × kg BW for light exercise and 0.07 g Ca × kg BW for moderate exercise. While a heavily exercising horse may have only a small increased need for extra calcium compared to a lightly exercising horse if the exercise intensity has been constant, these recommendations are established to minimize or eliminate problems as the intensity of exercise increases.

Phosphorus

Function

Like calcium, phosphorus (P) is a major constituent of bone, making up 14 to 17 percent of the skeleton (El Shorafa et al., 1979). In addition, it is required for many energy transfer reactions associated with adenosine diphosphate (ADP) and adenosine triphosphate (ATP), and for the synthesis of phospholipids, nucleic acids, and phosphoproteins.

Sources and Factors Influencing Absorption

True phosphorus absorption is quite variable and typically ranges from 30–55 percent. It varies depending upon other dietary constituents, how much and what type of phosphorus is fed, and the age of the horse. High calcium concentrations in the diet depress phosphorus absorption. In diets averaging 0.89 percent calcium, Pagan (1994) reported true phosphorus absorption to be around 25 percent. Similarly, phosphorus absorption of a high-phosphorus diet (0.125 g P/kg BW) decreased from 25 percent in horses receiving a diet containing 0.148 g Ca/kg BW/d to 11 percent and 13 percent when fed diets containing 0.316 and 0.535 g Ca/kg BW/d, respectively (van Doorn et al., 2004b). All horses were in positive phosphorus balance. High dietary phosphorus concentrations (1.19 percent phosphorus) have been shown to increase phosphorus retention and plasma phosphorus concentrations (Schryver et al., 1971b). Buchholz-Bryant et al. (2001) reported similar findings when examining the effect of calcium and phosphorus supplementation in young, mature, and aged horses with different training regimens. All groups retained phosphorus regardless of whether they were fed normal (0.24 percent) or high (0.57 percent) phosphorus diets. Increases in dietary sodium chloride from 1 percent to 5 percent increased phosphorus absorption from 28 to 40 percent (Schryver et al., 1987b). Despite concern with aluminum interference in phosphorus absorption, phosphorus absorption was not affected by feeding an aluminum (Al) supplement (931 ppm Al/kg feed or 12 mg of Al/kg BW/d) for 1 month (Roose et al., 2001).

Diets containing high concentrations of oxalates depress phosphorus retention (Blaney et al., 1981; McKenzie et al., 1981). Phytate phosphorus, the salt of phytic acid and a predominant form of phosphorus in plants, is poorly absorbed by horses, though some phytase exists in the hindgut (Hintz et al., 1973). To meet phosphorus requirements, inorganic phosphates are often added to the equine diet and this could be at least partially avoided if the absorbability of phytate phosphorus could be increased by an appropriate use of phytates (Eeckhout and De Paepe, 1994). Despite an abundance of research on the use of phytase to increase phosphorus availability in other species, Morris-Stoker et al. (2001) reported no benefit to horses of feeding phytase (200 units/g) at the rate of 1 g/kg of feed. Patterson et al. (2002) also found no improvement in phosphorus apparent digestibility with the addition of phytase up to 900 Phytase unit (FTU)/kg of diet. When horses were fed four different diets (Coasta Bermudagrass with whole oats, alfalfa cubes, a textured sweet feed, or a pelleted concentrate), Hainze et al. (2004) found phytase decreased fecal phosphorus only for the sweet feed-based diet, due largely to decreased fecal output of the insoluble fraction of phosphorus. Because horse manure contains a lower proportion of total phosphorus as the water-soluble phosphorus fraction compared with that from other farm animals, phosphorus in horse feces may be less prone to runoff in typical pasture-based management systems. Hainze et al. (2004) concluded that under normal feeding conditions, phytase probably has limited potential for decreasing concerns over environmental phosphorus contamination as the proportion of fecal phosphorus represented by the soluble fraction is increased. However, Warren (2003) cautioned that, though equine research has not shown phytase to be useful in reducing phosphorus excretion, evaluated diets have had sufficient phosphorus. A better test is to determine if phytase can increase phosphorus utilization by the horse when dietary phosphorus concentrations are below required amounts (Warren, 2003).

Phosphorus absorption is assumed to be higher by foals consuming milk than it is in mature horses, though Grace et al. (1999a) suggested creep feed be fed to nursing foals as milk may be insufficient in phosphorus (as well as calcium) for optimal growth of foals. A phosphorus absorption efficiency of 35 percent is used for mature horses (except for lactating mares) as they primarily consume plant sources of phosphorus. For lactating mares and growing horses, a 45-percent efficiency is used because their diets are often supplemented with inorganic phosphorus. Horses at 8 months were more efficient at utilizing phosphorus than horses at 12 months (Cymbaluk, 1990). Environment appears to influence phosphorus absorption as horses housed in a warm barn had greater true phosphorus digestibility than those housed in a cold barn (Cymbaluk, 1990). Similar to the findings for calcium, Stephens et al. (2001) reported the efficiency of absorption can vary with requirements. Absorption, at least to a degree, apparently increases when demand for phosphorus increases and may change with stage of training though more studies are needed.

Signs of Deficiency or Excess

Inadequate dietary phosphorus will, like calcium and vitamin D, produce rachitic-like changes in growing horses and osteomalacic changes in mature horses. Excess phosphorus reduces the rate of calcium absorption and leads to chronic calcium deficiency and nutritional secondary hyperparathyroidism (NSH). Clinically, NSH is characterized by shifting lameness and, in advanced cases, by enlargement of the upper and lower jaws and facial crest (Krook and Lowe, 1964). Savage et al. (1993a) reported that foals fed 388 percent of the 1989 NRC recommendation for phosphorus showed numerous, severe lesions of osteochondrosis but no clinical signs of NSH, though Savage et al. (1993b), in a histomorphometric assessment of bone biopsies from the foals, reported that the changes were consistent with NSH.

Both organic and inorganic phosphorus exist in serum, though serum inorganic phosphorus is derived entirely from inorganic compounds and is the value utilized in clinical practice (Lau, 1986). Serum inorganic phosphorus concentrations are high at birth and decline over several months to normal adult values. Serum inorganic phosphorus values may be more indicative of dietary phosphorus status than serum calcium is of calcium status because homeostatic mechanisms for phosphorus are less sensitive than for calcium (Schryver et al., 1970, 1971b). Caple et al. (1982) determined that horses excreting more than 15 μmol of P/mOsm of urine solute and having a phosphorus: creatinine clearance ratio greater than 4 had excessive phosphorus intake and were subject to NSH. It has been suggested that a maximum tolerable concentration of dietary phosphorus in horses fed adequate dietary calcium is 1 percent assuming an appropriate calcium:phosphorus ratio (NRC, 2005).

Calcium:Phosphorus Ratio

The absolute intakes of calcium and phosphorus by horses must be adequate, but secondarily, it is important to evaluate the calcium:phosphorus ratio of equine rations. If calcium intake is less than phosphorus intake (ratio less than 1:1), calcium absorption may be impaired. Even if the diet contains adequate calcium, excessive phosphorus intake may cause skeletal abnormalities (Schryver et al., 1971b). Nutritional secondary hyperparathyroidism is covered more completely in Chapter 12. This condition does not occur often in the United States, but Hintz (1997) cautioned that horse owners still need to be made aware of this potential problem, particularly if horses are fed large amounts of grain-based feedstuffs such as wheat bran or oats. While this condition is rare, it can still occur in situations when horses are fed grains not supplemented with calcium and are receiving forage relatively low in calcium or that contains substantial amounts of oxalates (Mason et al., 1988; Ronen et al., 1992; Luthersson et al., 2005). Though typically not a concern with forages, certain types, such as orchardgrass, can have inverted calcium:phosphorus ratios. With grains being naturally higher in phosphorus than calcium, it is quite easy to feed too much phosphorus in relation to calcium when raw grains or grain byproducts are fed in large quantities. Clinical signs vary depending on the degree of the imbalance of calcium to phosphorus, oxalate content of the diet, age of the horse, performance level, and environmental conditions (Ramirez and Seahorn, 1997). While a low calcium:phosphorus ratio can be quite detrimental, ratios as high as 6:1 in the growing horse may be acceptable if phosphorus intake is adequate (Jordan et al., 1975). The calcium:phosphorus ratio in milk has been reported to range between 1.8 and 2.5:1 between weeks 16 and 24 of lactation (Sonntag et al., 1996).

Recommendations

Endogenous losses of phosphorus by the mature horse have been estimated at 10 mg/kg BW/d (Schryver et al., 1971b). Combined with a 35 percent absorption efficiency, the 1989 NRC estimated the maintenance phosphorus requirements for a 500-kg horse to be 14.3 g (0.028 g P/kg BW). Using data from a number of studies, Pagan (1994) estimated endogenous phosphorus loss to be 4.7 g/d (R^2 = 0.33) for a 550-kg horse (about 8.5 mg/kg BW), which is slightly lower than the 1989 NRC estimates. The true digestibility of phosphorus was estimated to be 25.2 percent, which is also lower than the 35 percent used by the 1989 NRC. However, the resulting requirement for a 500-kg horse was estimated at 17 g P/d which, although slightly higher, is similar to 1989 NRC values. This emphasizes the importance of knowing the availability of a phosphorus source when formulating rations as the absorption efficiency can greatly influence the amount of phosphorus needed in the diet. Due to concerns with extra phosphorus being introduced into the environment, the subcommittee has chosen to remain with the lower estimate for phosphorus requirements.

As foals deposit about 8 g P/kg BW gain (Schryver et al., 1974), the 1989 NRC suggested growing horses require 17.8 g (8 g/0.45 percent efficiency) for each kg of gain in addition to the maintenance requirements. Thus, a 215-kg foal gaining 0.85 kg/d would require about 15.1 g of phosphorus (8 g/0.45 × 0.85 kg gain) in addition to its maintenance requirement of 4.8 g (215 kg × 10 mg/0.45). While Furtado et al. (2000) estimated endogenous fecal losses in growing horses to be 10.3 mg P/kg of BW/d, Pagan (1989) argued that endogenous phosphorus losses in young horses are double those used by the NRC (1989) in estimating dietary phosphorus requirement. This agrees with Cymbaluk et al. (1989), who estimated endogenous fecal phosphorus to be 18 mg/kg BW/d in growing Quarter horses. Using the higher estimate for endogenous loss (215 kg × 18 mg/0.45), the total phosphorus requirements would be increased to 23.7 g P/d. Grace et al. (1999b) suggested 21 g of P/d is the required amount compared to the 16 to 20 g recommended by the 1989 NRC for growing horses expected to reach 500 kg. Their calculations were based upon a 200-kg horse gaining 1 kg/d and using an absorption efficiency of 0.5. With a lower absorption efficiency, requirements would be even greater. The results of these studies suggest that the endogenous losses, and hence, maintenance phosphorus requirements, for young horses are greater than previously assumed and an endogenous loss of 18 mg/kg BW/d was used in determining the requirements. The requirement for growth recommended in this publication thus contains both a maintenance component (0.018 g/0.45 absorption efficiency × kg BW) and a growth component (8 g/0.45 percent absorption efficiency × kg gain). Phosphorus requirements increase during late gestation and lactation. Phosphorus requirements for the products of conception for mares in months 9, 10, and 11 of pregnancy have been estimated to be 7, 12, and 6.7 mg/kg BW/d, respectively (Drepper et al., 1982). At 35 percent absorption efficiency, the daily phosphorus requirements for a 500-kg mare for products of conception during gestation months 9, 10, and 11 would be 10, 17.1, and 9.6 g, respectively (mean 12.2 g/d). The mean daily phosphorus deposition for the last 3 months of gestation ((8.6 mg/kg BW)/0.35 absorption efficiency) was added to maintenance needs to determine the requirements. An average of maintenance and late gestation was used for the phosphorus requirements during months 7 and 8 to allow for fetal growth occurring during that period. Thus, to meet endogenous losses of 10 mg P/kg BW with an absorption rate of 35 percent and to meet fetal deposition rate of 4.3 mg P/kg BW with a 35 percent absorption rate, the requirement for pregnancy during months 7 and 8 is (0.028 g × kg BW) + (0.012 g × kg BW), or simply 0.04 g × kg BW. To meet endogenous losses of 10 mg P/kg BW with an absorption rate of 35 percent and to meet a fetal deposition rate of 8.6 mg P/kg BW with a 35 percent absorption rate during months 9, 10, and 11 of pregnancy, the requirement is (0.028 g × kg BW) + (0.0245 g × kg BW), or simply 0.0525 g × kg BW.

The phosphorus concentration of mares' milk ranges from 0.75 g/kg of fluid milk in early lactation to 0.50 g/kg of fluid milk in late lactation. If the absorption efficiency of lactating mares is 45 percent, the daily phosphorus requirements above maintenance (adjusted for the higher percent absorption) for lactation would be 26.7 g for a mare producing 16 kg milk/d in early lactation and 11.1 g for a mare producing 10 kg milk/d during late lactation. At these rates of milk production, a 500-kg mare would require 37.8 and 22.2 g P/d in early and late lactation, respectively. No data have been found suggesting the 1989 NRC recommendation for lactation should be changed other than to account for a revision of milk production estimates. To meet endogenous losses of 10 mg P/kg BW with an absorption rate of 45 percent and to meet milk production needs estimated at 0.032 kg milk/kg BW containing 0.75 g P/kg milk that is absorbed at a 45 percent rate, the phosphorus requirement for lactation from foaling to 3 months is (0.022 g × kg BW) + (0.032 × kg BW × 1.67 g). To meet endogenous losses of 10 mg P/kg BW with an absorption rate of 45 percent and to meet milk production needs estimated at 0.026 kg milk/kg BW containing 0.5 g P/kg milk that is absorbed at a 45 percent rate, the phosphorus requirement for lactation from 4 to 5 months is (0.022 g × kg BW) + (0.026 × kg BW × 1.11 g). To meet endogenous losses of 10 mg P/kg BW with an absorption rate of 45 percent and to meet milk production needs estimated at 0.020 kg milk/kg BW containing 0.5 g P/kg milk that is absorbed at a 45 percent rate, phosphorus requirement for lactation after 5 months is (0.022 g × kg BW) + (0.020 × kg BW × 1.11 g).

The influence of exercise on phosphorus requirements has been studied in combination with calcium. During the first 4 months of race training in 2-year-old Quarter horses, Nielsen et al. (1998b) reported phosphorus retention remained relatively constant over a range of phosphorus concentrations in the diet (0.21 to 0.30 percent on an as-fed basis). Likewise, 0.24 percent of the total diet (average amount fed to control group) appeared to be adequate and no apparent benefit was seen by feeding 0.29 percent, though both the minimum and maximum amounts are above the 1989 NRC recommended amount based upon a percentage of the diet. In similarly trained horses, Stephens et al. (2004) reported phosphorus requirements to be at least 66 mg/kg BW/d, which was 32 percent over the 1989 NRC recommendation. While feeding various amounts of calcium, phosphorus, and magnesium to horses in race training, Nolan et al. (2001) reported diminished mineralization of the third metacarpus when feeding phosphorus at the 1989 NRC suggested amount, even when additional calcium and magnesium was provided. Only when phosphorus was at 130 percent of the NRC recommendation (calcium and magnesium both above 150 percent) was mineralization increased. Furthermore, exercised horses had a higher phosphorus balance than did horses that were sedentary for 2 months and then exercised for 2 months (Elmore-Smith et al., 1999). Young et al. (1989) also found an increase in daily phosphorus retention when miniature horses were exercised. In contrast, Lawrence et al. (2003) reported no differences in phosphorus retention between exercising horses and sedentary horses in a review of studies reporting phosphorus intake and excretion. Likely, the majority of the horses from the studies that were reviewed were mature horses and undergoing a relatively constant training protocol in contrast to many of the studies reporting requirements higher than the 1989 NRC that were conducted in young horses just entering training. Like with calcium, any potentially higher requirements associated with exercise in the rapidly growing horse (typically under 24 months) should be met by the phosphorus requirements for growth that have been increased from the 1989 NRC. With no strong evidence to suggest mature exercising horses have a higher requirement than was suggested by the 1989 NRC, the requirements remain unchanged and are 0.058 g P × kg BW for heavy exercise, 0.042 g P × kg BW for moderate exercise, and 0.036 g P × kg BW for light exercise.

Magnesium

Function

Magnesium (Mg) constitutes approximately 0.05 percent of the body mass. Sixty percent of magnesium in the body is found in the skeleton and about 30 percent can be found in muscle (Grace et al., 1999b). Magnesium is an important ion in the blood, plays a role as an activator of many enzymes, and participates in muscle contractions.

Sources and Factors Influencing Absorption

Many commonly used feedstuffs contain 0.1–0.3 percent magnesium, and magnesium absorption from these feedstuffs appears to be 40–60 percent (Hintz and Schryver, 1972, 1973; Meyer, 1979). According to Harrington and Walsh (1980), inorganic supplemental sources such as magnesium oxide, magnesium sulfate, and magnesium carbonate appear to be essentially equivalent as supplemental dietary sources of magnesium for growing foals and have a higher absorption rate (70 percent) than the magnesium found in natural sources. Data from human studies indicate the absorption rate of magnesium oxide to be lower than magnesium citrate (Lindberg et al., 1990; Walker et al., 2003) and magnesium chloride, magnesium lactate, and magnesium aspartate (Firoz and Graber, 2001). Stadermann et al. (1992) reported apparent digestibility of magnesium was higher with alfalfa hay (51 percent) than with concentrate (31 percent). McKenzie et al. (1981) reported magnesium to be 42–45 percent digestible and not affected by oxalate. Supplemental phytase also did not affect magnesium absorption (van Doorn et al., 2004a). Further, van Doorn et al. (2004b) reported no differences in the apparent digestibility of magnesium (approximately 41–45 percent) when horses were fed rations ranging from 0.148–0.535 g Ca/kg BW/d. Excess phosphorus decreased magnesium absorption (Kapusniak et al., 1988), though the apparent digestibility of magnesium was still between 41 and 45 percent when mature ponies were fed excess phosphorus of approximately 125 mg P/kg BW/d (van Doorn et al., 2004b). In a small study, Weidenhaupt (1977) reported high potassium concentrations slightly decreased magnesium apparent digestibility. In contrast, high concentrations of aluminum did not alter magnesium absorption (Schryver et al., 1986a) and neither did varying the consumption of salt (Schryver et al., 1987b). Wall et al. (1992) reported that varying DCAD did not alter mean daily urinary excretion of magnesium. Schryver et al. (1987b) found that the calculated true absorption of magnesium was between 62 and 67 percent. Olsman et al. (2004) reported a diet rich in sugar beet pulp did not alter magnesium absorption even though pH of intestinal contents should have theoretically been lowered, resulting in increased mineral solubility. Pagan et al. (1998) reported that the apparent digestibility of magnesium in mature horses did not differ between exercised (28.5 percent) and nonexercised (35 percent) groups. Magnesium is absorbed from both the small and large intestine, though the majority appears to be absorbed from the small intestine (Kapusniak et al., 1988).

Signs of Deficiency or Excess

Meyer (1990) suggested that renal creatinine/magnesium quotients greater than 7.5 indicate an insufficient dietary supply. Stewart et al. (2004) reported that determination of urinary magnesium excretion during a 24-hour period was a better method to indicate decreased magnesium intake as compared to serum total and ionized magnesium, as well as muscle magnesium concentrations, but a spot sample of the fractional clearance of magnesium can be conveniently used to identify horses consuming a magnesium-deficient diet. Hypomagnesemia was reported in foals with magnesium intake at 7–8 mg/kg diet/d (Harrington, 1974). Assuming a feed intake equivalent to 3 percent BW, magnesium intake would have been only 0.2 mg/kg BW in comparison to the control animals receiving 390 mg/kg diet or 11.7 mg/kg BW. Clinical signs of magnesium deficiency include nervousness, muscle tremors, and ataxia, with the potential for collapse, hyperpnea, and death. Meyer and Ahlswede (1977) indicated that a magnesium intake of 5–6 mg/kg BW/d resulted in hypomagnesemia (less than 1.6 mg/dl serum) and a marked reduction in renal excretion of magnesium, whereas 20 mg of Mg/kg BW/d resulted in normal serum magnesium values of 1.6–2.0 mg/dl. Hypomagnesemia induces mineralization (focal calcium and phosphorus deposits) in the aorta. Histologic changes occur within 30 days of initiation of a low-magnesium diet (Harrington, 1974). The 1989 NRC indicated pastures that are conducive to magnesium deficiency, tetany, and death in ruminants do not affect horses similarly, though no evidence was found in the literature to provide support for this claim. However, while uncommon, tetany in transported horses has been attributed to hypocalcemia and potentially hypomagnesemia (Green et al., 1935; Merck Veterinary Manual, 2005).

Controlled studies evaluating the toxicity of magnesium in horses have not been done, though the maximum tolerable concentration has been estimated at 0.8 percent (NRC, 2005), up from 0.3 percent in the 1980 NRC. Some alfalfa hays with magnesium concentrations of 0.5 percent have been fed to horses without apparent ill effects (Lloyd et al., 1987). The source of magnesium may be important for horses, since mature ponies fed diets containing 0.86 percent magnesium for 1 month had no noted adverse effects when the magnesium source was magnesium oxide (Hintz and Schryver, 1973). Historically, magnesium sulfate was used intravenously as an anesthetic agent in horses prior to the advent of barbiturates and inhalation anesthetics (Kato et al., 1968). At normal dietary concentrations, there is no indication that magnesium sulfate has an anesthetic effect. However, magnesium sulfate is used as a saline laxative for treatment of intestinal impactions, but can cause magnesium toxicosis when overdosed, resulting in renal insufficiency, hypocalcemia, or a compromise of intestinal integrity (Henninger and Horst, 1997). Magnesium supplementation is a practice done to calm horses that could greatly influence magnesium intake if done often.

Normal serum magnesium concentrations in the horse range from 18–35 μg/dl (Puls, 1994). However, Edwards (2004) reported that serum magnesium concentrations in both Grant's and common zebras are reported to be 14 to 15 ppm.

Recommendations

Endogenous magnesium excretion was estimated at 6 mg/kg BW/d (NRC, 1989), though Pagan (1994), summarizing results from numerous studies, reported endogenous magnesium excretion of 2.2 mg/kg BW ($R^2 = 0.76$). A study by van Doorn et al. (2004b) reported magnesium retention to be around 4.4 mg/kg BW/d despite varying magnesium concentrations in the diet (from 31.4 to 38.4 mg/kg BW/d) as well as varying calcium concentrations (from 148 to 535 mg/kg BW/d). Using the initial value and a 40 percent absorption rate, a 500-kg horse at maintenance requires 7.5 g of dietary Mg/d or 15 mg/kg BW, which is lower than the 20 mg/kg BW proposed by Drepper et al. (1982). While magnesium requirements need to be better defined, Hintz (2000) suggested there are no strong reasons that the 1989 NRC magnesium requirements for maintenance are not satisfactory and that the Pagan (1994) data suggest they could potentially be lower. Requirements for gain range from 0.85 to 1.25 g Mg/kg BW gained per day (Schryver et al., 1974). Using the higher value, a 200-kg foal gaining 1 kg/d would need 1.25 g of magnesium for growth plus 3 g for endogenous fecal loss, for a total of 4.25 g/d. By comparison, using the factorial method, Grace et al. (1999b) calculated the dietary magnesium requirement of a 200-kg horse gaining 1 kg/d at 0.7 g Mg/kg DM intake. Assuming an intake of 3 percent BW, this would result in a similar intake of 4.2 g of magnesium. The magnesium requirement for growth consists of $0.015 \text{ g} \times \text{kg BW}$ to account for endogenous losses and 1.25 g magnesium for every kg of daily gain.

The magnesium requirement of the mare associated with products of conception has been estimated at 0.23, 0.31, and 0.36 mg/kg BW of the mare for months 9, 10, and 11, respectively (Drepper et al., 1982). To meet the magnesium requirement for these periods, and assuming an absorption rate of 40 percent, a 500-kg mare would need 287, 387, and 450 mg of dietary magnesium daily for fetal growth. Given that data on deposition rate of minerals in the fetus are very limited, a mean deposition rate of 0.30 mg/kg gain was used as the magnesium requirement for development of the products of conception for the last 3 months. Mean dietary magnesium required for fetal growth was added to maintenance needs for the same period to determine the requirement. This relatively minor increase in magnesium requirements for a mare during late gestation is supported by a similar finding in cattle (House and Bell, 1993). Little research is available to determine magnesium requirements during months 7 and 8 of gestation, but an additional amount between that of maintenance and late gestation was added to accommodate the growth of the products of conception. Thus, to meet endogenous losses of 6 mg Mg/kg BW with an absorption rate of 40 percent and to meet a fetal deposition rate of 0.08 mg Mg/kg BW with a 40 percent absorption rate, the magnesium requirement for months 7 and 8 of gestation is $(0.015 \text{ g} \times \text{kg BW}) + (0.0002 \text{ g} \times \text{kg BW})$, or simply $0.0152 \text{ g} \times \text{kg BW}$. To meet endogenous losses of 6 mg Mg/kg BW with an absorption rate of 40 percent and to meet fetal deposition rate of 0.12 mg Mg/kg BW with a 40 percent absorption rate, the magnesium requirement for months 9, 10, and 11 of gestation is $(0.015 \text{ g} \times \text{kg BW}) + (0.0003 \text{ g} \times \text{kg BW})$, or simply $0.0153 \text{ g} \times \text{kg BW}$.

Grace et al. (1999a) reported magnesium concentrations to be greater in colostrum (302 mg/L) than the average in milk from day 55 to day 150 (47 mg/L). Concentrations of magnesium in milk declined during the course of lactation (Schryver et al., 1986b) and concentrations during early lactation were double that of late lactation (NRC, 1989). Assuming a 40 percent absorption efficiency, a mare producing 16 kg of milk/day with a magnesium concentration of 90 μg/g of milk during early lactation would require an additional 3.6 g of dietary Mg/d for milk production in addition to her maintenance requirement of 7.5 g. Magnesium requirements for milk would be $(0.015 \text{ g} \times \text{kg BW}) + (0.032 \times \text{kg BW} \times 0.23)$ from foaling to 3 months to meet endogenous losses of 6 mg Mg/kg BW with an absorption rate of 40 percent and to meet milk production needs estimated at

0.032 kg milk/kg BW containing 0.09 g Mg/kg of milk that is absorbed at a 40 percent rate; (0.015 g × kg BW) + (0.026 × kg BW × 0.23) from 4 to 5 months to meet endogenous losses of 6 mg Mg/kg BW with an absorption rate of 40 percent and to meet milk production needs estimated at 0.026 kg milk/kg BW containing 0.09 g Mg/kg milk that is absorbed at a 40 percent rate; and (0.015 g × kg BW) + (0.020 × kg BW × 0.11) after 5 months to meet endogenous losses of 6 mg Mg/kg BW with an absorption rate of 40 percent and to meet milk production needs estimated at 0.020 kg milk/kg BW containing 0.045 g Mg/kg that is absorbed at a 40 percent rate.

Much of the work done with magnesium nutrition in exercising horses is confounded with varying concentrations of calcium and phosphorus. For instance, in a study comparing various concentrations of calcium, phosphorus, and magnesium in young horses, Nielsen et al. (1998b) found an increase in mineral content of the third metacarpus after 3 months of training in horses supplemented with extra calcium. Likewise, magnesium retention increased at that point in training. As substantial amounts of magnesium are found in bone mineral (Jee, 1988), it was hypothesized that the increased magnesium retention was caused by increased bone formation that was permitted by the additional calcium in the diet. The authors suggested that the 1989 NRC recommendations for magnesium in the young horse in training were too low and appear to be between 0.15 and 0.20 percent on an as-fed basis. Nolan et al. (2001) reported increased mineralization of the third metacarpus when the magnesium in the diet was above 150 percent of the NRC recommended amount, though their findings were also confounded with varying calcium and phosphorus concentrations. Stephens et al. (2004) reported an intake of 36 mg/kg BW/d resulted in maximal retention of magnesium at day 64 of race training in young horses fed varying amounts of calcium, phosphorus, and magnesium. These studies suggest the magnesium requirements during training are too low, though Pagan (1994) suggested that the requirement for magnesium may be about half of the NRC requirement. Most likely, exercise and stage of training influence magnesium requirements (Stephens et al., 2001), and this may explain the difference between conclusions of Pagan (1994) and those drawn from the other studies. Matsui et al. (2002) reported that in a cool ambient temperature, magnesium loss due to exercise-related sweating was small (less than 2 percent of the 1989 NRC requirement). Drepper et al. (1982) suggested that light to medium work increased magnesium requirements by 1 to 2 g/d for a 600-kg horse. Wolter et al. (1986) suggested supplementing 0.18 percent dietary magnesium for horses in training, especially if supplemental fat has been incorporated in the diet. In contrast to calcium and phosphorus, additional magnesium requirements associated with growth appear to be less than the extra requirements needed for exercise. While there is not sufficient evidence to support increasing magnesium requirements for mature horses above what was recommended in the 1989 NRC, the amount previously recommended for heavy exercise (0.030 g Mg × kg BW) and moderate exercise (0.023 g Mg × kg BW) were greater than what was recommended for both the long yearling and 2-year-old in training (0.022 g Mg × kg BW). Therefore, the recommendation for young horses (under 24 months) in training of any intensity is the same as the requirement for heavy exercise to accommodate increased needs associated with the onset of training.

To meet endogenous losses of 6 mg Mg/kg BW with an absorption rate of 40 percent and to meet additional requirement for light work of 1.6 mg Mg/kg BW with a 40 percent absorption rate, the magnesium requirement for light exercise is estimated at (0.015 g × kg BW) + (0.004 g × kg BW), or simply 0.019 g × kg BW. To meet endogenous losses of 6 mg Mg/kg BW with an absorption rate of 40 percent and to meet an additional requirement for moderate work of 3.2 mg Mg/kg BW with a 40 percent absorption rate, the magnesium requirement for moderate exercise is estimated at (0.015 g × kg BW) + (0.008 g × kg BW), or simply 0.023 g × kg BW. To meet endogenous losses of 6 mg Mg/kg BW with an absorption rate of 40 percent and to meet an additional requirement for heavy work of 6 mg Mg/kg BW with a 40 percent absorption rate, the magnesium requirement for heavy exercise is estimated at (0.015 g × kg BW) + (0.015 g × kg BW), or simply 0.030 g × kg BW.

Potassium

Function

As the major intracellular cation, potassium (K) is involved in maintenance of acid-base balance and osmotic pressure and is the most quantitatively important ion involved in neuromuscular excitability (Kronfeld, 2001). The total amount of body potassium in a 500-kg horse has been estimated to be about 28,000 mEq (Rose, 1990). Most of the body's potassium is found in skeletal muscle (Johnson, 1995), while less than 1.5 percent of the total body potassium is found in the extracellular fluid (Rose, 1990). Meyer (1987) estimated 75 percent of potassium is found in the skeletal muscle, 5 percent is in the skeleton, 5 percent is in the blood and skin, 4.5 percent is in the ingesta, and 10.5 percent is found in other tissues. After chronic potassium depletion, the greatest total amount of potassium lost was from muscle (7.5 percent of the body's total), while 3 percent of the body's total was lost from the skeleton (representing 60 percent of the skeleton's reserves).

Sources and Factors Influencing Absorption

Forages and oilseed meals generally contain 1–2 percent potassium on a dry matter basis, whereas cereal grains (corn, oats, wheat) contain 0.3–0.4 percent potassium. Normally, potassium intake greatly exceeds requirements due to the high potassium concentrations in most types of forage (Coenen, 2005). When potassium supplementation is required, potassium chloride and potassium carbonate are effective sources of supplemental potassium. Pagan and Jackson (1991b) reported the apparent digestibility of potassium to be between 61 and 65 percent, though it has been shown to be as high as 99.8 percent (Reynolds et al., 1998). Pagan (1994) estimated true potassium digestibility to be around 75 percent. Jansson et al. (1999) reported that in response to an increase in dietary potassium, urinary excretion is increased first, followed by an increase in fecal excretion. Hence, the equine kidney is particularly efficient at excreting extra potassium, but the horse may not be efficient at conserving potassium when intake is inadequate (Johnson, 1995). The body attempts to maintain a balance between dietary intake of electrolytes and excretion of them through the feces, urine, and sweat, though the amount of electrolytes excreted through the kidneys is the primary variable that can be controlled in an attempt to respond to varying intake (Coenen, 2005). The redistribution of electrolytes is needed during exercise and the gastrointestinal tract can serve as a temporary reservoir, but its capacity depends on diet and the time between feeding and exercise. If a diet containing lower concentrations of potassium is desired, feeding hay harvested from fields not heavily fertilized with potash may be advised (Hintz, 1995). Exercise in mature horses decreased apparent potassium digestibility from 74.3 percent to 66.3 percent (Pagan et al., 1998). McKenzie et al. (2002) reported that varying DCAD did not alter the daily balance of potassium.

Signs of Deficiency or Excess

Foals fed potassium-deficient, pelleted, purified diets gradually refused to eat and, therefore, lost weight, became unthrifty in appearance, and had moderately lowered serum potassium concentration (hypokalemia). On addition of potassium carbonate to the purified diet, an immediate resumption of normal feed intake occurred (Stowe, 1971). Given that fluid losses during exercise can reach 10 to 15 L per hour in the horse and that horse's sweat is hypertonic with respect to plasma, large amounts of sodium, chloride, and potassium can be lost during prolonged exercise (Flaminio and Rush, 1998). Hence, a deficiency in the exercising horse, particularly in the endurance horse, can develop. As sweat fluid losses are almost double when horses compete in a hot, humid climate as compared to a cool, dry climate (McCutcheon and Geor, 1996), dietary intake of potassium, sodium, and chloride may not be sufficient in hard working horses in warm, humid climates when supplementation is not provided. In cases of diarrhea in horses, it has been suggested that using an oral rehydration solution as an alternative to intravenous fluids may be a cost-effective method of restoring fluids and electrolytes (Ecke et al., 1998a,b; Schott, 1998). While most intravenous and oral fluid replacement products are higher in sodium than potassium, combined fecal and urinary losses resulted in greater potassium losses than sodium. As a result, potassium depletion can occur if horses are not eating. Metabolic acidosis can also occur due to an increase in plasma chloride concentrations resulting in a greater decrease in strong ion difference after oral rehydration therapy. Attention should be paid to these concerns when preparing such solutions.

Despite the NRC (2005) maximum tolerable concentration of potassium being listed as 1 percent of intake, many forages commonly fed to horses without any apparent problems have a much greater concentration of potassium. Thus, the true maximum concentration is likely much greater as excess dietary potassium is excreted readily, primarily via the urine, when water intake is unrestricted. Lewis (1995) concluded that if adequate water is not available, horses will refuse to eat if potassium concentrations are too great, in effect negating the likelihood of potassium toxicity. Additionally, the required potassium concentration in a purified-type diet for growing foals was estimated at 1 percent by Stowe (1971), further suggesting the maximum tolerable amount is greater than suggested by the 2005 NRC. However, Hintz and Schryver (1976) suggested the recommendation by Stowe to be excessive based upon studies of body composition and balance trials they conducted. The effects of excess potassium have not been studied in the horse; however, hyperkalemia, induced by parenteral administration of excess potassium, would be expected to cause cardiac arrest (Tasker, 1980), though hyperkalemia during exercise does not cause any cardiac issues. Horses with hyperkalemic periodic paralysis (HYPP) syndrome are sensitive to high potassium concentrations in their diet, but being afflicted with the problem does not seem to alter potassium balance (Reynolds et al., 1998). More information on HYPP can be found in Chapter 12.

The normal range for serum potassium concentrations has been given as 2.4 to 5.6 mEq/L by Puls (1994). The potassium concentration of the middle gluteal muscle in healthy adult horses was reported as 91.1 ± 3.0 µM potassium/g muscle (wet weight) but decreased ($P < 0.05$) to 73.6 ± 1.9 µM potassium/g muscle after 7 days of food deprivation (Johnson et al., 1991).

Recommendations

Drepper et al. (1982) estimated the daily potassium requirements for a 600-kg horse to be 22 g for maintenance (0.037 g/kg BW). Hintz and Schryver (1976), however, using a series of balance trials, calculated that mature ponies required 0.048 g of K/kg BW/d, though their data was derived only from fecal and urine losses and did not include sweat and dermal losses of potassium. As a result of not including sweat losses, Hintz and Schryver (1976) suggested that the maintenance requirement would actually be greater than 0.048 g K/kg of BW. Not being able to quantify loss of minerals (such as potassium, sodium, and chloride) through the sweat during digestibility trials tends to underestimate the requirements for those minerals by inadequately predicting the amount of mineral retained and the resulting calculated endogenous losses. An endogenous loss of 40 mg/kg BW/d with an absorption rate of 80 percent has been proposed by GEH (1994) and results in a maintenance requirement of 0.05 g K/kg BW. A 500-kg horse would thus require 25 g (500 kg × 0.05 g) of dietary potassium daily for maintenance. Since forages are usually high in potassium concentration and since forages usually constitute a major proportion of the horse's diet, requirements are typically easily satisfied.

For growth of foals with an anticipated mature body weight of 600 kg, Drepper et al. (1982) estimated the daily potassium requirements to be 11 g (about 0.05 g/kg BW) for months 3 to 6, 14 g for months 7 to 12 (about 0.04 g/kg BW), and 18 g for months 12 to 24 (about 0.03 g/kg BW). Jarrige and Martin-Rosset (1981) suggested 0.6 percent potassium in the diet of 6- to 12-month-old foals, and 0.8 percent for horses 18 to 24 months of age. Growing horses have been shown to deposit 1.5 g of K/kg gain (Schryver et al., 1974). Thus, a 215-kg foal gaining 0.85 kg BW/d and having a true potassium retention efficiency of 50 percent requires 2.6 g (1.5 g K × 0.85 kg BW/0.5) of dietary K/d for skeletal growth in addition to 10.8 g (0.05 g K × 215 kg BW) for maintenance. The 50 percent absorption rate, used by the 1989 NRC, may be low but helps to ensure that potassium will not be limited for the growing horse.

Pregnant mares require little additional potassium (Meyer and Ahlswede, 1978). Jarrige and Martin-Rosset (1981) indicated that the optimal dietary potassium concentration was 0.4 percent for late gestation. Drepper et al. (1982) indicated that the products of conception require 1.2, 1.7, and 2.2 mg of K/kg of mare weight during gestation months 9, 10, and 11, respectively. To determine requirements for late gestation, potassium for maintenance was added to an average of the amount needed for the product of conception. Hence, to meet endogenous losses of 40 mg K/kg BW with an 80 percent absorption rate and to meet a fetal deposition rate of 1.36 mg K/kg BW with an 80 percent absorption rate, the potassium requirement for months 9, 10 and 11 of gestation was estimated to be (0.05 g × kg BW) + (0.0017 g × kg BW), or simply 0.0517 g × kg BW.

Drepper et al. (1982) estimated the potassium requirement for a 600-kg mare to be 34 g during lactation, which is lower than recommended by the 1989 NRC. No research has demonstrated the requirement for lactation is different than that established by the 1989 NRC, so it was not changed. However, the percent absorption (50 percent) used to calculate the additional potassium needed for milk may be low. Additionally, new estimates of milk production are used to determine requirements. The recommended potassium requirement for lactating mares from foaling to 3 months is (0.05 g × kg BW) + (0.032 × kg BW × 1.4) to meet endogenous losses of 40 mg K/kg BW with an absorption rate of 80 percent and to meet milk production needs estimated at 0.032 kg milk/kg BW containing 0.7 g K/kg milk that is absorbed at a 50 percent rate. The requirement from 4 to 5 months is (0.05 g × kg BW) + (0.026 × kg BW × 0.8) to meet endogenous losses of 40 mg K/kg BW with an absorption rate of 80 percent and to meet milk production needs estimated at 0.026 kg milk/kg BW containing 0.4 g K/kg milk that is absorbed at a 50 percent rate. The requirement for lactation after 5 months is estimated to be (0.05 g × kg BW) + (0.020 × kg BW × 0.8) to meet endogenous losses of 40 mg K/kg BW with an absorption rate of 80 percent and to meet milk production needs estimated at 0.020 kg milk per kg BW containing 0.4 g K/kg milk that is absorbed at a 50 percent rate.

Renal excretion of potassium increases in reaction to exercise and, combined with heavy sweating losses, can lead to a potential potassium deficit (Meyer, 1987; Schott et al., 1991; Johnson, 1998). Jarrige and Martin-Rosset (1981) indicated that the optimal potassium concentrations of equine diets were 0.4 to 0.5 percent for light to medium work. Drepper et al. (1982) estimated the daily potassium requirements for a 600-kg horse to be 32 g for light work (0.053 g/kg BW), 43 g for medium work (0.072 g/kg BW), and 53 g (0.088 g/kg BW) for heavy work. When maintenance requirements are applied to the work of Drepper et al. (1982), the requirement for light, medium, and heavy work become 1.1, 1.4, and 1.8 times maintenance, respectively. This relationship has also been approximated by a potassium-to-DE relationship. Hoyt et al. (1995a) proposed diets for exercising horses should contain 4.5 g K/Mcal DE.

The main increase in requirements for the electrolytes potassium, sodium, and chloride associated with exercise is to replace the amounts lost in sweat. Typical equine diets contain excess potassium, so inclusion of potassium in electrolytes for horses may not be needed. Supplementation of an electrolyte mixture without potassium resulted in a similar completion rate to horses supplemented with a potassium-containing electrolyte mixture in an 80-km endurance ride (Hess et al., 2005). Exercise conditions greatly influence sweat production but quantifying sweat production in the field is not simple (Coenen, 2005). However, sweat losses account for about 90 percent of the changes in body weight during exercise (Meyer et al., 1990). Thus, Coenen (2005) proposed that, for practical purposes, the change in body weight during exercise can be used as an estimate of sweat losses. Using data from Meyer et al. (1990) and McCutcheon and Geor (1998), Coenen (2005) estimated equine sweat to contain 1.4 g K/L, so the potassium recommendation for exercise can be expressed as maintenance plus 2.8 g (1.4 g/0.50 percent absorption) for every kilogram of weight lost during exercise. Some weight loss obviously can occur through defecation and urination, but this amount is relatively small compared to sweat losses

(Butudom et al., 2002). An exception to this is when furosemide is administered, as furosemide greatly increases urine production (Hinchcliff et al., 1995) and likely increases urinary loss of electrolytes. This could result in an increased transient requirement associated with the estimated 700,000 doses given to Thoroughbred and Standardbred racehorses a year in the United States (Hinchcliff, 2005). While requiring weighing a horse before and after exercise, and though not applicable after furosemide administration, using weight loss as an estimate of sweat loss likely provides an accurate estimate of the additional potassium requirements associated with exercise. Because it is not always practical to weigh horses before and after exercise, estimates of sweat loss for horses performing different levels of exercise have been made in order to estimate the electrolyte requirements of exercising horses. It is important to note that sweat loss will be greatly influenced by environmental temperature and whether the animal is acclimated to the imposed exercise and the environmental conditions. A discussion of factors affecting sweat losses can be found in Chapter 7. McConaghy (1994) has suggested that 1 liter of sweat is necessary to dissipate 580 kcal of heat in the horse. Therefore, sweat loss may be approximated from heat production during exercise. The factors affecting heat production during exercise are discussed in Chapter 1. For the purposes of this document, daily sweat loss associated with work for horses in the light, moderate, heavy, and very heavy exercise categories are estimated at 0.25, 0.5, 1, and 2 percent of body weight, respectively. These estimates are based on weekly workloads expected for the horses in different categories and do not necessary account for losses associated with a strenuous competition, such as a race or a 3-day event. After a strenuous event, particularly in a hot environment, additional supplementation may be necessary to replace electrolyte losses. A sweat loss of 2.4 percent of body weight has been reported in horses becoming acclimated to and exercising in hot, humid conditions (McCutcheon et al., 1999). This percentage, greater than the estimate used for very heavy exercise, demonstrates the impact environmental conditions have on sweating rate and serves as a reminder that the estimates for sweat loss for varying intensities of work are only a guide and can be much greater.

Sodium

Function

Sodium (Na) is critical for normal function of the central nervous system, generation of action potentials in excitable tissues, and transport of many substances such as glucose across cell membranes (Johnson, 1995). Sodium is the major extracellular cation and the major electrolyte involved in maintenance of acid-base balance and osmotic regulation of body fluids. The average sodium concentration in the extracellular fluid is 138 to 140 mmol/L, which is about 14,000 mmol for a 500-kg horse with an extracellular fluid volume of 100 L (Rose, 1990). This is referred to as the exchangeable sodium. The skeleton contains 51.1 percent of the sodium in the body, the ingesta contains 12.4 percent, both blood and muscle contain 10.8 percent, the skin contains 8.5 percent, and the organs contain 2.1 percent, according to Meyer (1987). During chronic sodium completion, the greatest loss is from the ingesta (9.9 percent of the body's total sodium), with the next greatest loss coming from the skeleton (5.2 percent of the body's total).

Sources and Factors Influencing Absorption

The sodium concentration of natural feedstuffs for horses is often lower than 0.1 percent. Sodium chloride ((NaCl) common salt) is often added to concentrates at rates of 0.5 percent to 1 percent or fed free-choice as plain, iodized, cobalt-iodized, or trace-mineralized salt. In exercising horses, Jansson and Dahlborn (1999) reported sodium intake solely from a salt block was equal to or less (range from 0 to 62 mg/kg BW/d) than the maintenance requirement in four out of six horses, suggesting supplementation in feed may be required for some exercising horses to meet losses associated with sweating. Ingesta in the large intestine has been shown to be a reservoir for water, as well as for sodium, chloride, and potassium, when exercising (Meyer, 1996a,b), and may be why exercising horses rarely develop severe hyponatraemia despite losing substantial amounts of sodium through their sweat. Sosa Leon et al. (1998) concluded administration of electrolyte paste is advantageous over water alone in restoring fluid, electrolyte, and acid-base balance after fluid and electrolyte loss attributable to furosemide administration. Butudom et al. (2002) reported 0.45 and 0.9 percent saline solutions, offered during the first 5 minutes after completing exercise, were more effective in maintaining elevated plasma sodium concentrations and restoring body weight loss during exercise than was water alone. It was cautioned that this should be pursued after horses have been trained to drink salt water during and after exercise to prevent greater dehydration. Additionally, repeated oral administration of an electrolyte solution has been associated with an exacerbation of gastric ulcers (Holbrook et al., 2005). Urinary sodium loss is minimized when sodium is relatively deficient in the diet and temperatures are cool (Tasker, 1967), as well as after exercise (Jansson et al., 1995). Lindinger et al. (2000) also reported an improved conservation of sodium after heat acclimation and training. However, sodium excretion in the feces may exceed that in urine under some conditions (Alexander, 1977). When dietary sodium is increased, an increase in urinary excretion will maintain the total exchangeable sodium pool (Rose, 1990). Sodium concentrations have been reported to increase in equine sweat in response to exercise (McCutcheon and Geor, 1998; Jansson et al., 1999).

Schryver et al. (1987b) found 75–94 percent of ingested sodium was absorbed. Pagan et al. (1998) reported the apparent digestibility of sodium to be increased in four mature horses from 48.9–83.6 percent—presumably to meet the increased sodium needs that accompany additional sweat losses. Apparent absorption of sodium was 99.6 percent in mature broodmares (Reynolds et al., 1998).

Signs of Deficiency or Excess

Chronic sodium depletion results in decreased skin turgor, a tendency for horses to lick objects such as sweat-contaminated tool handles, a slowed rate of eating, decreased water intake, and eventually a cessation of eating (Meyer et al., 1984). In acute sodium deficiency, muscle contractions and chewing were uncoordinated and horses had an unsteady gait; serum sodium and chloride concentrations decreased markedly, whereas serum potassium increased (Meyer et al., 1984). As ambient temperatures and exercise intensity increased, sodium concentrations in sweat increased and sodium losses could result in relatively large ion deficits (McCutcheon and Geor, 1998). This can lead to alterations in skeletal muscle ion content and potentially muscular dysfunction. As long as sufficient water is available, excess sodium will typically be excreted in the urine. The maximum tolerable concentration of sodium chloride in the diet has been set at 6 percent of intake (NRC, 2005).

Recommendations

Optimal sodium concentrations for equine diets have been reported to be between 1.6 and 1.8 g/kg dry matter for growth, maintenance, and late gestation and 3.6 g/kg dry matter for moderate to heavy work (Jarrige and Martin-Rosset, 1981). Endogenous sodium loss in the idle adult horse has been estimated at 15 to 20 mg/kg BW/d (Meyer et al., 1984; Schryver et al., 1987b). If sodium is 90 percent absorbed, and using an endogenous loss of 18 mg/kg BW/d, the maintenance requirement is 0.02 g Na/kg BW daily. A 500-kg horse would meet that requirement by consuming 25 g NaCl/day.

Based upon whole body analyses of euthanized foals, Grace et al. (1999b) determined 0.85 g Na/d were deposited at an absorption rate of 80 percent, resulting in a calculated daily sodium requirement of 1 g sodium for a 200-kg horse gaining 1 kg/d. The requirement for growing horses has been set at $(0.02 \text{ g} \times \text{kg BW}) + (1.0 \text{ g} \times \text{average daily gain in kg})$ to meet endogenous losses of 18 mg Na/kg BW with a 90 percent absorption rate and to meet growth requirements of 0.85 g Na/kg BW gain with an 80 percent absorption rate.

Drepper et al. (1982) reported that the sodium requirement of pregnant mares, above maintenance, is approximately 1.9 mg/kg BW/d during the 10th month of gestation. The requirement for months 9, 10, and 11 of pregnancy has been estimated as $(0.02 \text{ g} \times \text{kg BW}) + (0.002 \text{ g} \times \text{kg BW})$, or simply $0.022 \text{ g} \times \text{kg BW}$, to meet endogenous losses of 18 mg Na/kg BW with a 90 percent absorption rate and to meet a fetal deposition rate of 1.9 mg Na/kg BW based upon the work of Drepper et al. (1982).

Schryver et al. (1986b) reported sodium concentrations during the first 3 months after foaling to average 180 mg/kg fluid milk, but had dropped to 115 mg/kg milk from 12 to 17 weeks. Grace et al. (1999a) reported sodium concentrations to average 130 mg/L milk in pasture-fed mares during the first 5 months after foaling, which would equate to about 126 mg/kg milk. Using an average of the two estimates and an absorption rate of 90 percent, each kg of milk would require 0.17 g sodium during the first 3 months of lactation and 0.14 g sodium after that. Thus, from foaling to 3 months, the sodium requirement for lactating mares is $(0.02 \text{ g} \times \text{kg BW}) + (0.032 \times \text{kg BW} \times 0.17)$ to meet endogenous losses of 18 mg Na/kg BW with an absorption rate of 90 percent and to meet milk production needs estimated at 0.032 kg milk/kg BW containing 0.153 g Na/kg milk that is absorbed at a 90 percent rate. From 4 to 5 months, the estimated requirement is $(0.02 \text{ g} \times \text{kg BW}) + (0.026 \times \text{kg BW} \times 0.14)$ to meet endogenous losses of 18 mg Na/kg BW with an absorption rate of 90 percent and to meet milk production needs estimated at 0.026 kg milk/kg BW containing 0.126 g Na/kg milk that is absorbed at a 90 percent rate. After 5 months, the sodium requirement for lactating mares is estimated as $(0.02 \text{ g} \times \text{kg BW}) + (0.020 \times \text{kg BW} \times 0.14)$ to meet endogenous losses of 18 mg Na/kg BW with an absorption rate of 90 percent and to meet milk production needs estimated at 0.020 kg milk/kg BW containing 0.126 g Na/kg milk that is absorbed at a 90 percent rate.

Even though sodium excretion has been shown to be reduced by as much as 73 percent during the early stages of training (McKeever et al., 2002), prolonged exercise and elevated temperatures increase the sodium requirement because sweat contains a notable amount of sodium. Sodium losses in sweat are estimated to range from 8.25 to 82.5 g (Meyer, 1987). Butudom et al. (2002) calculated sodium losses due to sweat losses during endurance exercise to be between 1,500 to 2,000 mmol (34.5 to 46 g), with an additional loss of 1,500 mmol (34.5 g) due to administration of furosemide, a diuretic. Meyer et al. (1984) reported that a negative sodium balance could be demonstrated transiently in nonexercised horses and ponies after initial restriction of sodium intake to 5 mg/kg BW/d. However, over time, these horses adapted to sodium restriction and, ultimately, could be in positive sodium balance while consuming only 1.6 mg Na/kg BW/day. Hoyt et al. (1995a) proposed diets for horses exercising in hot, humid conditions should contain 1.3 g Na/Mcal DE. Because of limited data on specific requirements for sodium and the influence of activity, adaptation, and environment on animal needs, precise recommendations cannot be made. However, the 1989 NRC suggested sodium concentration in the maintenance diet should be at least 0.1 percent. For intensely exercising horses in a hot climate, Hoyt et al. (1995b) indicated that 0.41 percent sodium in the diet of horses drinking tap water would be necessary to meet sodium demands and that adding 0.9 percent salt to the diet would meet those demands. This represents a large salt intake that would not normally be required under less stringent conditions. A more precise estimate of sodium requirements can be determined with exercising horses by measuring weight losses during exercise, and using weight loss as an estimate of sweat loss. Sweat contains 2.8 g Na/L (Coenen, 2005), so adding 3.1 g Na/kg weight loss during exercise to maintenance requirements provides a reasonable estimate of sodium requirements during exercise. Thus, the requirement for sodium in exercising horses has been estimated as (0.02 g × kg BW) + (3.1 g × BW loss in kg during exercise) to meet endogenous losses of 18 mg Na/kg BW with an absorption rate of 90 percent and to meet additional requirement for work associated with sweat loss of 2.8 g of Na/kg of BW loss as an estimate of sweat loss during exercise with a 90 percent absorption rate.

Chlorine

Function

Chlorine (Cl) normally accompanies sodium in the diet as the anion chloride. Chloride is an important extracellular anion involved in acid-base balance and osmotic regulation. It is an essential component of bile and is important in the formation of hydrochloric acid, a component of gastric secretions necessary for digestion.

Sources and Factors Influencing Absorption

Common salt is 61 percent chloride and is often used to meet chlorine needs. Some chloride concentrations of common equine feedstuffs range from 0.05 percent for corn and soybean meal to 3 percent for molasses (NRC, 1982). Schryver et al. (1987b) reported chloride absorption to be 100 percent and did not vary as dietary sodium chloride concentrations increased.

Signs of Deficiency or Excess

A chlorine deficiency is unlikely to occur without a sodium deficiency, although it could occur if horses were being administered sodium bicarbonate (Lewis, 1995). Chlorine deficiency was clearly correlated to metabolic alkalosis as observed in horses with minimized chlorine intake (Coenen, 1988, 1991) because of a compensatory increase in bicarbonate during the chlorine deficit (Tasker, 1980). Clinical signs of chlorine deficiency may be similar to those reported in ruminants, which include decreased food intake, weight loss, muscle weakness, decreased milk production, dehydration, constipation, and depraved appetite (Fettman et al., 1984).

Horses are considered tolerant of high concentrations of salt in their diets if they have free access to fresh drinking water. High salt concentrations in feeds are sometimes used to limit feed intake, especially of supplements. Parker (1984) reported that ponies consumed a 3-day grain ration over 3 days when the grain contained 16 percent salt but consumed the same ration in 1–2 days when the grain contained only 4–8 percent salt. The elevated dietary salt concentrations were associated with marked increases in water intake. Regulating the concentrate intake by salt addition is generally not as effective in horses as in ruminants. The maximum percentages of the daily salt requirements tolerated in drinking water for 450-kg working and lactating horses were estimated at 840 and 1,050 percent, respectively (NRC, 1974). Central nervous system manifestations of salt toxicity occur in some species. Horses can be expected to respond similarly, though it has not been documented.

Chloride concentrations in serum or plasma provide a good guide to chlorine balance (Rose, 1990). Normal range for plasma chloride concentrations in mature performance horses has been given as 94–104 mmol/L (Hodgson and Rose, 1994).

Recommendations

While the chlorine requirements of horses have not been strongly established, chlorine requirements are presumed to be adequate when the sodium requirements are met with sodium chloride. However, a review of studies by Coenen (1999) revealed fecal chlorine excretion to be 2.3 ± 1.2 mg/kg BW/d without any major influence of chlorine intake. Given that chloride absorption can be 100 percent (Schryver et al., 1987b), this likely represents the fecal endogenous losses. Coenen (1999) proposed using 3 mg Cl/kg BW to account for fecal endogenous losses, 2 mg/kg BW for renal endogenous losses, and 1 mg/kg BW for cutaneous endogenous losses for a total of 6 mg Cl/kg BW/d for total endogenous losses. Another 14 mg Cl/kg BW/d was suggested to replace that loss through perspiration for a total minimum maintenance requirement of 20 mg Cl/kg BW/d. However, 80 mg/kg BW/d were required to prevent changes in acid-base balance and hypochloremia and this likely represents the recommended minimum daily chlorine intake and has been set as the maintenance requirement.

Coenen (1999) suggested the requirements for growth up to 6 months of age equals maintenance plus 13 mg Cl/kg BW/d, and maintenance plus 5 mg Cl/kg BW/d for 6–12 months. Though specific requirements for growth from 12–24 months have not been specifically determined, an intermediate value between the long weanling and maintenance is used. Thus, the requirement for growing horses is estimated as (0.08 g × kg BW) + (0.013 g × kg BW), or simply 0.093 g Cl × kg BW, to meet maintenance requirements and to meet growth requirements. The requirement for growing horses 6 to 12 months of age is estimated to be (0.08 g × kg BW) + (0.005 g × kg BW), or simply 0.085 g Cl × kg BW, to meet maintenance requirements and to meet growth requirements. For growing horses 12 to 24 months, the requirement has been set at (0.08 g × kg BW) + (0.0025 g × kg BW), or simply 0.0825 g Cl × kg BW, to meet maintenance requirements and to meet growth requirements.

During the last 3 months of pregnancy, requirements equal maintenance plus 2 mg Cl/kg BW/d or simply 0.082 g Cl × kg BW. Lactation requirements are maintenance plus 11 mg Cl/kg BW/d (0.091 g Cl × kg BW) based upon data from literature related to milk composition (Coenen, 1999).

Hoyt et al. (1995a) proposed rations for exercising horses should contain 3.1 g Cl/Mcal DE. For a 500-kg horse consuming 24.6 Mcal DE, this would equate to 76.3 g Cl or 150 mg Cl/kg BW. Alternatively, Hoyt et al. (1995b) proposed intensely exercising horses in a hot climate consuming tap water would need 0.88 percent chlorine in the ration, which could be met by adding 1.14 percent salt to the ration. Alternatively, Coenen (1999) suggested chlorine requirements for exercising horses equal maintenance requirements plus 5.5 mg Cl/g sweat/kg BW. An average of 5.3 g Cl/L sweat was given later by Coenen (2005), and that average was used in establishing the requirement for horses based upon sweat loss. Thus, the requirement for exercise is (0.08 g × kg BW) + (5.3 g × BW loss in kg during exercise) to meet maintenance requirements and to meet the additional requirement for work associated with sweat loss assuming a concentration of 5.3 g Cl/kg sweat and using BW loss as an estimate of sweat loss during exercise with a 100 percent Cl absorption rate.

Sulfur

Function

Sulfur, in the form of sulfur-containing amino acids, B vitamins (thiamin and biotin), heparin, insulin, and chondroitin sulfate, makes up about 0.15 percent of the body weight. The sulfur-containing amino acids cysteine and methionine play a major role in the structural component of almost all proteins and enzymes in the body. Thiamin is involved in carbohydrate metabolism, biotin is a co-enzyme involved with intermediary metabolism, heparin serves as an anticoagulant, insulin helps regulate carbohydrate metabolism, and chondroitin sulfate is important to joint health.

Sources and Factors Influencing Absorption

Horses must meet their sulfur requirements from organic forms such as cystine and methionine. Although about 10–15 percent of total plant sulfur is inorganic, most of the sulfur in plants is organic sulfur present in the amino acids in the plant proteins (Georgievskii et al., 1982). Some dietary inorganic sulfur is incorporated into sulfur-containing microbial protein in the equine hindgut, but amino acid absorption from this region is limited. Inorganic forms of dietary sulfur are used in the synthesis of some sulfur-containing substances such as chondroitin sulfate, heparin, and insulin. Adequate, high-quality dietary protein (e.g., from soybean meal) usually provides at least 0.15 percent organic sulfur. No studies were found that specifically examined sulfur absorption rates, though Wall et al. (1992) reported that anaerobically exercised horses that had a sulfur intake of 16 g/d had urinary excretion of 22 g/d regardless of dietary cation-anion balance. While this suggests a tremendous loss of sulfur from the body is possible, the work also suggests sulfur absorption may be high.

Signs of Deficiency or Excess

Sulfur deficiency in horses has not been described. The maximum tolerable dietary sulfur concentration has been estimated at 0.5 percent from data in other species (NRC, 2005). Corke (1981), however, reported the effects of excess sulfur on 5- to 12-year-old horses that were accidentally fed between 200 and 400 g of flowers of sulfur (> 99 percent sulfur). The horses became lethargic within 12 hours, and colic often supervened. Other signs included a yellow, frothy discharge from the external nares, jaundiced mucous membranes, and labored breathing. Two of the 12 horses developed an expiratory snort and cyanosis; despite treatment, they died following convulsions. Chronic consumption of excess sulfur in ruminants depresses copper absorption and can induce secondary copper deficiencies. No evidence has been found that the equine species is subject to this effect of sulfur (Strickland et al., 1987).

Recommendations

The sulfur requirements of the horse have not been established, though the sulfur in high-quality dietary protein appears adequate to meet the sulfur requirements of the horse (NRC, 1978; Jarrige and Martin-Rosset, 1981). Until further studies verify the need for adjustment, the recommendations of the 1989 NRC (0.15 percent sulfur on a DM basis) remain unchanged.

MICROMINERALS

Cobalt

Function

Cecal and colonic microflora of horses use dietary cobalt (Co) in the synthesis of vitamin B_{12} (Davies, 1971; Salminen, 1975), and cobalt, in the form of vitamin B_{12}, is interrelated with iron and copper in hematopoiesis or blood cell formation (Ammerman, 1970).

Sources and Factors Influencing Absorption

Common horse feeds typically contain between 0.05 to 0.6 mg Co/kg dietary dry matter (DM). Cobalt-iodized salt often contains around 100 mg cobalt/kg DM. The lower Atlantic Coastal Plain and parts of New England have soils that are deficient in cobalt, as do other areas of the world including Australia, New Zealand, East Africa, and Norway (Ammerman, 1970). Information regarding the availability of various compounds is limited, but the carbonate, chloride, and sulfate forms of cobalt have been proposed as adequate sources for beef cattle (Cunha et al., 1964).

Signs of Deficiency or Excess

A cobalt deficiency would result in a vitamin B_{12} deficiency. However, no known cases of either a cobalt or vitamin B_{12} deficiency have been reported or experimentally induced in horses. A maximum tolerable concentration of 25 mg/kg DM intake has been set for cobalt from data in other species (NRC, 2005).

Recommendations

The cobalt requirements of horses have not been studied specifically. Filmer (1933) reported that horses remained in good health while grazing pastures that were inadequate in cobalt for ruminants. The 1989 NRC set the minimum recommended amount for horses at 0.1 mg cobalt/kg DM. Considering that the occurrence of deficiency symptoms in cattle and sheep were observed at concentrations of less than 0.04 to 0.07 mg/kg dietary DM, and considering that horses are tolerant of lower concentrations than cattle, the minimum recommended amount has been set at 0.05 mg/kg dietary DM. This should typically be met through the consumption of normal feedstuffs.

Copper

Function

Copper (Cu) is essential for several copper-dependent enzymes involved in the synthesis and maintenance of elastic connective tissue, mobilization of iron stores, preservation of the integrity of mitochondria, melanin synthesis, and detoxification of superoxide.

Sources and Factors Affecting Absorption

The copper concentration of common feedstuffs ranges widely from approximately 1 mg/kg for corn to 80 mg/kg for cane molasses. Although few controlled studies on comparative copper availability have been reported for the horse, salts such as cupric chloride, cupric sulfate, and cupric carbonate are effective supplemental copper sources in other nonruminants (Cromwell et al., 1978, 1984). Though Cymbaluk et al. (1981a) suggested the efficiency of copper absorption is inversely related to the dietary copper concentration, Lawrence (2004) did not find such a relationship when doing a retrospective analysis of nine studies reported between 1981 and 2003. It should be noted that the reviewed studies used a variety of copper sources, which may have confounded the results. Schryver et al. (1987b) reported copper absorption to range between 24 and 48 percent. Pagan (1994) estimated true copper digestibility to be around 40 percent in the mature horse (calculated endogenous loss estimated at 38 mg/d), while Pagan and Jackson (1991b) reported apparent digestibilities of copper ranging from 27.2–32.5 percent. Hudson et al. (2001) did not detect differences in true copper digestibility between sedentary horses (41.8 percent) and exercised horses (54.4 percent). Pagan and Jackson (1991a) reported apparent copper digestibility to be higher in a pelleted blend of alfalfa and Bermuda straw (36.2 percent) as compared to alfalfa hay (10 percent) or alfalfa pellets (9.2 percent). Wagner et al. (2005) reported the absorption of copper oxide, sulfate, and an organic-chelate to be 5.3, 6.6, and 2.8 percent, respectively, and these did not differ between sources. However, it was noted that these values were lower than previous studies. No differences on bone metabolism (Baker et al., 2003) or liver copper concentrations (Siciliano et al., 2001) were found between an inorganic copper source and a mix of organic and inorganic copper sources. However, Miller et al. (2003) reported an increase in copper retention and apparent digestibility of yearling horses supplemented with an organic copper source (proteinate) as compared to copper sulfate. In contrast, Baker et al. (2005) showed that apparent copper digestibility and retention were greater in mature horses supplemented with copper sulfate as compared to the same organic copper proteinate.

Several factors can influence copper metabolism. Copper interacts with many other minerals, including molybdenum, sulfur, zinc, selenium, silver, cadmium, iron, and lead (Underwood, 1981). There are limited quantitative studies in the horse that explore these relationships; however, some distinct species differences are known. Molybdenum intakes at 1 to 3 mg/kg of the ration interfered with copper utilization in ruminants (Underwood, 1981), but much higher concentrations of molybdenum were tolerated by the horse (Underwood, 1977; Cymbaluk et al., 1981b). Molybdenum at 20 mg/kg of the ration did not interfere with copper absorption (Rieker et al., 1999). Therefore, the likelihood of a molybdenum problem in the horse is minimal (Strickland et al., 1987). In contrast, a secondary copper deficiency was induced after 5 to 6 weeks in weanling foals fed a basic ration containing 7.7 mg Cu/kg of ration and containing either 1,000 or 2,000 mg zinc/kg of the ration, but not when the ration contained either 29.1 or 250 mg zinc/kg (Bridges and Moffitt, 1990).

Signs of Deficiency or Excess

Osteochondrosis and osteodysgenesis reportedly are associated with hypocupremia (Carbery, 1978; Bridges et al., 1984). When foals were fed a liquid milk-replacer diet containing 1.7 mg Cu/kg DM for 13–16 weeks, lameness was observed 2–6 weeks after serum copper concentrations had decreased to less than 0.1 µg/ml (Bridges and Harris, 1988). A decline in serum copper with increasing age of mares appeared to be related to the incidence of usually fatal rupture of the uterine artery in aged, parturient mares (Stowe, 1968). Feeding 8 ppm copper, as compared to 25 ppm, resulted in declining liver copper values, osteochondritis, epiphysitis, and limb deformities over a 6-month period (Hurtig et al., 1993). However, van Weeren et al. (2003) found no relationship between liver copper concentrations and osteochondrosis (see Chapter 12 for further discussion on the role of Cu in developmental orthopedic disease).

Horses are relatively tolerant of high dietary copper concentrations. Pony mares fed 791 mg of Cu/kg ration for 183 days had elevated liver copper, but no adverse clinical signs were observed in the mares or their foals (Smith et al., 1975). Single oral doses of 20 and 40 mg of Cu/kg BW (as copper sulfate) were administered to mature ponies without apparent adverse effects (Stowe, 1980). The maximum tolerable concentration of copper for horses has been estimated to be approximately 250 mg/kg ration (NRC, 2005), though the report by Smith et al. (1975) provided evidence that it may be substantially higher. Other dietary factors such as zinc or iron concentrations, as well as the source of copper, can influence this also.

Bathe and Cash (1995) suggested serum copper concentrations may be of limited clinical usefulness in assessing copper status. Mee and McLaughlin (1995) reported a wide range in what is considered to be "normal" serum copper concentrations, depending upon what procedures are used and whether the population of horses being routinely sampled is supplemented or not. Auer et al. (1989) reported an increase in plasma copper concentrations in response to an acute reaction after localized injury, suggesting another limitation of sampling blood to assess dietary copper status. Suttle et al. (1996) proposed a threshold value for serum copper of 16 µmol/L to distinguish normal from subnormal copper status and 11.5 µmol/L as an interim threshold to distinguish a deficient from a marginal copper status. Newborn foals have low serum copper concentrations as compared to mature horses (Cymbaluk et al., 1986). Additionally, an apparent sedimentation of ceruloplasmin copper occurs during clot retraction resulting in lower serum copper concentrations than obtained for using plasma (Paynter, 1982). Meyer and Tiegs (1995) proposed that liver copper concentrations in the 10- and 11-month-old fetus of greater than 300 µg Cu/g DM and in newly born foals of greater than 400 µg of Cu/g DM reflect an adequate copper supply of their dams.

Recommendations

Jarrige and Martin-Rosset (1981) and Drepper et al. (1982) recommended 10 mg Cu/kg ration for all ages of horses, regardless of degree of work or stage of production, though Jeffcott and Davies (1998) suggested that there are differences in copper requirements for horses of different breed, age, sex, and pregnancy status. Hudson et al. (2001) showed endogenous copper losses to be 15.7 mg/d (0.029 mg Cu/kg BW with a true copper digestibility of 41.8 percent) for sedentary horses and 20.3 mg/d (0.038 mg Cu/kg BW with a true copper digestibility of 54.5 percent) for exercising horses averaging 534 kg, with a resultant requirement ranging from 35 to 44 mg Cu/d (0.066 to 0.083 mg Cu/kg BW/d). By comparison, in evaluating the results of many prior studies, Pagan (1994) estimated endogenous copper loss to be about 0.069 mg/kg BW and the true digestibility of copper to be 40 percent. The resulting requirement for a 500-kg horse would be 86 mg Cu/d or 0.172 mg Cu/kg BW. Assuming an intake of 2 percent of BW, this would result in a dietary copper concentration of 8.6 mg/kg DM feed, suggesting the 10 mg/kg DM requirement given in the 1989 NRC is adequate for maintenance. Noting the lower copper absorption rate in various feedstuffs, a 35 percent absorption rate was used with the endogenous copper losses estimated by Pagan (1994) to ensure adequate dietary copper with the resultant copper requirement for maintenance being 0.2 mg/kg BW/d.

Only one study could be found that made an attempt at factoring out the true copper requirement for growth based on whole body analysis. Grace et al. (1999b) determined 1 mg Cu/d was deposited at an estimated absorption rate of 30 percent for gain of 1 kg/d in 200-kg foals. The result would increase requirements over maintenance by only 0.017 mg Cu/kg BW/d. That would result in a requirement of 0.217 mg Cu/kg BW for growing horses. If that were converted to a concentration basis assuming a 2.5 percent feed intake, it would result in a recommendation of 8.68 mg Cu/kg DM intake. Satisfactory growth was attained by foals fed 9 mg Cu/kg ration (Cupps and Howell, 1949), whereas normal copper homeostasis was maintained in mature ponies fed 3.5 mg of Cu/kg ration (Cymbaluk et al., 1981a). Knight et al. (1985) reported a negative correlation between the copper concentrations of weanling rations and a perceived degree of affliction with metabolic bone disease. The 1989 NRC subcommittee reviewed the data by Knight et al. (1985) and a follow-up study by Knight et al. (1988) that reported histologic lesions without statistical inference. The subcommittee considered the data to be inconclusive and left the copper requirements for growth, pregnancy, and lactation unchanged from the previous NRC (1978). In support of this, Kronfeld et al. (1990) pointed out that the correlation reported by Knight et al. (1985) becomes nonsignificant (P > 0.05) if two outlier values (32 and 40 ppm of copper) were eliminated from the 19 points.

Subsequently, Knight et al. (1990) published greater details of the 1988 study. Mares were fed either 13 ppm or 32 ppm during the last 3 to 6 months of gestation and the first 3 months of lactation. Their respective foals were fed a pelleted concentrate containing 15 ppm or 55 ppm and were then euthanized at 3 or 6 months and necropsied. Foals receiving the ration containing the lower copper concentration had more lesions than did the ones receiving supplementation at the higher rate though one foal in the low copper group accounted for a disproportional percentage of the lesions. Similarly, Hurtig et al. (1993) reported defective cartilage and bone growth in foals fed 8 ppm as compared to those receiving 25 ppm. Though the information may be useful, the animals in that study were housed by treatment in two pens so the experimental number is arguably only one (n = 1), thus, the statistical inference lacks validity. Supplementation with copper at the rate of 0.5 mg Cu/kg BW to foals on pasture containing 4.4 to 8.6 ppm copper had no effect on bone or cartilage parameters, but similar supplementation of mares decreased radiographic indices of physitis in the distal third metatarsal bone of their foals at 150 days and the prevalence of articular cartilage lesions (Pearce et al., 1998a). These results led the investigators to conclude that mare supplementation probably had an effect on foal skeletal development in utero rather than through the provision of greater copper stores in the liver of neonates. (It should be noted that the zinc:copper ratio appears to be over three times greater in the unsupplemented group than in the supplemented group [Pearce et al., 1998c], and the horses in the study also had low calcium and phosphorus intakes, as well as calcium:phosphorus ratios below 1 for 6 of the 11 months of the trial [Pearce et al., 1998a], and these factors certainly could have influenced the results). Gee et al. (2000) reported parenteral copper supplementation of broodmares in late gestation had no effect on liver copper concentration of foals at birth, though copper liver concentrations can be increased through supplementation beginning after birth (Pearce et al., 1998b). Though all the broodmares were consuming the same pasture, Van Weeren et al. (2003) reported that foals born with low liver copper concentrations had worsening osteochondrosis scores from 5 to 11 months, while foals born with higher liver copper concentrations showed improvement. This finding led them to propose that copper may be involved in the repair process of existing lesions during growth.

Interestingly, Voges et al. (1990) found copper concentrations in equine bone increase up to age 8 and then begin to decrease. It was proposed that the lower amount in older horses may be the result of differences in feeding horses in more recent years, when supplementation is more frequent, providing some support for the greater incorporation of copper into the skeleton if it is available. This finding raises the question as to whether increased copper concentrations in the ration are efficacious in reducing the incidence of osteochondrosis. Despite most commercially prepared feeds for growing horses typically containing substantially higher amounts of copper than the amount recommended by the 1989 NRC, the incidence of osteochondrosis remains high in certain populations of horses. Interestingly, Gabel (2005) reported that the optimum concentration of copper from a follow-up study of the farms used in the Knight et al. (1985) study appeared to be 25 ppm. However, Gabel (2005) reported that in the follow-up study, yearlings were consuming 160 percent of the protein requirements and 120 percent of the energy requirements recommended by the NRC. Savage (1992) reported that when 48 foals were fed 11.1 to 11.7 ppm Cu, there was no increase in osteochondrosis provided the DE and phosphorus content were similar to what was suggested by the 1989 NRC. These studies emphasized the apparent need to feed a balanced ration rather than simply increase the concentration of a single nutrient. Furthermore, in a study using 629 Hanoverian foals from 83 farms, Winkelsett et al. (2005) reported no relationship between copper intake of the pregnant mare and osteochondrosis in the foals. Though the requirement, based upon the replacement of endogenous losses and an allotment for growth, may be slightly lower, a recommendation has been set at 0.25 mg/kg BW for growing horses as studies have indicated potential problems when the concentration of copper is under 10 ppm. Assuming an intake of 2.5 percent of BW, this recommendation will meet that minimum. As there is some evidence that additional copper may be useful in the pregnant mare in increasing fetal copper stores, which may be of use after birth, the requirement for the pregnant mare during months 9, 10, and 11 of gestation has been set at 0.25 mg/kg BW, which would work out to a concentration of 12.5 mg/kg DM for a mare consuming 2 percent of her body weight. Further studies in a tightly controlled setting will need to be conducted to determine the adequacy of this recommendation.

Anderson (1992) reported milk copper concentration as 0.155 mg/kg milk. Grace et al. (1999a) determined milk copper concentrations to be 0.23 mg/L milk during the first 3 months after gestation and 0.18 mg/kg during months 4 and 5, which would equate to about 0.22 and 0.17 mg/L milk, respectively. Milk copper concentrations ranged from a high of 0.6 mg/kg milk at birth to about 0.17 mg/kg milk for weeks 3 to 8 postpartum and was not influenced by dietary copper concentration (Breedveld et al., 1987). Likewise, foal blood mineral concentrations also were not influenced by the copper concentration of the mare's ration. Similar results were reported by Baucus et al. (1987). Using an average of the three milk concentrations (0.185 mg Cu/kg milk) and an absorption rate of only 35 percent, the estimated milk production of 3.2 percent of body weight used during the first 3 months of lactation results in an increased requirement of only 0.017 mg Cu/kg BW more than maintenance. The resulting 0.217 mg Cu/kg BW would result in a need for 108.5 mg copper for a 500-kg lactating mare. If that mare were consuming 2.5 percent of her body weight, the resulting concentration would be 8.68 mg/kg DM. As feeding rations containing about 9 ppm copper to broodmares result in milk with normal copper concentrations (Hintz, 1987b), and since no increases in either milk concentrations or foal serum concentrations are reported with additional supplementation, the amount recommended by the 1989 NRC appears to be adequate. Assuming a 2.5 percent intake for the lactating mare, the recommended daily copper allotment is 0.25 mg/kg BW.

The lack of data for copper requirements in mature, exercising horses precludes any changes to recommendations and remains at 10 mg/kg of dietary DM. Assuming a 2 percent of BW intake for light exercise, this would result in a copper intake of 0.2 mg/kg BW; assuming a 2.25 percent of BW intake for moderate exercise, an intake of 0.225 mg/kg BW; for heavy exercise with an assumed intake of 2.5 percent of BW, an intake of 0.25 mg/kg BW.

Iodine

Function

Most of the body's iodine (I) is found in the thyroid gland (Schryver, 1990). Iodine is necessary for the synthesis of thyroxine (T_4) and triiodothyronine (T_3), which are thyroid hormones that regulate basal metabolism. In the thyroid glands and in peripheral tissues, T_4 is deiodinated to T_3. An increase in either results in decreased thyroid stimulating hormone (TSH) secretion and an increase in metabolic rate. Both deficiencies and toxicities of iodine may result in hypothyroidism. When an iodine deficiency is present, sufficient thyroid hormones are unable to be produced. If excess iodine is present, it can directly inhibit the synthesis and release of thyroid hormones. In both situations, TSH production is increased in an attempt to elevate the reduced concentrations of thyroid hormones and alleviate the hypothyroidism. The resultant increase in TSH causes an increase in the size of the thyroid gland in a condition known as goiter.

Dietary iodine and selenium have also been shown to interact to affect thyroid hormone metabolism (Hotz et al., 1997). A high iodine intake, when selenium is deficient, may permit thyroid tissue damage as a result of low thyroidal selenium-dependent glutathione peroxidase (GSH-px) activity during thyroid stimulation, whereas a moderately low selenium intake normalized circulating T_4 concentration in the presence of iodine deficiency.

Sources and Factors Influencing Absorption

Laboratory analyses of feedstuffs usually do not report iodine concentrations, though iodine concentrations in most common feedstuffs vary from 0 to 2 mg/kg DM (NRC, 1989). This depends on the concentrations of iodine in the soil on which the feedstuffs were grown. Kelp and other seaweed are sometimes fed to horses and can have concentrations as high as 1,850 mg of I/kg DM (Baker and Lindsey, 1968). Ethylenediaminedihydroiodide (EDDI) is used as an equine antifungus supplement and can contribute to excess dietary iodine. Typically, iodine supplementation is accomplished by feeding iodized or trace mineralized salts that often contain 70 mg of I/kg DM. Cobalt-iodized salt is not required, nor is it detrimental. Potassium iodate is more stable and, hence, is preferred to potassium iodide. Digestibility of iodine appears to be quite high as renal excretion goes up linearly with increasing iodine intake while fecal excretion remained relatively low, but constant, with only a small increase in response to increased iodine intake (Wehr et al., 2002).

Signs of Deficiency or Excess

The classic symptom of either a severe deficiency or excess of iodine in the ration is hypothyroidism resulting in thyroid gland hypertrophy or goiter. As concentrations of iodine in the newborn foal are determined by the maternal intake (Meyer, 1996c), reproduction of the mare and health of foals can be affected when iodine concentrations in the ration are inappropriate, even when goiter is not present in broodmares. Meyer and Klug (2001) indicated that both a deficiency and excess of iodine depressed the viability of foals and probably influenced embryonic and fetal development. In 1935, Rodenwold and Simms reported losing about 50 percent of foals born to mares receiving iodine-deficient feedstuffs with the foals showing signs of goiter. Supplementation of 15 grains per week of potassium iodide (equivalent to about 100 mg I/day) during the second half of gestation ended the problem, while supplementation with 5 grains per week was not effective. Iodine content below 0.2 mg/kg DM in the majority of feedstuffs fed to horses on a Japanese farm without supplementation resulted in seven foals showing bilateral thyroid enlargement, and four of the seven had extensive flexion of the lower forelegs (Osame and Ichijo, 1994). Stillborn foals, or foals born weak with difficulty in standing to suckle, can result if broodmares are fed an iodine-deficient ration even when the symptom of thyroid gland enlargement is not present in the mare. Likewise, iodine-deficient mares have been reported to have abnormal estrous cycles (Kruzhova, 1968). Feedstuffs such as uncooked soybeans, cabbage, kale, and mustard are known to have an anti-thyroid activity (goitrogens) that can also cause goiter (Jackson and Pagan, 1996). Supplemental iodine is not particularly effective at inhibiting the goitrogenic response, but heating these feedstuffs can inactivate the enzyme responsible for this action.

The maximum tolerable concentration of iodine has been set at 5 mg/kg of dietary intake (NRC, 2005), though the Merck Veterinary Manual (2005) indicated iodine toxicities in mares have been reported at an intake as low as 40 mg/d. Toxicities seem to be more common than deficiencies in recent years (Hintz, 1989). An iodine toxicity usually results only when iodine is oversupplemented or when animals are receiving feeds containing unusually high amounts of iodine such as some types of seaweed. Silvia et al. (1987) reported that excess iodine supplementation of 700 mg inorganic iodine in foals and of more than 350 mg in pregnant and lactating mares caused a high incidence of goiters in the newborn, as well as causing abortions and foal mortality. Eroksuz et al. (2004) reported goiter in newborn foals whose mares had been supplemented with 299 mg I/d during the last 24 weeks of pregnancy. Iatrogenic iodism and an associated alopecia were reported in a horse being treated with 90 g/d for 18 days of EDDI for dermatophilosis (Fadok and Wild, 1983). An increase is susceptibility to infectious disease may also occur with excessive dietary iodine (Baker and Lindsey, 1968).

Wehr et al. (2002) reported the renal excretion of iodine was nearly equivalent to iodine intake when iodine supplementation ranged from 0 to 80 μg/kg BW/d. No changes were seen in concentrations of thyroid hormones. Hence, urinary iodine can be used to estimate the amount of iodine being fed. As the clinical signs of an iodine deficiency or toxicity appear similar, a simple evaluation of the ration should reveal whether iodine concentrations are excessive or deficient and the appropriate corrections can then be made.

Recommendations

Using data from other species, a range of 0.1 to 0.6 mg/kg ration was used in the second printing of the 1989 NRC for all classes of horses. It has been proposed that a 500-kg horse at light work requires 1.75 mg of iodine, 2.5 mg for moderate work, and 2.7 to 3 mg/d for intense work (Jackson, 1997), but research to support the higher requirements for work have not been substantiated. Likewise, Donoghue et al. (1990) suggested that, like in humans, requirements during the third trimester of pregnancy may be slightly increased. As feed intake increases to meet the increased caloric demand of work, daily intake of iodine would be increased if concentrations in the ration remained constant. However, insufficient iodine may be consumed when iodine intake depends on free-choice iodized salt intake. This was reported as the possible cause of iodine deficiency in some pregnant mares whose foals were born with leg abnormalities (McLaughlin and Doige, 1981; McLaughlin et al., 1986). This does not suggest that the recommended range is too low, but does reflect the limitations of depending upon the intake of one nutrient to guarantee the intake of another. For calculating iodine requirements of horses, endogenous iodine losses were assumed to be 7 μg/kg BW/d (Wehr et al., 2002). Given that Osame and Ichijo (1994) reported foals developed goiter when fed feedstuffs that were generally below 0.2 mg I/kg DM, with only alfalfa hay at 0.6 mg I/kg DM, and that the foals were returned to normal by oral administration of 2 mg I/d (approximately 0.33 mg I/kg DM) for 2–4 weeks, it is questionable whether the concentration of 0.1 mg I/kg DM is sufficient. Thus, the average (0.35 mg I/kg DM) of the range (0.1 to 0.6 mg I/kg DM) given in the second printing of the 1989 NRC is likely a safe minimum recommendation. Assuming a near 100 percent absorption, the maintenance requirement would be 0.007 mg/kg BW (which would account for the endogenous losses suggested by Wehr et al. in 2002) or 0.35 mg/kg DM assuming 2 percent of BW intake. Due to limited data from equine studies, this dietary concentration is used with all classes except for the broodmare in late gestation. The increased amount allotted for humans during the final trimester of pregnancy (Donoghue et al., 1990) appears to be prudent and the dietary concentration has been set at 0.4 mg I/kg DM.

Iron

Function

Iron (Fe) is contained in hemoglobin, myoglobin, cytochromes, and many enzyme systems. Iron plays a critical role in oxygen transport and cellular respiration (Schryver, 1990). The body of a 500-kg horse contains about 33 g of iron. The approximate distributions are hemoglobin (60 percent), myoglobin (20 percent), storage and transport forms (20 percent), and cytochromic and other enzymes (0.2 percent) (Moore, 1951).

Sources and Factors Influencing Absorption

Forage and by-product ingredients commonly contain 100–250 mg Fe/kg DM. Grains usually contain less than 100 mg/kg DM, some milled concentrates can have greater than 500 to 1,400 mg/kg DM, and calcium and phosphorus supplements often contain 2–3 percent iron. Dietary iron absorption in nonruminants fed adequate iron is likely to be 15 percent or less. Iron is absorbed more efficiently in newborn animals. A small amount of orally administered iron may exceed the iron-binding capacity of the serum, resulting in free iron reaching the liver and causing liver necrosis and failure (Schryver, 1990). Iron utilization increases in iron-deficient rations and diminishes with higher than normal intakes of cadmium, cobalt, copper, manganese, and zinc (Underwood, 1977).

Signs of Deficiency or Excess

The primary sign of iron deficiency is a microcytic, hypochromic anemia. Although young, milk-fed foals are most susceptible to this anemia, iron deficiency is not a practical problem in foals or mature horses at any performance level if they have access to soil. This is true, in part, because the body efficiently salvages and retains iron derived from the catabolism of body constituents. However, Brommer and Sloet van Oldruitenborgh-Oosterbaan (2001) reported lowered hemoglobin concentrations and packed cell volumes in exercised and unexercised, box-stalled weanlings compared to foals raised on pasture. Blood iron concentrations were also lower ($P < 0.05$) in the two box-stalled groups (101 ± 61 µg/dL and 123 ± 67 µg/dL) as compared to the pastured group (212 ± 67 µg/dL) though serum ferritin, a better indicator of dietary iron status, was not reported. This occurred even though box-stalled foals received fresh-cut grass harvested from the same pastures that the pastured foals were grazing. Additionally, box-stalled foals appeared to be listless compared to pastured foals. Oral supplementation of iron increased hemoglobin concentrations and packed cell volumes and the stabled foals became as active as the pastured foals. It was concluded that the pastured foals likely had increased iron consumption due to the consumption of soil that contained high concentrations of iron, while stalled horses had no such opportunity due to the concrete flooring of their stalls. Of interest, the iron concentration of the grass being fed was sampled twice and the iron concentration was found to be 186 and 310 mg/kg DM—well above the minimum amount required. Thus, it is unclear whether an iron deficiency truly existed or if the timing of the oral supplementation and resultant change in behavior was confounded with other factors. Kohn et al. (1990) reported four doses (248 mg each) of supplemental oral iron during the second and third weeks after birth in foals had no beneficial effects on hematologic variables. They concluded that most foals apparently have sufficient body iron stores at birth and sufficient intake to support demands for iron during early foalhood.

From data in other species, the maximum tolerable concentration of iron has been set at 500 mg/kg ration (NRC, 2005). Some feedstuffs, particularly forages such as sorghum hay, contain more than this concentration of iron, but there are no reports of iron toxicity from feeding these feeds to horses. Although various iron supplements have been ineffective in improving the hemoglobin or oxygen-carrying capacity of red blood cells under natural feeding programs (Kirkham et al., 1971), some iron supplements have been implicated in chronic iron toxicity when fed at 0.6 mg Fe/kg BW/d in the form of ferrous sulphate (Edens et al., 1993). Clinical signs disappeared after discontinuation of the iron supplement. However, Edens et al. (1993) suggested that other factors such as iron amount in the primary feed source, inaccurate reporting of dosage amount, or some other underlying problem may be the reason for such a small amount to be toxic. In comparison, ponies given 50 mg Fe/kg of BW/d from ferrous sulfate did not show signs of poisoning, and it was concluded that administration of that concentration for a period of less than 8 weeks would not cause iron toxicosis (Pearson and Andreasen, 2001). High concentrations of supplemental dietary iron (500 and 1,000 mg/kg feed) fed to ponies had no effect on feed intake, daily gain, red blood cell count, hemoglobin concentration, packed cell volume, or serum iron, calcium, copper, and manganese (Lawrence, 1986; Lawrence et al., 1987). The higher dietary iron concentration, however, depressed both serum and liver zinc. Johnson and Murphy (1988) also reported that high iron concentrations decreased copper absorption in copper-deficient rats. Mills and Marlin (1996) concluded that possible adverse effects of excessive iron might outweigh any supposed advantages. It should be noted that supplemental iron can be toxic to newborn foals and iron injections are dangerous to horses, often resulting in severe reactions or death.

Excess iron is especially toxic to young animals, and deaths among foals have been attributed to oral administration of digestive inocula containing supplemental iron (Mullaney and Brown, 1988). Foals dosed according to manufacturer's recommendations received 350 mg of elemental iron as ferrous fumarate at birth and at 3 days of age. Prior to death, these foals exhibited diarrhea, icterus, dehydration, and coma. Morphologic changes included erosion of jejunal villi, pulmonary hemorrhage, massive iron deposition in the liver, and liver degeneration. Since the removal in the 1980s of products containing ferrous fumarate for administration to neonates, iron poisoning has become less common (Casteel, 2001). Ferrous fumarate toxicity in a mature horse has been reported by Arnbjerg (1981). Serum iron concentrations exceeding 400 µg/dL suggest acute toxicosis (Puls, 1994). Because serum iron content can be affected secondarily by several disorders, Smith et al. (1986) reported that serum ferritin content seems to be the best indicator of iron status in horses. Smith et al. (1984) reported serum ferritin ranging from 70 to 250 ng/ml with a mean of 152 ± 55 for normal horses.

Recommendations

Daily endogenous losses of iron have not been reported for horses, and the dietary iron requirement is estimated to be 50 mg/kg DM for growing foals or pregnant and lactating mares and 40 mg/kg DM for mature horses. Common feedstuffs should meet the iron requirements. According to Meyer (1986), approximately 37, 38, and 92 mg of iron are deposited each day in the fetus and placental membranes during months 9, 10, and 11 of gestation, respectively. For a 500-kg mare, this equates to 74, 76, and 184 µg Fe/kg mare weight. The iron content of mare's milk ranges from 1.3 µg/g at parturition to 0.49 µg/g at 4 months postpartum (Ullrey et al., 1974), though an average of 0.22 µg/g has also been reported (Anderson, 1992). A mare producing 15 kg milk/d would require approximately 130 mg of iron daily for milk production in early lactation and 32.6 mg of iron for 10 kg milk/d in late lactation, in addition to the iron requirement for maintenance. Iron loss through sweat is small having been reported to be only 0.6 percent of intake, so it would not contribute appreciably to iron requirements for exercise (Inoue et al., 2003). Without an accurate estimate of endogenous losses, and hence maintenance requirements, the 1989 NRC requirements are unchanged.

Manganese

Function

Manganese (Mn) is essential for carbohydrate and lipid metabolism and for synthesis of the chondroitin sulfate necessary in cartilage formation.

Sources and Factors Influencing Absorption

Forages contain 40 to 140 mg of Mn/kg DM, and most concentrates (except corn) contain 15 to 45 mg/kg DM. Wagner et al. (2005) reported the absorption of manganese oxide, sulfate, and an organic-chelate to be 13.6, 8.6, and 15.5 percent, respectively, and these did not differ between sources. Siciliano et al. (2001) found no difference in liver manganese concentrations between horses supplemented with manganese-oxide or a combination of half manganese-oxide and half manganese-methionine. Pagan and Jackson (1991b) reported the apparent digestibility of manganese to range from 4.7–10.6 percent, while Pagan (1994) reported true manganese digestibility to be around 28.5 percent in mature horses. Exercise has been shown to decrease true digestibility of manganese from 58 percent to 40 percent (Hudson et al., 2001). The variation in reported digestibilities results in difficulties in precisely determining requirements.

Signs of Deficiency or Excess

Manganese deficiency in other species results in abnormal cartilage development. This is due to failure of chondroitin sulfate synthesis, which results in bone malformation. The crooked limbs of newborn calves have been associated with manganese deficiency (Howes and Dyer, 1971). Similar afflictions (congenitally enlarged joints, twisted legs, and shortened forelimb bones) have been associated with "smelter smoke syndrome" in Oklahoma (Cowgill et al., 1980); the extensive liming required to offset the acidic effects of smelter effluent on the soil was thought to markedly reduce manganese availability. It has been suggested since, but not proven, that manganese deficiency may be associated with limb abnormalities and congenital contractures in newborn foals. However, no direct evidence exists to support this theory. Manganese is among the least toxic of the trace elements (Underwood, 1977), and there are no known instances of manganese intoxication in horses (Schryver, 1990). However, large amounts of manganese in the ration can interfere with phosphorus absorption. The 2005 NRC has suggested 400 ppm of dietary manganese may be the maximum tolerable amount based upon interspecies extrapolation.

Recommendations

The manganese requirements of horses have not been firmly established; however, based upon data from other species, 40 mg Mn/kg DM (Rojas et al., 1965) was considered adequate by the 1989 NRC. Hudson et al. (2001) calculated endogenous losses in horses averaging 534 kg to be between 164 ± 68 and 305 ± 95 mg/d (0.31 and 0.57 mg/kg BW) with a resultant requirement ranging from 408 ± 107 to 529 ± 167 mg/d (0.76–0.99 mg Mn/kg BW or 380–495 mg of Mn/d for a 500-kg horse). Pagan (1994) estimated endogenous manganese loss to be 110 mg/d (about 0.2 mg/kg BW) though the R^2 for the calculation was only 0.40. The true digestibility of manganese was estimated to be 28.5 percent. The resulting requirement for a 500-kg horse (350 mg of Mn/d) is lower than the 1989 NRC recommendation (400 mg Mn/d) assuming a 2 percent of BW intake; however, the Pagan (1994) horses consumed less total feed. The results of the Pagan (1994) report do provide at least some evidence that the requirements established by the 1989 NRC subcommittee should adequately meet the requirements of the horse. Sobota et al. (2001) reported decreased growth rates in yearlings receiving only 35.8 mg Mn/kg ration compared to yearlings receiving 101 mg Mn/kg ration. Though not substantially lower than the 1989 NRC recommendation, Sobota et al. (2001) concluded that the decreased growth rates seen when feeding 35.8 mg Mn/kg ration provide support for the minimum requirement of 40 mg Mn/kg ration. Milk manganese concentrations in mares have reported to be 0.255 µmol/L or 0.014 ppm (Anderson, 1992). Until further studies are conducted that suggest a need to increase the previous recommendations, or that they can be decreased without causing problems, the recommendation remains at 40 mg Mn/kg DM.

Selenium

Function

Selenium (Se) is an essential component of selenium-dependent glutathione peroxidase (Rotruck et al., 1973), which aids in detoxification of lipo- and hydrogen peroxides that are toxic to cell membranes. Selenium also plays a role in the control of thyroid hormone metabolism (Hotz et al.,

1997). The deiodinating enzyme, which produces most of the circulating T_3, type I iodothyronine 5-deiodinase, is a selenoenzyme with most of the activity occurring in liver, kidney, and thyroid.

Sources and Factors Influencing Absorption

The concentration of selenium in feedstuffs commonly ranges from 0.01 to 0.3 mg/kg and is influenced by variations in soil selenium and pH. Alkaline soils are more conducive to plants accumulating selenium. Drought conditions also encourage deeper root growth where selenium concentrations in the soil may be greater. Drought conditions can also encourage animals to eat accumulator plants that might otherwise be ignored. Accumulator plants may store high concentrations of selenium and can result in toxicities when consumed (Finley, 2005). Selenium in forages and seed grains is normally present as organic selenium in the form of selenocystine, selenocysteine, and selenomethionine. Sodium selenite and sodium selenate are common inorganic sources of supplemental selenium, and no differences in bioavailability between the two sources were observed by Podoll et al. (1992). Pagan et al. (1999) reported a trend ($P < 0.1$) for the apparent absorption of selenium from selenium-enriched yeast to be greater than from sodium selenite (57.3 vs. 51.1 ± 1.4 percent). Janicki et al. (2001) reported greater serum selenium concentrations in mares receiving supplementation of 3 mg/d of selenium as selenium-yeast compared to mares receiving either 1 or 3 mg Se/d as sodium selenite. Selenium in the colostrum and milk was also greater in the mares receiving the supplemental organic selenium. By comparison, Richardson et al. (2006) reported no clear difference in various markers of selenium status (e.g., selenium concentration of plasma and middle gluteal muscle; GSH-px activity of plasma, red blood cells, and middle gluteal muscle) was identified in 18-month-old nonexercised horses fed diets containing either zinc-L-selenomethionine or sodium selenite (0.45 mg Se/kg DM) over a 56-d experimental period. Selenium is absorbed more efficiently in nonruminants than in ruminants (77 compared to 29 percent: Wright and Bell, 1966). Selenium concentration of milk was shown to be one-fourth of that in colostrum 1 day postpartum and was considered a minor source of selenium regardless of the selenium status of their mares during gestation (Lee et al., 1995). Although the Food and Drug Administration (FDA) has approved maximal selenium supplementation at 0.3 mg/kg DM in complete feeds for cattle, sheep, and swine (FDA, 1987), selenium supplementation of equine feeds in the United States is not covered and is restricted only by nutritional recommendations and industry practices (Ullrey, 1992). By comparison, the Feed Additive Directive 70/524/EC allows maximal selenium supplementation of 0.5 mg/kg in complete feeds (assuming 88 percent dry matter). Selenized salt blocks are available to provide supplemental selenium (Hintz, 1999). These contain up to 120 ppm selenium. Shellow et al. (1985) reported blood selenium concentrations increased linearly for 5–6 weeks and then were unchanged for the remainder of a 12-week study when supplemental selenium was fed to horses receiving a basal ration of 0.06 ppm selenium. Hayes et al. (1987) reported that dietary selenium concentrations often did not correlate with blood selenium concentrations. In a small survey of farms, the farm having the highest concentration of dietary selenium had inadequate blood concentrations in the animals tested, leading the authors to conclude that interactions with other minerals may have been influencing absorption of selenium or that breed differences may have played a role in the ability to absorb selenium. Besides other dietary minerals, knowledge of the vitamin E status of the animals is also important.

Signs of Deficiency or Excess

Through veterinary and laboratory surveys of every state, Edmonson et al. (1993) reported selenium-deficiency diseases in 46 states. Deficiencies were an important livestock problem in regions of 37 states, but deficiencies in wildlife were reported in only 10 states. By comparison, natural occurring toxicosis is rare and was only reported in 7 states even though oversupplementation was reported in 15 states. Acute, subacute, and chronic forms of selenium deficiency in horses have been reported in China (Jiong et al., 1987). The myopathy results in weakness, impaired locomotion, difficulty in suckling and swallowing, respiratory distress, and impaired cardiac function (Dill and Rebhun, 1985). Serum changes include elevations in creatine kinase, aspartate aminotransferase, potassium, and blood urea nitrogen (Dill and Rebhun, 1985). Elevated aspartic-pyruvic transaminase and gamma-glutamyltransferase have also been associated with the vitamin E/selenium-response disease. Occurrence of the tying-up syndrome did not correlate with vitamin E or selenium status (Lindholm and Asheim, 1973; Gallagher and Stowe, 1980; Blackmore et al., 1982). The clinical and morphologic manifestations of selenium deficiency are affected by the concomitant vitamin E status. Perkins et al. (1998) reported on four cases of neonatal foals with rhabdomyolysis due to selenium deficiency both with and without vitamin E deficiency. Nutritional myopathy (white muscle disease or vitamin E/selenium-responsive disease) involves skeletal and cardiac muscles and is associated with glutathione peroxidase (GSH-px) values lower than 25 enzyme units (EU)/dl (Caple et al., 1978) and with serum selenium values lower than 60 ng/ml (Blackmore et al., 1982). Though low selenium serum concentrations are often used as evidence of a selenium deficiency, if no other clinical problems are evident, it is questionable whether a deficiency is truly present. For example, Vervuert et al. (2001) reported Icelandic horses had low plasma selenium concentrations (66.7 ± 47.2 ng Se/ml) with no health problems and suggested those horses had an efficient metabolism that allowed them to compensate for a low selenium supply. Likewise, GSH-px activity was not correlated with selenium intake or selenium plasma concentrations in a field study of 106 horses (Wichert et al., 2002a). Without other symptoms of a selenium deficiency, low concentrations of selenium in the blood and low GSH-px activity should not be taken as a clear sign that a selenium deficiency is present.

Based upon studies with other species, the maximum tolerable concentration of selenium in horses has been estimated at 5 mg/kg DM (NRC, 2005). However, the 1989 NRC recognized that maximum tolerable concentration of selenium to be 2 mg/kg DM and this seems to be a more advisable upper limit. The LD_{50} for orally administered selenium is considered to be approximately 3.3 mg of Se (as sodium selenite)/kg BW (Miller and Williams, 1940). The chemical form of selenium can influence its toxicity, with organic selenium compounds found in plants (selenocystine, selenocysteine, and selenomethionine) being the most toxic (Schryver, 1990). Horses appear to be more susceptible to selenium toxicity than are cattle (Rogers et al., 1990). Copper pretreatment can increase the LD_{50} markedly (Stowe, 1980). Acute selenium toxicity—blind staggers—is characterized by apparent blindness, head pressing, perspiration, abdominal pain, colic, diarrhea, increased heart and respiration rates, and lethargy (Rosenfeld and Beath, 1964). Hair loss and changes in hooves could also be expected after an acutely high dose of selenium (Fan and Kizer, 1990). Chronic selenium toxicity—alkali disease—is characterized by alopecia, especially about the mane and tail, as well as cracking of the hooves around the coronary band (Rosenfeld and Beath, 1964; Traub-Dargatz et al., 1986). Orally administering mixtures of sulphates that antagonize selenium are a suggested cure for chronic toxicity (Rogers et al., 1990). There are anecdotal accounts of immediate death after administration of injectable vitamin E/selenium preparations. These deaths appear due to an anaphylactoid sensitivity of the horse to a carrier ingredient in the injectable preparations and not to the toxicity of selenium or vitamin E. As a result of chronically elevated selenium intake, it is believed that sulfur is replaced by selenium in such sulfur-containing tissues as keratin, potentially resulting in weakened hooves and hair (Merck Veterinary Manual, 2005). Therefore, even though below toxic amounts, there appears to be no justification for feeding selenium at a concentration greater than 0.5 mg Se/kg DM.

The selenium status of horses can be evaluated by measuring serum, plasma, or whole blood selenium by the sensitive fluorometric selenium assay (Whetter and Ullrey, 1978). Selenium-dependent GSH-px of serum and erythrocytes can also be measured (Paglia and Valentine, 1967); however, sample storage time and temperature are critical. Serum selenium concentrations of 100–500 µg/dl have been found in chronic selenosis and 2,000–2,500 µg/dl in acute intoxication (Traub-Dargatz et al., 1986). Whole blood appears to be a more preferable indicator of serum status than serum (McLaughlin and Cullen, 1986). The serum selenium of foals from selenium-adequate mares is typically much lower than their dams and ranges from 70 to 80 ng of selenium per ml of serum (Stowe, 1967). If, according to Blackmore et al. (1982), serum selenium values below 65 ng/ml are indicative of deficiency, young foals may be prone to nutritional muscular dystrophy, especially if their vitamin E status is low. Carmel et al. (1990) reported that of 202 randomly sampled horses in Maryland, blood selenium concentrations ranged from 50–266 ng/ml. Stowe and Herdt (1992) expected serum selenium values to increase gradually with age from starting ranges for newborn foals of 70–90 ng/ml with expected or "normal" values for the adult horses to range from 130–160 ng/ml. Normal liver selenium concentrations are considered to range between 1.2 and 2.0 µg/g on a dry weight basis, regardless of age (Stowe and Herdt, 1992).

Recommendations

The selenium requirement of the horse was estimated at 0.1 mg/kg ration (Stowe, 1967). This is consistent with the report of Shellow et al. (1985), who found that plasma selenium concentrations of mature horses reached a plateau at about 140 ng/ml in horses fed either 0.14 or 0.23 mg of Se/kg ration. They concluded that there was no advantage in supplementing the mature idle horse with more than 0.1 mg Se/kg ration and that 140 ng of Se/ml plasma (or serum) was adequate to prevent problems associated with selenium deficiency. A similar selenium supplementation rate, 1 mg/d for horses 1 to 6 years of age, was reported by Maylin et al. (1980) to increase blood selenium from 45 to 123 ng/ml over an 11-week period. The higher blood selenium value was considered well above the concentration associated with myodegeneration. Glutathione peroxidase values for racing Standardbred horses were reported to be 17 EU/mg hemoglobin (Gallagher and Stowe, 1980). Maylin et al. (1980) and Roneus and Lindholm (1983) confirmed a strong relationship between selenium intake and GSH-px activity and noted that the GSH-px response to oral selenium was much lower than to parenteral selenium. Wichert et al. (2002b) reported selenium intake in over half of 106 horses sampled was below 1.25 µg/kg BW without signs of selenium deficiency. This amount was almost half of what was recommended by the 1989 NRC, so there is a possibility that the minimum requirement may be somewhat overestimated. It can be concluded the true requirement for selenium is unknown, though a recommendation (0.1 mg/kg DM) can be given that is known to prevent a classical deficiency. However, Janicki et al. (2001) found greater influenza antibodies in foals from mares receiving 3 mg Se/d as compared to

1 mg Se/d suggesting that selenium intake necessary for optimum immune function could be greater than that needed to prevent classical deficiency symptoms.

Zinc

Function

Zinc (Zn) is present in the body as a component of more than 100 enzymes including many metalloenzymes such as carbonic anhydrase, alkaline phosphatase, and carboxypeptidase. The highest concentrations of zinc occur in the choroid and iris of the eye and in the prostate gland. Intermediate concentrations of zinc are present in skin, liver, bone, and muscle, whereas low concentrations are found in blood, milk, lungs, and brain.

Sources and Factors Influencing Absorption

Many feedstuffs contain 15–40 mg Zn/kg DM. Sources of supplemental zinc include zinc sulfate, zinc oxide, zinc chloride, zinc carbonate, and various organic sources of zinc chelates. Zinc absorption is regulated by the zinc status of the animal and is typically in the 5–15 percent range. Pagan and Jackson (1991b) reported the apparent digestibility to be between 7.8 and 11.5 percent. Pagan (1994) reported an apparent digestibility of 9.4 percent and a true digestibility of nearly 21 percent. A study by Hudson et al. (2001) showed true zinc digestibility to decrease to 14 percent when horses were exercised compared to 25 percent in sedentary horses. Wagner et al. (2005) found the absorption of zinc oxide, sulfate, and an organic-chelate to be 13.9, 12.8, and 10.6 percent, respectively, in mature horses. Baker et al. (2005) also reported mature horses retained more zinc when supplemented with zinc oxide as compared to organically chelated zinc. No difference was found between an inorganic source and a combination of organic and inorganic sources of zinc fed at higher than required concentrations on bone metabolism (Baker et al., 2003) or liver zinc concentrations (Siciliano et al., 2001), though Miller et al. (2003) reported an increased zinc retention in yearlings fed the organic zinc as compared to the inorganic zinc. Wichert et al. (2002c) reported higher bioavailability of inorganic zinc sulfate and zinc sulfate chelate than zinc oxide after a high single dose. These conflicting data make it hard to claim that organic or inorganic zinc forms are better absorbed. When comparing organic vs. inorganic minerals, cost is often an important consideration besides digestibility.

Signs of Deficiency or Excess

Zinc deficiency has been produced in foals fed 5 mg of Zn/kg purified diet (Harrington et al., 1973). Zinc deficiency in foals is accompanied by inappetence, reduced growth rate, parakeratosis (especially on the lower limbs), alopecia, reduced serum and tissue zinc concentrations, and decreased alkaline phosphatase (Harrington et al., 1973). Horses appear quite tolerant of excess dietary zinc and a maximum tolerable concentration has been set at 500 mg/kg ration based upon interspecies extrapolation (NRC, 2005). Except when homeostatic mechanisms that act on absorption are overwhelmed, zinc generally does not accumulate with continued exposure (Casteel, 2001). No detrimental effects were observed in mares or foals fed rations containing up to 700 mg Zn/kg feed (Graham et al., 1940). However, Messer (1981) reported tibiotarsal effusion in three Arabian fillies that had marked elevations in serum zinc. Foals fed 90 g Zn/d (equal to about 2 percent of the ration) developed enlarged epiphyses, stiffness of gait, lameness, and increased tissue zinc (Graham et al., 1940). Similar signs were observed by Eamens et al. (1984) in four young horses grazed near industrial plants where the pasture contained high zinc concentrations and by Gunson et al. (1982) in two young foals raised near a zinc smelter. The cause appeared to be a secondary copper deficiency induced by zinc toxicosis. Similarly, Bridges and Moffitt (1990) reported foals fed rations containing zinc (supplemented in the form of zinc oxide) at 1,000 and 2,000 mg/kg BW became hypocupremic within 5–6 weeks and were lame within 6 weeks because of cartilage defects. The ratio of copper to zinc should be considered, as zinc is believed to compete for the same transport mechanisms as copper and is a potent inducer of metallothionein synthesis, which binds copper. Thus, the amount of zinc necessary to cause a deficiency in copper is dependent on the reserve amount of copper present in the liver and other tissues (Bridges et al., 1984; Cymbaluk and Smart, 1993; Campbell-Beggs et al., 1994). As a result, dietary zinc excess or high dietary zinc:copper ratios may create a copper deficiency. By altering zinc:copper ratios from 6.3 to 3, Caure et al. (1998) was able to reduce osteochondrosis scores on one of two French farms, though they were not able to alter the prevalence of the lesions. It should be noted that this study was not controlled and alterations in other nutrients were also made. Young et al. (1987) and Coger et al. (1987) were unable to alter the copper absorption in growing and mature ponies fed rations containing 580 or 1,200 mg Zn/kg feed. Therefore, the purported effect of elevated zinc intake on copper metabolism may involve postabsorptive events rather than the actual site of absorption.

Time between blood collection and separation, in addition to the contamination of blood samples from rubber stoppers, makes evaluation of zinc status from blood difficult (English and Hambidge, 1988; Casteel, 2001). Concentrations of zinc in the serum or plasma, while often used for evaluating zinc intake, can vary from low to high within the same herd and are not a good indicator of zinc status. Likewise, serum zinc concentrations have been found to be quite variable with respect to age (Bell et al., 1987).

Recommendations

Harrington et al. (1973) demonstrated that 40 mg Zn/kg purified-type diet was sufficient to prevent zinc deficiency in foals. Schryver et al. (1974) reported that foals fed 41 mg Zn/kg natural diet grew at acceptable rates and maintained normal body stores of zinc. Drepper et al. (1982) and Jarrige and Martin-Rosset (1981) indicated that 50 mg Zn/kg dry matter was adequate for all classes of horses. According to Knight et al. (1985), based on farm surveys, the optimal dietary zinc concentration in equine rations to minimize the incidence of metabolic bone disease approaches 90 mg/kg feed. Although these workers suggested that the 1978 NRC recommendations on zinc requirements be reevaluated, no controlled studies support a dietary zinc requirement greater than 50 mg/kg ration DM and the 1989 NRC did not change the recommendations from 40 mg/kg dietary DM. Likewise, Wichert et al. (2002b) reported that only 42 percent of 106 sampled horses had zinc intake of 1 mg/kg BW and 25 percent of the horses were fed < 0.5 mg Zn/kg BW with none of the horses showing signs of zinc deficiency. Mare's milk contains 1.8–3.2 mg Zn/kg fluid milk (NRC, 1989; Anderson, 1992). Thus, foals drinking 15 kg of milk/d would consume 27–48 mg of Zn/d. On a dry matter basis, this is equivalent to 17–30 mg Zn/kg DM intake. The zinc in milk is assumed to be highly available. Kavazis et al. (2002) concluded that supplementing late gestating and lactating mares with zinc at higher concentrations than recommended by the 1989 NRC did not have any influence on foal growth and development or the zinc concentrations of mare milk or foal serum.

Pagan (1994) estimated endogenous zinc loss to be 54 mg/d for a 550-kg horse (about 0.1 mg/kg BW), which is similar to Hudson et al. (2001). They estimated endogenous zinc losses to be between 65 and 70 mg Zn/d for horses averaging 534 kg (about 0.12–0.13 mg Zn/kg BW). Pagan (1994) calculated the true digestibility of zinc to be 20.8 percent. The resulting requirement for a 500-kg horse (236 mg Zn/d) is much lower than the 1989 NRC recommendation assuming a 2 percent of BW intake (400 mg/d). However, until studies are performed demonstrating lower amounts can be fed without problems for longer periods, the decision was made to keep the requirements the same at 40 mg/kg of DM.

OTHER MINERALS OF INTEREST

Chromium

Chromium plays a role in carbohydrate and lipid metabolism. It acts as a potentiator of insulin to facilitate glucose clearance and is considered an essential nutrient in humans (Mertz, 1992).

Trivalent and hexavalent are the two most common forms of chromium. Organic chromium appears to be more bioavailable than inorganic forms. Absorption of inorganic forms have been reported to range from 0.4–3 percent (Anderson, 1987), while chromium from sources such as brewer's yeast has been reported to be absorbed at rates as high as 10–25 percent by rats (Underwood, 1977).

While no evidence has been found of a chromium deficiency in horses, a chromium deficiency leads to symptoms associated with adult-onset diabetes and cardiovascular disease in humans (Vincent, 1999). From data in other species, the maximum tolerable concentration of chromium in the ration of horses is set at 3,000 mg/kg DM for the oxide form and 100 mg/kg DM for the chloride form of the trivalent forms of chromium (NRC, 2005). The hexavalent forms of chromium appear to be much more toxic (NRC, 1997). Chromosome damage in hamsters has been noted after treatment with chromium picolinate but not with chromium nicotinate, nicotinic acid, and trivalent chromium chloride hexahydrate at the same doses (Stearns et al., 1995).

At this time, insufficient information is available to determine if there is a chromium requirement for horses, though the recommended safe and adequate daily intake for humans is 50–200 µg/d (Anderson and Kozlovsky, 1985). Jackson (1997) suggested chromium requirements may be higher for exercising horses than for sedentary horses. While not strongly supported by research in horses, this is supported by Lukaski (2000) for humans in endurance training. Pagan et al. (1995) reported that exercising horses supplemented with 5 mg of chromium from a chromium yeast product had lower plasma glucose concentrations during several stages of a standardized exercise test. Likewise, supplemented horses had lower blood insulin 1 hour after grain feeding than did control horses. In contrast, Pagan et al. (1995) indicated no response to supplementation in untrained, sedentary horses. Ott and Kivipelto (1999) reported chromium tripicolinate supplementation resulted in peak plasma glucose concentrations decreasing more rapidly following an intravenous insulin sensitivity test. Likewise, mean glucose fractional turnover rate values increased in response to the chromium tripicolinate supplementation. Gentry et al. (1997) reported chromium tripicolinate supplementation had only a marginal effect on metabolic, hormonal, and immune responses. Vervuert et al. (2005b) reported that horses supplemented with a chromium yeast product did not have improved glucose "handling" capabilities. Chromium-supplemented horses also had higher heart rates and blood lactate at the end of a standardized exercise test suggesting that the exercise capacity of chromium-supplemented horses was compromised. Supplementation of chromium-L-methionine to geriatric mares for a period of 4 weeks did not alter most immune parameters (Dimock et al., 1999). In addition, 4 mg/d of chromium propionate supplementation did not alleviate elevations in plasma leptin and insulin or alter glucose dynamics and insulin sensitivity in horses with a high body condition (Cartmill et al., 2005). While it has been suggested that dietary supplementation with chromium can calm horses and may be beneficial in horses with recurrent exertional rhabdomyolysis, because horses with polysaccharide storage myopathy display abnormal sensitivity to insulin, chromium supplementation may be counterproductive in those animals (Valberg, 2005). Porter et al. (1999) suggested that, at least in humans, routine use of chromium supplements is not warranted based upon current data.

Fluorine

Fluorine (F) is known to be involved in bone and teeth development, but its dietary necessity for horses has not been established.

Forages often contain between 2 and 16 mg F/kg DM and cereal grains usually contain between 1 and 3 mg fluoride/kg DM (NRC, 1980). Phosphorus supplements that have not been adequately defluorinated are a common source of excess dietary fluorine.

A fluorine deficiency is not known to have been reported in horses. Horses appear to be more tolerant than cattle of excess fluorine (Buck et al., 1976). Fluorine intoxication may result from long-term ingestion of feed or water contaminated by certain industrial operations or from consumption of water or mineral supplements that contain high concentrations of fluorine (Schryver, 1990). Excess intake results in discolored teeth (fluorosis), bone lesions, lameness, and unthriftiness. Shupe and Olson (1971) indicated horses can tolerate 50 mg F/kg ration for extended periods without detrimental effects, but the maximum tolerable concentration of fluorine has been set at 40 mg/kg DM intake based upon data with other species (NRC, 2005).

An equine requirement for fluorine has not been established, but given the concentrations of fluorine in normal feedstuffs, any potential requirement is likely met and additional supplementation is not suggested.

Silicon

Despite silicon being the second most common element of Earth's crust (Carlisle, 1972), surprisingly little is known about the nutritional importance of it in the diet of mammalian species. Silicon is involved in the formation of new bone (Carlisle, 1970) and is an important component of connective tissue, hyaluronic acid, and articular cartilage (Carlisle, 1974).

Grains are high in silicon content (Pennington, 1991). However, silicon in the environment is naturally found as silica (SiO_2) and is not easily absorbed. Sodium zeolite A (SZA) is a silicon source that is converted into orthosilicic acid ($Si(OH)_4$) in the stomach, which can then be absorbed. Nielsen et al. (1993) reported race horses supplemented with SZA at 1.86 percent of total feed intake (providing about 150 mg of silicon) had higher plasma silicon concentrations, were able to go nearly twice the distance in training before experiencing an injury compared to nonsupplemented control animals, and had fewer injuries compared to controls. Feeding a natural zeolite, as compared to the synthetic SZA, did not increase plasma silicon (Mazzella et al., 2005). Greater rates of bone formation (Lang et al., 2001b) and lower rates of bone resorption (Lang et al., 2001a) as compared to the control horses were reported in SZA-supplemented horses, suggesting an overall increase in bone production. Turner et al. (2005) reported an increase in bone turnover in calves fed SZA and hypothesized that the reduction in injuries reported previously was due to rapid repair of subclinical injuries. These studies suggested benefits associated with supplemental available silicon. Silicon appears to reduce aluminum absorption and toxicity (Jugdaohsingh et al., 2000), though it is not certain to what degree each element inhibits the absorption of each other.

The relative abundance of silicon makes the deficiency of this element difficult to achieve. Likewise, silicon naturally found in the environment is not very absorbable and thus is not likely to cause toxic effects through dietary intake. The NRC (2005) did not set a maximum tolerable concentration for silicon in horses, but set one at 0.2 percent for cattle and sheep.

As a result of research demonstrating silicon can interact with other nutrients for apparent beneficial effects (Nielsen, 1991), the American Institute of Nutrition reformulated its published formulas of purified diets for experimental rodents and added silicon to the required nutrient profile at the rate of 5 mg/kg ration (Reeves, 1997). Difficulty in producing a silicon-deficient purified diet for horses will make determining a minimum requirement difficult, though a need for silicon in the ration likely exists for the equine.

Other Elements

Further elements are, in principle, accepted as essential constituents in a mammalian diet (e.g., boron, nickel, and vanadium). Based on the current status of knowledge, their natural occurrence is sufficient to ensure the required very small amounts of these elements. The supplementation of these elements, including the rare earth elements, is not based on scientifically elaborated, valid data and has the potential to be dangerous to horses.

REFERENCES

Alexander, F. 1977. Diuretics and faecal electrolytes in horses. Br. J. Pharmacol. 60:589–593.

Ammerman, C. B. 1970. Recent developments in cobalt and copper in ruminant nutrition: A review. J. Dairy Sci. 53:1097–1106.

Anderson, R. A. 1987. Chromium in animal tissues and fluids. Pp. 225–244 in Trace Elements in Human and Animal Nutrition, Vol. 1, 5th ed., W. Mertz, ed. New York: Academic Press.

Anderson, R. A., and A. S. Kozlovsky. 1985. Chromium intake, absorption and excretion of subjects consuming self-selected diets. Am. J. Clin. Nutr. 41:1177–1183.

Anderson, R. R. 1992. Comparison of trace elements in milk of four species. J. Dairy Sci. 75:3050–3055.

Arnbjerg, J. 1981. Poisoning in animals due to oral application of iron with description of a case in a horse. Nord. Veterinaermed. 33:71–76.

Asano, R., K. Suzuki, T. Otsuka, M. Otsuka, and H. Sakurai. 2002. Concentrations of toxic metals and essential minerals in the mane hair of healthy racing horses and their relation to age. J. Vet. Med. Sci. 64:607–610.

Asano, R., K. Suzuki, M. Chiba, K. Sera, T. Matsumoto, R. Asano, and T. Sakai. 2005. Influence of the coat color on the trace elemental status measured by particle-induced X-ray emission in horse hair. Biol. Trace Elem. Res. 103:169–176.

Auer, D. E., J. C. Ng, H. L. Thompson, S. Inglis, and A. A. Seawright. 1989. Acute phase response in horses: changes in plasma cation concentrations after localized tissue injury. Vet. Rec. 124:235–239.

Baker, H. J., and J. R. Lindsey. 1968. Equine goiter due to excess dietary iodine. J. Am. Vet. Med. Assoc. 153:1618.

Baker, L. A., D. R. Topliff, D. W. Freeman, R. G. Teeter, and B. Stoecker. 1998. The comparison of two forms of sodium and potassium and chloride versus sulfur in the dietary cation-anion difference equation: effects on acid-base status and mineral balance in sedentary horses. J. Equine Vet. Sci. 18:389–395.

Baker, L. A., T. Kearney-Moss, J. L. Pipkin, R. C. Bachman, J. T. Haliburton, and G. O. Veneklasen. 2003. The effect of supplemental inorganic and organic sources of copper and zinc on bone metabolism in exercised yearling geldings. Pp. 100–105 in Proc. 18th Equine Nutr. Physiol. Soc. Symp., East Lansing, MI.

Baker, L. A., M. R. Wrigley, J. L. Pipkin, J. T. Haliburton, and R. C. Bachman. 2005. Digestibility and retention of inorganic and organic sources of copper and zinc in mature horses. Pp. 162–167 in Proc. 19th Equine Sci. Soc., Tucson, AZ.

Bathe, A. P., and R. Cash. 1995. Overestimation of copper deficiency in horses? Vet. Rec. 25:203–204.

Baucus, K. L., S. L. Ralston, V. A. Rich, and E. L. Squires. 1987. The effect of dietary copper and zinc supplementation on composition of mare's milk. Pp. 179–184 in Proc. 10th Equine Nutr. Physiol. Soc. Symp., Fort Collins, CO.

Bell, J. U., J. M. Lopez, and K. D. Bartos. 1987. The postnatal development of serum zinc, copper and ceruloplasmin in the horse. Comp. Biochem. Physiol. A. 87:561–564.

Bell, R. A., B. D. Nielsen, K. Waite, D. Rosenstein, and M. Orth. 2001. Daily access to pasture turnout prevents loss of mineral in the third metacarpus of Arabian weanlings. J. Anim. Sci. 79:1142–1150.

Blackmore, D. J., C. Campbell, D. Cant, J. E. Holden, and J. E. Kent. 1982. Selenium status of Thoroughbreds in the United Kingdom. Equine Vet. J. 14:139–143.

Blaney, B. J., R. J. W. Gartner, and R. A. McKenzie. 1981. The inability of horses to absorb calcium oxalate. J. Agr. Sci. Camb. 97:639–641.

Brama, P. A. J., J. M. TeKoppele, R. A. Bank, A. Barneveld, and P. R. VanWeeren. 2002. Biochemical development of subchondral bone from birth until age eleven months and the influence of physical activity. Equine Vet. J. 34:143–149.

Breedveld, L., S. G. Jackson, and J. P. Baker. 1987. The determination of a relationship between the copper, zinc and selenium levels in mares and those in their foals. Pp. 159–164 in Proc. 10th Equine Nutr. Physiol. Soc. Symp., Fort Collins, CO.

Breidenbach, A., C. Schlumbohm, and J. Harmeyer. 1998. Peculiarities of vitamin D and of the calcium and phosphate homeostatic system in horses. Vet. Res. 29:173–186.

Bridges, C. H., and E. D. Harris. 1988. Experimentally induced cartilaginous fractures (osteochondritis dissecans) in foals fed low-copper diets. J. Am. Vet. Med. Assoc. 193:215–221.

Bridges, C. H., and P. G. Moffitt. 1990. Influence of variable content of dietary zinc on copper metabolism of weanling foals. Am. J. Vet. Res. 51:275–280.

Bridges, C. H., J. E. Womack, E. D. Harris, and W. L. Scrutchfield. 1984. Considerations of copper metabolism in osteochondrosis of suckling foals. J. Am. Vet. Med. Assoc. 185:173.

Brommer, H., and M. M. Sloet van Oldruitenborgh-Oosterbaan. 2001. Iron deficiency in stabled Dutch warmblood foals. J. Vet. Intern. Med. 15:482–485.

Bronner, F. 1993. Nutrient bioavailability, with special reference to calcium. J. Nutr. 123:797–802.

Buchholz-Bryant, M. A., L. A. Baker, J. L. Pipkin, B. J. Mansell, J. C. Haliburton, and R. C. Bachman. 2001. The effect of calcium and phosphorus supplementation, inactivity, and subsequent aerobic training on the mineral balance in young, mature, and aged horses. J. Equine Vet. Sci. 21:71–77.

Buck, W. B., G. D. Osweiler, and G. A. Van Gelder. 1976. Pp. 345–354 in Clinical and Diagnostic Veterinary Toxicology. Dubuque, IA: Kendall/Hunt.

Bushinsky, D. A., and R. D. Monk. 1998. Calcium. Lancet 352(9124): 306–311.

Butudom, P., H. C. Schott II, M. W. Davis, C. A. Kobe, B. D. Nielsen, and S. W. Eberhart. 2002. Drinking salt water enhances rehydration in horses dehydrated by frusemide administration and endurance exercise. Equine Vet. J. Suppl. 34:513–518.

Campbell-Beggs, C. L., P. J. Johnson, N. T. Messer, J. C. Lattimer, G. Johnson, and S. W. Casteel. 1994. Osteochondritis dissecans in an Appaloosa foal associated with zinc toxicosis. J. Equine Vet. Sci. 14:546–550.

Cape, L., and H. F. Hintz. 1982. Influence of month, color, age corticosteroids and dietary molybdenum on mineral concentration of equine hair. J. Am. Vet. Med. Assoc. 43:1132–1136.

Caple, I. W., S. J. A. Edwards, W. M. Forsyth, P. Whiteley, R. H. Selth, and L. J. Fulton. 1978. Blood glutathione peroxidase activity in horses in relation to muscular dystrophy and selenium nutrition. Austral Vet. J. 54:57–60.

Caple, I. W., J. M. Bourke, and P. G. Ellis. 1982. An examination of the calcium and phosphorus nutrition of Thoroughbred racehorses. Austral Vet. J. 58:132–135.

Carbery, J. T. 1978. Osteodysgenesis in a foal associated with copper deficiency. N. Z. Vet. J. 26:279–280.

Carlisle, E. M. 1970. Silicon: a possible factor in bone calcification. Science 167:279.

Carlisle, E. M. 1972. Silicon: an essential element for the chick. Science 178:619–621.

Carlisle, E. M. 1974. Silicon as an essential element. Fed. Proc. 33:1758.

Carmel, D. K., M. V. Crisman, W. B. Ley, M. H. Irby, and G. H. Edwards. 1990. A survey of whole blood selenium concentrations of horses in Maryland. Cornell Vet. 80:251–258.

Cartmill, J. A., D. L. Thompson, Jr., W. A. Storer, N. K. Huff, and C. A. Waller. 2005. Effects of chromium supplementation on plasma insulin and leptin in horses with elevated concentrations of leptin. P. 353 in Proc. 19th Equine Sci. Soc., Tucson, AZ.

Casteel, S. W. 2001. Metal toxicosis in horses. Vet. Clin. N. Am. Equine Pract. 17:517–527.

Caure, S., G. Tourtoulou, J. Valette, A. Cosnier, and P. Lebreton. 1998. Prat. Vet. Equine. 30:49–59.

Cheng, I., I. Qureshi, N. Chattopadhyay, A. Qureshi, R. R. Butters, A. E. Hall, R. R. Cima, K. V. Rogers, S. C. Hebert, J. P. Geibel, E. M. Brown, and D. I. Soybel. 1999. Expression of an extracellular calcium-sensing receptor in rat stomach. Gastroenterology 116:118–126.

Coenen, M. 1988. Effects of an experimental induced chloride deficiency in the horse. Z. Tierphysiol., Tierernahr. Futtermittelkd. 60:37–38.

Coenen, M. 1991. Chlorine metabolism in working horses and the improvement of chlorine supply. Pp. 91–92 in Proc. 12th Equine Nutr. Physiol. Soc. Symp., Calgary, Alberta.

Coenen, M. 1999. Basics for chloride metabolism and requirement. Pp. 353–354 in Proc. 16th Equine Nutr. Physiol. Soc. Symp., Raleigh, NC.

Coenen, M. 2005. Exercise and stress: impact on adaptive processes involving water and electrolytes. Livest. Prod. Sci. 92:131–145.

Coger, L. S., H. F. Hintz, H. F. Schryver, and J. E. Lowe. 1987. The effect of high zinc intake on copper metabolism and bone development in growing horses. P. 173 in Proc. 10th Equine Nutr. Physiol. Soc. Symp., Fort Collins, CO.

Cooper, S. R., K. H. Kline, J. H. Foreman, H. A. Brady, and L. P. Frey. 1998. Effects of dietary cation-anion balance on pH, electrolytes, and lactate in Standardbred horses. J. Equine Vet. Sci. 18:662–666.

Cooper, S. R., D. R. Topliff, D. W. Freeman, J. E. Breazile, and R. D. Geisert. 2000. Effect of dietary cation-anion difference on mineral balance, serum osteocalcin concentration and growth in weanling horses. J. Equine Vet. Sci. 20:39–44.

Corke, M. J. 1981. An outbreak of sulphur poisoning in horses. Vet. Rec. 109:212–213.

Cowgill, U. M., S. J. States, and J. E. Marburger. 1980. Smelter smoke syndrome in farm animals and manganese deficiency in northern Oklahoma, USA. Environ. Pollut. (Ser. A) 22:259–272.

Cromwell, G. L., V. W. Hays, and T. L. Clark. 1978. Effects of copper sulfate, copper sulfide, and sodium sulfide on performance and copper liver stores of pigs. J. Anim. Sci. 46:692–698.

Cromwell, G. L., T. S. Stahly, and H. J. Monegue. 1984. Effects of level and source of copper (sulfate vs. oxide) on performance and lever copper levels of weanling pigs. J. Anim. Sci. 59(Suppl. 1):267.

Crozier, J. A., V. G. Allen, N. E. Jack, J. P. Fontenot, and M. A. Cochran. 1997. Digestibility, apparent mineral absorption, and voluntary intake by horses fed alfalfa, tall fescue, and caucasian bluestem. J. Anim. Sci. 75:1651–1658.

Cuddeford, D., A. Woodhead, and R. Muirhead. 1990. Potential of alfalfa as a source of calcium for calcium deficient horses. Vet. Rec. 126:425–429.

Cunha, T. J., R. L. Shirley, H. L. Chapman, Jr., C. B. Ammerman, G. K. Davis, W. G. Kirk, and J. F. Hentges, Jr. 1964. Minerals for beef cattle in Florida. Florida Agr. Exp. Sta. Bull. 683.

Cupps, P. T., and C. E. Howell. 1949. The effects of feeding supplemental copper to growing foals. J. Anim. Sci. 8:286–289.

Cymbaluk, N. F. 1990. Cold housing effects on growth and nutrient demand on young horses. J. Anim. Sci. 68:3152–3162.

Cymbaluk, N. F., and M. E. Smart. 1993. A review of possible metabolic relationships of copper to equine bone disease. Equine Vet. J. 16(Suppl.):19–26.

Cymbaluk, N. F., H. F. Schryver, and H. F. Hintz. 1981a. Copper metabolism and requirements in mature ponies. J. Nutr. 111:87–95.

Cymbaluk, N. F., H. F. Schryver, H. F. Hintz, D. F. Smith, and J. E. Lowe. 1981b. Influence of dietary molybdenum on copper metabolism in ponies. J. Nutr. 111:96–106.

Cymbaluk, N. F., F. M. Bristol, and D. A. Christensen. 1986. Influence of age and breed of equid on plasma copper and zinc concentrations. Am. J. Vet. Res. 47:192–195.

Cymbaluk, N. F., G. I. Christison, and D. H. Leach. 1989. Nutrient utilization by limit- and *ad libitum*-fed growing horses. J. Anim. Sci. 67:414–425.

Davies, M. E. 1971. The production of B12 in the horse. Br. Vet. J. 127:34.

De Behr, V., D. Daron, A. Gabriel, B. Remy, I. Dufrasne, D. Serteyn, and L. Istasse. 2003. The course of some bone remodeling plasma metabolites in healthy horses and in horses offered a calcium-deficient diet. J. Anim. Physiol. Anim. Nutr. 87:149–159.

Dill, S. G., and W. C. Rebhun. 1985. White muscle disease in foals. Comp. Cont. Ed. 7:S627.

Dimock, A. N., S. L. Ralston, K. Malinowski, and D. W. Horohov. 1999. The effect of supplemental dietary chromium on the immune status of geriatric mares. Pp. 10–11 in Proc. 16th Equine Nutr. Physiol. Soc. Symp., Raleigh, NC.

Donoghue, S., T. N. Meacham, and D. S. Kronfeld. 1990. A conceptual approach to optimal nutrition of brood mares. Vet. Clin. North Am. Equine Pract. 6:373–390.

Drepper, K., J. O. Gutte, H. Meyer, and F. J. Schwarz. 1982. Energie- und Nahrstoffbedarf landwirtschaftlicher Nutztiere. Nr. 2 Empfehlungen zur Energie- und Nahrstoffversorgung der Pferde. Frankfurt am Main, Germany: DLG Verlag.

Dufner, M. M., P. Kirchhoff, C. Remy, P. Hafner, M. K. Muller, S. X. Cheng, L.-Q. Tang, S. C. Hebert, J. P. Geibel, and C. A. Wagner. 2005. The calcium-sensing receptor acts as a modulator of gastric acid secretion in freshly isolated human gastric glands. Am. J. Physiol. Gastrointest. Liver. Physiol. 289:G1084–G1090.

Eamens, G. J., J. F. Macadam, and E. A. Laing. 1984. Skeletal abnormalities in young horses associated with zinc toxicity and hypocuprosis. Austral Vet. J. 61:205–207.

Ecke, P., D. R. Hodgson, and R. J. Rose. 1998a. Induced diarrhoea in horses. Part 1: Fluid and electrolyte balance. Vet. J. 155:149–159.

Ecke, P., D. R. Hodgson, and R. J. Rose. 1998b. Induced diarrhoea in horses. Part 2: Response to administration of an oral rehydration solution. Vet. J. 155:161–170.

Edens, L. M., J. L. Robertson, and B. F. Feldman. 1993. Cholestatic hepatopathy, thrombocytopenia and lymphopenia associated with iron toxicity in a Thoroughbred gelding. Equine Vet. J. 25:81–84.

Edmondson, A. J., B. B. Norman, and D. Suther. 1993. Survey of state veterinarians and state veterinary diagnostic laboratories for selenium deficiency and toxicosis in animals. J. Am. Vet. Med. Assoc. 202:865–872.

Edwards, M. S. 2004. Aspects of equine nutrition and management at the zoological society of San Diego. Proc. Comp. Nutr. Soc. Pp. 30–38.

Eeckhout, W., and M. De Paepe. 1994. Total phosphorus, phytate-phosphorus and phytase activity in plant feedstuffs. Anim. Feed Sci. Technol. 47:19–29.

El Shorafa, W. M., J. P. Feaster, and E. A. Ott. 1979. Horse metacarpal bone: age, ash content, cortical area, and failure-stress interrelationships. J. Anim. Sci. 49:979–982.

Elmore-Smith, K. A., J. L. Pipkin, L. A. Baker, W. J. Lampley, J. C. Haliburton, and R. C. Bachman. 1999. The effect of aerobic exercise after a sedentary period on serum, fecal, and urine calcium and phosphorus concentrations in mature horses. Pp. 106–107 in Proc. 16th Equine Nutr. Physiol Soc. Symp., Raleigh, NC.

English, J. L., and K. M. Hambidge. 1988. Plasma and serum zinc concentrations: effect of time between collection and separation. Clin. Chim. Acta. 175:211–216.

Eroksuz, H., Y. Eroksuz, A. Ozer, A. O. Ceribasi, I. Yaman, and N. Ilhan. 2004. Equine goiter associated with excess dietary iodine. Vet. Hum. Toxicol. 46:147–149.

Fadok, V. A., and S. Wild. 1983. Suspected cutaneous iodinism in a horse. J. Am. Vet. Med. Assoc. 183:1104–1106.

Fan, A. M., and K. W. Kizer. 1990. Selenium: nutritional, toxicologic, and clinical aspects. West. J. Med. 153:160–167.

FDA (Food and Drug Administration). 1987. Food additives permitted in feed and drinking water of animals. Fed. Reg. 52 (Part 573, No. 65):10887. April 6.

Fettman, M. J., L. E. Chase, J. Bentinck-Smith, C. E. Coppocdk, and S. A. Zinn. 1984. Effects of dietary chloride restriction in lactating dairy cows. J. Am. Vet. Med. Assoc. 185:167.

Filmer, J. F. 1933. Enzootic marasmus of cattle and sheep. Austral. Vet. J. 9:163–179.

Finley, J. W. 2005. Selenium accumulation in plant foods. Nutr. Rev. 63:196–202.

Firoz, M., and M. Graber. 2001. Bioavailability of US commercial magnesium preparations. Magnes. Res. 14:257–262.

Flaminio, M. J., and B. R. Rush. 1998. Fluid and electrolyte balance in endurance horses. Vet. Clin. North Am. Equine Pract. 14:147–158.

Furtado, C. E., H. Tosi, D. M. S. S. Vitti. 2000. Endogenous loss and true absorption of phosphorus in the diet for growing horses. Pesq. Agropec. Bras. 35:1023–1028.

Gabel, A. 2005. Metabolic bone disease to developmental orthopedic disease. J. Equine Vet. Sci. 25:94.

Gallagher, K., and H. D. Stowe. 1980. Influence of exercise on serum selenium and peroxide reduction system of racing Standardbreds. Am. J. Vet. Res. 41:1333–1335.

Garcia-Lopez, J. M., P. J. Provost, J. E. Rush, S. C. Zicker, H. Burmaster, and L. M. Freeman. 2001. Prevalence and prognostic importance of hypomagnesia and hypocalcemia in horses that have colic surgery. Am. J. Vet. Res. 62:7–12.

Gee, E. K., N. D. Grace, E. C. Firth, and P. F. Fennessy. 2000. Changes in liver copper concentration of Thoroughbred foals from birth to 160 days of age and the effect of prenatal copper supplementation of their dams. Austral. Vet. J. 78:347–353.

GEH (Gesellschaft fur Ernahrungsphysiologie der Haustiere). 1994. Energie- und Nahrstoffbedarf landwirtschaftlicher Nutztiere, Nr. 2: Empfehlungen zur Energie- und Nahrstoffverssorgung der Pferde. Frankfurt am Main: DLG-Verlag, pp. 67.

Gentry, L. R., D. L. Thompson, Jr., J. M. Fernandez, L. A. Kincaid, D. W. Horohov, and B. S. Leise. 1997. Effects of chromium tripicolinate supplementation on hormone and metabolite concentrations and immune function in mares. Pp. 151–152 in Proc. 15th Equine Nutr. Physiol Soc. Symp., Ft. Worth, TX.

Georgievskii, V. I., B. N. Annenkov, and V. T. Samokhin. 1982. The physiological role of macroelements. Pp. 159–170 in Mineral Nutrition in Animals. London: Butterworth.

Glade, M. J. 1993. Effects of gestation, lactation, and maternal calcium intake on mechanical strength of equine bone. J. Am. College Nutr. 12:372–377.

Grace, N. D., S. G. Pearce, E. C. Firth and P. F. Fennessy. 1999a. Concentration of macro- and micro-elements in the milk of pasture-fed Thoroughbred mares. Austral Vet. J. 77:177–180.

Grace, N. D., S. G. Pearce, E. C. Firth and P. F. Fennessy. 1999b. Content and distribution of macro- and micro-elements in the body of pasture-fed young horses. Austral Vet. J. 77:172–176.

Grace, N. D., C. W. Rogers, E. C. Firth, T. L. Faram, and H. L. Shaw. 2003. Digestible energy intake, dry matter digestibility and effect of increased calcium intake on bone parameters of grazing Thoroughbred weanlings in New Zealand. N. Z. Vet. J. 51:165–173.

Graham, R., J. Sampson, and H. R. Hester. 1940. The results of feeding zinc to pregnant mares and foals. Vet. Rec. 97:41–47.

Gray, J., P. Harris, and D. H. Snow. 1988. Preliminary investigations into the calcium and magnesium status of the horse. Pp. 307–317 in Animal Clinical Biochemistry—the Future, D. J. Blackmore, ed. Cambridge, MA: Cambridge University Press.

Green, H. H., W. M. Allcroft, and R. F. Montgomerie. 1935. Hypomagnesaemia in equine transit tetany. J. Comp. Pathol. 48:74–79.

Gunson, D. E., D. F. Kowalczyk, C. R. Shoop, and C. F. Ramberg. 1982. Environmental zinc and cadmium pollution associated with generalized osteochondrosis, osteoporosis, and nephrocalcinosis. J. Am. Vet. Med. Assoc. 180:295.

Hainze, M. T. M., R. B. Muntifering, C. W. Wood, C. A. McCall, and B. H. Wood. 2004. Faecal phosphorus excretion from horses fed typical diets with and without added phytase. Anim. Feed Sci. Tech. 117:265–279.

Harmeyer, J., and C. Schlumbohm. 2004. Effects of pharmacological doses of Vitamin D3 on mineral balance and profiles of plasma Vitamin D3 metabolites in horses. J. Steroid Biochem. Mol. Biol. 89–90;595–600.

Harrington, D. D. 1974. Pathological features of magnesium deficiency in young horses fed purified rations. Am. J. Vet. Res. 35:503–513.

Harrington, D. D., and J. J. Walsh. 1980. Equine magnesium supplements: evaluation of magnesium sulphate and magnesium carbonate in foals fed purified diets. Equine Vet. J. 12:32–33.

Harrington, D. D., J. Walsh, and V. White. 1973. Clinical and pathological findings in horses fed zinc deficient diets. P. 51 in Proc. 3rd Equine Nutr. Physiol. Soc. Symp., Gainesville, FL.

Hayes, J. W., C. G. Stiner, M. J. Holmes, and S. A. Mackenzie. 1987. Comparison of selenium blood levels and dietary selenium in three breeds of horses. Equine Pract. 9:25–29.

Henninger, R. W., and J. Horst. 1997. Magnesium toxicosis in two horses. J. Am. Vet. Med. Assoc. 211:82–85.

Hess, T. M., D. S. Kronfeld, C. A. Williams, J. N. Waldron, P. M. Graham-Thiers, K. Greiwe-Crandell, M. A. Lopes, and P. A. Harris. 2005. Effects of oral potassium supplementation on acid-base status and plasma ion concentrations of horses during endurance exercise. Am. Vet. Res. 66:466–473.

Highfill, J. L., G. D. Potter, E. M. Eller, P. G. Gibbs, B. D. Scott, and D. M. Hood. 2005. Comparative absorption of calcium fed in varying chemical forms and effects on absorption of phosphorus and magnesium. Pp. 37–42 in Proc. 19th Equine Sci. Soc., Tucson, AZ.

Hinchcliff, K. W. 2005. Exercise-induced pulmonary hemorrhage. P. 51 in Proc. Am. Assoc. Equine Pract., Seattle, WA.

Hinchcliff, K. W., K. H. McKeever, W. W. Muir, and R. A. Sams. 1995. Pharmacologic interaction of furosemide and phenylbutazone in horses. Am. J. Vet. Res. 56:1206–1212.

Hiney, K. M., B. D. Nielsen, and D. S. Rosenstein. 2004. Short-duration exercise and confinement alters bone mineral content and shape in weanling horses. J. Anim. Sci. 82:2313–2320.

Hintz, H. F. 1987a. Self-selection of calcium by horses. Equine Pract. 9:5–6.

Hintz, H. F. 1987b. Effect of diet on copper content of milk. Equine Pract. 9:6–7.

Hintz, H. F. 1989. Iodine toxicosis. Equine Pract. 11:5–6.

Hintz, H. F. 1995. Lowered potassium forage. Equine Pract. 17:6–7.

Hintz, H. F. 1996. Mineral requirements of growing horses. Pferdeheilkunde. 12:303–306.

Hintz, H. F. 1997. Straight from the horse's mouth: nutritional secondary hyperparathyroidism still happens. Equine Pract. 19:5–6.

Hintz, H. F. 1999. Sources of selenium for grazing horses. Equine Pract. 21:6.

Hintz, H. F. 2000. Macrominerals-calcium, phosphorus and magnesium. Adv. Equine Nutr., Proc. 2000 Equine Nutr. Conf. Feed Manuf.: 121–131.

Hintz, H. F., and H. F. Schryver. 1972. Magnesium metabolism in the horse. J. Anim. Sci. 35:755.

Hintz, H. F., and H. F. Schryver. 1973. Magnesium, calcium, and phosphorus metabolism in ponies fed varying levels of magnesium. J. Anim. Sci. 37:927–930.

Hintz, H. F., and H. F. Schryver. 1976. Potassium metabolism in ponies. J. Anim. Sci. 42:637–643.

Hintz, H. F., A. J. Williams, J. Rogoff, and H. F. Schryver. 1973. Availability of phosphorus in wheatbran when fed to ponies. J. Anim. Sci. 36:522–525.

Hintz, H. F., H. F. Schryver, J. Doty, C. Lakin, and R. A. Zimmerman. 1984. Oxalic acid content of alfalfa hays and its influence on the availability of calcium, phosphorus, and magnesium to ponies. J. Anim. Sci. 58:939–942.

Hodgson, D. R., and R. J. Rose. 1994. The Athletic Horse. Philadelphia: W. B. Saunders, pp. 67.

Hoekstra, K. E., B. D. Nielsen, M. W. Orth, D. S. Rosenstein, H. C. Schott, and J. E. Shelle. 1999. Comparison of bone mineral content and bone metabolism in stall- versus pasture-reared horses. Equine Vet. J. Suppl. 30:601–604.

Hoffman, R. M., L. A. Lawrence, D. S. Kronfeld, W. L. Cooper, D. J. Sklan, J. J. Dascanio, and P. A. Harris. 2000. Dietary carbohydrates and fat influence radiographic bone mineral content of growing horses. J. Anim. Sci. 77:3330–3338.

Hoffman, R. M., J. A. Wilson, L. A. Lawrence, D. S. Kronfeld, W. L. Cooper, and P. A. Harris. 2001. Supplemental calcium does not influence radiographic bone mineral content of growing foals fed pasture and a fat-and-fiber supplement. P. 122 in Proc. 17th Equine Nutr. Physiol. Soc. Symp., Lexington, KY.

Holbrook, T. C., R. D. Simmons, M. E. Payton, and C. G. MacAllister. 2005. Effect of repeated oral administration of hypertonic electrolyte solution on equine gastric mucosa. Equine Vet. J. 37:501–504.

House, W. A., and A. W. Bell. 1993. Mineral accretion in the fetus and adnexa during late gestation in Holstein cows. J. Dairy Sci. 76:2999–3010.

Hotz, C. S., D. W. Fitzpatrick, K. D. Trick, and M. R. L'Abbe. 1997. Dietary iodine and selenium interact to affect thyroid hormone metabolism. J. Nutr. 127:1214–1218.

Howes, A. D., and I. A. Dyer. 1971. Diet and supplemental mineral effects on manganese metabolism in newborn calves. J. Anim. Sci. 32:141–145.

Hoyt, J. K., G. D. Potter, L. W. Greene, M. M. Vogelsang, and J. G. Anderson, Jr. 1995a. Electrolyte balance in exercising horses fed a control and a fat-supplemented diet. J. Equine Vet. Sci. 15:429–435.

Hoyt, J. K., G. D. Potter, L. W. Greene, J. G. Anderson, Jr. 1995b. Mineral balance in resting and exercised miniature horses. J. Equine Vet. Sci. 15:310–314.

Hudson, C., J. Pagan, K. Hoekstra, A. Prince, S. Gardner, and R. Geor. 2001. Effects of exercise training on the digestibility and requirements of copper, zinc and manganese in Thoroughbred horses. Pp. 138–140 in Proc. 17th Equine Nutr. Physiol Soc. Symp., Lexington, KY.

Hurtig, M., S. L. Green, H. Dobson, Y. Mikuni-Takagaki, and J. Choi. 1993. Correlative study of defective cartilage and bone growth in foals fed a low-copper diet. Equine Vet. J. 16:66–73.

Inoue, Y., A. Matsui, Y. Asai, F. Aoki, K. Yoshimoto, T. Matsui, and H. Yano. 2003. Effects of exercise on iron metabolism in Thoroughbred horses. P. 268 in Proc. 18th Equine Nutr. Physiol. Soc. Symp., East Lansing, MI.

Jackson, S. G. 1997. Trace minerals for the performance horses: known biochemical roles and estimates of requirements. Irish Vet. J. 50:668–674.

Jackson, S. G., and J. D. Pagan. 1996. Nutrition and productivity: practical problems related to nutrition. Pp. 131–148 in Proc. 18th Aust. Equine Vet. Assoc. Bain Memorial Lect., Glenelg, South Australia.

Janicki, K. M., L. M. Lawrence, T. Barnes, and C. J. Stine. 2001. The effect of dietary selenium source and level on selenium concentration, glutathione peroxidase activity, and influenza titers in broodmares and their foals. Pp. 43–44 in Proc. 17th Equine Nutr. Physiol Soc. Symp., Lexington, KY.

Jansson, A., and K. Dahlborn. 1999. Effects of feeding frequency and voluntary salt intake on fluid and electrolyte regulation in athletic horses. J. Appl. Physiol. 86:1610–1616.

Jansson, A., S. Nyman, K. Morgan, C. Palmgren-Karlsson, A. Lindholm, and K. Dahlborn. 1995. The effect of ambient temperature and saline loading on changes in plasma and urine electrolytes (Na^+ and K^+) following exercise. Equine Vet. J. Suppl. 20:147–152.

Jansson, A., A. Lindholm, J. E. Lindberg, and K. Dahlborn. 1999. Effects of potassium intake on potassium, sodium and fluid balances in exercising horses. Equine Vet. J. Suppl. 30:412–417.

Jarrige, R., and W. Martin-Rosset. 1981. Le cheval: Reproduction, selection, alimentation, exploitation. XIII Journees du Grenier de Theix. Paris: Institut National de la Recherche Agronomique.

Jee, W. S. S. 1988. The skeletal tissues. P. 207 in Histology: Cell and Tissue Biology, 5th ed., L. Weiss, ed. New York: Elsevier Biomedical.

Jeffcott, L. B., and M. E. Davies. 1998. Copper status and skeletal development in horses: still a long way to go. Equine Vet. J. 30:183–185.

Jiong, Z., C. Zeng-Cheng, L. Su-Mei, D. Yin Jie, Z. Kang-Nan, and Z. Xu-Jiu. 1987. Selenium deficiency in horses (1981–1983). P. 843 in Selenium in Biology and Medicine, Part B, G. F. Combs, J. E. Spallholz, O. A. Levander, and J. E. Oldfields, eds. New York: Van Nostrand Reinhold.

Johnson, M. A., and C. L. Murphy. 1988. Adverse effects of high dietary iron and ascorbic acid on copper status in copper-deficient and copper-adequate rats. Am. J. Clin. Nutr. 47:96–101.

Johnson, P. J. 1995. Electrolyte and acid-base disturbances in the horses. Vet. Clin. North Am. Equine Pract. 11:491–514.

Johnson, P. J. 1998. Physiology of body fluids in the horse. Vet. Clin. North Am. Equine Pract. 14:1–22.

Johnson, P. J., T. E. Goetz, J. H. Foreman, R. S. Vogel, W. E. Hoffman, and G. J. Baker. 1991. Effect of whole-body potassium depletion on plasma, erythrocyte, and middle gluteal muscle potassium concentrations of healthy, adult horses. Am. J. Vet. Res. 52:1676–1683.

Jones, H., and G. H. Rasmusson. 1980. Recent advances in the biology and chemistry of vitamin D. Pp. 63–111 in Progress in the Chemistry of Organic Natural Products, vol. 39, W. Herz, H. Griesbach, and G. W. Kirby, eds. Berlin: Springer.

Jordan, R. M., V. S. Meyers, B. Yoho, and F. A. Spurrell. 1975. Effect of calcium and phosphorus levels on growth, reproduction, and bone development of ponies. J. Anim. Sci. 40:78–85.

Jugdaohsingh, R., D. M. Reffitt, C. Oldham, J. P. Day, L. K. Fifield, R. P. H. Thompson, and J. J. Powell. 2000. Oligomeric but not monomeric silica prevents aluminum absorption in humans. Am. J. Clin. Nutr. 71:944–949.

Kapusniak, L. J., L. W. Greene, and G. D. Potter. 1988. Calcium, magnesium and phosphorus absorption from the small and large intestine of ponies fed elevated amounts of aluminum. Equine Vet. Sci. 8:305–309.

Kato, G., J. S. Kelly, K. Drnjevic, and G. Somjen. 1968. Anaesthetic action of magnesium ions. Can. Anaesth. Soc. J. 15:539.

Kavazis, A. N., J. Kivipelto, and E. A. Ott. 2002. Supplementation of broodmares with copper, zinc, iron, manganese, cobalt, iodine, and selenium. J. Equine Vet. Sci. 22:460–464.

Kirkham, W. W., H. Guttridge, J. Bowden, and G. T. Edds. 1971. Hematopoietic responses to hematinics in horses. J. Am. Vet. Med. Assoc. 159:1316–1318.

Knight, D. A., A. A. Gabel, S. M. Reed, L. R. Bramlage, W. J. Tyznik, and R. M. Embertson. 1985. Correlation of dietary mineral to incidence and severity of metabolic bone disease in Ohio and Kentucky. P. 445 in Proc. 31st Am. Assoc. Equine Pract., F. J. Milne, ed. Lexington, KY: Am. Assoc. Equine Pract.

Knight, D. A., S. E. Weisbrade, L. M. Schmall, and A. A. Gavel. 1988. Copper supplementation and cartilage lesions in foals. Pp. 191–194 in Proc. 33rd Conv. Am. Assoc. Equine Pract., New Orleans.

Knight, D. A., S. E. Weisbrode, L. M. Schmall, S. M. Reed, A. A. Gabel, L. Bramlage. 1990. The effects of copper supplementation on the prevalence of cartilage lesions in foals. Equine Vet. J. 22:426–432.

Kohn, C. W., R. M. Jacobs, D. Knight, W. Hueston, A. A. Gabel, and S. M. Reed. 1990. Microcytosis, hypoferremia, hypoferritemia, and hypertransferrinemai in Standardbred foals from birth to 4 months of age. Am. J. Vet. Res. 51:1198–1205.

Kronfeld, D. S. 2001. Body fluids and exercise: replacement strategies. J. Equine Vet. Sci. 21:368–375.

Kronfeld, D. S., T. N. Meacham, and S. Donoghue. 1990. Dietary aspects of developmental orthopedic disease in young horses. Vet. Clin. North Am.: Equine Pract. 6:451–465.

Krook, L., and J. E. Lowe. 1964. Nutritional secondary hyperparathyroidism in the horse. Pathol. Vet. 1(Suppl. 1):98.

Krook, L., and G. A. Maylin. 1988. Fractures in Thoroughbred race horses. Cornell Vet. 98(Suppl. 11):5–133.

Kruzhova, E. 1968. Mikroelementy i vosproizvoditel'naja funkeija kobyl. Tr. Vses. Inst. Konevodstvo. 2:28 (as cited in Nutr. Abstr. Rev. 39:807, 1968).

Lang, K. J., B. D. Nielsen, K. L. Waite, J. Link, G. M. Hill, and M. W. Orth. 2001a. Increased plasma silicon concentrations and altered bone resorption in response to sodium zeolite A supplementation in yearling horses. J. Equine Vet. Sci. 21:550–555.

Lang, K. J., B. D. Nielsen, K. L. Waite, G. M. Hill, and M. W. Orth. 2001b. Supplemental silicon increases plasma and milk silicon concentrations in horses. J. Anim. Sci. 79:2627–2633.

Lau, K. 1986. Phosphate disorders. Pp 398–471 in Fluids and Electrolytes, J. P. Kokko and R. L. Tannen, eds. Philadelphia: W. B. Saunders Co.

Lawrence, L. 1986. The use of non-invasive techniques to estimate bone mineral content and bone strength in the horse. Ph.D. dissertation. University of Florida.

Lawrence, L. 2004. Trace minerals in equine nutrition: assessing bioavailability. Pp. 84–91 in Proc. Conf. Equine Nutr. Res., Texas A&M University.

Lawrence, L. A., E. A. Ott, R. L. Asquith, and G. J. Miller. 1987. Influence of dietary iron on growth, tissue mineral composition, apparent phosphorus absorption, and chemical properties of bone. Pp. 563 in Proc. 10th Equine. Nutr. Physiol. Soc. Symp., Fort Collins, CO.

Lawrence, L., J. Bicudo, J. Davis, and E. Wheeler. 2003. Relationships between intake and excretion for nitrogen and phosphorus in horses. Pp. 306–307 in Proc. 18th Equine Nutr. Physiol. Soc. Symp., East Lansing, MI.

Lee, J., E. S. McAllister, and R. W. Scholz. 1995. Assessment of selenium status in mares and foals under practical management conditions. J. Equine Vet. Sci. 15:240–245.

Lewis, L. D. 1995. Equine Clinical Nutrition: Feeding and Care. Media, PA: Williams & Wilkins.

Lindberg, J. S., M. M. Zobitz, J. R. Poindexter, and C. Y. Pak. 1990. Magnesium bioavailability from magnesium citrate and magnesium oxide. J. Am. Coll. Nutr. 9:48–55.

Lindholm, A., and A. Asheim. 1973. Vitamin E and certain muscular enzymes in the blood serum of horses. Acta Agr. Scand. Suppl. 19:40–42.

Lindinger, M. I., L. J. McCutcheon, G. L. Ecker, and R. J. Geor. 2000. Heat acclimation improves regulation of plasma volume and plasma Na(+) content during exercise in horses. J. Appl. Physiol. 88:1006–1013.

Lloyd, K., H. F. Hintz, J. D. Wheat, and H. F. Schryver. 1987. Enteroliths in horses. Cornell Vet. 77:172–186.

Lloyd, T., M. A. Petit, H.-M. Lin, and T. J. Beck. 2004. Lifestyle factors and the development of bone mass and bone strength in young women. J. Pediatr. 144:776–782.

Lopez, I., J. C. Estepa, F. J. Mendoza, R. Mayer-Valor, and E. Aguilera-Tejero. 2006. Fractionation of calcium and magnesium in equine serum. Am. J. Vet. Res. 67:463–466.

Lukaski, H. C. 2000. Magnesium, zinc, and chromium nutriture and physical activity. Am. J. Clin. Nutr. 72:585S–593S.

Luthersson, N., S. Chunekamrai, J. C. Estepa, and E. Aguilera-Tejero. 2005. Secondary nutritional hyperparathyroidism in ponies in Northern Thailand. Pferdeheilkunde. 21:97–98.

Mansell, B. J., L. A. Baker, J. L. Pipkin, M. A. Buchholz, G. O. Veneklasen, D. R. Topliff, and R. C. Bachman. 1999. The effects of inactivity and subsequent aerobic training, and mineral supplementation on bone remodeling in varying ages of horses. Pp. 46–51 in Proc. 16th Equine Nutr. Physiol. Soc. Symp., East Lansing, MI.

Martin, K. L., R. M. Hoffman, D. S. Kronfeld, W. B. Ley, and L. D. Warnick. 1996. Calcium decreases and parathyroid hormone increases in serum of periparturient mares. J. Anim. Sci. 74:834–839.

Mason, D. K., K. L. Watkins, and J. T. McNie. 1988. Diagnosis, treatment and prevention of nutritional secondary hyperparathyroidism in Thorough-bred race horses in Hong Kong. Equine Pract. 10:10–17.

Matsui, A., T. Osawa, H. Fujikawa, Y. Asai, T. Matsui, and H. Yano. 2002. Estimation of total sweating rate and mineral loss through sweat during exercise in 2-year-old horses at cool ambient temperature. J. Equine Sci. 13:109–112.

Maylin, G. H., D. S. Rubin, and D. H. Lein. 1980. Selenium and vitamin E in horses. Cornell Vet. 70:272.

Mazzella, G., R. Godbee, W. Schurg, and M. Arns. 2005. Plasma silicon concentrations in weanling horses fed sodium zeolite A or azomite A. P. 353 in Proc. 19th Equine Sci. Soc. Symp., Tucson, AZ.

McConaghy, F. 1994. Thermoregulation. In The Athletic Horse, R. Hodgson and R. J. Rose, eds. Philadelphia: W. B. Saunders.

McCutcheon, L. J., and R. J. Geor. 1996. Sweat fluid and ion losses in horses during training and competition in cool vs. hot ambient conditions: implications for ion supplementation. Equine Vet. J. Suppl. 22:54–62.

McCutcheon, L. J., and R. J. Geor. 1998. Sweating. Fluid and ion losses and replacement. Vet. Clin. North Am. Equine Pract. 14:75–95.

McCutcheon, L. J., R. J. Geor, G. L. Ecker, and M. I. Lindinger. 1999. Equine sweating responses to submaximal exercise during 21 days of heat acclimation. J. Appl. Physiol. 87:1843–1851.

McKeever, K. H., R. Scali, S. Geiser, and C. F. Kearns. 2002. Plasma aldosterone concentration and renal excretion are altered during the first days of training. Equine Vet. J. Suppl. 34:524–531.

McKenzie, E. C., S. J. Valberg, S. M. Godden, J. D. Pagan, G. P. Carlson, J. M. MacLeay, and F. D. DeLaCorte. 2002. Plasma and urine electrolyte and mineral concentrations in Thoroughbred horses with recurrent exertional rhabdomyolysis after consumption of diets varying in cation-anion balance. Am. J. Vet. Res. 63:1053–1060.

McKenzie, E. C., S. J. Valberg, S. M. Godden, J. D. Pagan, G. P. Carlson, J. M. MacLeay, and F. D. DeLaCorte. 2003. Comparison of volumetric urine collection versus single-sample urine collection in horses consuming diets varying in cation-anion balance. Am. J. Vet. Res. 64:284–291.

McKenzie, R. A., B. J. Blaney, and R. J. W. Gartner. 1981. The effect of dietary oxalate on calcium, phosphorus and magnesium balances in horses. J. Agr. Sci. Camb. 97:69–74.

McLaughlin, B. G., and C. E. Doige. 1981. Congenital musculoskeletal lesions and hyperplastic goiter in foals. Can. Vet. J. 22:130–133.

McLaughlin, B. G., C. E. Doige, and P. S. McLaughlin. 1986. Thyroid hormone levels in foals with congenital musculoskeletal lesions. Can. Vet. J. 27:264–267.

McLaughlin, J. G., and J. Cullen. 1986. Clinical cases of chronic selenosis in horses. Irish Vet. J. 40:136–138.

Mee, J. F., and J. McLaughlin. 1995. "Normal" blood copper levels in horses. Vet. Rec 136:275.

Mello, J. R. B. 2003. Calcinosis—calcinogenic plants. Toxicon. 41:1–12.

Merck Veterinary Manual. 2005. 9th ed. Whitehouse Station, NJ: Merck & Co.

Mertz, W. 1992. Chromium: history and nutritional importance. Biol. Trace Min. Res. 32:3–8.

Messer, N. T. 1981. Tibiotarsal effusion associated with chronic zinc intoxication in three horses. J. Am. Vet. Med. Assoc. 178:294–297.

Meyer, H. 1979. Magnesiumstoffwechsel und Magnesiumbedarf des Pferdes (Magnesium metabolism and magnesium requirement in the horse). Übersichten Tierernährung 7:75–92.

Meyer, H. 1986. Mineral requirements of riding horses. Paper presented at IV World Congress of Animal Feeding, Madrid, June 30–July 4.

Meyer, H. 1987. Nutrition of the equine athlete. Pp. 644–673 in Equine Exercise Physiology II, J. R. Gillespie and W. E. Robinson, eds. Davis, CA: ICEEP Publ.

Meyer, H. 1990. Assessing of the mineral supply of horses by urine analysis. Pp. 86–97 in Contributions to water and mineral metabolism of the horse, Animal Nutrition 21, H. Meyer and B. Stadermann, eds. Adv. Anim. Physiol.

Meyer, H. 1996a. Influence of feed intake and composition, feed and water restriction, and exercise on gastrointestinal fill in horses, Part 1. Equine Pract. 18:26–29.

Meyer, H. 1996b. Influence of feed intake and composition, feed and water restriction, and exercise on gastrointestinal fill in horses, Part 3. Equine Pract. 18:25–28.

Meyer, H. 1996c. The newly born foal—everything clear? Pferdeheilkunde. 3:171–178.

Meyer, H., and L. Ahlswede. 1977. Untersuchungen zum Mg-Stoffwechsel des Pferdes. Zentralbl. Veterinacrmed. 24:128–139.

Meyer, H., and L. Ahlswede. 1978. The intrauterine growth and body composition of foals and the nutrient requirements of pregnant mares. Anim. Res. Dev. 8:86.

Meyer, H., and E. Klug. 2001. Dietary effects on the fertility of mares and the viability of newly born foals. Pferdeheilkunde. 1:47–62.

Meyer, H., and W. Tiegs. 1995. Liver Cu-concentration in the fetus and newly born foal. Pp. 8–12 in Proc. 14th Equine Nutr. Physiol. Soc. Symp., Ontario, CA.

Meyer, H., M. Schmidt, A. Lindner, and M. Pferdekamp. 1984. Beitrage zur Verdauungsphysiologie des Pferdes. 9. Einfluss einer marginalen Na-Versorgung auf Na-Bilanz. Na-Gehalt im Schweiss sowie klinische Symptome. Z. Tierphysiol. Tierernahr. Futtermittelkd. 51: 182–196.

Meyer, H., M. Heilemann, A. Hipp-Quarton, and H. Perez-Noriega. 1990. Amount and composition of sweat in ponies. Pp. 21–34 in Contributions to water and mineral metabolism of the horse, Animal Nutrition 21. H. Meyer and B. Stadermann, eds. Adv. Anim. Physiol.

Michael, E. M., G. D. Potter, K. J. Maathiason-Kochan, P. G. Gibbs, E. L. Morris, L. W. Greene, and D. Topliff. 2001. Biochemical markers of bone modeling and remodeling in juvenile racehorses fed differing levels of minerals. Pp. 117–121 in Proc. 17th Equine Nutr. Physiol. Soc. Symp., Lexington, KY.

Miller, W. T., and K. T. Williams. 1940. Minimal lethal dose of selenium as sodium selenite in horses, mules, cattle, and swine. J. Agr. Res. 60:163–173.

Miller, E. D., L. A. Baker, J. L. Pipkin, R. C. Bachman, J. T. Haliburton, and G. O. Veneklasen. 2003. The effect of supplemental inorganic and organic forms of copper and zinc on digestibility in yearling geldings in training. Pp. 107–112 in Proc. 18th Equine Nutr. Physiol. Soc. Symp., East Lansing, MI.

Mills, P. C., and D. J. Marlin. 1996. Plasma iron in elite horses at rest and after transport. Vet. Rec. 139:215–217.

Moffett, A. D., S. R. Cooper, D. W. Freeman, and H. T. Purvis II. 2001. Response of yearling Quarter Horses to varying concentrations of dietary calcium. Pp. 62–68 in Proc. 17th Equine Nutr. Physiol. Soc. Symp., Lexington, KY.

Moore, C. V. 1951. Iron metabolism and nutrition. Harvey Lect. 55:67.

Morris-Stoker, L. B., L. A. Baker, J. L. Pipkin, R. C. Bachman, and J. C. Haliburton. 2001. The effect of supplemental phytase on nutrient digestibility in mature horses. Pp. 48–52 in Proc. 17th Equine Nutr. Physiol. Soc. Symp., Lexington, KY.

Mullaney, T., and C. Brown. 1988. Iron toxicity in neonatal foals. Equine Vet. J. 20:119–124.

Nielsen, B. D. 2005. What do markers of bone formation tell us in equine nutritional studies? Pferdeheilkunde 21:99–100.

Nielsen, B. D., G. D. Potter, E. L. Morris, T. W. Odom, D. M. Senor, J. A. Reynolds, W. B. Smith, M. T. Martin, and E. H. Bird. 1993. Training distance to failure in young racing Quarter Horses fed sodium zeolite A. J. Equine Vet. Sci. 13:562–567.

Nielsen, B. D., G. D. Potter, E. L. Morris, T. W. Odom, D. M. Senor, J. A. Reynolds, W. B. Smith, and M. T. Martin. 1997. Changes in the third metacarpal bone and frequency of bone injuries in young Quarter Horses during race training—observations and theoretical considerations. J. Equine Vet. Sci. 17:541–549.

Nielsen, B. D., G. D. Potter, L. W. Greene, E. L. Morris, M. Murray-Gerzik, W. B. Smith, and M. T. Martin. 1998a. Characterization of changes related to mineral balance and bone metabolism in the young racing Quarter Horse. J. Equine Vet. Sci. 18:190–200.

Nielsen, B. D., G. D. Potter, L. W. Greene, E. L. Morris, M. Murray-Gerzik, W. B. Smith, and M. T. Martin. 1998b. Response of young horses in training to varying concentrations of dietary calcium and phosphorus. J. Equine Vet. Sci. 18:397–404.

Nielsen, F. H. 1991. Nutritional requirements for boron, silicon, vandium, nickel, and arsenic: current knowledge and speculation. FASEB J. 5:2661–2667.

Nolan, M. M., G. D. Potter, K. J. Mathiason, P. G. Gibbs, E. L. Morris, L. W. Greene, and D. Topliff. 2001. Bone density in the juvenile racehorse fed differing levels of minerals. Pp. 33–38 in Proc. 17th Equine Nutr. Physiol. Soc. Symp., Lexington, KY.

NRC (National Research Council). 1974. Nutrients and Toxic Substances in Water for Livestock and Poultry. Washington, DC: National Academy Press.

NRC. 1978. Nutrient Requirements of Horses, 4th rev. ed. Washington, DC: National Academy Press.

NRC. 1980. Mineral Tolerance of Domestic Animals. Washington, DC: National Academy Press.

NRC. 1982. United States-Canadian Tables of Feed Composition. Washington, DC: National Academy Press.

NRC. 1989. Nutrient Requirements of Horses. Washington, DC: National Academy Press.

NRC. 1997. The Role of Chromium in Animal Nutrition. Washington, DC: National Academy Press.

NRC. 2005. Mineral Tolerance of Animals, 2nd rev. ed. Washington, DC: The National Academies Press.

O'Connor, C. I., and B. D. Nielsen. 2006. Handling method influences equine urinary calcium and nitrogen. J. Anim. Vet. Adv. 5:165–167.

Olsman, A. F. S., C. M. Huurdeman, W. L. Jansen, J. Haaksma, M. M. Sloet van Oldruitenborgh-Oosterbaan, and A. C. Beynen. 2004. Macronutrient digestibility, nitrogen balance, plasma indicators of protein metabolism and mineral absorption in horses fed a ration rich in sugar beet pulp. J. Anim. Physiol. Anim. Nutr. 88:321–331.

Osame, S., and S. Ichijo. 1994. Clinicopathological observations on Thoroughbred foals with enlarged thyroid gland. J. Vet. Med. Sci. 56:771–772.

Ott, E. A., and J. Kivipelto. 1999. Influence of chromium triplicolinate on growth and glucose metabolism in yearling horses. J. Anim. Sci. 77:3022–3030.

Pagan, J. D. 1989. Calcium, hindgut function affect phosphorus needs. Feedstuffs 61(35):1–2.

Pagan, J. D. 1994. Nutrient digestibility in horses. Feeding the performance horse. Pp. 127–136 in Proc. KER Short Course for Feed Manufacturers, Lexington, KY.

Pagan, J.D., and S.G. Jackson. 1991a. Digestibility of long-stem alfalfa, pelleted alfalfa or an alfalfa/bermuda straw blend pellet in horses. Pp. 29–32 in Proc. 12th Equine Nutr. Physiol. Soc. Symp., Calgary, Alberta.

Pagan, J. D., and S. G. Jackson. 1991b. Distillers dried grains as a feed ingredient for horse rations: a palatability and digestibility study. Pp. 49–54 in Proc. 12th Equine Nutr. Physiol. Soc. Symp., Calgary, Alberta.

Pagan, J. D., Rotmensen, T., and S. G. Jackson. 1995. The effect of chromium supplementation on metabolic response to exercise in Thoroughbred horses. Pp. 96–101 in Proc. 14th Equine Nutr. Physiol. Soc. Symp., Ontario, CA.

Pagan, J. D., P. Harris, T. Brewster-Barnes, S. E. Duran, and S. G. Jackson. 1998. Exercise affects digestibility and rate of passage of all-forage and mixed diets in thoroughbred horses. J. Nutr. 128:2704S–2707S.

Pagan, J. D., P. Karnezos, M. A. P. Kennedy, T. Currier, and K. E. Hoekstra. 1999. Effect of selenium source on selenium digestibility and retention in exercised Thoroughbreds. Pp. 135–140 in Proc. 16th Equine Nutr. Physiol. Soc. Symp., Raleigh, NC.

Paglia, D. E., and W. H. Valentine. 1967. Studies on the quantitative and qualitative characterization of erythrocyte glutathione peroxidase. J. Lab. Clin. Med. 70:158.

Parker, M. I. 1984. Effect of sodium chloride in feed preference and on control of feed and water intake in ponies. M.S. Thesis. Cornell University.

Patterson, D. P., S. R. Cooper, D. W. Freeman, and R. G. Teeter. 2002. Effects of varying levels of phytase supplementation on dry matter and phosphorus digestibility in horses fed a common textured ration. J. Equine Vet. Sci. 22:456–459.

Paynter, D. I. 1982. Differences between serum and plasma ceruloplasmin activities and copper concentrations: investigations of possible contributing factors. Aust. J. Biol. Sci. 35:353–361.

Pearce, S. G., E. C. Firth, N. D. Grace, and P. F. Fennessy. 1998a. Effect of copper supplementation on the evidence of developmental orthopaedic disease in pasture-fed New Zealand Thoroughbreds. Equine Vet. J. 30:211–218.

Pearce, S. G., N. D. Grace, E. C. Firth, J. J. Wichtel, S. A. Holle, and P. F. Fennessy. 1998b. Effect of copper supplementation on the copper status of pasture-fed young thoroughbreds. Equine Vet. J. 30:204–210.

Pearce, S. G., N. D. Grace, J. J. Wichtel, E. C. Firth, and P. F. Fennessey. 1998c. Effect of copper supplementation on copper status of pregnant mares and foals. Equine Vet. J. 30:200–203.

Pearson, E. G., and C. B. Andreasen. 2001. Effect of oral administration of excessive iron in adult ponies. J. Am. Vet. Med. Assoc. 218:400–404.

Pennington, J. A. T. 1991. Silicon in foods and diets. Food Add. Contam. 8:97–118.

Perkins, G., S. J. Valberg, J. M. Madigan, G. P. Carlson, and S. L. Jones. 1998. Electrolyte disturbances in foals with severe rhabdomyolysis. J. Vet. Intern. Med. 12:173–177.

Podoll, K. L., J. B. Bernard, D. E. Ullrey, S. R. DeBar, P. K. Ku, and W. T. Magee. 1992. Dietary selenate versus selenite for cattle, sheep, and horses. J. Anim. Sci. 70:1965–1970.

Porr, C. A., D. S. Kronfeld, L. A. Lawrence, R. S. Pleasant, and P. A. Harris. 1998. Deconditioning reduces mineral content of the third metacarpal bone in horses. J. Anim. Sci. 76:1875–1879.

Porter, D. J. 1999. Chromium: friend or foe? Arch. Family Med. 8:386–390.

Puls, R. 1994. Mineral Levels in Animal Health. Clearbrook, British Columbia: Sherpa International.

Ramirez, S., and T. L. Seahorn. 1997. How to manage nutritional secondary hyperparathyroidism in horses. Vet. Med. 92:980–985.

Reeves, P. G. 1997. Components of the AIN-93 diets as improvements in the AIN-76A diet. J. Nutr. 127:838S–841S.

Reynolds, J. A., G. D. Potter, L. W. Greene, G. Wu, G. K. Carter, M. T. Martin, T. V. Peterson, M. Murray-Gerzik, G. Moss, and R. S. Erkert. 1998. Genetic-diet interactions in the hyperkalemic periodic paralysis syndrome in Quarter Horses fed varying amounts of potassium: I. Potassium and sodium balance, packed cell volume and plasma potassium and sodium concentrations. J. Equine Vet. Sci. 18:591–600.

Richardson, S. M., P. D. Siciliano, T. E. Engle, C. K. Larson, and T. L. Ward. 2006. Effect of selenium supplementation and source on the selenium status of horses. J. Anim. Sci. 84:1742–1748.

Rieker, J. M., D. R. Topliff, D. W. Freeman, R. G. Teeter, and S. R. Cooper. 1999. The effects of supplemental molybdenum on copper balance in mature geldings. Pp. 365–370 in Proc. 16th Equine Nutr. Physiol. Soc. Symp., Raleigh, NC.

Rodenwold, B. W., and B. T. Simms. 1935. Iodine for broodmares. Proc. Am. Soc. Anim. Prod. 34:89–92.

Rogers, P. A. M., S. P. Arora, G. A. Fleming, R. A. P. Crinion, and J. G. McLaughlin. 1990. Selenium toxicity in farm animals: treatment and prevention. Irish Vet. J. 43:151–153.

Rojas, M. A., I. A. Dyer, and W. A. Cassatt. 1965. Manganese deficiency in bovine. J. Anim. Sci. 22:664–667.

Ronen, N., J. Van Heerden, and S. R. Van Amstel. 1992. Clinical and biochemistry findings and parathyroid hormone concentrations in three horses with secondary hyperparathyroidism. J. South Afr. Vet. Assoc. 63:134–136.

Roneus, B. O., and B. Lindholm. 1983. Glutathione peroxidase activity in blood of healthy horses given different selenium supplementation. Nord. Veterinaermed. 35:337.

Roose, K. A., K. E. Hoekstra, J. D. Pagan, and R. J. Goer. 2001. Effect of an aluminum supplement on nutrient digestibility and mineral metabolism in Thoroughbred horses. Pp. 364–369 in Proc. 17th Equine Nutr. Physiol. Soc. Symp., Lexington, KY.

Rose, R. J. 1990. Electrolytes: clinical application. Vet. Clin. North Am. Equine Pract. 6:281–294.

Rosenfeld, I., and O. A. Beath. 1964. Selenium: Geobotany, Biochemistry, Toxicity, and Nutrition. New York: Academic Press.

Rotruck, J. T., A. L. Pope, H. E. Ganther, A. M. Swanson, D. G. Hafeman, and W. G. Hoekstra. 1973. Selenium: biochemical role as a component of glutathione peroxidase. Science 179:588–590.

Salimen, K. 1975. Cobalt metabolism in horses: serum level and biosynthesis of vitamin B12. Acta Vet. Scand. 16:84.

Savage, C. J. 1992. The influence of nutrition on skeletal growth and induction of osteochondrosis (dyschondroplasia) in horses. Ph.D. Thesis. University of Melbourne, Australia.

Savage, C. J., R. N. McCarthy, and L. B. Jeffcott. 1993a. Effects of dietary phosphorus and calcium on induction of dyschondroplasia in foals. Equine Vet. J. Suppl. 16:80–83.

Savage, C. J., R. N. McCarthy, and L. B. Jeffcott. 1993b. Histomorphometric assessment of bone biopsies from foals fed diets high in phosphorus and digestible energy. Equine Vet. J. Suppl. 16:80–83.

Schott, H. C. 1998. Oral fluids for equine diarrhoea: an underutilized treatment for a costly disease? Vet. J. 155:119–121.

Schott, H. C., D. R. Hodgson, W. Bayly, and P. D. Gollnick. 1991. Renal response to high intensity exercise. Equine Exercise Physiology. 3:361–367.

Schryver, H. F. 1990. Mineral and vitamin intoxication in horses. Vet. Clin. North Am. Equine Pract. 6:295–318.

Schryver, H. F., P. H. Craig, and H. F. Hintz. 1970. Calcium metabolism in ponies fed varying levels of calcium. J. Nutr. 100:955–964.

Schryver, H. F., H. F. Hintz, and P. H. Craig. 1971a. Calcium metabolism in ponies fed high phosphorus diet. J. Nutr. 101:259–264.

Schryver, H. F., H. F. Hintz, and P. H. Craig. 1971b. Phosphorus metabolism in ponies fed varying levels of phosphorus. J. Nutr. 101:1257–1263.

Schryver, H. F., H. F. Hintz, J. E. Lowe, R. L. Hintz, R. B. Harper, and J. T. Reid. 1974. Mineral composition of the whole body, liver, and bone of young horses. J. Nutr. 104:126–132.

Schryver, H. F., H. F. Hintz, and J. E. Lowe. 1978. Calcium metabolism, body composition, and sweat losses of exercised horses. Am. J. Vet. Res. 39:245–248.

Schryver, H. F., D. L. Mills, L. V. Soderholm, J. Williams, and H. F. Hintz. 1986a. Metabolism of some essential minerals in ponies fed high levels of aluminum. Cornell Vet. 76:354–360.

Schryver, H. F., O. T. Oftedal, J. Williams, L. V. Soderholm, and H. F. Hintz. 1986b. Lactation in the horse: the mineral composition of mare's milk. J. Nutr. 116:2142–2147.

Schryver, H. F., D. W. Meakim, J. E. Lowe, J. Williams, L. V. Soderholm, and H. F. Hintz. 1987a. Growth and calcium metabolism in horses fed varying levels of protein. Equine Vet. J. 19:280–287.

Schryver, H. F., M. T. Parker, P. D. Daniluk, K. I. Pagan, J. Williams, L. V. Soderholm, and H. F. Hintz. 1987b. Salt consumption and the effect of salt on mineral metabolism in horses. Cornell Vet. 77:122–131.

Shellow, J. S., S. G. Jackson, J. P. Baker, and A. H. Cantor. 1985. The influence of dietary selenium levels on blood levels of selenium and glutathione peroxidase activity in the horse. J. Anim. Sci. 61:590–594.

Shupe, J. L., and A. E. Olson. 1971. Clinical aspects of fluorosis in horses. J. Am. Vet. Med. Assoc.158:167–174.

Siciliano, P. D., K. D. Culley, and T. E. Engle. 2001. Effect of trace mineral source (inorganic vs organic) on trace mineral status in horses. Pp. 419–420 in Proc. 17th Equine Nutr. Physiol. Soc. Symp., Lexington, KY.

Silvia, C. A. M., H. Merkt, P. N. L. Bergamo, S. S. Barros, C. S. L. Barros, M. N. Santos, H. O. Hoppen, P. Heidemann, and H. Meyer. 1987. Intoxication of iodine in Thoroughbred foals. Pferdeheilkunde. 5:271–276.

Smith, J. D., R. M. Jordan, and M. L. Nelson. 1975. Tolerance of ponies to high levels of dietary copper. J. Anim. Sci. 41:1645–1649.

Smith, J. E., K. Moore, J. E. Cipriano, and P. G. Morris. 1984. Serum ferritin as a measure of stored iron in horses. J. Nutr. 114:677–681.

Smith, J. E., J. E. Cipriano, R. DeBowes, and K. Moore. 1986. Iron deficiency and pseudo-iron deficiency in hospitalized horses. J. Am. Vet. Med. Assoc. 188:285–287.

Smith, N. J., G. D. Potter, E. M. Michael, P. G. Gibbs, B. D. Scott, H. S. Spooner, and M. Walker. 2005. Influence of dietary protein quality on calcium balance and bone quality in immature horses. Pp. 127–128 in Proc. 19th Equine Sci. Soc., Tucson, AZ.

Sobota, J. S., E. A. Ott, E. Johnson, L. McDowell, A. N. Kavazis, and J. Kivipelto. 2001. Influence of manganese on yearling horses. Pp. 136–137 in Proc. 17th Equine Nutr. Physiol. Soc. Symp., Lexington, KY.

Sonntag, A. C., H. Enbergs, L. Ahlswede, and K. Elze. 1996. Components in mare's milk in relation to stage of lactation and environment. Pferdeheilkunde 12:220–222.

Sosa Leon, L. A., D. R. Hodgson, G. P. Carlson, and R. J. Rose. 1998. Effects of concentrated electrolytes administered via a paste on fluid, electrolyte, and acid base balance in horses. Am. J. Vet. Res. 59:898–903.

Spooner, H. S., G. D. Potter, E. M. Michael, P. G. Gibbs, B. D. Scott, N. J. Smith, and M. Walker. 2005. Influence of protein intake on bone density in immature horses. Pp. 11–16 in Proc. 19th Equine Sci. Soc., Tucson, AZ.

Stadermann, B., T. Nehring, and H. Meyer. 1992. Calcium and magnesium absorption with roughage or mixed feed. Pferdeheilkunde. 1:77–80.

Stearns, D. M., J. J. Belbruno, and K. E. Wetterhahn. 1995. Chromium (III) picolinate produces chromosome damage in Chinese hamster ovary cells. FASEB J. 9:1643–1648.

Stephens, T. L., G. D. Potter, K. J. Mathiason, P. G. Gibbs, E. L. Morris, L. W. Green, and D. Topliff. 2001. Mineral balance in juvenile horses in race training. Pp. 26–31 in Proc. 17th Equine Nutr. Physiol. Soc. Symp., Lexington, KY.

Stephens, T. L., G. D. Potter, P. G. Gibbs, and D. M. Hood. 2004. Mineral balance in juvenile horses in race training. J. Equine Vet. Sci. 24:438–450.

Stewart, A. J., J. Hardy, C. W. Kohn, R. E. Toribio, K. W. Hinchcliff, and B. Silver. 2004. Validation of diagnostic tests for determination of magnesium status in horses with reduced magnesium intake. Am. J. Vet. Res. 65:422–430.

Stowe, H. D. 1967. Serum selenium and related parameters of naturally and experimentally fed horses. J. Nutr. 93:60–64.

Stowe, H. D. 1968. Effects of age and impending parturition upon serum copper of Thoroughbred mares. J. Nutr. 95:179–183.

Stowe, H. D. 1971. Effects of potassium in a purified equine diet. J. Nutr. 101:629–633.

Stowe, H. D. 1980. Effects of copper pretreatment upon the toxicity of selenium in ponies. Am. J. Vet. Res. 41:1925–1928.

Stowe, H. D., and T. H. Herdt. 1992. Clinical assessment of selenium status of livestock. J. Anim. Sci. 70:3928–3933.

Strickland, K., F. Smith, M. Woods, and J. Jason. 1987. Dietary molybdenum as a putative copper agonist in the horse. Equine Vet. J. 19:50–54.

Sturgeon, L. S., L. A. Baker, J. L. Pipkin, J. C. Haliburton, and N. K. Chirase. 2000. The digestibility and mineral availability of matua, bermudagrass, and alfalfa hay in mature horses. J. Equine Vet. Sci. 20:45–48.

Suttle, N. F., J. N. W. Small, E. A. Collins, D. K. Mason, and K. L. Watkins. 1996. Serum and hepatic copper concentrations used to define normal, marginal and deficient copper status in horses. Equine Vet. J. 28:497–499.

Swartzman, J. A., H. F. Hintz, and H. F. Schryver. 1978. Inhibition of calcium absorption in ponies fed diets containing oxalic acid. Am. J. Vet. Res. 3:1621–1623.

Tasker, J. B. 1967. Fluid and electrolyte studies in the horse. III. Intake and output of water, sodium, and potassium in normal horses. Cornell Vet. 57:649–657.

Tasker, J. B. 1980. Fluids, electrolytes, and acid-base balance. P. 425 in Clinical Biochemistry of Domestic Animals, 3rd ed., J. J. Kaneko, ed. New York: Academic Press.

Toribio, R. E., C. W. Kohn, D. J. Chew, R. A. Sams, and T. J. Rosol. 2001. Comparison of serum parathyroid hormone and ionized calcium and magnesium concentrations and fractional urinary clearance of calcium and phosphorus in healthy horses and horses with enterocolitis. Am. J. Vet. Res. 62:938–947.

Traub-Dargatz, J. L., A. P. Knight, and D. W. Hamar. 1986. Selenium toxicity in horses. Comp. Cont. Vet. Ed. 8:771–776.

Turner, K. K., B. D. Nielsen, C. I. O'Connor, D. S. Rosenstein, B. P. Marks, and M. W. Orth. 2005. Bone characteristics and turnover after silicon supplementation. Pp. 31–36 in Proc. 19th Equine Sci. Soc., Tucson, AZ.

Ullrey, D. E. 1992. Basis for regulation of selenium supplements in animal diets. J. Anim. Sci. 70:3922–3927.

Ullrey, D. E., W. T. Ely, and R. L. Covert. 1974. Iron, zinc, and copper in mare's milk. J. Anim. Sci. 38:1276–1277.

Underwood, E. J. 1977. Trace elements in human and animal nutrition. 4th ed. New York: Academic Press.

Underwood, E. J. 1981. The Mineral Nutrition of Livestock. 2nd ed. Slough, UK: Commonwealth Agricultural Bureaux.

Valberg, S. 2005. Equine exertional rhabdomyolysis. Part I. Management of sporadic and recurrent exertional rhabdomyolysis. Pp 197–203 in Proc. 3rd Mid-Atlantic Nutr. Conf., Univ. Maryland.

van Doorn, D. A., H. Everts, H. Wouterse, and A. C. Beynen. 2004a. The apparent digestibility of phytate phosphorus and the influence of supplemental phytase in horses. J. Anim. Sci. 82:1756–1763.

van Doorn, D. A., M. E. van der Spek, H. Everts, H. Wouterse, and A. C. Beynen. 2004b. The influence of calcium intake on phosphorus digestibility in mature ponies. J. Anim. Physiol. Anim. Nutr. 88:412–418.

Van Weeren, P. R., J. Knaap, and E. C. Firth. 2003. Influence of liver copper status of mare and newborn foal on the development of osteochondrotic lesions. Equine Vet. J. 35:67–71.

Vervuert, I., M. Coenen, and S. Braun. 2001. Nutrition and health status in Icelandic Horses in Iceland and after importation. Pp. 194–195 in Proc. 17th Equine Nutr. Physiol. Soc. Symp., Lexington, KY.

Vervuert, I., M. Coenen, and J. Zamhofer. 2005a. Effects of draught load exercise and training on calcium homeostasis in horses. J. Anim. Phys. Anim. Nutr. 89:134–139.

Vervuert, I., D. Cuddeford, and M. Coenen. 2005b. Effects of two levels of a chromium supplement on selected metabolic responses in resting and exercising horses. Pferdeheilkunde 21:109–110.

Vincent, J. B. 1999. Mechanisms of chromium action: low-molecular-weight chromium-binding substance. J. Am. College Nutr. 18:6–12.

Voges, F., E. Kienzele, and H. Meyer. 1990. Investigations on the composition of horse bones. Equine Vet. Sci. 10:208–214.

Wagner, E. L., G. D. Potter, E. M. Eller, P. G. Gibbs, and D. M. Hood. 2005. Absorption and retention of trace minerals in adult horses. Prof. Anim. Scientist 21:207–211.

Walker, A. F., G. Marakis, S. Christie, and M. Byng. 2003. Mg citrate found more bioavailable than other Mg preparations in a randomised, double-blind study. Magnes. Res. 16:183–191.

Wall, D. L., D. R. Topliff, and D. W. Freeman. 1997. The effect of dietary cation-anion balance on mineral balance in growing horses. Pp. 145–150 in Proc. 15th Equine Nutr. Physiol. Soc. Symp., Ft. Worth, TX.

Wall, D. L., D. R. Topliff, D. W. Freeman, D. G. Wagner, J. W. Breazile, and W. A. Stutz. 1992. Effect of dietary cation-anion balance on urinary mineral excretion in exercised horses. J. Equine Vet. Sci. 12: 168–171.

Warren, L. K. 2003. Conquering Mount Manure: the need for education, outreach, and research in the horse industry. Pp. 220–229 in Proc. 18th Equine Nutr. Physiol. Soc. Symp., East Lansing, MI.

Wehr, U., B. Englschalk, E. Kienzle and W. A. Rambeck. 2002. Iodine balance in relation to iodine intake in ponies. J. Nutr. 132:1767S–1768S.

Weidenhaupt, K. 1977. Potassium metabolism in the horse. Prat. Vet. Equine. 28:85–96.

Whetter, P. A., and D. E. Ullrey. 1978. Improved fluorometric method for determining selenium. J. Assoc. Off. Anal. Chem. 61:927–930.

Whitlock, R. H., H. F. Schryver, L. Krook, H. F. Hintz, and P. H. Craig. 1970. The effects of high dietary calcium for horses. P. 127 in Proc. 16th Am. Assoc. Equine Pract., F. J. Milne, ed. Lexington, KY: Am. Assoc. Equine Pract.

Wichert, B., T. Frank, and E. Kienzle. 2002a. Supply with the trace elements zinc, copper and selenium in horses in the south of Bavaria. Tierärztliche Praxis Großtiere 30:107–114.

Wichert, B., T. Frank, and E. Kienzle. 2002b. Zinc, copper and selenium intake and status of horses in Bavaria. J. Nutr. 132:1776S–1777S.

Wichert, B., K. Kreyenberg, and E. Kienzle. 2002c. Serum response after oral supplementation of different zinc compounds in horses. J. Nutr. 132:1769S–1770S.

Winkelsett, S., I. Vervuert, M. Granel, A. Borchers, and M. Coenen. 2005. Feeding practice in Warmblood mares and foals and the incidence to osteochondrosis. Pferdeheilkunde 21:124–126.

Wright, P. L., and M. C. Bell. 1966. Comparative metabolism of selenium and tellurium in sheep and swine. Am. J. Physiol. 211:6–10.

Wolter, R., J. P. Valette, and J. M. Marion. 1986. Magnesium et effort d'endurance chez le poney. Ann. Zootech. 35:255–263.

Young, J. K., G. D. Potter, L. W. Greene, S. P. Webb, J. W. Evans, and G. W. Webb. 1987. Copper balance in miniature horses fed varying amounts of zinc. P. 173 in Proc. 10th Equine Nutr. Physiol. Soc. Symp., Fort Collins, CO.

Young, J. K., G. D. Potter, L. W. Greene, and J. W. Evans. 1989. Mineral balance in resting and exercised miniature horses. P. 79 in Proc. 11th Equine Nutr. Physiol. Soc. Symp., Stillwater, OK.

6

Vitamins

INTRODUCTION

Vitamins are defined as a group of complex unrelated fat- and water-soluble organic compounds present in minute amounts in natural foodstuffs. They are essential to normal metabolism and their lack in the diet causes deficiency diseases (McDowell, 2000). Vitamin requirements of horses have been estimated using several response variables (e.g., prevention of specific deficiency symptoms, maximizing tissue stores, and optimization of various biological functions). It should be noted that the requirement for a vitamin may differ depending upon the response variable used. For example, 0.233 international units (IU) of vitamin E/kg body weight (BW) was determined to be the minimum requirement necessary to maintain erythrocyte stability in growing horses (Stowe, 1968a), whereas approximately 1 IU/kg BW was reported to have an immunostimulatory effect in adult horses when compared to controls fed approximately 0.315 IU/kg BW (Baalsrud and Overnes, 1986).

Requirements for vitamins A, D, E, thiamin, and riboflavin have been estimated. The basis for these estimates is discussed below along with information regarding dietary sources and consequences of deficiency and toxicity. Although limited, information regarding vitamin nutrition for vitamin K, niacin, biotin, folate, vitamin B_{12}, vitamin B_6, pantothenic acid, and vitamin C (ascorbic acid) is discussed. However, insufficient information exists to estimate dietary requirements of these vitamins for horses. In addition to requirements, an attempt was made to estimate the presumed upper safe levels of intake for each vitamin. The presumed upper safe level is defined as the estimated (based on literature) upper range of vitamin intake that can be presumed to be safe, and is not necessarily the maximum tolerance level of vitamin intake (NRC, 1987).

Many of the vitamin requirements in the previous revision of this document were expressed per unit of dry matter (DM) intake, and have been transformed to a BW basis in the current revision. The transformation assumes a (DM) intake of 2 percent of BW for maintenance, breeding, gestation, and light work; 2.25 percent of BW for moderate work; and 2.5 percent of BW in DM intake for all other feeding classes. For example, the vitamin E requirement for lactation in the previous revision is 80 IU/kg DM and has been transformed to 2 IU/kg BW, assuming a DM intake of 2.5 percent of BW (i.e., 80 IU vitamin D/kg DM × 2.5 kg DM/100 kg BW).

VITAMIN A

Function

The classical function of vitamin A is its role in night vision (Wald, 1968). Vitamin A in the form of 11-*cis*-retinal combines with opsin to produce rhodopsin, which breaks down in the presence of light-yielding energy that is transported to the brain by the optic nerve in the process of sight. Vitamin A functions in cell differentiation by the regulation of gene expression via nuclear retinoic acid receptors, and as a result plays crucial roles in reproduction and embryogenesis (Solomons, 2001). Additionally, vitamin A is important for maintaining the innate and adaptive immune response to infection (Stephensen, 2001).

Dietary Sources

Vitamin A refers to a subgroup of retinoids possessing the biological activity of all-*trans*-retinol (Solomons, 2001). Retinol does not occur naturally in feedstuffs commonly used for horses (e.g., forages, cereal grains, plant protein supplements), but is derived from pro-vitamin A compounds (carotenoids). Retinol is present in vitamin A supplements as retinyl-ester (e.g., retinyl-acetate, retinyl-palmitate).

The biological activity of various retinoids and pro-vitamin A compounds differs and must be taken in account when evaluating and formulating equine diets. The international unit is used to express vitamin A activity of different sources on an equivalent basis. One IU of vitamin A is equivalent to the biological activity of 0.300 μg of all-*trans*-retinol.

Beta-carotene is the primary naturally occurring provitamin A source in feedstuffs used for horses. Beta-carotene can be metabolized into a retinyl ester (retinyl-palmitate or retinyl-stearate) within the mucosa of the small intestine, and the liver to some extent (Ullrey, 1972; Napoli, 2000). Retinyl esters formed in the small intestinal mucosa are then transported to the liver for storage or distributed to other tissues for further metabolism. Previous NRC publications have assumed 1 mg of β-carotene is equivalent to no more than 400 IU of vitamin A (NRC, 1989). Different conversion rates for pregnant mares and growing horses have been suggested (1 mg β-carotene = 555 and 333 IU vitamin A, respectively) based on an extrapolation of conversion rates established in rats (McDowell, 1989). The aforementioned conversion efficiencies are higher than reported for other monogastric species. In typical swine diets 1 mg total carotene was calculated to be equivalent to 267 IU vitamin A (Ullrey, 1972). Reference dietary intakes used for humans consider 1 mg β-carotene equivalent to 275 IU vitamin A activity. Additionally the effect of β-carotene intake can influence the conversion rate. An inverse relationship between the amount of β-carotene metabolized into vitamin A and β-carotene intake has been reported for several species (Ullrey, 1972; Solomons, 2001), but has not been investigated in horses. Clearly more work is necessary to establish accurate estimates of the vitamin A value of naturally occurring β-carotene and other carotenoids.

Beta-carotene concentrations derived from back-calculation of vitamin A values published in NRC (1989) (i.e., 400 IU of vitamin A is equivalent to 1 mg β-carotene) vary widely among forages. Forages contain from 30–385 mg β-carotene/kg DM. Pasture (nondormant) contains the greatest concentration of β-carotene, while mature grass hay has the lowest concentrations. Several factors, such as degree of maturity, conditions at harvest, and length of storage, can influence β-carotene concentrations of forages (Ullrey, 1972). Among cereal grains, corn contains the greatest concentration of β-carotene (approximately 6 mg/kg DM), which is considerably less than that of forages.

Synthetic β-carotene has been evaluated as a source of provitamin A. Watson et al. (1996) suggested that a water-dispersible form of β-carotene was not well absorbed by ponies as indicated by a lack of effect on plasma β-carotene concentration following supplementation, but vitamin A status of the ponies was not evaluated. Greiwe-Crandell et al. (1997), using this same form of β-carotene, found it was not effective at maintaining vitamin A status in mares over a 20-month period as compared to retinyl-palmitate or naturally occurring β-carotene from pasture and hay. However, it should be noted that the β-carotene used in this study was administered in two large doses per week rather than daily, which may have influenced the conversion of β-carotene to vitamin A. The amount of β-carotene metabolized into vitamin A is dependent upon β-carotene intake (Ullrey, 1972; Solomons, 2001). Kienzle et al. (2002) found a water-dispersible β-carotene source, different from the aforementioned studies, was effective at increasing plasma β-carotene concentration, but vitamin A status was not measured. Interestingly the dosage of β-carotene used by Kienzle et al. was approximately half that (0.8 vs. 1.8 mg β-carotene/kg BW) used by Watson et al. (1996). Therefore, effectiveness of synthetic β-carotene as sources of pro-vitamin A for horses remains to be determined.

Retinyl-palmitate and -acetate are supplemental forms of vitamin A used in diets for horses (NRC, 1989). These esterified forms are more stable than retinol making them less vulnerable to degradation during storage as compared to unesterified forms (McDowell, 2000). Retinyl-esters are hydrolyzed within the lumen of the small intestine to retinol, which is then absorbed. One IU of vitamin A is equivalent to the biological activity of 0.550 μg of all-*trans*-retinyl palmitate, or 0.344 of all-*trans*-retinyl acetate.

Deficiency

Night blindness is a classical vitamin A deficiency symptom reported in horses, as well as other species (McDowell, 1989). Extremely low vitamin A intake is necessary for the condition to occur. Induction of night blindness in Percheron horses occurred after rations consisting of barley, oats, bran, and straw containing low concentrations of total carotene (5 to 10 μg/kg BW; no more than 2 to 4 IU vitamin A/kg BW) were fed for 265 to 627 days (Guilbert et al., 1940). Semi-purified diets devoid of vitamin A activity were necessary to induce clinical signs of vitamin A deficiency in orphaned foals (Stowe, 1968b). Greiwe-Crandell (1997) reported no clinical signs of vitamin A deficiency and a plateau effect in vitamin A status in mares consuming hay, previously stored for 2 years, containing less than 4 mg β-carotene/kg DM for 22 months. The authors interpreted the results as an adaptive response to very low levels of carotene intake. These results suggest that horses are somewhat resilient to vitamin A deficiency, at least when common clinical deficiency symptoms are used as indicators of deficiency. Impaired growth and hematopoiesis were reported in growing ponies fed rations marginally deficient in vitamin A (Donoghue et al., 1981). Therefore, parameters associated with growth and hematopoiesis appear to be more sensitive indicators of vitamin A deficiency as compared to clinical symptoms such as night blindness.

In addition to clinical signs, serum total vitamin A concentration has been used as an indicator of vitamin A deficiency. Total serum vitamin A concentration of less than 10 μg/dl is considered deficient (Lewis, 1995). However, total serum vitamin A is not a sensitive indicator of marginal vitamin A status due to mobilization of retinol from the liver into blood in response to inadequate vitamin A intake (Jarrett and Schurg, 1987). The relative dose response test (RDR), an indirect measure of liver vitamin A stores, has been suggested as a more accurate indicator of marginal vitamin A status in horses than either serum total vitamin A or serum retinol (Greiwe-Crandell et al., 1995). The RDR is expressed as the percentage increase in serum retinol following oral administration of a vitamin A bolus. The time period between the initial and final measures of serum retinol used to determine its percent increase coincide with peak serum retinol concentration. The basis for the RDR is that during vitamin A sufficiency, a relatively large proportion of newly absorbed vitamin A is stored in the liver due to relatively low production and concentration of retinol binding protein (RBP), which is necessary for transport of vitamin A from the liver to peripheral tissues. In contrast, during vitamin A deficiency, RBP synthesis and concentration increase and newly absorbed vitamin A is transported from the liver to peripheral tissues resulting in a relative increase in serum retinol concentration after administration of an oral bolus; therefore, RDR increases. Relative dose response values greater than 20 percent have been observed in horses consuming rations deficient in vitamin A (Greiwe-Crandell et al., 1995; Lewis, 1995; Greiwe-Crandell et al., 1997). However, an RDR ranging from 20–30 percent was reported in reproductively sound mares with no clinical symptoms of vitamin A deficiency (Greiwe-Crandell et al., 1997), suggesting more work is necessary to define exact thresholds for vitamin A deficiency using RDR. Since vitamin A can be stored in the liver (McDowell, 2000), it is possible that the lack of clinical deficiency symptoms were due to liver stores of vitamin A covering dietary deficits.

Immunity and reproduction are two other physiological functions influenced by vitamin A status. Respiratory infection in weanlings was associated with low vitamin A status as measured by RDR (Greiwe-Crandell et al., 1995). Impaired function of the immune system during vitamin A deficiency has been documented in several species (McDowell, 1989; Stephensen, 2001). Vitamin A deficiency in swine has been shown to increase early embryonic mortality (McDowell, 1989). The effect of vitamin A status on both immunity and reproduction in horses require further study.

Toxicity

Vitamin A toxicity has been reported to result in bone fragility, hyperostosis, exfoliated epithelium and teratogenesis (NRC, 1987). In addition, excess vitamin A has been implicated in developmental orthopedic disease in growing horses (Donoghue et al., 1981; Kronfeld et al., 1990). The presumed upper safe level of vitamin A in the diet is 16,000 IU/kg DM (NRC, 1987). Plasma total vitamin A concentrations greater than 40–60 μg/dl are indicative of toxicosis (Lewis, 1995). Retinyl-ester concentration of plasma increases relative to retinol during toxicosis and may also be an indicator of excess vitamin A consumption (Donoghue et al., 1981; Jarrett and Schurg, 1987). Toxicity due to β-carotene has not been reported. Additionally, it should be noted that the previously mentioned assumption that 1 mg of β-carotene contains 400 IU of vitamin A may yield vitamin A concentrations above the presumed upper safe level of 16,000 IU/kg DM, which is most likely erroneous based on the absence of toxicity in horses consuming these amounts.

Requirements

Vitamin A requirements for horses of different physiological states are not well defined. Limited information exists regarding vitamin A nutrition as it pertains to maintenance (Guilbert et al., 1940), reproduction (Stowe, 1967), gestation (Greiwe-Crandell et al., 1997; Maenpaa et al., 1988a,b), lactation (Stowe, 1982; Schweigert and Gottwald, 1999), growth (Donoghue et al., 1981), and work (Abrams, 1979).

Maintenance

The vitamin A requirement for horses with maintenance-only requirements is based on the intake of vitamin A necessary to prevent night blindness, plus an allowance deemed sufficient to maximize tissue storage (NRC, 1989). This recommendation is based on the work of Guilbert et al. (1940) and has been the basis for maintenance vitamin A requirements since the first publication on recommended nutrient allowances for horses in 1949. Guilbert et al. (1940) used 9 Percheron horses ranging in age from 119–444 days in a depletion-repletion experiment that was aimed at determining the minimum intake of either total carotene or vitamin A, from alfalfa and cod-liver oil, respectively, which was necessary to prevent clinical signs of night blindness. Daily consumption of 17–22 IU/kg BW was the minimum necessary to prevent clinical signs of night blindness. However, previous work conducted by these authors on rats indicated that 3 times the minimum vitamin A requirement, or 51–66 IU/kg BW, was necessary for significant tissue storage.

Using data from the manuscript of Guilbert et al. (1940), mean vitamin A intakes (± SD) of horses showing no signs of night blindness, partial night blindness, and total night blindness were calculated to be 22.9 ± 5.1 (n = 10), 17.5 ± 2.6 (n = 5), and 4 ± 2.7 (n = 10) IU vitamin A/kg BW, respectively. When the mean vitamin A intake of horses showing no signs of night blindness is increased by two standard deviations, the vitamin A intake is 33.1 IU/d, which is approximately equal to NRC (1989) requirement for maintenance (30 IU/kg BW). Based on this information, 30 IU/kg BW is recommended as the maintenance vitamin A requirement.

Growth

The role of vitamin A in the growing horse is not well studied. Daily vitamin A requirements for growth in the second through fourth revisions of the NRC publications (NRC, 1966, 1973, 1978) remained the same at 40 IU/kg BW, but were increased slightly in the fifth revision (NRC, 1989) to 45 IU/kg BW. The basis for this change in vitamin A requirement was unclear. Guilbert et al. (1940) observed growth and development was normal in horses consuming 22.9 ± 5.1 IU vitamin A/kg BW and ranging in age from 119–444 days. Donoghue et al. (1981) suggested that a range from 60–200 IU/kg BW resulted in optimization of seven different response variables, which included growth rate, serum biochemistry, and hematologic criteria in ponies ranging in age from 4–12 months. However, the authors noted that this conclusion is based on interpolation and requires further definition in growing horses. Interpolation was made across an extremely wide range, i.e., 12–1,200 µg retinol/kg BW/d, which may detract from the accuracy of the estimate. Stowe (1968b) reported a minimum vitamin A requirement in growing horses (9.5–11 IU/kg BW) that was considerably less than that of Donoghue et al. (1981), albeit using younger horses (orphaned foals) and different response variables (maintenance of appetite). Based on the information available, there is no justification for changing the requirement from that established by previous NRC committees, i.e., 45 IU/kg BW. This value is similar to average values required by finishing swine (NRC, 1998).

Breeding, Gestation, and Lactation

The vitamin A requirement for pregnant and lactating mares was reported to be 60 IU/kg BW (NRC, 1989). Barren Standardbred mares supplemented orally with 100,000 IU vitamin A/day + 100 IU vitamin E/day had improved reproductive status (e.g., more serviced heats, greater number of live foals) compared to unsupplemented controls, or horses consuming either 100,000 IU vitamin A/day or 100 IU vitamin E/day (Stowe, 1967). The vitamin A activity of the unsupplemented control ration was not reported. However, this experiment was somewhat biased because mares receiving the control ration and vitamin A-only ration were older than the other two groups. The average age of mares in the control, vitamin A only, vitamin E only, and vitamins A plus E was 19.8, 16.5, 14, and 14.8 years, respectively. However, a separate experiment reported in the manuscript by Stowe (1967), where age of the mares was balanced across treatments, indicated that a parenteral dose of vitamins A and E, approximately equivalent to the oral dose used in the first experiment, also resulted in improved reproductive status. These results suggest an interaction between vitamins A and E may enhance reproductive status. Seasonal variation in vitamin A status has been reported in broodmares in several studies (Maenpaa et al., 1988a,b; Greiwe-Crandell et al., 1997). Some of the seasonal variation was most likely due to change in diet (i.e., pasture vs. preserved forage) and deterioration of β-carotene in preserved forage (Fonnesbeck and Symons, 1967). However, Maenpaa (1988a) stated the seasonal decline in pregnant mares was greater than previously reported in nonpregnant adult horses (Maenpaa et al., 1987: approximately 36 and 8.9 percent, respectively) and suggested the difference may be due to increased utilization of vitamin A during gestation. Interestingly, supplementation with 18–36 IU vitamin A/kg BW (source not reported) did not prevent the seasonal decline in the pregnant mares (Maenpaa et al., 1988b). Seasonal declines in vitamin A status have been reported in broodmares maintained in a drylot setting both with retinyl-palmitate supplementation (125 IU vitamin A/kg BW) and without vitamin A supplementation (< 0.8 IU/kg BW) (Greiwe-Crandell et al., 1997), which supports the idea that the seasonal decline in vitamin A status is not completely due to changes in vitamin A intake and may be influenced by gestation. Stowe (1982) provided evidence that metabolism of vitamin A increases at parturition due to increased secretion of vitamin A in colostrum. Greiwe-Crandell et al. (1997) also reported that mares maintained on pasture with no other vitamin A supplementation (i.e., β-carotene from pasture was the only source of vitamin A activity) had a greater vitamin A status (as measured by a relative dose response test) than mares maintained on dry-lot and receiving a dose of vitamin A equivalent to 125 IU /kg BW/d from retinyl-palmitate. It was further suggested that if the vitamin A status of horses on pasture is viewed as optimum, then supplementation with approximately twice the NRC (1989) requirement is below optimum. However, it should also be noted that horses used in this study were only supplemented with vitamin A two times per week using a vitamin A dose equivalent to a daily supplementation of 125 IU/kg BW/d. Although vitamin A status of unsupplemented mares without access to pasture declined in these studies, no negative effects due to declining status were reported in these mares. At present, no evidence suggests vitamin A requirements for broodmares are different from those previously recommended, i.e., 60 IU/kg BW (NRC, 1989).

Several studies have investigated the hypothesis that β-carotene, or provitamin A, improves reproductive status, but results are equivocal (Watson et al., 1996). Some have suggested the water-dispersible form of β-carotene used in these studies was not well absorbed and does not increase blood concentrations of β-carotene or retinol (Watson et al., 1996; Greiwe-Crandell et al., 1997), while others provided evidence to the contrary (Kienzle et al., 2002). Therefore the effect of β-carotene, independent of vitamin A activity, on reproduction in mares remains uncertain.

Work

Vitamin A requirements specific to work have not been established. Previous editions of the NRC nutrient requirements of horses consider the requirement for work to be somewhere between maintenance (30 IU/kg BW) and that for gestation and lactation (60 IU/kg BW). The fifth edition of the NRC (1989) *Nutrient Requirements of Horses* stated the vitamin A requirement for work as 45 IU/kg BW.

In a search of the literature, only one report dealing with vitamin A supplementation to working horses was identified. Abrams (1979) hypothesized that vitamin A supplementation to Thoroughbred racehorses in training would assist in the maintenance of connective tissue integrity, thereby reducing tendon injury. Horses were supplemented with 50,000 IU/d (approximately 111–125 IU/kg BW/d; source not provided) over a 2-year period. Vitamin A-supplemented horses completed more races with a greater number of wins and a lower incidence of tendon injuries as compared to controls. However, the design of the experiment precludes definitive conclusions in that the opportunity to race was not afforded equally to all horses.

In conclusion, additional experiments are required to establish vitamin A requirements specific to work. Vitamin A requirements for exercising horses in this edition are unchanged from the previous addition (i.e., 45 IU/kg BW) due to the lack of new information.

VITAMIN D

Function

Vitamin D plays an important role in calcium homeostasis. Vitamin D_3 does not possess any direct biological activity, but is metabolized into 25 $(OH)D_3$, 1,25 $(OH)_2D_3$, and 24,25 $(OH)_2D_3$. The classical target organs for vitamin D action are intestine, kidney, and bone. Vitamin D facilitates calcium absorption from the intestine and reabsorption of calcium from the kidney, and influences both mobilization and accretion of calcium (and phosphorus) from bone. Vitamin D's role in calcium homeostasis is its most well-recognized function; however, vitamin D has also been demonstrated to influence cell growth and differentiation (Norman, 2001).

Dietary Sources

Vitamin D is found in both plants (ergocalciferol, vitamin D_2) and animals (cholecalciferol, vitamin D_3). However, its presence in feeds commonly used for horses is relatively low. Some vitamin D_2 is found in sun-cured hay, particularly alfalfa (McDowell, 2000). Vitamin D is synthesized in the skin from the ultraviolet irradiation of 7-dehydrocholesterol (McDowell, 2000). Vitamin D_3 is the most common supplemental form of vitamin D for horses.

Deficiency

Rickets, a disease characterized by bone deformities resulting from decreased concentration of calcium (Ca) and phosphorus (P) in the organic matrices of cartilage and bone, is the classical vitamin D deficiency symptom in animals and humans (McDowell, 2000). Bone growth and development were affected in ponies deprived of sunlight and dietary vitamin D as compared to two other groups of ponies either fed diets containing 1,000 IU/d and having no exposure to sunlight, or fed diets containing no supplemental vitamin D and having exposure to sunlight; however, externally visible bone deformities typifying rickets were not evident (Elshorafa et al., 1979). Although vitamin D status of horses has been reported to be low relative to other species (Maenpaa et al., 1988a), and supplemental vitamin D has been reported to promote calcium and phosphorus absorption in horses (Hintz et al., 1973), there are no reports of vitamin D deficiency to date in horses maintained in practical settings with some exposure to sunlight.

Toxicity

Toxicity of vitamin D is associated with calcification of soft tissue (Harrington, 1982; Harrington and Page, 1983) and death (Hintz et al., 1973). The presumed upper safe level is 44 IU/kg BW/d (NRC, 1987).

Requirements

In the first edition of the NRC (1949), it was stated that

Under normal farm conditions, where horses are worked regularly and are exposed to sunshine, they probably do not need added amounts of vitamin D. Where they are confined or where exposure to sunshine is restricted, or if they are fed for rapid growth and development of bone such as for racing at an early age, there may be some basis for supplying extra amounts of vitamin D. Experimental information on the requirements of the horse for vitamin D is not available. On the basis of information on other species 300 I.U. of vitamin D per 100 pounds live weight daily should be adequate to meet the needs of horses.

Although a true minimum vitamin D requirement for horses exposed to sunshine is unknown, the value of 300 IU vitamin D/100 lb BW was maintained through subsequent revisions, albeit expressed as 6.6 IU/kg BW in the third edition (NRC, 1973) and expressed as 300 IU/kg DM in the fifth revision. The fifth revision qualifies this recommendation further by stating in footnote b of Table 5-3 that "recommendations are for horses not exposed to sunlight or to artificial light with an emission spectrum of 280–315 nm." This recommendation (6.6 IU/kg BW) is maintained in the present edition for all feeding classes except growing horses. In the fifth revision (NRC, 1989), additional information from an experiment conducted in growing ponies deprived of sunlight (Elshorafa et al., 1979) was used to estimate vitamin D requirements of 800 IU/kg DM for horses in the early stages of growth deprived of sunlight, but indicated that 500 IU/kg DM may be sufficient for later stages of growth. Using BW, mature BW, average daily gain (ADG), and month of age values, from Tables 5-1A-G (NRC, 1989), and the NRC (1989) model software; vitamin D requirements for growing horses were estimated across a range of BW, mature BW, and ages. These estimates were then converted from a diet concentration (i.e., IU/kg DM) to a BW basis (i.e., IU/kg BW). The converted estimates are as follows: 22.2, 17.4, 15.9, and 13.7 IU/kg BW for 0–6, 7–12, 13–18, and 19–24 months of age, respectively. In conclusion, the true minimum dietary vitamin D requirement for horses exposed to sunlight has not been defined. The metabolic requirement for vitamin D is assumed to be met by exposure to sunlight. The above estimates may be useful for horses with limited exposure to sunlight (e.g., horses maintained predominantly indoors).

VITAMIN E

Function

Vitamin E's most widely accepted function is that of a biological antioxidant (Sies, 1993). Its lipophilic nature allows it to incorporate into cell membranes where it serves to protect unsaturated lipids and other susceptible membrane components against oxidative damage. Vitamin E donates a hydrogen atom from its phenolic group to lipid peroxyl radicals produced during auto-oxidation of membrane polyunsaturated fatty acids forming a more stable lipid peroxide and stable tocopheryl radical. The subsequent lipid peroxides are further degraded by selenium-dependent glutathione peroxidase. A detailed description of vitamin E's antioxidant function is described by Pryor (2001).

Dietary Sources

Vitamin E activity originates from eight different naturally occurring compounds, four tocopherols (α, β, γ, δ) and four tocotrienols (α, β, γ, δ). Both tocopherols and tocotrienols consist of a chromanol ring and a 16-C side chain. Tocopherols have a saturated side chain, whereas tocotrienols contain an unsaturated side chain. The α, β, γ, and δ forms differ due to placement and number of methyl groups on the chromanol ring, which accounts for some of the differences in vitamin E activity among the different forms (Lynch, 1996a). The side chain of α-tocopherol contains three asymmetric carbons resulting in eight different stereoisomers. Naturally occurring tocopherols exist as the $2R\ 4'R\ 8'R$ (commonly referred to as *RRR*) stereoisomer. Naturally occurring *RRR*-α-tocopherol contains the greatest biological activity (1.49 IU/mg) of the different vitamin E forms. Concentration of naturally occurring vitamin E activity varies considerably in typical feeds used for horses (NRC, 1989; Lynch, 1996b). Fresh forages and those harvested at an immature state generally contain the highest concentrations of vitamin E activity (30–100 IU/kg DM), while grains (e.g., corn, oats, and barley) tend to have lesser concentrations (20–30 IU/kg DM). Naturally occurring vitamin E declines over time in stored feeds. For example, losses of 54–73 percent of vitamin E have been reported in alfalfa stored at 33°C for 12 weeks (Lynch, 1996b). Therefore, the intake of vitamin E can vary considerably depending on the horse's diet. Many commercial horse feeds account for this variation and are formulated with supplemental vitamin E (generally, all-*rac*-α-tocopheryl acetate) to compensate for potentially limiting concentrations in forages and other raw ingredients used in horse feed manufacture. Supplemental vitamin E used in commercial feeds and vitamin supplements are esters of α-tocopherol (e.g., α-tocopheryl acetate) and is termed natural-source or synthetic depending upon whether it exists as the *RRR* stereoisomer (e.g., *RRR*-α-tocopheryl acetate) or a racemic mixture of the eight stereoisomers (e.g., all-*rac*-α-tocopheryl acetate). The natural-source *RRR*-α-tocopheryl acetate contains 1.36 IU/mg, whereas the synthetic all-*rac*-α-tocopheryl acetate contains 1 IU/mg. Natural-source vitamin E appears more efficient at increasing serum α-tocopherol as compared to synthetic vitamin E. Gansen et al. (1995) reported a similar increase in serum α-tocopherol in horses fed diets for 6 weeks supplemented with natural-source vitamin E (212 mg *RRR*-α-tocopheryl acetate, 252 mg *RRR*-γ-tocopheryl acetate, and 116 mg *RRR*-δ-tocopheryl acetate) as compared to those fed diets supplemented with a synthetic form (672 mg all-*rac*-α-tocopheryl acetate), but they noted that the natural source contained approximately one-third the α-tocopherol as compared to the synthetic form. Pagan et al. (2005) reported that a synthetic source of vitamin E (all-*rac*-α-tocopheryl acetate) was less effective at elevating plasma α-tocopherol concentrations than natural-source vitamin E and that natural-source micellized vitamin E was superior at elevating plasma α-tocopherol during short-term administration (~ 14 d) as compared to either the synthetic or natural-source vitamin E.

Deficiency

White muscle disease (also known as nutritional muscular dystrophy) is a noninflammatory degenerative disease that affects skeletal and cardiac muscle of foals ranging in age from birth to 11 months of age (Lofstedt, 1997). Although vitamin E deficiency has been implicated in white muscle disease (Schougaard et al., 1972; Wilson et al., 1976), available evidence points to selenium deficiency as the primary cause rather than vitamin E deficiency (Lofstedt, 1997). However, vitamin E along with selenium has been used in treatment of white muscle disease.

Equine degenerative myeloencephalopathy (EDM) is an idiopathic, diffuse, degenerative disease of the spinal cord and selected parts of the brain in young horses (generally < 2 years of age) that results in gait deficits (Blythe and Craig, 1997). Some evidence suggests a role for vitamin E in the pathophysiology of EDM (Liu et al., 1983; Mayhew et al., 1987; Gandini et al., 2004); however, an unidentified familial factor is a prerequisite of the disease (Blythe et al., 1991). Based on this evidence, EDM does not appear to be a primary vitamin E deficiency symptom.

Equine motor neuron disease (EMND) is a neurodegenerative disorder of the somatic lower motor neurons affecting horses 2 years of age and older (Divers, 2005). Clinical findings include an acute onset of trembling, almost constant shifting of weight in the rear legs when standing, prolonged recumbency, and muscle wasting (Divers, 2005), as well as ocular manifestations (Riis et al., 1999). Several lines of evidence support the hypothesis that EMND occurs following a prolonged period of vitamin E deficiency (Divers, 2005). Evidence includes serum α-tocopherol concentration in affected horses that is often < 1 µg/ml, and induction of equine motor neuron disease in horses fed diets low in vitamin E (concentration not reported, but it was < 50 to 80 IU/kg DM) for 18–22 months.

Serum α-tocopherol is commonly used as an indicator of vitamin E status. Craig et al. (1992) found single serum samples an unsatisfactory indicator of vitamin E status in horses, and stated this finding may have clinical application in the evaluation of horses suspected to be affected with EDM, or other vitamin E-related conditions. Within horse serum, α-tocopherol concentrations fluctuated considerably over a 72-hour period in 12 different horses (25 samples/horse taken at 3-hour intervals). The mean coefficient of variation (CV) for α-tocopherol in all horses was 12 percent and ranged from 7–17 percent in individuals. In some instances, serum α-tocopherol within an individual horse fluctuated over a 72-hour period from concentrations considered by the authors as adequate (> 2 µg/ml) through those considered marginal (1.5–2 µg/ml) and deficient (< 1.5 µg/ml).

Addition of dietary fat containing relatively high concentrations of polyunsaturated fatty acids (PUFA, such as corn oil and soybean oil) has been suggested to decrease vitamin E status in several species (Muggli, 1989; McDowell, 2000). Based on work in animals and humans, a ratio of 0.6 mg α-tocopherol to 1 g PUFA was predicted as a minimum to protect against vitamin E deficiency (Harris and Embree, 1963); however, as the degree of fatty acid unsaturation increases, the ratio of α-tocopherol:PUFA may be even greater (Muggli, 1989). Information regarding the relationship between vitamin E status and PUFA in horses is limited. Addition of soybean oil (6.4 percent of the total diet; approximately 20 percent of the total DE intake) to the diet did not negatively affect serum α-tocopherol concentrations in 2-year-old horses over a 90-day period, and, in fact, mean serum α-tocopherol concentration was greater on day 90 in ditionally, some dietary sources of PUFA contain relatively high concentrations of vitamin E (Hoffman et al., 1998).

Vitamin C and selenium status may also influence vitamin E status and subsequent requirements. Evidence from species other than horses suggests vitamin C status can influence vitamin E status (Halpner et al., 1998; Lauridsen and Jensen, 2005). The mechanism by which vitamin C influences vitamin E status may involve either recycling of the α-tocopheroxyl radical back to α-tocopherol, or a sparing effect whereby vitamin C quenches free radicals that would otherwise consume α-tocopherol (Halpner et al., 1998). Selenium is a component of the antioxidant enzyme glutathione peroxidase and has also been demonstrated to spare vitamin E (Combs, 1996). However, the effect of vitamin C and selenium status on vitamin E status in horses remains to be determined.

Toxicity

Vitamin E does not appear to be toxic to horses even at relatively high intakes, and the upper safe diet concentration is set at 1,000 IU/kg DM (NRC, 1987). However, this presumed upper safe level is based on observations in other species. Coagulopathy and impaired bone mineralization have been reported in other species consuming diets above the upper safe level (1,000 IU/kg DM) (NRC, 1987).

Requirements

Maintenance

The first published vitamin E requirement for horses was 15 IU vitamin E/kg diet DM (NRC, 1978), and was based on concentrations required to maintain erythrocyte stability in vitamin E-deficient foals (i.e., 0.233 IU/kg BW) (Stowe, 1968a). In the fifth revision (NRC, 1989), the maintenance vitamin E requirement was increased to 50 IU/kg DM or approximately 1 IU/kg BW, based on a report of enhanced humoral immune function in mature horses supplemented with 1 IU vitamin E/kg BW (Baalsrud and Overnes, 1986). The change in vitamin E requirement was also supported by the finding of Roneus et al. (1986) that 1.4–4.4 IU vitamin E/kg BW was necessary to maximize tissue stores of vitamin E. To date there is no new information suggesting maintenance vitamin E requirement is different from that of the fifth revision of this document (NRC, 1989).

Growth

Vitamin E requirements specific to growth have not been defined. A vitamin E requirement of 0.233 IU/kg BW was estimated for foals using erythrocyte stability as a response variable (Stowe, 1968a), which is approximately 11 IU vitamin E/kg DM assuming a DM intake of 2.5 percent of BW. Nutritional muscular dystrophy was identified in neonatal foals whose dams consumed diets containing low concentrations of vitamin E (approximately 6–8 IU vitamin E/kg DM); however, this finding was confounded by low selenium intake in the mares (Wilson et al., 1976).

More work is necessary to determine the requirements for vitamin E specific to growth. Based on the information available, 80 IU/kg DM recommended in the 1989 NRC is more than adequate for growing horses. Vitamin E requirements of growing horses in the current revision are expressed as IU/kg BW (2 IU/kg BW), which is equivalent to 80 IU/kg DM assuming 2.5 percent BW as DM intake.

Breeding, Gestation, and Lactation

Stowe (1967) reported a beneficial effect of a low level of oral vitamin E supplementation (100 IU/d, approximately 10 percent of the current requirement) on reproduction in barren mares. Ott and Asquith (1981) did not find any advantage of supplementing 46 IU of additional vitamin E/d to a ration already containing vitamin E concentration equivalent to NRC (1978) requirements (i.e., 15 IU/kg DM) on rebreeding efficiency in foaling mares. Supplementation of 200–400 IU vitamin E/d to gestating mares was ineffective at maintaining serum α-tocopherol concentrations of mares fed a base diet of preserved forage (Maenpaa et al., 1988b), yet no outward signs of deficiency were reported. Libido and seminal characteristics were not affected when stallions were supplemented with 5,000 IU vitamin E/d, as compared to an unsupplemented ration consisting of grain mix and grass hay (Rich et al., 1983). These results suggest that even the maintenance requirement for vitamin E recommended in the NRC (1989), i.e., 50 IU/kg DM, is sufficient for reproduction in both stallions and mares. Therefore, the requirement for reproduction remains unchanged from the previous revision (i.e., 50 IU/kg DM or 1 IU/kg BW assuming a DM intake of 2 percent of BW).

Hoffman et al. (1999) reported that foals suckling mares fed diets containing approximately 160 IU vitamin E/kg DM, or twice that recommended for broodmares (NRC, 1989), tended to have greater serum immunoglobulin G (IgG) titers than those suckling mares fed 80 IU vitamin E/kg DM. This response was thought to be a reflection of the significantly greater IgG concentration of the colostrum from those mares. Vitamin E used in the aforementioned experiment was supplied both from the base ration (mixed grass hay plus a grain-mix-concentrate) and from a supplemental source containing all-*rac*-α-tocopheryl acetate. Whether or not the difference in antibody titers reported in these foals results in improved health remains to be determined. The current vitamin E requirement for lactation is unchanged from the previous revision (i.e., 80 IU/kg DM or 2 IU/kg BW assuming a DM intake of 2.5 percent BW).

Work

Interest in the vitamin E requirement for work was stimulated by a possible relationship between vitamin E status and exertional rhabdomyolysis, and the potential for oxidative damage to skeletal muscle during exercise.

A relationship between vitamin E (and selenium) deficiency and exertional rhabdomyolysis was initially suggested (Hill, 1962); however, subsequent studies did not support this idea (Roneus and Hakkarainen, 1985) and pointed to multifactorial etiologies (Beech, 1994).

The relationship between vitamin E and exercise-induced oxidative stress has been investigated in horses. There is evidence that exercise induces some degree of lipid oxidation in horses (McMeniman and Hintz, 1992; Williams et al., 2004a,b), yet its contribution toward oxidative damage of tissues and subsequent health of the horse is uncertain (McMeniman and Hintz, 1992; Siciliano et al., 1997). Exercise conditioning has been demonstrated to influence vitamin E status. Petersson et al. (1991) reported that plasma, but not middle gluteal muscle, vitamin E concentration was lower over a 4-month period in exercised horses compared with nonexercised controls when they consumed a diet deficient in vitamin E (NRC, 1989) consisting of grain (7.8 IU E/kg DM) and free choice straw (18.5 IU E/kg DM). When the ration was supplemented with vitamin E (grain and straw containing 85.6 and 17 IU E/kg DM, respectively), there was no difference in plasma vitamin E between exercised and nonexercised groups. Additionally, there was a trend toward an inverse relationship between middle gluteal muscle vitamin E concentration and an indicator of lipid oxidation (thiobarbituric acid reactive substances) in skeletal muscle. Although these horses were fed a vitamin E-deficient diet over a 4-month period, no clinical signs of vitamin E deficiency were observed, nor were blood variables indicative of deficiency altered (red cell hemolysis, muscle enzyme leakage). It should be noted that the exercise protocol used in this experiment was relatively light. Vitamin E status of horses performing rigorous endurance type exercise was improved with levels of supplementation exceeding the current NRC requirement (240 IU/kg DM or approximately 6 IU/kg BW assuming DM intake of 2.5 percent of BW: Hoffman et al., 2001; 11.1 IU/kg BW: Williams et al., 2004b). Siciliano et al. (1997) reported a decline in both serum (approximately 30 percent) and middle gluteal muscle vitamin E concentration (approximately 20 percent) over a 90-day exercise conditioning period when horses were fed a basal diet (15–44 IU/kg DM, or 0.3–0.88 IU/kg BW) or 80 IU/kg DM (1.6 IU/kg BW), but not in horses fed 300 IU/kg DM (6 IU/kg BW). This result suggests that dietary concentrations of vitamin E greater than 80 IU/kg DM and potentially approaching 300 IU/kg DM are necessary to maintain blood and skeletal muscle concentrations undergoing exercise conditioning. This finding is in agreement with Saastamoinen and Juusela (1993), who found that approximately 150–250 IU of vitamin E/kg DM was necessary to prevent serum vitamin E concentration from declining in horses receiving regular exercise. Vitamin E supplementation (5,000 IU/d or approximately 11.1 IU/kg BW) decreased white blood cell apoptosis and plasma creatine kinase activity during and after a treadmill-simulated 55-km endurance race (Williams et al., 2004b).

Although the above findings suggest that vitamin E supplementation exceeding current recommendations may improve vitamin E status of exercising horses in some situations, more work using varied dietary vitamin E concentrations and differing exercise protocols is required to establish optimum requirements necessary to maintain vitamin E status during exercise. The current requirements are unchanged from the previous revision, but are expressed per unit of BW assuming a DM intake of 2, 2.25, and 2.5 percent of BW for light, moderate, and all other levels of work, respectively (i.e., 80 IU/kg DM is equivalent to 1.6, 1.8, and 2 IU/kg BW for light, moderate, and all other levels of work, respectively).

VITAMIN K

Function

Vitamin K serves as a cofactor for vitamin K-dependent carboxylase, which catalyzes the post-translational synthesis of γ-carboxyglutamic acid (Gla) from glutamic acid residues contained in precursor proteins (Ferland, 2001). The resulting vitamin K-dependent proteins, also referred to as Gla-proteins, are involved in blood clotting, bone metabolism, and vascular health (Dowd et al., 1995; Vermeer et al., 1996, 2004). Vitamin K has also been suggested to play a role in brain sphingolipid metabolism through mechanisms that are not well understood (Denisova and Booth, 2005).

Dietary Sources

Vitamin K occurs naturally as phylloquinone (K_1; 2-methyl-3-phytyl-1,4-napthoquinone) and the group of compounds known as menaquinone (K_2; 2-methyl-1,4-napthoquinones) (Ferland, 2001). Phylloquinone is the form of vitamin K found in plants. Menaquinone is produced by intestinal bacteria. Menadione (K_3) is a synthetic form of vitamin K used as a feed supplement and is metabolized in the body to an active form, i.e., menaquinone-4.

Among typical feedstuffs used for horses, forages contain the greatest concentration of vitamin K (2.73–21.6 mg/kg DM) and cereals contain relatively low concentrations (0.2–0.4 mg/kg DM) (McDowell, 1989; Siciliano et al., 2000a). Menaquinones produced by intestinal bacteria may also provide the horse with some vitamin K, but the exact contribution is unknown. Menaquinones derived from intestinal bacteria can be absorbed in humans and rodents, but the overall contribution toward meeting vitamin K requirements may be limited by the capacity for absorption in the lower bowel (Suttie, 1995) and may be inadequate to maintain optimum status in humans (Ferland, 2001).

Deficiency

Vitamin K deficiency results in the production of undercarboxylated Gla-proteins, such as undercarboxylated osteocalcin, that lack biological activity. Impairment of blood coagulation is the major clinical sign of vitamin K deficiency in all species (McDowell, 1989). Vitamin K deficiency has also been implicated in diseases affecting bone and vascular health in humans (Vermeer et al., 2004).

Vitamin K deficiency in horses due to inadequate vitamin K consumption has not been identified. Vitamin K antagonists such as dicumarol and other coumarin derivatives (e.g., warfarin) can impair vitamin K metabolism and result in deficiency symptoms. Dicumarol is produced in moldy sweet clover hay and has been reported to impair blood coagulation, according to a single report in one horse (McDonald, 1980). Additionally, therapeutic administration of warfarin to horses can interfere with vitamin K metabolism and impair blood coagulation. Prothrombin time increased in horses receiving warfarin administration (0.08 mg/kg BW/d for 4–5 days) and was restored in 24 hours by either intravenous or subcutaneous administration of 300–500 mg vitamin K_1 (Byars et al., 1986).

Toxicity

Excess intake of phylloquinone appears to be essentially innocuous. Molitor and Robinson (1940) administered 25 g/kg BW orally or parenterally to laboratory animals with no adverse effect. Menaquinones and menadione in the diet probably also have low toxicity. The NRC (1987) proposed that oral toxic levels are at least 1,000 times the dietary requirement. However, Rebhun et al. (1984) administered single doses of menadione bisulfite to horses in amounts of 2.1–8.3 mg/kg BW via intramuscular or intravenous routes. These dosages conformed to manufacturer's recommendations, but resulted in renal colic, hematuria, azotemia, and electrolyte abnormalities consistent with acute renal failure. At necropsy, lesions of renal tubular nephrosis were found. Because phylloquinone injectables appear safer than menadione injectables for the human newborn (American Academy of Pediatrics, 1971), use of the former seems preferable when parenteral vitamin K is administered to the horse.

Requirements

Dietary vitamin K requirements have not been determined for the horse (NRC, 1989). Phylloquinone content of pasture, hay, or both, along with menaquinones synthesized by intestinal bacteria, presumably meet requirements in all but the most unusual of circumstances.

Limited reports exist regarding factors influencing vitamin K requirements of horses. Vitamin K status, as measured by undercarboxylated osteocalcin, was not affected by the initiation of exercise training in young horses (18–24 months of age) while consuming a diet containing 2.73 mg phylloquinone/kg DM, nor was it correlated to exercise associated changes in bone mineral or bone pathology (Siciliano et al., 2000a). Vitamin K status, as measured by undercarboxylated osteocalcin, of foals and weanlings increased with age possibly reflecting increased forage consumption and increased capacity for intestinal microbial synthesis of menaquinone (Siciliano et al., 2000b). Serum undercarboxylated osteocalcin was not correlated with medial radiographic bone density in these foals and weanlings. The effect of lower vitamin K status on bone health in foals remains to be determined.

THIAMIN

Function

Thiamin is required by pyruvate dehydrogenase, α-ketoglutarate dehydrogenase, and transketolase, all of which are involved in carbohydrate metabolism (Bates, 2001). Pyruvate dehydrogenase and α-ketoglutarate dehydrogenase are involved in the metabolism of substrates used for adenosine triphosphate (ATP) synthesis (e.g., glucose), whereas transketolase is involved in the pentose phosphate pathway.

Dietary Sources

Thiamin is found in relatively high concentrations in cereal grains (e.g., corn, 3.5; oats, 5.2; wheat, 5.5; barley, 5.7 mg/kg DM), cereal grain byproducts (wheat bran, 8; wheat middlings, 12; rice bran, 23 mg/kg DM), protein supplements (e.g., cottonseed meal, 6.4; peanut meal, 12 mg/kg DM), and is particularly high in brewer's yeast (95.2 mg/kg) (McDowell, 1989). Thiamin is supplemented as either thiamin hydrochloride or mononitrate.

Deficiency

The classical deficiency symptom for thiamin is beriberi (Bates, 2001). Anorexia, bradycardia, muscle fasciculations, and ataxia have been reported in cases of thiamin deficiency in horses (Carroll et al., 1949; Roberts et al., 1949; Cymbaluk et al., 1978). Carroll et al. (1949) reported thiamin deficiency symptoms in two horses fed semi-purified diets containing approximately 1.1 mg/kg for a 16-week period. Thiamin deficiency symptoms have been reported in horses due to ingestion of bracken fern (Roberts et al., 1949) and the coccidiostat amprolium (Cymbaluk et al., 1978), both of which interfere with thiamin metabolism. Thiamin deficiency in horses fed typical feed ingredients, in the absence of interfering substances, has not been reported.

Toxicity

Thiamin toxicity in horses does not seem likely and has not been reported (NRC, 1989).

Requirements

The NRC (1989) requirement for thiamin is 5 mg/kg DM for working horses and 3 mg/kg DM for all others, and was based on diet concentrations necessary to maintain appetite (Carroll et al., 1949), increase growth rate (Jordan, 1979), improve thiamin balance, and improve biochemical measures reflective of thiamin function in exercising horses (Topliff et al., 1981).

Carroll et al. (1949) provided evidence of microbial thiamin synthesis in the gastrointestinal tract of horses, particularly the anterior portion of the large colon. In a follow-up experiment, evidence indicated microbial thiamin synthesis alone was inadequate to prevent deficiency symptoms as thiamin deficiency symptoms (e.g., loss of appetite, weight loss, ataxia) were reported in two Percheron horses (2 years of age, approximately 600-kg BW) fed the same semi-purified diet containing 1.1 mg thiamin/kg DM (total DM intake approximately 1.25–1.5 percent of BW) over a 16-week period (Carroll et al., 1949). One horse died following 19 weeks of the low-thiamin diet and the other improved over a 12-week period when supplemented with 30 mg thiamin/d (approximately 5.5 mg thiamin/100 kg BW).

Jordan (1979) reported that weanling ponies (110–130 days of age) fed diets containing 6.6 mg thiamin/kg DM (70 percent corn, 30 percent alfalfa meal) gained more BW (89.5 percent increase) as compared to those consuming the basal diet only. Feed intake was not different between the two groups. No clinical signs of thiamin deficiency were reported in the unsupplemented group.

Topliff et al. (1981) concluded that 3 mg thiamin/kg DM may not be adequate for exercising horses. This conclusion was based on the finding that the mean blood thiamin concentrations of horses fed diets containing either 4 or 28 mg thiamin/kg DM were greater than in horses fed diets containing 2 mg thiamin/kg DM. Additionally, an indicator of pyruvate dehydrogenase activity suggested greater activity following 30 minutes of exercise in horses fed diets containing 4 or 28 mg thiamin/kg DM as compared to 2 mg thiamin/kg DM.

There is no new evidence to suggest that thiamin requirements are different from NRC (1989). Thiamin requirements in the previous revision, expressed per kg DM, have been transformed to a BW basis assuming a DM intake of 2 percent of BW for maintenance, breeding stallions, gestation, and light work; 2.25 percent of BW for moderate work; and 2.5 percent of BW for all other feeding classes. For example, a maintenance requirement previously expressed as 3 mg/kg DM is now expressed as 0.06 mg/kg BW (i.e., 3 mg/kg DM × 2 kg DM/100 kg BW).

RIBOFLAVIN

Function

Riboflavin is a precursor to the coenzymes flavin adenine dinucleotide (FAD) and flavin mononucleotide (FMN). Both FAD and FMN are involved in oxidation-reduction reactions used in ATP synthesis, drug metabolism, lipid metabolism, and antioxidant defense mechanisms (i.e., glutathione redox cycle) (Rivlin, 2001).

Dietary Sources

Relative to dietary requirements for horses, values published in the U.S. Canadian Feed tables suggest that riboflavin is found in high concentration in legumes such as alfalfa and clover (13–17 mg/kg DM). However, slightly lesser concentrations are found in some grass hays (7–10 mg/kg DM), and relatively low concentrations occur in cereal grains (1.4–1.7 mg/kg DM) (NRC, 1982). Naturally occurring riboflavin present in feedstuffs is generally in the form of FAD and FMN, both of which are coenzyme derivatives of riboflavin.

Riboflavin synthesis in the intestine of the adult horse or pony has been demonstrated by Jones et al. (1946), Carroll et al. (1949), and Linerode (1966). When Carroll and colleagues (1949) fed a riboflavin-deficient diet containing 0.4 mg of riboflavin/kg DM, riboflavin concentrations (mg/kg ingesta DM) in the various intestinal sections were as follows: duodenum, 3.8; ileum, 1.1; cecum, 7; anterior large colon, 9.2; and anterior small colon, 12.2. The increased concentrations occurring in the cecum and large colon relative to the foregut are indicative of microbial riboflavin synthesis.

Deficiency

Although riboflavin deficiency has not been described in horses, signs in other species include rough hair coat; atrophy of the epidermis, hair follicles, and sebaceous glands; dermatitis; vascularization of the cornea; catarrhal conjunctivitis; photophobia; and excess lacrimation. Some years ago, it was suggested that periodic ophthalmia (recurrent uveitis or moon blindness) is a consequence of riboflavin deficiency (Jones, 1942; Jones et al., 1945). However, the linkage between the two is not substantial, and invasions of the cornea by leptospira (Roberts, 1958) or microfilaria (*Onchrocera cervicalis*) (Cello, 1962) have been implicated in the production of periodic ophthalmia.

Toxicity

Little evidence exists of oral toxicity of riboflavin in any species. Schumacher et al. (1965) reported a reduction in pups born to rats supplemented with 104 mg of riboflavin/kg diet. Estimates of the rat LD_{50} for intraperitoneal, subcutaneous, and oral administration are 0.56, 5, and more than 10 g of riboflavin/kg BW, respectively.

Requirements

The first NRC riboflavin allowance estimated for horses was 2.2 mg/kg air-dried feed (NRC, 1949). This estimate was based on the work of Pearson et al. (1944a,b) who reported that 44 µg riboflavin/kg BW (approximately 2.2 mg/kg air dried feed) was adequate based on measurements of growth and whole body riboflavin status in Shetland ponies. However, in another report two horses fed a ration low in B vitamins containing 0.4 mg/kg air-dried feed for 19 weeks did not demonstrate deficiency symptoms attributed to the low-riboflavin content of the diet (Carroll et al., 1949). In the fifth NRC revision (1989), the requirement remained similar and was suggested to be no more than 2 mg/kg DM air-dried feed. At the time of this writing, no new information regarding riboflavin requirements of horses exists. Horses fed forage-based diets should have a riboflavin intake well above 2 mg/kg air-dried feed based on estimates of riboflavin concentration in feedstuffs previously discussed. Riboflavin requirements in the previous revision, expressed per kg DM, have been transformed to a BW basis assuming a DM intake of 2 percent of BW for maintenance, breeding stallions, gestation, and light work; 2.25 percent for moderate work; and 2.5 percent of BW for all other feeding classes. For example, a maintenance requirement previously expressed as 2 mg/kg DM is now expressed as 0.04 mg/kg BW (i.e., 2 mg/kg DM × 2 kg DM/100 kg BW).

NIACIN

Function

Niacin is essential for the coenzymes nicotinamide adenine dinucleotide (NAD) and nicotinamide adenine dinucleotide phosphate (NADP), which are involved in many important biological oxidation-reduction reactions. Additionally, NAD has been reported to provide the substrate for three classes of enzymes that transfer ADP-ribose units to proteins involved in DNA processing, cell differentiation, and cellular calcium mobilization (Jacob, 2001).

Dietary Sources

Niacin is a generic term for nicotinic acid (pyridine-3-carboxylic acid) and nicotinamide (nicotinic acid amide). Both nicotinic acid and nicotinamide are equivalent in terms of their vitamin activity.

Naturally occurring niacin present in feedstuffs is in the form of NAD and NADP (Jacob, 2001). Both NAD and NADP are hydrolyzed in the intestinal mucosa to yield nicotinamide. Niacin is widely distributed in the diet, but varies in availability depending upon whether it is in a bound form (NRC, 1982; McDowell, 1989). Corn, oats, and barley have been reported to contain 28, 16, and 94 mg niacin/kg DM, respectively; however, 85–90 percent may be in an unavailable bound form. Therefore, McDowell (1989) suggested niacin from cereal grain sources should be ignored or at least given a value of no greater than one-third of the total niacin. Other reported niacin concentrations for feedstuffs include: soybean meal, 31 mg/kg DM; alfalfa, 42 mg/kg DM; and timothy hay, 24 mg/kg DM (NRC, 1982). Approximately 40 percent of niacin in oilseeds is in a bound form (McDowell, 1989). No estimate of the percentage of bound niacin is available for soybean meal or forages commonly fed to horses.

Niacin appears to be produced by microbial fermentation in the hindgut of the horse. Carroll et al. (1949) fed a diet containing 3 mg of nicotinic acid/kg DM and found the following nicotinic acid concentrations (mg/kg DM) in ingesta: duodenum, 55; ileum, 58; cecum, 121; anterior large colon, 96; and anterior small colon, 119. Linerode (1966) also concluded that appreciable microbial niacin synthesis occurs in the cecum and colon of the adult pony.

Niacin can be synthesized from tryptophan in the horse's hepatic tissues (Schweigert et al., 1947). The Food and Nutrition Board (1998) uses a tryptophan to niacin conversion of 60 mg tryptophan to 1 mg niacin.

Deficiency

Niacin deficiency has not been described in the horse. Niacin deficiency in other species results in severe metabolic disorders that manifest as lesions of the skin (e.g., pellagra) and digestive system (McDowell, 1989).

Toxicity

Effects of niacin excess have not been described in the horse. However, high oral intakes of nicotinic acid have produced vasodialation, itching, sensations of heat, nausea, vomiting, headaches, and occasional skin lesions in humans (Robie, 1967; Hawkins, 1968). In addition, Winter and Boyer (1973) reported hepatotoxicity from high nicotinamide intake. Research with laboratory animals suggests that daily oral intake greater than 350 mg of nicotinic acid equivalents/kg BW can be toxic (NRC, 1987). Nicotinic acid may be tolerated somewhat better than nicotinamide. Limits for parenteral administration could be lower than those for oral intake.

Because niacin toxicity has been reported to inhibit the mobilization of free fatty acids (FFA) from adipose tissue of humans during exercise (Heath et al., 1993; Murray et al., 1995), Parker et al. (1997) investigated the effect of 6 weeks of nicotinic supplementation (3 g/d) on niacin status and plasma FFA concentrations associated with a standardized exercise test. Niacin status was not affected by either nicotinic acid supplementation or exercise conditioning, nor was plasma FFA concentration associated with a standardized exercise test affected by nicotinic acid supplementation. Interestingly niacin number (the ratio of NAD to NADP) used as an indicator of niacin status in this experiment ranged from 75 to 100, which is lower than the reference range for healthy humans (i.e., 127 to 223) (Jacob, 2001).

Requirements

No dietary requirement for niacin has been established for horses.

BIOTIN

Function

Biotin is a co-enzyme for four carboxylase enzymes: acetyl-CoA carboxylase, pyruvate carboxylase, propionyl-CoA carboxylase, and β-methylcrotonyl-CoA carboxylase (Zempleni, 2001). These carboxylase enzymes are involved in fatty acid synthesis (acetyl-CoA carboxylase), gluconcogenesis (pyruvate carboxylase), amino acid metabolism (propionyl-CoA carboxylase and β-methylcrotonyl-CoA carboxylase), and metabolism of cholesterol and odd-chain fatty acids (propionyl-CoA carboxylase). As a result biotin plays an important role in intermediary metabolism.

Biotin is essential for cell proliferation. Biotin's role in intermediary metabolism (i.e., carboxylase enzymes), along with roles in gene expression and biotinylation of histones, have been suggested as the basis for the role of biotin in cell proliferation (Zempleni and Mock, 2001).

Dietary Sources

Biotin is 2-keto-3, 4-imadazilido-2-tetrahydrothiophene-valeric acid and has eight possible isomers of which only d-biotin contains vitamin activity (McDowell, 1989). Information regarding biotin concentration of feedstuffs for horses is limited. That which is available indicates relatively high concentrations for alfalfa (0.2 mg/kg DM, hay; 0.49 mg/kg DM, fresh); intermediate concentrations for oats (0.11–0.39 mg/kg DM), barley (0.13–0.17 mg/kg DM), and soybean meal (0.18–0.5 mg/kg DM); and low concentrations for corn (0.06–0.1 mg/kg DM) (NRC, 1982; McDowell, 1989). Biotin availability has not been assessed for horses, but that for poultry and swine suggests corn and soybean meal are relatively high at 75–100 percent and 100 percent, respectively (Baker, 1995). Most naturally occurring biotin exists in a form bound to protein, i.e., ε-N-biotinyl-L-lysine (biocytin), making availability dependent upon digestibility of the specific binding proteins (Baker, 1995).

Biotin is also synthesized by intestinal microbes. Carroll et al. (1949) fed a diet containing less than 0.01 mg of biotin/kg DM and found the following biotin concentrations in ingesta (mg/kg of DM): duodenum, less than 0.1; ileum, 0.1; cecum, 0.2; anterior large colon, 3.8; and anterior small colon, 2.3.

Deficiency

Severe dermatitis is the most common deficiency symptom seen in livestock (McDowell, 1989). No unequivocal evidence of biotin deficiency in the horse has been published. Signs in other species include inflammation and cracks of the plantar surface of the feet (Cunha et al., 1946, 1948).

Biotin deficiency has been implicated in some populations of horses chronically affected with poor hoof quality, such as soft white line and crumbling, fissured horn at the bearing border of the hoof wall (Josseck et al., 1995; Zenker et al., 1995). Daily supplementation with 20 mg biotin improved hoof wall integrity (via macroscopic assessment) following at least 9 months of supplementation, but not growth rate (Josseck et al., 1995), and improved hoof structure (via histological assessment) and hoof wall tensile strength following 33 and 38 months of supplementation (Zenker et al., 1995). Previous observations from uncontrolled field studies suggested 10–30 mg biotin/d for not less than 6–9 months improved hardness and integrity of hooves previously of poor quality (Comben et al., 1984; Kempson, 1987). Using scanning electron microscopy, Kempson (1987) identified two types of defects in hoof samples from horses having thin friable horn. The first type of defect was characterized by a loss of structure and horn in the stratum externum of the hoof wall, whereas the second was characterized by a loss of tubular structure in the inner layers of the hoof wall. The first defect appeared responsive to biotin supplementation (~ 15 mg/d). The second defect, which consisted of approximately 94 percent of the affected horses studied, was thought due to dietary protein and calcium deficiency. This work suggests that some horses with thin friable hoof wall may benefit from dietary biotin supplementation, while others may not.

Buffa et al. (1992) reported increased hoof wall growth rate and hoof hardness in Thoroughbred and Thoroughbred-cross horses fed 15 mg biotin/d for 10 months as compared to controls fed 0.81 mg biotin/d. Reilly et al. (1998) reported a 15 percent higher hoof wall growth rate in ponies supplemented with 0.12 mg biotin/kg BW/d for 5 months as compared to controls fed 0.0015 mg naturally occurring biotin/kg BW/d.

Toxicity

Effects of excess biotin have not been described in the horse. Fetal resorption has been reported in rats injected subcutaneously with 50 to 100 mg biotin/kg BW. Poultry and swine can tolerate at least 4 to 10 times their dietary requirement and probably much more (NRC, 1987).

Requirements

No controlled studies have been published establishing a dietary biotin requirement above that supplied by intestinal synthesis. As stated in the deficiency section, there is some evidence that biotin supplementation may be useful in improving hoof integrity in certain horse populations, particularly those affected with poor hoof quality. However, no definitive requirement for biotin has been determined.

FOLATE

Function

Folate is required for numerous biosynthetic pathways involving transfer and utilization of single carbon units. Among them are reactions necessary for DNA, purine, and methionine synthesis (Bailey et al., 2001). Therefore, folate is particularly important for tissues in which rapid cell growth, turnover, or some combination is occurring.

Dietary Sources

Folate is a generic term referring to folic acid and naturally occurring folate (Bailey et al., 2001). Folic acid is the synthetic form of folate and consists of a pteridene bicyclic ring system, p-aminobenzoic acid and glutamic acid. Naturally occurring dietary folate differs from folic acid in that it contains 5 to 8 glutamic acids joined in γ-peptide linkages, i.e., polyglutamate form.

Reported values for folate concentration of typical horse feed ingredients are limited. Those available are for alfalfa (2.5–4.1 mg/kg DM), timothy hay (2.3 mg/kg DM), and cereal grains (corn, 0.3; oats, 0.4; barley, 0.6 mg/kg DM) (NRC, 1982). Horses consuming fresh forage have greater serum folate concentrations compared to horses consuming preserved forages, grains, and grain byproducts, which presumably reflects greater folate concentrations of fresh forage.

Folic acid appears to be produced in the digestive tract by microbial synthesis. Carroll et al. (1949) fed a diet containing less than 0.1 mg folic acid/kg DM and found the following folic acid concentrations in ingesta (mg/kg of DM): duodenum, 0.9; ileum, 0.5; cecum, 3; anterior large colon, 4.7; and anterior small colon, 2.7.

Bioavailability estimates of folic acid and naturally occurring dietary folate in humans are 85 and 50 percent, respectively (Food and Nutrition Board, 1998). However, Allen (1984) found that orally administered folic acid was absorbed poorly in the horse.

Deficiency

Folate deficiency has not been described in the horse (NRC, 1989). Megaloblastic anemia and leukopenia are common findings in other species. In addition, tissues having a rapid rate of cell growth or tissue regeneration (e.g., gastrointestinal tract epithelial lining, epidermis, and bone marrow) are also affected (McDowell, 1989). Folate deficiency in pregnant women is associated with increased risk of preterm delivery, infant low birth weight, fetal growth retardation, and neural tube defects (Bailey et al., 2001).

Sulfadiazine and pyrimethamine are antimicrobials used to treat equine protozoal myeloencephalitis (EPM). Both of these drugs can impair folate status. Sulfadiazine inhibits microbial synthesis of folate by preventing dihydroteroic acid formation from para-aminobenzoic acid. Pyrimethamine inhibits dihydrofolate reductase, which is necessary for folate absorption and metabolism. Colahan et al. (2002) reported a 2 ng/ml reduction in serum folate (5-methyltetrahydrofolate) from approximately 8 to 6 ng/ml following 4 days of sulfadiazine and pyrimethamine administration. Piercy et al. (2002) reported clinical findings compatible with folate deficiency in a horse treated with sulfadiazine and pyrimethamine for EPM over a 9-month period. The findings included hematological defects, hypoplastic bone marrow, and dysphagia caused by oral ulceration and glossitis. Serum folate concentration was approximately 4.5 ng/ml. Folic acid supplementation (19.2 mg/d) accompanied the treatment and was hypothesized to exacerbate the deficiency by competing for absorption with the active, reduced form of folate (5-methyl tetrahydrofolate). A similar hypothesis was put forth and supported by the finding of congenital defects in newborn foals born of mares treated with sulfadiazine and pyrimethamine for equine protozoal myeloencephalitis during pregnancy, and also supplemented with folic acid (40 mg/day) for periods ranging from the last 3 months of gestation to 2 years (Toribio et al., 1998).

Toxicity

Folate is generally regarded as nontoxic (NRC, 1987). However, single parenteral doses about 1,000 times greater than the dietary requirement have been reported to induce epileptic convulsion and renal hypertrophy in the rat.

As discussed above, folic acid supplementation is not recommended in horses treated with dihydrofolate reductase inhibitors (e.g., pyrimethamine) (Toribio et al., 1998; Piercy et al., 2002).

Requirements

Folate requirements of horses have not been determined. Folate originating from microbes in the gastrointestinal tract and that occurring naturally in feeds appears to meet the needs of most horses. However, Seckington et al. (1967) reported lower serum folate concentration in stabled Thoroughbred racehorses and postpartum mares (mean 7.5 and 7.4 ng/ml, respectively) as compared to mature horses at pasture (mean 11.5 ng/ml). Likewise, serum folate was lower in race horses undergoing training for 6 months without access to pasture (range 1.5–6.1 ng/ml) as compared to unexercised horse and pony mares maintained on pasture (range 6.4–15.8 and 7.4–16.6 ng/ml, for horses and ponies, respectively: Allen, 1978). Roberts (1983) also reported serum folate concentration of horses on pasture was approximately 3-fold that of stabled horses fed preserved forage and suggested that exercise may increase folate needs of some horses in training.

The effect of folate status on athletic performance is relatively uninvestigated. Physiological response to exercise and time to fatigue during a stepwise exercise test carried out to exhaustion on a high-speed treadmill was not influenced when serum folate was decreased from 8 to 6 ng/ml following oral administration of sulfadiazine and pyrimethamine (Colahan et al., 2002). The duration of this experiment was relatively short (i.e., 4 days of sulfadiazine and pyrimethamine administration) and longer term effects of sulfadiazine and pyrimethamine administration on folate status and exercise performance were not evaluated.

Ordakowski-Burk et al. (2005) reported folate status in mares and foals from foaling through 6 months of lactation and concluded folate supplementation was not necessary. The mares consumed folate from natural sources only (pasture, hay, and supplemental feed) in amounts ranging from 30–80 mg folate/d.

The current lack of information regarding folate requirements of horses precludes accurate estimation of a true requirement. Based on the absence of reports of folate deficiency in horses maintained in practical settings, naturally occurring folate in feeds and that of microbial origin appear to satisfy the requirement. However, further investigation of folate requirements for horses not having access to pasture is warranted, particularly for horses with potentially high requirements, e.g., gestation, lactation, growth, and intense exercise.

OTHER B-VITAMINS

Information regarding dietary requirements for vitamin B_{12}, pantothenic acid, and vitamin B_6 of horses is either extremely limited or not available (NRC, 1989). All of these vitamins appear to be synthesized in the gastrointestinal tract of horses (Carroll et al., 1949; Linerode, 1966; Alexander and Davies, 1969; Davies, 1971).

Vitamin B_{12} (cyanocobalamin) is a component of several enzyme systems involved in purine and pyrimidine synthesis, transfer of methyl groups, protein synthesis, carbohydrate, and fat metabolism (McDowell, 2000). Vitamin B_{12} is not present in plants, but is synthesized by microorganisms present in the digestive tract. Synthesis of vitamin B_{12} requires the trace mineral cobalt. Supplemental cobalt (15 mg cobalt chloride) has been reported to influence serum and fecal vitamin B_{12} concentrations (Alexander and Davies, 1969). Stillions et al. (1971b) fed adult horses a semipurified diet containing about 1 μg of vitamin B_{12} and about 5 mg cobalt/kg air-dry feed. Although serum vitamin B_{12} concentration and daily urinary vitamin B_{12} excretion were lower than with a diet containing 90 μg of vitamin B_{12}/kg, daily vitamin B_{12} excretion was about 500 μg or five times greater than intake on the low- or high-vitamin B_{12} diet, respectively. No evidence of vitamin B_{12} deficiency was seen, and hemoglobin and hematocrit values were normal over an experimental period of 11 months. Horses have remained in good health while grazing pastures so low in cobalt that ruminants confined to them have died (Filmer, 1933). Evidence of absorption of vitamin B_{12} from the cecum and colon was reported by Stillions et al. (1971b) and Salminen (1975). Caple et al. (1982) examined several hundred horses and reported plasma vitamin B_{12} concentrations of 1.8–7.3 µg/L. Intramuscular injections of vitamin B_{12} were cleared rapidly from the plasma, and large amounts were excreted in the feces via the bile when vitamin B_{12} was administered intravenously in foals. Colostrum contributed significantly to the vitamin B_{12} status of the foal during the first 24 hours after birth. Much of the vitamin was stored in the liver. In a survey of 88 horses in various states of physiology and training, Roberts (1983) found no evidence of vitamin B_{12} deficiency based on serum vitamin B_{12} concentrations or cellular hematology. No evidence of a dietary vitamin B_{12} requirement above that supplied by intestinal synthesis has been reported. Vitamin B_{12} deficiency or toxicity has not been described in the horse (NRC, 1989).

Pantothenic acid is a constituent of coenzyme A and acyl-carrier protein, which are involved in numerous metabolic pathways involving carbohydrates, proteins, lipids, neurotransmitters, steroid hormones, porphyrins, and hemoglobin (McDowell, 2000). Pantothenic acid is widely distributed in the diet (McDowell, 2000). No signs of deficiency were observed in adult horses fed diets containing 0.8 mg of pantothenic acid or less than 0.2 mg pantothenic acid/kg DM (Carroll et al., 1949). Likewise, no signs of deficiency were observed by Pearson and Schmidt (1958) in growing ponies fed a diet containing 3.2 mg pantothenic acid/kg air-dried feed. No dietary pantothenic acid requirement has been established for horses, nor has a deficiency or toxicity been reported in horses (NRC, 1989).

Vitamin B_6 is a component of numerous enzymes involved in the metabolism of protein, fats, and carbohydrates, and it is widely distributed in the diet (McDowell, 2000). No dietary vitamin B_6 requirement has been established, nor has a deficiency or toxicity been reported in horses (NRC, 1989).

VITAMIN C

Function

Vitamin C functions as a biological antioxidant within the redox system and as a cofactor for mixed function oxidases involved in the synthesis of collagen, carnitine, and norepinephrine (Johnston, 2001).

Dietary and Other Sources

Vitamin C activity originates from two compounds, L-ascorbic acid and dehydro-L-ascorbic acid, which are equivalent in biological activity (McDowell, 1989; Johnston, 2001). Vitamin C concentrations of typical feedstuffs for horses are not available.

Ascorbic acid, ascorbyl palmitate, and calcium ascorbyl-2-monophosphate have been used as vitamin C supplements for horses. Ascorbyl palmitate has been reported to be more efficient at raising plasma ascorbic acid concentration than ascorbyl-2-monophosphate (Deaton et al., 2003) or ascorbic acid (Snow and Frigg, 1987, 1990).

Vitamin C can be synthesized from glucose in several species (Chatterjee, 1973). Horses also appear to have the ability to synthesize vitamin C from glucose (Pearson et al., 1943; Stillions et al., 1971a).

Deficiency

Scurvy, resulting from impaired collagen synthesis, is the classical vitamin C deficiency symptom. Classic vitamin C deficiency has not been reported in horses. However, some authors have reported a relationship between decreased blood ascorbic acid concentrations in horses and several diseases, including post-operative and post-traumatic wound infections, epistaxis, strangles, acute rhinopneumonia, and performance insufficiency (Jaeschke and Keller, 1978b; Jaeschke, 1984). Serum ascorbic acid concentrations reflective of deficiency have not been established in horses; however, several values for healthy horses have been reported. Jaeschke and Keller (1978a) reported mean serum ascorbic acid concentration of 488 healthy adult horses was 5.9 ± 1.4 µg/ml. Snow et al. (1987) reported mean plasma ascorbic acid concentrations in a group of approximately 20 unsupplemented Thoroughbred racehorses over the period from February to October ranged from 2–4.2 µg/ml. Mean plasma ascorbic acid concentrations reported in endurance racing horses ranged from 0.8–4.6 µg/ml (Hargreaves et al., 2002; Marlin et al., 2002; Williams et al., 2004a). Pearson et al. (1943) reported a mean plasma ascorbic acid concentration of 3.2 ± 1.3 µg/ml in unsupplemented Shetland ponies.

Toxicity

Excess ascorbic acid intakes in humans and laboratory animals have been reported to produce allergic responses, oxaluria, uricosuria, and interference with mixed function oxidase systems; however, there is insufficient information on the tolerance and toxicity of ascorbic acid in most domestic animals (NRC, 1987). Daily doses of 20 g (approximately 44 mg ascorbic acid/kg BW) have been administered to horses over a period of approximately 8 months with no apparent negative effect (Snow et al., 1987).

Requirements

Dietary vitamin C requirements for the horse have not been determined and are assumed to be met by endogenous synthesis (Pearson et al., 1943; Stillions et al., 1971a). Several factors, including disease (Jaeschke, 1984), transport

(Baucus et al., 1990a,b), recurrent airway obstruction (Deaton et al., 2004), old age (> 20 years of age: Ralston et al., 1988), and endurance exercise (Hargreaves et al., 2002; Marlin et al., 2002) have been demonstrated to decrease plasma or serum concentrations of ascorbic acid in horses, which may suggest an increased consumption of ascorbic acid pools within the body in the presence of these factors. However, it is important to note that others have reported an increase in plasma ascorbic acid concentration (adjusted for changes in plasma volume) following endurance exercise (Williams et al., 2004a), or transient increases over a 12-week period in physically conditioned Thoroughbred racehorses (de Moffarts et al., 2005), and no apparent difference between aged and younger horses (Deaton et al., 2004). Further investigation is required to determine whether endogenous ascorbic acid synthesis is adequate to meet requirements for all horses.

REFERENCES

Abrams, J. T. 1979. The effect of dietary vitamin A supplements on the clinical condition and track performance of racehorses. Bibliotheca Nutritio et Dieta 27:113–120.

Alexander, F., and M. E. Davies. 1969. Studies on vitamin B_{12} in horse. Br. Vet. J. 125:169–176.

Allen, B. V. 1978. Serum folate levels in horses, with particular reference to the English Thoroughbred. Vet. Rec. 103:257–259.

Allen, B. V. 1984. Dietary intake and absorption of folic acid in the horse. P. 118 in Proc. Assoc. Vet. Clin. Pharmacol. Ther.

American Academy of Pediatrics, Committee on Nutrition. 1971. Vitamin K supplementation for infants receiving milk substitute infant formulas and for those with fat malabsorption. Pediatrics 48:483–487.

Baalsrud, K. J., and G. Overnes. 1986. Influence of vitamin E and selenium supplement on antibody production in horses. Equine Vet. J. 18:472–474.

Bailey, L. B., S. Moyers, and J. F. Gregory III. 2001. Folate. P. 214 in Present Knowledge in Nutrition, B. A. Bowman and R. M. Russel, eds. Washington, DC: ISLI Press.

Baker, D. H. 1995. Vitamin bioavailability. P. 399 in Bioavailability of Nutrients for Animals: Amino Acids, Minerals, Vitamins, C. B. Ammerman, D. H. Baker, and A. J. Lewis, eds. New York: Academic Press.

Bates, C. J. 2001. Thiamin. P. 184 in Present Knowledge in Nutrition, B. A. Bowman and R. M. Russel, eds. Washington, DC: ISLI Press.

Baucus, K. L., S. L. Ralston, C. F. Nockels, A. O. McKinnon, and E. L. Squires. 1990a. Effects of transportation on early embryonic death in mares. J. Anim. Sci. 68:345–351.

Baucus, K. L., E. L. Squires, S. L. Ralston, A. O. McKinnon, and T. M. Nett. 1990b. Effect of transportation on the estrous cycle and concentrations of hormones in mares. J. Anim. Sci. 68:419–426.

Beech, J. 1994. Treating and preventing chronic intermittent rhabdomyolysis. Vet. Med. 89:458–461.

Blythe, L. L., and A. M. Craig. 1997. Degenerative myeloencephalopathy. P. 319 in Current Therapy in Equine Medicine, N. E. Robinson, ed. Philadelphia: W. B. Saunders.

Blythe, L. L., A. M. Craig, E. D. Lassen, K. E. Rowe, and L. H. Appell. 1991. Serially determined plasma alpha-tocopherol concentrations and results of the oral vitamin E absorption test in clinically normal horses and in horses with degenerative myeloencephalopathy. Am. J. Vet. Res. 52:908–911.

Buffa, E. A., S. S. Vandenberg, F. J. M. Verstraete, and N. G. N. Swart. 1992. Effect of dietary biotin supplement on equine hoof horn growth-rate and hardness. Equine Vet. J. 24:472–474.

Byars, T. D., C. E. Greene, and D. T. Kemp. 1986. Antidotal effect of vitamin-K-1 against warfarin-induced anticoagulation in horses. Am. J. Vet. Res. 47:2309–2312.

Caple, I. W., G. G. Halpin, J. K. Azuolas, G. F. Nugent, and R. J. Cram. 1982. Studies of selenium, iodine and vitamin B_{12} nutrition of horses in Victoria. Pp. 57–68 in Proc. 4th Bain-Fall Memorial Lecture. Sydney, Australia: Sydney University.

Carroll, F. D., H. Goss, and C. E. Howell. 1949. The synthesis of B vitamins in the horse. J. Anim. Sci. 8:290–299.

Cello, R. M. 1962. Recent findings in periodic ophthalmia. P. 39 in 8th Annu. Assoc. Equine Practitioners, San Francisco, CA.

Chatterjee, I. B. 1973. Evolution and biosynthesis of ascorbic-acid. Science 182:1271–1272.

Colahan, P. T., J. E. Bailey, M. Johnson, B. L. Rice, C. C. Chou, J. P. Cheeks, G. L. Jones, and M. Yang. 2002. Effect of sulfadiazine and pyrimethamine on selected physiological and performance parameters in athletically conditioned Thoroughbred horses during an incremental exercise stress test. Vet. Ther. 3:49–63.

Comben, N., R. J. Clark, and D. J. B. Sutherland. 1984. Clinical observations on the response of equine hoof defects to dietary supplementation with biotin. Vet. Rec. 115:642–645.

Combs, G. F. 1996. Nutritional interrelationship of vitamin E and selenium. Pp. 37 in Vitamin E in Animal Nutrition and Management, 2nd rev. ed., M. B. Coelho, ed. Mount Olive, NJ: BASF.

Craig, A. M., L. L. Blythe, K. E. Rowe, E. D. Lassen, R. Barrington, and K. C. Walker. 1992. Variability of alpha-tocopherol values associated with procurement, storage, and freezing of equine serum and plasma samples. Am. J. Vet. Res. 53:2228–2234.

Cunha, T. J., D. C. Lindley, and M. E. Ensminger. 1946. Biotin deficiency syndrome in pigs fed desiccated egg white. J. Anim. Sci. 5:219–225.

Cunha, T. J., R. W. Colby, L. K. Bustad, and J. F. Bone. 1948. The need for and interrelationship of folic acid, anti-pernicious anemia liver extract, and biotin in the pig. J. Nutr. 36:215–229.

Cymbaluk, N. F., P. B. Fretz, and F. M. Loew. 1978. Amprolium-induced thiamine deficiency in horses: clinical features. Am. J. Vet. Res. 39:255–261.

Davies, M. E. 1971. Production of vitamin-B_{12} in horse. Br. Vet. J. 127:34–36.

Deaton, C. M., D. J. Marlin, N. C. Smith, C. A. Roberts, P. A. Harris, F. J. Kelly, and R. C. Schroter. 2003. Pulmonary bioavailability of ascorbic acid in an ascorbate-synthesising species, the horse. Free Radical Res. 37:461–467.

Deaton, C. M., D. J. Marlin, N. C. Smith, P. A. Harris, C. A. Roberts, R. C. Schroter, and F. J. Kelley. 2004. Pulmonary epithelial lining fluid and plasma ascorbic acid concentrations in horses affected by recurrent airway obstruction. Am. J. Vet. Res. 65:80–87.

De Moffarts, B., N. Kirschvink, T. Art, J. Pincemail, and P. Lekeux. 2005. Effect of oral antioxidant supplementation on blood antioxidant status in trained Thoroughbred horses. Vet. J. 169:65–74.

Denisova, N. A., and S. L. Booth. 2005. Vitamin K and sphingolipid metabolism: evidence to date. Nutr. Rev. 63:111–121.

Divers, T. J. 2005. Equine motor neuron disease. J. Equine Vet. Sci. 25:238–240.

Donoghue, S., D. S. Kronfeld, S. J. Berkowitz, and R. L. Copp. 1981. Vitamin A nutrition of the equine: growth, serum biochemistry and hematology. J. Nutr. 111:365–374.

Dowd, P., S. W. Ham, S. Naganathan, and R. Hershline. 1995. The mechanism of action of vitamin K. Annu. Rev. Nutr. 15:419–440.

Elshorafa, W. M., J. P. Feaster, E. A. Ott, and R. L. Asquith. 1979. Effect of vitamin-D and sunlight on growth and bone-development of young ponies. J. Anim. Sci. 48:882–886.

Ferland, G. 2001. Vitamin K. P. 164 in Present Knowledge in Nutrition, B. A. Bowman and R. A. Russel, eds. Washington, DC: ILSI Press.

Filmer, J. F. 1933. Enzootic marasmus of cattle and sheep. Austral Vet. J. 9:163.

Fonnesbeck, P. V., and L. D. Symons. 1967. Utilization of the carotene of hay by horses. J. Anim. Sci. 26:1030–1038.

Food and Nutrition Board. 1998. Dietary reference intakes for thiamin, riboflavin, niacin, vitamin B_6, folate, vitamin B_{12}, pantothenic acid, biotin, and choline. Washington, DC: National Academy Press.

Gandini, G., R. Fatzer, M. Mariscoli, A. Spadari, M. Cipone, and A. Jaggy. 2004. Equine degenerative myeloencephalopathy in five Quarter horses: clinical and neuropathological findings. Equine Vet. J. 36:83–85.

Gansen, S., A. Lindner, and A. Wagener. 1995. Influence of a supplementation with natural and synthetic vitamin E on serum α-tocopherol content and V_4 of Thoroughbred horses. Page 68 in Proc. 14th Equine Nutr. Physiol. Soc. Symp., Ontario, CA.

Greiwe-Crandell, K. M., D. S. Kronfeld, L. A. Gay, and D. Sklan. 1995. Seasonal vitamin A depletion in grazing horses is assessed better by the relative dose response test than by serum retinol concentration. J. Nutr. 125:2711–2716.

Greiwe-Crandell, K. M., D. S. Kronfeld, L. S. Gay, D. Sklan, W. Tiegs, and P. A. Harris. 1997. Vitamin A repletion in Thoroughbred mares with retinyl palmitate or beta-carotene. J. Anim. Sci. 75:2684–2690.

Guilbert, H. R., C. E. Howell, and G. H. Hart. 1940. Minimum vitamin A and carotene requirements of mammalian species. J. Nutr. 19:91–103.

Halpner, A. D., G. J. Handelman, J. M. Harris, C. A. Belmont, and J. B. Blumberg. 1998. Protection by vitamin C of loss of vitamin E in cultured rat hepatocytes. Arch. Biochem. Biophys. 359:305–309.

Hargreaves, B. J., D. S. Kronfeld, J. N. Waldron, M. A. Lopes, L. S. Gay, K. E. Saker, W. L. Cooper, D. J. Sklan, and P. A. Harris. 2002. Antioxidant status of horses during two 80-km endurance races. J. Nutr. 132:1781S–1783S.

Harrington, D. D. 1982. Acute vitamin-D_2 (ergocalciferol) toxicosis in horses—case-report and experimental studies. J. Am. Vet. Med. Assoc. 180:867–873.

Harrington, D. D., and E. H. Page. 1983. Acute vitamin-D3 toxicosis in horses—Case-reports and experimental studies of the comparative toxicity of vitamin-D_2 and vitamin-D_3. J. Am. Vet. Med. Assoc. 182:1358–1369.

Harris, P. L., and N. D. Embree. 1963. Quantitative consideration of the effect of polyunsaturated fatty acid content of the diet upon the requirements for vitamin E. Am. J. Clin. Nutr. 13:385–392.

Hawkins, D. R. 1968. Treatment of schizophrenia based on the medical model. J. Schiz. 2:3.

Heath, E. M., A. R. Wilcox, and C. M. Quinn. 1993. Effects of nicotinic-acid on respiratory exchange ratio and substrate levels during exercise. Med. Sci. Sports Exer. 25:1018–1023.

Hill, H. E. 1962. Selenium-vitamin E treatment of tying up in horses. Mod. Vet. Pract. 43:66.

Hintz, H. F., H. F. Schryver, J. E. Lowe, J. King, and L. Krook. 1973. Effect of vitamin-D on Ca and P metabolism in ponies. J. Anim. Sci. 37:282 (Abstr.).

Hoffman, R. M., D. S. Kronfeld, J. H. Herbein, W. S. Swecker, W. L. Cooper, and P. A. Harris. 1998. Dietary carbohydrates and fat influence milk composition and fatty acid profile of mare's milk. J. Nutr. 128:2708S–2711S.

Hoffman, R. M., K. L. Morgan, M. P. Lynch, S. A. Zinn, C. Faustman, and P. A. Harris. 1999. Dietary vitamin E supplemented in the periparturient period influences immunoglobulins in equine colostrum and passive transfer in foals. P. 96 in Proc. 16th Equine Nutr. Physiol. Soc. Symp., Raleigh, NC.

Hoffman, R. M., K. L. Morgan, A. Phillips, J. E. Dinger, S. A. Zinn, and C. Faustman. 2001. Dietary vitamin E and ascorbic acid influence nutritional status of exercising polo ponies. P. 129 in Proc. 17th Equine Nutr. Physiol. Soc. Symp., Lexington, KY.

Jacob, R. A. 2001. Niacin. P. 199 in Present Knowledge in Nutrition, B. A. Bowman and R. M. Russel, eds. Washington, DC: ILSI.

Jaeschke, G. 1984. Influence of ascorbic acid on physical development and performance of racehorses. P. 139 in Proc. of Ascorbic Acid in Domestic Animals, I. Wegger, F. J. Tagwerker, and J. Moustgaard, eds. Copenhagen: Danish Agriculture Society.

Jaeschke, G., and H. Keller. 1978a. Ascorbic-acid status of horses. 1. Methods and normal values. Berliner und Munchener Tierarztliche Wochenschrift 91:279–286.

Jaeschke, G., and H. Keller. 1978b. Ascorbic-acid status in horses. 2. Clinical aspects and deficiency symptoms. Berliner und Munchener Tierarztliche Wochenschrift 91:375–379.

Jarrett, S. H., and W. A. Schurg. 1987. Use of a modified relative dose response test for determination of vitamin A status in horses. Nutr. Rep. Int. 35:733–742.

Johnston, C. S. 2001. Vitamin C. P. 175 in Present Knowledge in Nutrition, B. A. Bowman and R. M. Russel, eds. Washington, DC: ILSI Press.

Jones, T. C. 1942. Equine periodic ophthalmia. Am. J. Vet. Res. 3:45–71.

Jones, T. C., F. D. Maurer, and T. O. Roby. 1945. The role of nutrition in equine periodic ophthalmia. Am. J. Vet. Res. 6:67–80.

Jones, T. C., T. O. Roby, and F. D. Maurer. 1946. The relation of riboflavin to equine periodic ophthalmia. Am. J. Vet. Res. 7:403–416.

Jordan, R. M. 1979. Effect of thiamin and vitamin A and D supplementation on growth of weanling ponies. P. 67 in Proc. 6th Equine Nutr. Physiol. Soc. Symp., College Station, TX.

Josseck, H., W. Zenker, and H. Geyer. 1995. Hoof horn abnormalities in Lipizzaner horses and the effect of dietary biotin on macroscopic aspects of hoof horn quality. Equine Vet. J. 27:175–182.

Kempson, S. A. 1987. Scanning electron microscope observations of hoof horn from horses with brittle feet. Vet. Rec. 120:568–570.

Kienzle, E., C. Kaden, P. P. Hoppe, and B. Opitz. 2002. Serum response of ponies to beta-carotene fed by grass meal or a synthetic beadlet preparation with and without added dietary fat. J. Nutr.132:1774S–1775S.

Kronfeld, D. S., T. N. Meacham, and S. Donoghue. 1990. Dietary aspects of developmental orthopedic disease in young horses. P. 451 in Vet. Clinics NA: Equine Pract., H. F. Hintz, ed. Philadelphia: W. B. Saunders.

Lauridsen, C., and S. K. Jensen. 2005. Influence of supplementation of all-rac-α-tocopheryl acetate preweaning and vitamin C postweaning on α-tocopherol and immune responses of piglets. J. Anim. Sci. 83:1274–1286.

Lewis, L. D. 1995. Equine Clinical Nutrition: Feeding and Care. Philadelphia: Williams and Wilkins.

Linerode, P. A. 1966. Studies on the synthesis and absorption of B-complex vitamins in the horse. Am. Assoc. Equine Practitioners 13:283.

Liu, S. K., E. P. Dolensek, C. R. Adams, and J. P. Tappe. 1983. Myelopathy and vitamin E deficiency in six Mongolian wild horses. J. Am. Vet. Med. Assoc. 183:1266–1268.

Lofstedt, J. 1997. White muscle disease of foals. Vet. Clin. North Am Equine Pract. 13:169–185.

Lynch, G. L. 1996a. Vitamin E structure and bioavailability. P. 1 in Vitamin E in Animal Nutrition and Management, M. B. Coelho, ed. Mount Olive, NJ: BASF.

Lynch, G. L. 1996b. Natural occurrence and content of vitamin E in feedstuffs. P. 51 in Vitamin E in Animal Nutrition and Management, M. B. Coelho, ed. Mount Olive, NJ: BASF.

Maenpaa, P. H., R. Lappetelainen, and J. Virkkunen. 1987. Serum retinol, 25-hydroxyvitamin D and alpha-tocopherol of racing trotters in Finland. Equine Vet. J. 19:237–240.

Maenpaa, P. H., T. Koskinen, and E. Koskinen. 1988a. Serum profiles of vitamins A, E and D in mares and foals during different seasons. J. Anim. Sci. 66:1418–1423.

Maenpaa, P. H., A. Pirhonen, and E. Koskinen. 1988b. Vitamin A, E and D nutrition in mares and foals during the winter season: effect of feeding two different vitamin-mineral concentrates. J. Anim. Sci. 66:1424–1429.

Marlin, D. J., K. Fenn, N. Smith, C. D. Deaton, C. A. Roberts, P. A. Harris, C. Dunster, and F. J. Kelly. 2002. Changes in circulatory antioxidant status in horses during prolonged exercise. J. Nutr. 132:1622S–1627S.

Mayhew, I. G., C. M. Brown, H. D. Stowe, A. L. Trapp, F. J. Derksen, and S. F. Clement. 1987. Equine degenerative myeloencephalopathy: a vitamin E deficiency that may be familial. J. Vet. Intern. Med. 1:45–50.

McDonald, G. K. 1980. Moldy sweet clover poisoning in a horse. Can. Vet. J. 21:250–251.

McDowell, L. R. 1989. Vitamins in Animal Nutrition. 1st ed. New York: Academic Press.

McDowell, L. R. 2000. Vitamins in Animal and Human Nutrition. 2nd ed. Ames: Iowa State Press.

McMeniman, N. P., and H. F. Hintz. 1992. Effect of vitamin E status on lipid peroxidation in exercised horses. Equine Vet. J. 24:482–484.

Molitor, H., and H. J. Robinson. 1940. Oral and parenteral toxicity of vitamin K-1, Phthiocol and 2 methyl 1, 4, naphthoquinone. Proc. Soc. Exp. Biol. Med. 43:125–128.

Muggli, R. 1989. Dietary fish oils increase the requirement for vitamin E in humans. P. 201 in Health Effects of Fish and Fish Oils, R. K. Chandra, ed., St. John's, Newfoundland: ARTS Biomedical Publisher and Distributors.

Murray, R., W. P. Bartoli, D. E. Eddy, and M. K. Horn. 1995. Physiological and performance responses to nicotinic-acid ingestion during exercise. Med. Sci. Sports Exer. 27:1057–1062.

Napoli, J. L. 2000. A gene knockout corroborates the integral function of cellular retinol-binding protein in retinoid metabolism. Nutr. Rev. 58:230–236.

Norman, A. W. 2001. Vitamin D. P. 146 in Present Knowledge in Nutrition, B. A. Bowman and R. M. Russell, eds. Washington, DC: ILSI Press.

NRC (National Research Council). 1949. Recommended Nutrient Allowances for Horses. Washington, DC: National Academy Press.

NRC. 1966. Nutrient Requirements of Horses, 2nd ed. Washington, DC: National Academy Press.

NRC. 1973. Nutrient Requirements of Horses, 3rd ed. Washington, DC: National Academy Press.

NRC. 1978. Nutrient Requirements of Horses, 4th ed. Washington, DC: National Academy Press.

NRC. 1982. Nutritional Data for United States and Canadian Feeds. Washington, DC: National Academy Press.

NRC. 1987. Vitamin Tolerance of Animals. Washington, DC: National Academy Press.

NRC. 1989. Nutrient Requirements of Horses, 5th ed. Washington, DC: National Academy Press.

NRC. 1998. Nutrient Requirements of Swine, 10th ed. Washington, DC: National Academy Press.

Ordakowski-Burk, A. L., D. S. Kronfeld, C. A. Williams, L. S. Gay, and D. J. Sklan. 2005. Temporal folate status during lactation in mares and growth in foals. Am. J. Vet. Res. 66:1214–1221.

Ott, E. A., and R. L. Asquith. 1981. Vitamin and mineral supplementation of foaling mares. P. 44 in Proc. 7th Equine Nutr. Physiol. Soc. Symp., Warrenton, VA.

Pagan, J. D., E. Kane, and D. Nash. 2005. Form and source of tocopherol affects vitamin E status in Thoroughbred horses. Pferdeheilkunde 21:101–102.

Parker, A. L., L. M. Lawrence, S. Rokuroda, and L. K. Warren. 1997. The effects of niacin supplementation on niacin status and exercise metabolism in horses. P. 19 in Proc. 15th Equine Nutr. Physiol. Soc. Symp., Ft. Worth, TX.

Pearson, P. B., and H. Schmidt. 1958. Pantothenic acid studies with the horse. J. Anim. Sci. 7:78.

Pearson, P. B., M. K. Sheybani, and H. Schmidt. 1943. The metabolism of ascorbic acid in the horse. J. Anim. Sci. 2:175–180.

Pearson, P. B., M. K. Sheybani, and H. Schmidt. 1944a. Riboflavin in the nutrition of the horse. Arch. Biochem. 3:467–474.

Pearson, P. B., M. K. Sheybani, and H. Schmidt. 1944b. The B-vitamin requirements of the horse. J. Anim. Sci. 3:166–174.

Petersson, K. H., H. F. Hintz, H. F. Schryver, and J. G. F. Combs. 1991. The effect of vitamin E on membrane integrity during submaximal exercise. P. 315 in Equine Exercise Physiology 3, G. B. Persson, A. Lindholm, and L. B. Jeffcott, eds. Davis, CA: ICEEP Publications.

Piercy, R. J., K. W. Hinchcliff, and S. M. Reed. 2002. Folate deficiency during treatment with orally administered folic acid, sulphadiazine and pyrimethamine in a horse with suspected equine protozoal myeloencephalitis (EPM). Equine Vet. J. 34:311–316.

Pryor, W. A. 2001. Vitamin E. P. 156 in Present Knowledge in Nutrition, B. A. Bowman and R. M. Russell, eds. Washington, DC: ILSI Press.

Ralston, S. L., C. F. Nockels, and E. L. Squires. 1988. Differences in diagnostic-test results and hematologic data between aged and young horses. Am. J. Vet. Res. 49:1387–1392.

Rebhun, W. C., B. C. Tennant, S. G. Dill, and J. M. King. 1984. Vitamin K3-induced renal toxicosis in the horse. J. Am. Vet. Med. Assoc. 184:1237–1239.

Reilly, J. D., D. F. Cottrell, R. J. Martin, and D. J. Cuddeford. 1998. Effect of supplementary dietary biotin on hoof growth and hoof growth rate in ponies: a controlled trial. Equine Vet. J. Suppl. 26:51–57.

Rich, G. A., D. E. McGlothlin, L. D. Lewis, E. L. Squires, and B. W. Pickett. 1983. Effect of vitamin E supplementation on stallion seminal characteristics and sexual behavior. P. 85 in Proc. 8th Equine Nutr. Physiol. Soc. Symp., Lexington, KY.

Riis, R. C., C. Jackson, W. Rebhun, M. L. Katz, E. Low, B. Summers, J. Cummings, A. de Lahunta, T. Divers, and H. Mohammed. 1999. Ocular manifestations of equine motor neuron disease. Equine Vet. J. 31:99–110.

Rivlin, R. S. 2001. Riboflavin. P. 191 in Present Knowledge in Nutrition, B. A. Bowmen and R. A. Russel, eds. Washington, DC: ILSI Press.

Roberts, H. E., E. T. Evans, and W. C. Evans. 1949. The production of bracken staggers in the horse and its treatment by B1 therapy. Vet. Rec. 61:549.

Roberts, M. C. 1983. Serum and red cell folate and serum vitamin B_{12} levels in horses. Austral Vet. J. 60:106–111.

Roberts, S. J. 1958. Sequelae of leptospirosis in horses on a small farm. J. Am. Vet. Med. Assoc. 133:189–194.

Robie, T. R. 1967. Cyproheptadine: an excellent antidote for niacin-induced hyperthermia. J. Schiz. 1:133.

Roneus, B., and J. Hakkarainen. 1985. Vitamin-E in serum and skeletal-muscle tissue and blood glutathione-peroxidase activity from horses with the azoturia-tying-up syndrome. Acta Vet. Scand. 26:425–427.

Roneus, B. O., R. V. Hakkarainen, C. A. Lindholm, and J. T. Tyopponen. 1986. Vitamin E requirements of adult Standardbred horses evaluated by tissue depletion and repletion. Equine Vet. J. 18:50–58.

Saastamoinen, M. T., and J. Juusela. 1993. Serum Vitamin-E concentration of horses on different vitamin-E supplementation levels. Acta Agric. Scand. Section A-Anim. Sci. 43:52–57.

Salminen, K. 1975. Cobalt metabolism in horse. Serum level and biosynthesis of vitamin B_{12}. Acta Vet. Scand. 16:84–94.

Schougaard, H., M. G. Simesen, A. Basse, and G. Gissel-Nielsen. 1972. Nutritional muscular–dystrophy (NMD) in foals. Nordisk. Veterinaer. Medicin. 24:67–84.

Schumacher, M. F., M. A. Williams, and R. L. Lyman. 1965. Effect of high intakes of thiamine, riboflavin, and pyridoxine on reproduction in rats and vitamin requirements of the offspring. J. Nutr. 86:343–349.

Schweigert, B. S., P. B. Pearson, and M. C. Wilkening. 1947. The metabolic conversion of tryptophan to nictinic acid and to N-methylnicotinamide. Arch. Biochem. 12:139.

Schweigert, F. J., and C. Gottwald. 1999. Effect of parturition on levels of vitamins A and E and of beta-carotene in plasma and milk of mares. Equine Vet. J. 31:319–323.

Seckington, O. R., R. G. Huntsman, and G. C. Jenkins. 1967. The serum folic acid levels of grass-fed and stabled horses. Vet. Rec. 81:158–161.

Siciliano, P. D., and C. H. Wood. 1993. The effect of added dietary soybean oil on vitamin E status of the horse. J. Anim. Sci. 71:3399–3402.

Siciliano, P. D., A. L. Parker, and L. M. Lawrence. 1997. Effect of dietary vitamin E supplementation on the integrity of skeletal muscle in exercised horses. J. Anim. Sci. 75:1553–1560.

Siciliano, P. D., C. E. Kawcak, and C. W. McIlwraith. 2000a. The effect of initiation of exercise training in young horses on vitamin K status. J. Anim. Sci. 78:2353–2358.

Siciliano, P. D., L. K. Warren, and L. M. Lawrence. 2000b. Changes in vitamin K status of growing horses. J. Equine Vet. Sci. 20:726–729.

Sies, H. 1993. Strategies of antioxidant defense. Eur. J. Biochem. 215:213–219.

Snow, D. H., and M. Frigg. 1987. Oral administration of different formulations of ascorbic acid to the horse. P. 617 in Proc. 10th Equine Nutr. Physiol. Soc. Symp., Fort Collins, CO.

Snow, D. H., and M. Frigg. 1990. Bioavailability of ascorbic-acid in horses. J. Vet. Pharmacol. Ther. 13:393–403.

Snow, D. H., S. P. Gash, and J. Cornelius. 1987. Oral-administration of ascorbic-acid to horses. Equine Vet. J. 19:520–523.

Solomons, N. W. 2001. Vitamin A and carotenoids. P. 127 in Present Knowledge in Nutrition, B. A. Bowman and R. M. Russell, eds. Washington, DC: ILSI Press.

Stephensen, C. B. 2001. Vitamin A, infection, and immune function. Annu. Rev. Nutr. 21:167–192.

Stillions, M. C., S. M. Teeter, and W. E. Nelson. 1971a. Ascorbic acid requirement of mature horses. J. Anim. Sci. 32:249–251.

Stillions, M. C., S. M. Teeter, and W. E. Nelson. 1971b. Utilization of dietary vitamin B12 and cobalt by mature horses. J. Anim. Sci. 32:252–255.

Stowe, H. D. 1967. Reproductive performance of barren mares following vitamin A and E supplementation. P. 81 in Proc. 13th Am. Assoc. Equine Pract., New Orleans, LA.

Stowe, H. D. 1968a. Alpha-tocopherol requirements for equine erythrocyte stability. Am. J. Clin. Nutr. 21:135–142.

Stowe, H. D. 1968b. Experimental equine avitaminosis A and E. P. 27 in Proc. 1st Equine Nutr. Res. Soc. Lexington: University of Kentucky.

Stowe, H. D. 1982. Vitamin A profiles of equine serum and milk. J. Anim. Sci. 54:76–81.

Suttie, J. W. 1995. The importance of menaquinones in human nutrition. Annu. Rev. Nutr. 15:399–417.

Topliff, D. R., G. D. Potter, J. L. Kreider, and C. R. Creagor. 1981. Thiamin supplementation of exercising horses. P. 167 in Proc. 7th Equine Nutr. Physiol. Soc. Symp., Warrenton, VA.

Toribio, R. E., F. T. Bain, D. R. Mrad, N. T. Messer, R. S. Sellers, and K. W. Hinchcliff. 1998. Congenital defects in newborn foals of mares treated for equine protozoal myeloencephalitis during pregnancy. J. Am. Vet. Med. Assoc. 212:697–701.

Ullrey, D. E. 1972. Biological activity of fat-soluble vitamins: vitamin A and carotene. J. Anim. Sci. 35:648–657.

Vermeer, C., B. L. Gijsbers, A. M. Craciun, M. M. Groenen-vanDooren, and M. H. Knapen. 1996. Effects of vitamin K on bone mass and bone metabolism. J. Nutr. 126:S1187–S1191.

Vermeer, C., M. J. Shearer, A. Zittermann, C. Bolton-Smith, P. Szulc, S. Hodges, P. Walter, W. Rambeck, E. Stocklin, and P. Weber. 2004. Beyond deficiency: potential benefits of increased intakes of vitamin K for bone and vascular health. Eur. J. Nutr. 43:325–335.

Wald, G. 1968. Molecular basis of visual excitation. Science 162:230–239.

Watson, E. D., D. Cuddeford, and I. Burger. 1996. Failure of beta-carotene absorption negates any potential effect on ovarian function in mares. Equine Vet. J. 28:233–236.

Williams, C. A., D. S. Kronfeld, T. M. Hess, K. E. Saker, J. N. Waldron, K. M. Crandell, R. M. Hoffman, and P. A. Harris. 2004a. Antioxidant supplementation and subsequent oxidative stress of horses during an 80-km endurance race. J. Anim. Sci. 82:588–594.

Williams, C. A., D. S. Kronfeld, T. M. Hess, K. E. Saker, and P. A. Harris. 2004b. Lipoic acid and vitamin E supplementation to horses diminishes endurance exercise induced oxidative stress, muscle enzyme leakage and apoptosis. Pp. 105–119 in The Elite Race and Endurance Horse, Arno Lindner, ed. Oslo, Norway: CESMAS.

Wilson, T. M., H. A. Morrison, N. C. Palmer, G. G. Finley, and A. A. Vandreumel. 1976. Myodegeneration and suspected selenium-vitamin-E deficiency in horses. J. Am. Vet. Med. Assoc. 169:213–217.

Winter, S. L., and J. L. Boyer. 1973. Hepatic toxicity from large doses of Vitamin-B_3 (Nicotinamide). New Eng. J. Med. 289:1180–1182.

Zempleni, J. 2001. Biotin. Pg. 241 in Present Knowledge in Nutrition., B. A. Bowman and R. M. Russel, eds. Washington, DC: ILSI Press.

Zempleni, J., and D. M. Mock. 2001. Biotin homeostasis during the cell cycle. Nutr. Res. Rev. 14:45–63.

Zenker, W., H. Josseck, and H. Geyer. 1995. Histological and physical assessment of poor hoof horn quality in Lipizzaner horses and a trial with biotin and a placebo. Equine Vet. J. 27:183–191.

7

Water and Water Quality

INTRODUCTION

Water is essential for body fluid balance, digestive function, and gastrointestinal health. Water, as a universal solvent, can contribute beneficial and/or detrimental nutrients to the diet of the horse. Horses tolerate water restriction for extended periods, particularly in the absence of feed (Tasker, 1967a). However, a total lack of water is more rapidly fatal to horses than a lack of feed. Therefore, health and diet assessments of individual or groups of horses should include evaluation of water criteria, including the quality and volume of imbibed water.

BODY FLUID COMPARTMENTS

Water must be consumed to maintain fluid balance. Total body water (TBW) is partitioned into several main compartments: extracellular fluid (ECF), which includes plasma, interstitial fluid, transcellular fluid, and lymph, and intracellular fluid (ICF). Total body water in adult horses has been estimated at 62–68 percent: ECF at 21–25 percent, plasma volume (PV) at 4 percent, and ICF at 36–46 percent of body mass or body weight (BW) (Andrews et al., 1997; Forro et al. 2000; Fielding et al., 2004). Total body water decreases linearly as horses age (Agabriel et al., 1984). Empty body water in foals aged 1, 4, and 8 weeks decreased from 70.6, to 69.1, to 66.2 percent, respectively, concomitant to increases in body fat content (Doreau et al., 1986). Because of the higher TBW content, disruption of the fluid supply to foals creates a more urgent health threat than in adults.

WATER LOSSES

Water balance in the horse is achieved by equalizing body water loss with water intake. Water intake occurs directly by drinking liquid water and eating moist feed, and indirectly through metabolism of carbohydrates, protein, and fats. All horses lose fluid by four routes—fecal, urinary, respiratory, and cutaneous losses. Lactating mares also lose fluid through milk secretion. Specific physiologic and husbandry conditions of the horse, such as lactation and cold weather, elicit different water needs.

Fecal Losses

The intestinal tract is the main water reserve for the horse; consequently, the main route of water loss by the horse at maintenance occurs through fluid excreted in feces. Daily fecal water losses by idle, mature horses fed alfalfa hay and pregnant mares fed hay-grain diets ranged from 3–3.8 L fluid/100 kg BW (Tasker, 1967a; Freeman et al., 1999). Horses fed highly digestible grain-based feeds had drier feces (66 percent moisture) than those fed hay (72–85 percent) (Cymbaluk, 1989, 1990a; Zeyner et al., 2004). Moist feces (72–85 percent moisture) are common in horses fed all-forage diets, and excretion of fecal water by horses fed hay diets represents 55–63 percent of their daily water intake (Cymbaluk, 1989; Freeman et al., 1999; Warren et al., 1999). Fecal water content and output was positively correlated to DM and intake (Cymbaluk, 1989, 1990a). Fecal moisture was not only affected by the amount of dietary fiber, but also by the type of fiber. Feces of horses fed diets high in soluble fiber were 5–11 percent wetter than those fed low-soluble fiber diets (Warren et al., 1999). After 72 hours of water deprivation, absolute fecal moisture values decreased 7 percent but renormalized within 24 hours of rehydration (Sneddon et al., 1993a). Normal horses deprived of water and feed for 8 days decreased fecal output and fecal water excretion to 3 percent of normal output (0.4 L/100 kg BW: Tasker 1967b). Surprisingly, diarrhea occurred after several days of water and feed deprivation.

Clinical abnormalities that impair water reabsorption from the gastrointestinal tract increase water loss through feces (Tasker, 1967c). Horses with induced diarrhea had fecal moisture exceeding 90 percent and lost twice the volume of water in feces (5.15 mL/kg BW·hr^{-1} or 12.2 L/100 kg BW·d⁻¹) than did control horses (Ecke et al., 1998). Plainly, fluid loss by diarrheic horses can greatly exceed maintenance water intake. Failure to replenish these fluids will result in dehydration.

Urine Losses

The kidney regulates body fluid homeostasis in horses. When fluid intake greatly exceeds needs, high volumes of dilute urine are produced. Conversely, when water intakes just meet or are below needs, small volumes of concentrated urine are excreted. With the exception of renal failure, the kidney continues to produce small amounts of urine even under conditions of total water deprivation. This is the baseline or obligatory urine loss, which in horses was determined to be about 0.5 L/100 kg BW (Tasker, 1967c).

Urine volume is typically higher and more variable than obligatory losses as a result of differences in dietary composition, water or fluid availability, and metabolic variations in response to changes in ambient temperature, exercise load, or gastrointestinal health. Healthy pregnant mares fed mature grass hay-grain diets with continuous access to water produced 0.6–0.68 L urine/100 kg BW (Freeman et al., 1999). By comparison, alfalfa-fed nonpregnant horses produced 2.9 L urine /100 kg BW (Rumbaugh et al., 1982). In the latter study, when these horses were deprived of feed and water for 3 days, their urine output decreased to 1.24 L/100 kg BW after 24 hours, 0.65 L/100 kg BW by 48 hours, and plateaued at 0.63 L/100 kg BW after 72 hours of water deprivation. Exercise has an unpredictable impact on urine volume. Urine volumes increased in horses performing submaximal exercise (Hinchcliff et al., 1990), but notably decreased in horses that were maximally exercised (Schott et al., 1995).

Urine excretion is dynamic and volume changes can be dramatic and immediate in response to variations in nutrient intake. Donkeys fed wheat straw, then given alfalfa hay, which increased their nitrogen intake by 8-fold, had a quadruple increase in urine flow rates (Izraely et al., 1989). Low dietary cation-anion difference (DCAD) (85 mEq/kg DM) increased urine volume 72–110 percent above moderate (190 mEq/kg DM) and high DCAD (380 mEq/kg DM) (McKenzie et al., 2003). High potassium diets (5.4 mmol potassium/kg BW) increased urine volume in horses by 26–30 percent compared to diets that supplied 4.1 mmol potassium/kg BW (Jansson et al., 1999). A potassium-chloride paste given to dehydrated horses increased their water intake but also increased urine flow and glomerular filtration rate (Schott et al., 2002). Thus, any changes to renal solute load, particularly by feeding excess protein, sodium, or potassium, can increase urine volume and increase water intake.

Total Evaporative Fluid Losses

Heat loss in horses, as in other species, is facilitated through vaporization of water. Evaporative heat losses and, therefore, fluid losses occur passively through the skin (diffusion) and lungs. Sweating is an active process, involving secretion of fluid by sweat glands, and is initiated by increases in body core temperature. Cutaneous fluid losses in horses increased exponentially above ambient temperatures of 20°C (Morgan et al., 1997). In horses participating in long-duration, low-intensity exercise, an estimated 23 percent of evaporative metabolic heat loss occurs through the respiratory tract, whereas 70 percent or more occurs through sweating (Kingston et al., 1997).

Daily evaporative losses for horses kept in a thermoneutral environment were estimated at 10 ± 2.7 L/d with a range of 1.7–3.3 L/100 kg BW (Groenendyk et al., 1988). The hourly evaporative loss by horses housed at temperatures between −3°C and 20°C was relatively constant at 48 W/m² (71 mL fluid/m²) but exceeded 250 W/m² (370 mL fluid/m²) at 37°C (Morgan et al., 1997). Based on the equation (q_{evap} = 48 + 1.02 × 10⁻⁴ t^4_{air}) derived for evaporative heat loss by the authors, a 500-kg heat-unadapted horse had an hourly evaporative heat loss of 0.48 L at 20°C and 1.5 L at temperatures 35°C or higher. Daily evaporative losses could total 11.5 L at temperatures of 20°C or lower, but could exceed 36 L if temperatures of 35°C were sustained. Extended exposure to temperatures of 35°C or more is uncommon in temperate climates, and even if protracted, adaptation is likely within 2–3 weeks with concomitant reduction in evaporative losses (Geor et al., 1996, 2000).

Sweat Losses

Passive cutaneous evaporative loss for idle horses at thermoneutrality (between 5–20°C) is predicted at 6 L/d or less. Elevated body core temperatures as a result of muscular activity or high ambient temperatures and solar radiation initiate sweating. Total evaporative fluid losses of worked or exercised horses depend on duration and intensity of exercise, environmental conditions, and acclimation of the horse to its climatic environment. Sweating increased dramatically during the first 20–30 minutes of exercise, then plateaued thereafter (Kingston et al., 1997). Sweat losses may account for 70–92 percent of total evaporative loss by horses during exercise (Hodgson et al., 1993; Kingston et al., 1997). Total body water losses of 20.4 L were reported for horses following a cross-country event (Ecker and Lindinger, 1995) and body mass losses of 33.8 kg, considered to be largely fluid losses, were recorded in horses performing long-duration, low-intensity activity (Kingston et al., 1997). High ambient temperatures alone caused evaporative fluid losses to quadruple (Morgan et al., 1997), where-as increasing ambient temperature from mild (20°C) to hot (35°C) elevated evaporative fluid losses of Standardbred horses by 45 percent (Jansson, 1999).

Training or conditioning and temperature acclimation increase temperature tolerance and thereby impact water intake. Training alone altered the sweating rate of horses, but imposing conditions of high humidity and high ambient temperatures further intensified sweating and respiratory fluid losses (McCutcheon and Geor, 1999, 2000). In cool, dry temperatures (20°C, 50 percent relative humidity [RH]), Thoroughbreds performing mild exercise lost 1.5 L sweat/100 kg BW, which was 82 percent and 73 percent lower than unacclimated horses doing the same exercise in hot, dry conditions (34°C, 55 percent RH) or hot, humid conditions (36°C, 86 percent RH), respectively (McCutcheon and Geor, 2000; Geor et al., 2000). Horses partially acclimate within 2 weeks of intermittent daily or prolonged exposure to temperature extremes, but full acclimation required 3 weeks (Geor et al., 2000). Following 3 weeks of acclimation to hot, humid conditions, sweating rates of Thoroughbred horses were 18 percent lower than during initial exposure. Acclimation to the environment, however, does not mean the horse is resistant to dehydration. Hypohydrated horses, which had lost in excess of 8.5 percent of total body water, continued to sweat with continued exercise (Kingston et al., 1997). This underscores the need for vigilant monitoring of hydration status of working horses.

Dehydration occurs when fluid losses exceed fluid absorbed. Clinically, signs of dehydration are detected by assessing skin turgor, capillary refill, and heart rate; Collastos (1999) described severe dehydration at fluid deficits of 8–10 percent.

Respiratory Losses

Respiratory heat losses and, consequently, fluid loss through vaporization accounted for 19–30 percent of the total heat produced by horses performing mild to intense exercise, with absolute fluid losses via the lung of 0.8–2.1 L (Hodgson et al., 1993; Kingston et al., 1997). These values would be likely to increase in warm or tropical environments. Acclimation to high heat was accomplished through increased sweating and elevated respiratory rates (Geor et al., 2000). Fluid losses through the respiratory tract are difficult to quantitate. Respiratory heat loss and, therefore, respiratory fluid loss vary with duration and intensity of the exercise, ambient temperature, and other environmental conditions imposed during exercise.

Lactational Losses

During the first 2 months of lactation, primiparous and multiparous Quarter horse mares produced about 1.8 and 2 L milk/100 kg BW daily, respectively, which declined thereafter (Pool-Anderson et al., 1994). Earlier studies with Quarter horse mares had reported daily milk volumes up to 2.1 L/100 kg BW over 150 days (Gibbs et al., 1982). Notably higher daily milk volumes were reported for primiparous and multiparous heavy and light mares, which produced 2.4 and 2.8 L milk/100 kg BW, respectively (Doreau et al., 1991) and for Australian stock horses, which were reported to produce 3.7–3.8 L milk/100 kg BW daily (Martin et al., 1992). Evidently, milking ability can differ among breeds of mares and with mare parity. Based on these data, lactating mares kept in thermoneutral environments can be predicted to increase water intake by at least 37–74 percent above maintenance needs solely to meet lactational demands. These water increases are only for milk production. Coupled with milk production, lactating mares also have an increased feed intake which further elevates water demand during lactation (see Pregnancy and Lactation Requirements).

WATER INTAKE

Horses obtain water by drinking liquid water, from water in feed, and from water generated by metabolic breakdown of dietary carbohydrates, protein, and fat. On pasture, grass can contribute a substantial amount of water, but in a typical hay-grain feeding program, the feed and metabolic water contribute little to the daily water requirements of horses. Metabolic water production by Thoroughbred horses fed hay was estimated at 0.2–0.25 L/hr (van den Berg et al., 1998). Daily metabolic water production by Standardbred horses fed alfalfa hay in thermoneutral conditions was estimated at 2.9 ± 0.4 L/d or about 0.68 L/100 kg BW (Groenendyk et al., 1988).

All feeds contain water, but the water content depends on the feed source. Dry feeds such as hay and grain may contain 10–15 percent moisture, so in a typical diet these feeds contribute only 1–2 L fluid/d (Freeman et al., 1999). Fresh forage (pasture), however, can be very high in moisture content and can contribute a large portion of the daily water needs of the horse. A vegetative perennial ryegrass pasture containing 79.6 percent moisture was reportedly consumed in amounts of 61–75 kg by pregnant mares and 39.5 kg by nonpregnant mares (Marlow et al., 1983). Although based on a small sample of horses, these data indicate that fresh pasture contributed between 31–60 kg fluid, an amount that approaches the mares' water requirements (Table 7-1).

Dietary Effects

Diet influences water intake by horses depending on the amount eaten and by the composition of the consumed feed. Total DM intake and composition directly affect the amount of water consumed by mature ponies and weaned foals (Cymbaluk, 1989, 1990b). Horses fed forage diets ate 19 percent more DM to provide a similar caloric intake to those fed a mixed diet and, consequently, drank 26 percent more water (Pagan et al., 1998). Likewise, horses fed 5.8 kg of a hay-only diet drank 17.8 kg water compared to 10.1 kg water consumed by horses fed 1.8 kg grain plus 1.3 kg hay (Danielsen et al., 1995), perhaps because of a lower DM intake as well as a different dietary composition. During transportation, horses greatly reduced their feed intake

TABLE 7-1 Estimated Water Needs of Horses[a]

Class	Ambient Temperature (°C)	Exercise Duration (hr)	Diet (kg /100 kg BW) Amount	Diet Type	Water Intake (L/100 kg BW)	Body Weight (kg)	Average Total Water Intake (L/d)	Estimated Range of Water Intakes[b] (L/d)
Idle, mature	20	—	1.5		5	500	25	21–29
	30	—	1.5	Hay only	9.6		48	42–54
	20	—	2.0		6.7		33.5	30–38
Idle, mature	20	—	2.0	Hay-grain	6.2	500	31	27–35
	−20	—	2.5	Hay only	8.4		42	37–47
Pregnancy	20	—	2.0	Hay-grain	6.2	500	31	27–35
Lactating	20	—	3.0	Hay only	11.9–13.9	500	65	52–78
	20	—	2.5	Hay-grain	9.2–11.2		51	40–63
Moderate exercise	20	1 hr	2.2	Hay-grain	8.2	500	41	36–46
	35 (daily average)	1 hr	2.2		16.4		82	72–92
Yearling	−10	—	2.0	Hay-grain	6.0	300	18	16–20
	20	—	2.0		6.3		19	17–21

[a]Based on a horse with a mature weight of 500 kg.
[b]Values are averages and specific water intakes by individual horses may be lower or higher depending on the individual horse's baseline, its clinical health, and variations in environmental conditions.
Calculations are based as follows:
1. Maintenance water intake by idle, adult horses is 5 L/100 kg BW when diet is fed at 1.5 kg/100 kg BW.
2. Temperature effects above 20°C (5–20 used as thermoneutral) used the equation of Morgan et al. (1997) to calculate hourly evaporative heat loss (q_{evap} = 48 + 1.02 × 10^{-4} t^4_{air}) where t_{air} is the ambient temperature measured in °C and q_{evap} is measured in W/m^2, which is converted to mL water based on the conversion factor of 2,428 J evaporate 1 g (mL) of water. Temperature effects on feed-water intake relationships of yearling horses were based on the equation derived by Cymbaluk (1990b) in which Y = 2.25 + 0.016T (Y = L water/kg DM intake; T = ambient temperature measured in °C). Hence, temperature effects are incorporated into the dietary component for yearlings.
3. Fluid losses in milk were based on published data indicating that milk production ranges from 1.8–3.8 L/100 kg BW.
4. Sweat and respiratory heat losses during exercise were based on Geor et al. (2000) in which horses lost 1.5 L/100 kg BW fluid at thermoneutral temperatures and 2.5 L/100 kg BW fluid at temperatures above 30°C.
5. Dietary effects assumed that for each 1 kg/100 kg BW of an all-hay diet eaten above 1.5 kg/100 kg BW, water intake would increase 3.4 L/100 kg BW and would increase 2.4 L/100 kg BW for hay-grain diets.

with attendant reductions in water intake (Smith et al., 1996).

Although diet affects water intake, the converse is also true; limiting water intake reduces feed intake. Gradual water restriction reduced feeding activity by 4–29 percent (Houpt et al., 2000). After 72 hours of total water deprivation, horses continued to eat concentrate at a near constant rate, but hay intake dropped by 45 percent (Sneddon et al., 1993a). Feed consumption, however, did not decrease until after 48 hours of water deprivation. Ponies and donkeys deprived of water for 36 hours reduced their feed intake by 32 percent and 13 percent, respectively (Mueller and Houpt, 1991). Donkeys were tolerant of water deprivation through water conservation strategies that incurred only modest reductions in feed intake.

Dietary composition—notably fiber, protein, and specific minerals such as sodium and potassium—can alter water intake by the horse, generally through increased urinary excretion. Water:feed ratios for mature ponies fed grass or alfalfa hay or high-grain complete pellets were 3.2, 3.3, and 2, respectively (Cymbaluk, 1989). Similarly, water:feed ratios of 3.4, 3.3, and 2.6 were reported for horses fed alfalfa-beet pulp, 77 percent hay-oats, and other forage-grain diets, respectively (Warren et al., 1999). The higher water intakes when the predominantly forage diets were fed were attributed to higher intakes of total fiber (Warren et al., 1999).

Water intake has a positive, linear correlation to salt intake (y = 36.5 + 0.22x where y = daily water intake in mL/kg BW and x = daily sodium intake in mg/kg BW: Jansson and Dahlborn, 1999). Yet, salt added to the diet at 1, 3, and 5 percent did not affect water intake or urine volume of horses (Schryver et al., 1987). Diets containing 5.4 mmol potassium k/kg BW/d increased water intake 6.8 percent compared to diets containing 4.1 mmol K/kg BW to offset the elevated urine output associated with elimination of excess potassium (Jansson et al., 1999).

Temperature Effects

Ambient temperatures that fluctuate radically from thermoneutrality influence water intake. Cold weather reduced water intake by 6–14 percent (Cymbaluk, 1990b). At −8°C and −17°C, weaned foals drank 2.3 and 2.1 L water/100 kg BW compared to cohorts housed at temperatures above 8°C, which drank 2.4 L water/100 kg BW. Free water intake was directly related to ambient temperatures in the range of −20 to 20°C by the equation Y = 2.25 + 0.016T where Y = L water/kg DM intake and T = ambient temperature in °C

(Cymbaluk, 1990b). Compared to water intakes (5.15 L/100 kg BW) during exercise in a thermoneutral environment (20° C and 45–50 percent RH), daily water intake increased 79 percent when horses were exercised at high temperatures (33–35°C) coupled with high humidity (80–85 percent) for 4 hours (Geor et al., 1996).

Water temperature influences water intake depending on environmental temperature. Cold weather alone reduces water intake, but horses also drink less cold water than warm water during cold weather. At 0–5°C, pastured, lactating mares drank infrequently, but as temperatures increased so did drinking frequency. During hot weather (30–35°C), mares drank every 1.8 hours (Crowell-Davis et al., 1985). Pony stallions kept outdoors or indoors at cool ambient temperatures drank 38–41 percent less near-frozen water than water heated to an average temperature of 19°C (Kristula and McDonnell, 1994). Yet, pony stallions kept indoors at warm ambient temperatures (15–29°C) drank similar amounts of warm (average 23°C) or icy (0–1°C) water (McDonnell and Kristula, 1996). Horses given a saline solution immediately after exercise on a treadmill in a room kept at 25°C at a relative humidity of 60 percent preferred a lukewarm solution (20°C) to a cool solution (10°C) or warm solution (30°C) (Butudom et al., 2004).

MAINTENANCE REQUIREMENTS

In typical horse management settings, horses consume most of their daily water needs by drinking liquid water. Body weight is the main determinant of the total volume of water imbibed. Maintenance water intake of adult horses fed a dry diet approaches values of about 5 L/100 kg BW. Free water intake by normal, nonworking horses fed alfalfa-timothy or alfalfa hay ad libitum was 5.1–5.6 L/100 kg BW (Tasker, 1967a; Groenendyk et al., 1988). Likewise, water intakes of 4.4–4.8 L/100 kg BW were reported for stabled, grass-fed Namib and Boerperd horses (Sneddon et al., 1993b). Stabled, mature ponies fed grass or alfalfa hay at maintenance rates drank 5–5.5 L water/100 kg BW/d (Cymbaluk, 1989). Average maintenance water intakes are about 5 L/100 kg BW/d, but individual horses of similar weight fed similar diets can have very different water intakes. Not only are differences evident among horses, but also the same individual has very different day-to-day water intakes (Groenendyk et al., 1988). Absolute water intake by pregnant mares fed identical diets varied by 16–20 percent and weight-scaled water intake varied by 11–13 percent from the average (Freeman et al., 1999). Similarly, individual Standardbred horses had absolute water intakes that deviated 21–25 percent from the average (Nyman et al., 2002), whereas Thoroughbred mares had weight-scaled water intakes that varied 64 percent (Smith et al., 1996). Daily variation in water intake by the same horse has been attributed to variation in voluntary DM intake or variation in intake of other dietary components such as salt (Jansson and Dahlborn, 1999). Although breed differences in water intake have not been identified in horses, donkeys appear to drink less water then ponies. Donkeys housed and fed similarly to ponies drank 30 percent less water (5 L/100 kg BW) than the ponies (6.5 L/100 kg BW) but also consumed 16 percent less feed (Mueller and Houpt, 1991). Based on these data, the estimated maintenance requirement for water by a 500-kg horse kept at thermoneutral temperatures fed hay at 1.5 kg/100 kg BW ranges from 21–29 L/day.

Suckling Foal Requirements

Nursing and orphan foals drink water in addition to the fluid obtained from the dam's milk or liquid milk replacer. Thus, accessible water should be available to dam and foal at all times. Pastured, suckling foals drank 3.9 kg of water at 1 month of age in addition to suckling 17.4 kg milk and continued to increase water intake up to 5.5 kg/d during the next month of growth with no concurrent decreases in milk intake (Martin et al., 1992). Orphan foals drank a total of 14.8–15.9 L fluid (water and liquid milk replacer)/100 kg BW beginning at 1 week of age, which progressively declined to 10.2–10.8 L/100 kg BW by 7 weeks of age as reliance on formula decreased and creep feed intake increased (Cymbaluk et al., 1993).

Pregnancy and Lactation Requirements

Pregnancy does not appear to impose increases in water intakes above maintenance except in response to diet type or imposition of exercise. Pregnant, idle mares kept indoors at thermoneutral temperatures fed a grass hay-grain diet at 2.2 percent of body weight drank 4.5–5.9 L water/100 kg BW, irrespective of whether water was provided intermittently or ad libitum (Freeman et al., 1999). Both absolute and weight-scaled water intakes declined slightly during pregnancy. Higher water intakes (6.9 L/100 kg BW) were reported for pregnant Thoroughbred mares fed hay-only diets (Houpt et al., 2000). Total daily water intakes by pregnant mares weighing 500 kg depend in part on diet but are expected to be in the range of 27–38 L.

Few water intake data are available for lactating mares, but water intakes may increase significantly above maintenance and pregnancy because mares lose additional fluid through lactation and eat considerably more feed to sustain milk production (Doreau et al., 1992). Dry matter intake by draft mares after 2 weeks lactation exceeded 3 kg DM/100 kg BW whether the mares were fed a high-forage or high-concentrate diet (Doreau et al., 1992). Adult horses typically ate 2 kg DM/100 kg BW (Dulphy et al., 1997) and pregnant mares ate 1.7–1.8 kg DM/100 kg BW (Doreau et al., 1991). Consequently, water intake by lactating mares would be expected to increase by 50–75 percent to compensate for a higher feed intake. Coupled with an increase of 37–74 percent in water intake to offset milk secretion, lactating mares would be expected to drink 1.8–2.5-fold more water than consumed at maintenance in thermoneutral conditions. Total water intakes will vary with diet and ambient temperature but volumes of 40–78 L/d are predicted for a 500-kg lactating mare, or approximately 2- to 3-fold greater than at maintenance.

Work or Exercise Requirements

Water needs of working or competitive horses are difficult to predict. Water loss and water intake depend on environmental conditions (mainly ambient temperature, humidity, and solar radiation), duration and intensity of the work, and fitness and acclimation of the horse to specific environmental conditions. Light activity causes only marginal increases in water intake. Lightly trained horses drank 24 L water by bucket or 17 L from an automatic water bowl (Nyman et al., 2002), which are within a maintenance range. However, in actual performance, fluid losses can be extensive depending on exercise duration and intensity and environmental conditions. Body weight losses of Arabian horses after an 80- or 160-km endurance ride averaged 15 ± 2.2 kg, with a maximum loss of 28.2 kg (Schott et al., 1997). Weight losses were considered to be largely fluid and represented losses of 3.6–7.7 percent of BW. To calculate water needs of exercised horses, both weather conditions and exercise load must be considered. In hot weather, unexercised horses sustained hourly sweat losses of 1.5 L/100 kg BW. In hot, humid conditions, horses performing submaximal exercise lost fluid through sweat at rates of 2–2.5 L/100 kg BW·hr^{-1} compared to 1.5 L/100 kg BW·hr^{-1} in cool, dry environments (Geor et al., 2000). Based on these data, water intake by exercised horses can increase 2- to 3-fold over maintenance depending on the duration and conditions of exercise. Total water intakes by a 500-kg horse could range from 36–92 L per day depending on conditions of exercise (Table 7-1).

For most forms of horse activity, liquid water is sufficient to offset fluid losses. Special considerations are needed for horses involved in intense physical work or exercise, especially when exercise is performed in hot, humid, sunny conditions. Water, although certainly the most available fluid source, may not be the preferred fluid of choice during exercise or during recovery of the work-exhausted horse. Compared to giving no fluid during exercise, providing water or electrolyte solution was beneficial in reducing the extent of the fluid loss but neither solution prevented hypohydration (Geor and McCutcheon, 1998). In all cases, the choice of fluid for rehydrating exhausted horses should always be made in conjunction with a clinician.

Transportation of horses creates its own unique water drinking requirements and behaviors. Horses that were offered water during transport showed a diurnal water intake pattern consuming less water during the cool periods of the day. During transportation, both water and feed intake decreased (Smith et al., 1996). Horses transported for longer than 30 hours without water became unfit for further transport, whereas those given water were able to tolerate an additional 2 hours of transportation (Friend, 2000).

DRINKING BEHAVIOR OF HORSES

Water consumption by horses is episodic and circadian. Drinking patterns are modified by water source, water availability, and age of the horse. Each drinking episode is biphasic: a long single draught is followed by sips of shorter duration. Normal drinking behavior for housed, adult horses has the following characteristics: episodes occur 2–8 times per day and last 10–60 seconds per episode with a cumulative daily total drinking duration of 1–8 minutes (McDonnell et al., 1999). The number of drinking bouts reported for horses watered through pressure-valve water bowls, float-valve water bowls, and buckets ranged from 16–21 episodes daily with drinking durations of 10–52 seconds per episode (Nyman and Dahlborn, 2001). In the first 5 minutes after exercise, horses had 6, 10, and 11 drinking episodes when saline was offered at temperatures of 10, 20, and 30°C, respectively (Butudom et al., 2004). During the subsequent hour of recovery, drinking episodes of water decreased (4–4.6) and were unaffected by temperature of the offered water.

The duration of a drinking episode by horses is brief. Suckling foals spent little total time drinking water and drinking bouts were short, only lasting 0.34 ± 0.06 minutes (Crowell-Davis et al., 1985). The daily frequency of drinking episodes by pregnant mares fed dry feed and housed indoors ranged from 18–39 times and each drinking episode lasted from 0.22–0.44 minutes (McDonnell et al., 1999). Drinking bouts by lactating mares on pasture were remarkably similar, lasting 0.39 ± 0.02 minutes (Crowell-Davis et al., 1985). Drinking bouts by bucket-watered pony geldings lasted 12.2–24.2 seconds (Sweeting and Houpt, 1987), similar to mean values of 11–28 seconds observed for group-transported horses (Gibbs and Friend, 2000). Thus, the total time during the day a horse spends drinking is remarkably small. Pregnant heavy and light mares with ad libitum access to water drank for 6.2 min/d compared to 5.7–10.7 min/d when offered water at regular intervals using a float-type water bowl (McDonnell et al., 1999; Flannigan, 2001). Likewise, Standardbred geldings spent a total daily drinking time of 3–15 minutes irrespective of whether the water was supplied in buckets or by water bowls equipped with either a float valve or pressure valve (Nyman and Dahlborn, 2001). Longer daily drinking times (21–27 min/d) were reported for ponies fed and watered ad libitum (Sufit et al., 1985).

The type of water bowl and watering method can influence duration of drinking and volume of water consumed. Bowls holding water 2.5–5 cm deep appeared to increase the drinking duration of horses, because the depth may have restricted the horse's ability to ingest water quickly (McDonnell et al., 1999). In a preference test comparing water bowls to buckets, horses favored drinking from buckets and drank 98 percent of their daily intake from buckets and only 2 percent from a pressure-valve bowl or a float-valve bowl (Nyman and Dahlborn, 2001). As seen with shallow water bowls (McDonnell et al., 1999), horses spent more time drinking from the pressure-valve waterer but consumed less water than when water was supplied by bucket or float waterers (Nyman et al., 2002).

Horses drink when they eat (Sufit et al., 1985; McDonnell et al., 1999; Nyman and Dahlborn, 2001). Drinking was periprandial (less than 2 hours after eating) for 75–89 percent of the drinking episodes observed in ponies fed ad libitum and horses fed four times daily (Sufit et al., 1985; Nyman and Dahlborn, 2001). Prandial drinking was felt to occur as a response to an increased plasma osmolality or total serum protein associated with the consumption of feed (Sufit et al., 1985; Pagan and Harris, 1999). Water intake relative to the time of grain feeding was significantly altered when hay was fed at the same time, 2 hours before or 4 hours after feeding grain (Pagan and Harris, 1999). However, peak water intakes fell within the 2-hour periprandial period of hay feeding. By contrast, daily water intake patterns of Standardbred horses offered similar amounts of hay-oats diets either two or six times per day did not differ (Jansson and Dahlborn, 1999). Total water intake was unaffected by feeding frequency, but water consumed at each feeding period was not uniform through the day. Horses drank more water in the afternoon and evening than in the morning (Jansson and Dahlborn, 1999). Pastured, lactating mares drank 86.4 percent of their daily water intake between 9:00 am and 9:00 pm (Crowell-Davis, 1985).

Stall-housed horses are commonly observed to dip hay or wet hay in the manger (McDonnell et al., 1999). Although hay dipping and unlimited access to water can create hygiene problems in mangers (Freeman et al., 1999), this behavior was felt to be a normal way to moisten dry feed to make it more palatable and easier to masticate (McDonnell et al., 1999).

The behavioral manifestations of water restriction are less dramatic than those of horses totally deprived of water. In water-restricted horses, the only behavioral changes recorded were a reduction in time spent eating and an increase in time spent mouthing the watering buckets (Houpt et al., 2000). Horses deprived of water for 8 days showed remarkably few behavioral changes except a loss of skin turgor and a tucked-up appearance (Tasker, 1967c).

WATER MANAGEMENT

Regardless of how water intake measurements are made, interpretation of adequacy of water intake must integrate information related to BW, age, diet, exercise intensity and duration, lactation needs, ambient temperature, and gastrointestinal health. Adequacy of water intake can be evaluated directly or indirectly. Water source and availability can be readily assessed. Direct measure of water intake is the simplest and most reliable way to measure volume of water drunk by the horse. Water intakes are easily attained for bucket-watered horses. Simple water meters can be grafted into water lines of automatic watering systems. Water intakes are recorded over a period of days, and then daily water intakes can be interpreted as appropriate for the horse's weight, diet, function, and ambient housing temperature.

Water can be provided in various ways. The simplest guideline for watering horses is to provide fresh, clean water at all times, but often this is neither possible nor hygienic. Obvious limitations exist where horses graze on extensive pastures and must walk considerable distances to get to water, or in unheated riding stables where cold temperatures freeze water lines, thereby precluding use of automatic watering systems. Intermittent provision of water in voluntary amounts supplied horses with their maintenance water needs (Freeman et al., 1999), so the use of buckets for watering as appears to be the practice in many horse barns is acceptable as long as sufficient water is provided. Buckets are still commonly used in horse husbandry and are not only preferred by horses (Nyman et al., 1997) but, along with bulk water tanks and automatic waterers, are associated with significantly lower risks of colic (Kaneene et al., 1997).

WATER QUALITY FOR HORSES

Water quality refers to both the suitable and unsuitable characteristics of water that determine whether it is acceptable for a specific purpose or use. Acceptable water standards may vary regionally, nationally, and internationally. The upper limits and acceptable concentrations of substances in water that are currently used in the United States are largely based on the summary of data described by an NRC (1974) document. Individual states may or may not have updated livestock water quality criteria since that publication. Many water quality criteria can be cross-referenced at the extensive database available through the USDA Cooperative State Research, Education, and Extension Service (CSREES) National Water Quality Network (http://www.usawaterquality.org) and the United States Geological Survey (http://waterdata.usgs.gov/nwis/). Maximum acceptable concentrations, interim acceptable concentrations, and aesthetic objectives of chemical components for livestock were recently updated for Australia and New Zealand (ANZECC, 2000) and Canada (CCME, 2002). A vast body of water research has been accumulated since the NRC publication in 1974, yet water quality data for livestock consumption appear to have received less attention than water contamination by livestock. The absence of controlled studies on water quality for horses makes it necessary to adapt water quality standards for horses from safety indexes used for other domestic livestock or for humans.

Horses do not drink pure water. Horses drink ground (deep or shallow aquifers) and surface water (streams, lakes, ponds, dugouts, and sloughs), which acquires all the aspects of the geochemistry, runoff, evaporation, precipitation, farming practices, and human and animal activity in its surroundings. Because of these numerous influences, water characteristics from wells and surface waters are constantly changing. Thus, a single water analysis is not representative of the chemical attributes of the water ingested by the horse throughout the year.

Ground water is a source of free water whose water composition can be altered by dissolution, precipitation, ion exchange, or reduction or oxidation of compounds percolating through soil and rock. A near linear relationship exists between mineralization and the depth of the ground water. Generally, the principal anion in shallow wells is bicarbonate, followed by sulphate in deeper wells, while chlorides dominate in the deepest wells. Calcium is the major cation in water of shallow wells, followed by magnesium then transitioning to sodium in deeper wells. These are generalizations: specific wells may have quite different cation and anion distributions.

Physical Criteria

Physical criteria used to describe water quality are turbidity, total dissolved solids (TDS), odor, color, and temperature. Turbidity assesses water clarity but is a seldom-used criterion. Turbidity in water may increase significantly after extreme rainfall and runoff events (Kistemann et al., 2002). Odor may affect water palatability for horses, but this is not a test frequently conducted on livestock water. Distinctive odors in water are attributed to sulfates, tannins, manure, rotting vegetation, and algal and microbial byproducts (Hargesheimer and Watson, 1996). There are no controlled studies to assess the impact of odoriferous water on intake by horses, but clean water may be important. Transported horses drank notably less water from a trough contaminated with feces (Friend, 2000). Color does not usually affect water quality or horse health but can affect human perception of quality for their horses. Pigments that give color to water can originate from suspended soil particles, tannins arising from organic matter, or iron-fixing bacteria. The latter are not uncommon in inconsistently cleaned water bowls.

Temperature not only affects the palatability of water for horses, but also it can affect growth of bacteria and certain algae. At cool ambient temperature, horses drank 34–41 percent less icy water than warm water (Kristula and McDonnell, 1994), but when ambient temperatures were warm, their intakes did not differ between icy or warm water (McDonnell and Kristula, 1996).

Chemical Criteria

Water quality is most commonly associated with its chemical characteristics. For livestock, water suitability is often based on TDS or total soluble salts (TSS) (Table 7-2). TDS is a measure of the aggregate composition of the ions in the water but does not discern the type of ions present—only the concentration of ions present in the water sample. Depending on type of ion present, water may or may not be palatable. Water has been described in terms of TDS concentrations. A TDS of less than 1,500 mg/L indicates fresh water, 1,500–5,000 mg/L indicates brackish water, 5,000–30,000 mg/L is saline water, 30,000–100,000 mg/L is seawater, and greater than 100,000 mg/L is brine (NRC, 1974). Typically, surface water has a lower TDS than groundwater.

Australian and New Zealand livestock quality guidelines (ANZECC, 2000) suggest that water with a TDS of 0–4,000 mg/L causes no adverse effects in horses, water with 4,000–6,000 mg/L TDS might affect initial intake until adaptation occurs, but waters with greater than 6,000 mg/L may affect health and productivity. These guidelines, however, were not confirmed with studies using horses. Generally, TDS is low (< 350 mg/L) in waters found on both coasts of North America. High TDS (> 2,500 mg/L) are found only in small areas of Texas (NRC, 1974).

Hardness is the total cationic effect of calcium and magnesium in water. Past methods of analysis equated hardness with calcium carbonate equivalents. Water quality in terms of hardness is given in Table 7-3. Calcium, magnesium, and sodium are mainly derived from mineral deposits, and potassium from soil organic matter. A detailed description of the mineral sources associated with specific water cations has been described (NRC, 2005). For example, water calcium is typically associated with carbonate, gypsum, feldspar, pyroxene, and amfibole. Hard water typically contains high concentrations of calcium and magnesium. However, neither water calcium nor magnesium is felt to contribute significant amounts to the dietary balance of these minerals to the horse.

The pH of water shows the hydrogen ion concentration and is an indication of the reactivity of the water with other dissolved compounds in the water and with containers. The most important anions in water that contribute to alkalinity

TABLE 7-2 Guidelines for Total Dissolved Solids (TDS) or Total Soluble Salts (TSS)[a]

< 1,000	Safe and should pose no health problems
1,000–2,999	Generally safe but may cause a mild temporary diarrhea in unaccustomed animals
3,000–4,999	Water may be refused when first offered to animals or may cause temporary diarrhea. Animal performance may be less than optimum because water intake is not optimized
5,000–6,999	Avoid these waters for pregnant or lactating animals.
7,000	This water should not be offered. Health problems or poor production may occur.

[a]SOURCE: NRC (1974).

TABLE 7-3 Water Hardness Guidelines[a]

Descriptor	Hardness (mg/L)
Soft	0–60
Moderately hard	61–120
Hard	121–180
Very hard	>180

[a]SOURCE: NRC (1974).

are carbonate, bicarbonate, and hydroxyl ions. The acidity or alkalinity of the water will also determine the biota that will survive therein. For example, pH values of 5–9 are accepted for domestic water, and values of 6.5–8.5 are acceptable for marine and freshwater aquatic life.

The cationic elements in water that affect its quality depend directly on the area and its constituent geological bedrock and soils (McLeese et al., 1991; Betcher et al., 1995). Sodium tends to dominate in saline lakes, alkali lakes, and ground sources. In alkali areas of the Canadian Prairies, sodium content of water in pig barns averaged as high as 258 mg/L with a range of 4–1,390 mg/L (McLeese et al., 1991). Two unconventional sources of sodium contamination of water are water softening agents and road de-icing salt. In rural and urban locations, cation exchange water softeners often use sodium chloride to reduce water hardness. Softened household water contained 278 ± 186 mg sodium/L (range 46–1219 mg/L) compared to untreated municipal water, which had 110 ± 98 mg sodium/L (range 0–253 mg/L) (Yarows et al., 1997). The second unusual source of extraneous water sodium occurs in northern geographical areas, which use de-icing salt to melt roadway ice in winter. During the spring thaw, residues of de-icing salt in ditch water have been shown to contaminate waterways not only with sodium, but also with other heavy metals including cadmium, copper, lead, and zinc (Backstrom et al., 2004).

A water sodium concentration of about 350 mg/L will provide sufficient sodium to meet the daily sodium requirements of a horse drinking maintenance amounts of water (5 L/100 kg BW). The upper limits of sodium concentrations (1,390 mg/L) detected in some Prairie waters (McLeese et al., 1991) would provide four times the sodium needed by an idle horse. In other livestock, high water sodium may reduce the palatability and voluntary intake of the water and may be a potential cause of dehydration. High sodium content in water has implications regarding voluntary intake of block or loose salt and/or water by horses. A decreased salt intake could impact horse health if salt is the only mechanism of providing trace minerals to the horse. The sodium content of the regional water supply should be considered during ration formulation.

Bicarbonate, carbonate, sulphate, and chloride are the principal anions in water. Bicarbonate (carbonate) water is common in Africa and western Canada. Carbonate and bicarbonate determine the pH and "alkalinity" of water. Chloride waters occur throughout the world, while sulphate waters occur in central and western North America. Chloride content is used to evaluate wastewater usability for agricultural purposes.

Sulphate in water is important in ruminants, especially if feed molybdenum is high, because the copper-thiomolybdate complex that forms reduces copper availability (Spears, 2003). To date, there is no evidence that high sulphate water impairs copper utilization in horses. High sulphate concentrations in water may cause metal corrosion. A "salty" taste may be detected typically due to the sodium, the cation most commonly associated with sulphate.

Although few studies have examined individual cation and anion toxicities in horses, Table 7-4 provides an estimate of generally considered safe upper level concentrations of some potentially toxic elements for horses. This summary is an amalgam of past and more recent livestock water guidelines. The data have generally not been derived from studies using horses.

Nitrate

High water nitrate and nitrite concentrations are a concern for humans, particularly infants and the elderly (Fan and Steinberg, 1996). The upper limit for nitrate-nitrogen in water for livestock has been specified at 100 mg/L and for nitrite-nitrogen at 10 mg/L (NRC, 1974; CCME, 2002). Australian water guidelines use trigger values of 400 mg nitrate/L and 30 mg nitrite/L (ANZECC, 2000) or about 90 mg/L nitrate-nitrogen and 9 mg/L nitrite-nitrogen. Nitrate and nitrite concentrations in water analyses are converted to their respective nitrogen values (nitrate-nitrogen and nitrite-nitrogen) by dividing by 4.43 and 3.29. Of the two components, nitrite is 10–15 times more toxic than nitrate. Nitrate, however, can be converted to nitrite by bacterial reduction in the rumen of cattle or sheep and to a lesser extent in the cecum of the horse. Nitrite creates its toxic effects by displacing oxygen on the hemoglobin molecule to form methemoglobin. Methemoglobin reduces oxygen transport to tissue, which results in the typical respiratory symptoms of nitrite (nitrate) poisoning. Few cases of nitrite- or nitrate-induced methemoglobinemia in horses are reported in the literature. A recent report in which diets containing 1.74–1.85 percent nitrate were fed to nonpregnant mares observed that neither methemoglobin, oxygenated haemoglobin, reduced haemoglobin, or hematocrit were significantly changed after 13 days of feeding despite significant elevations in blood nitrate/nitrite concentrations (Burwash et al., 2005). This suggests that horses may have a different threshold of nitrate and nitrite tolerance than ruminants. Generally, feed nitrate is a larger risk than water nitrate, but the cumulative effects of high feed and water nitrate (nitrite) intakes should be avoided.

The nitrate concentration of water has been described in a multivariable relationship with the following significant

TABLE 7-4 Generally Considered Safe Upper Level Concentrations (mg/L) of Some Potentially Toxic Nutrients and Contaminants in Water for Horses

Element	Upper Limit (NRC, 1974)	Upper Limit (NRC, 1989)	Livestock Water Guidelines (ANZECC, 2000)	Livestock Water Guidelines (CCME, 2002)
Aluminum	—	—	5	5
Arsenic	0.2	0.2	0.5	0.025
Boron	—	—	5	5
Cadmium	0.05	0.05	0.01	0.08
Chromium	1	1	—	0.05
Cobalt	1	1	—	1
Copper	0.5	0.5	0.5–5[a]	0.5–5[a]
Fluoride	2	2	2	1–2
Lead	0.1	0.1	0.1	0.1
Mercury	0.01	0.01	0.002	0.03
Molybdenum	Not established		0.15	0.5
Nickel	1	1	1	1
Selenium	—	—	0.02	0.05
Vanadium	0.1	0.1	—	0.1
Zinc	25	25	20	50

[a]Lower limits for sheep and cattle; higher values for pigs and poultry.

factors: nitrogen fertilizer loading, extent of cropland or pasture, human population density, well-drained soils, depth to the seasonally high water table, and presence or absence of unconsolidated sand and gravel aquifers (Nolan et al., 2002). Manure and agricultural fertilizers are usually felt to be the main sources of nitrate in water. In agricultural counties of upstate New York, 10 percent of small farms (100 acres or less) and 23 percent of large farms (501 acres or more) had water nitrate exceeding 10 mg/L (Gelberg et al., 1999). Wells less than 15 meters deep, and springs located on large farms, had higher water nitrate concentrations during summer and fall. Agricultural activities, however, differ from season to season and consequently skew the nitrate concentration upward or downward during those periods (Ridder et al., 1974). Scottish streams had the highest fluxes of ammonia and nitrate-nitrogen during autumn and winter but acute elevations occurred during or following storm events (Petry et al., 2002).

Protozoa

Two common pathogenic protozoa in water are *Cryptosporidium* and *Giardia* but neither protozoal organism typically causes significant disease in horses. The oocysts of both *Giardia* and *Cryptosporidium* increase markedly in tributaries draining agricultural lands following extreme rainfalls and flooding (Kistemann et al., 2002) and in the United Kingdom were highest in fall and winter coinciding with the calving season (Bodley-Tickell et al., 2002). *Giardia* and *Cryptosporidium* oocysts are not uncommon in feces of domestic livestock, especially in calves (Olson et al., 1997; Rose, 1997; Sturdee et al., 2003) in which diarrhea is the most common clinical sign. In North America, an average prevalence of infection with *Cryptosporidium* in horses is 16 percent, 50 percent in dairy calves, and 78 percent in sheep (Rose, 1997). *Cryptosporidium* oocyst numbers in feces of British horses varied annually, but the average prevalence rate was 8.9 percent (Sturdee et al., 2003). The prevalence of infection in horses with *Giardia* and *Cryptosporidium* in west-central Canada and the Yukon was 20 percent and 17 percent, respectively (Olson et al., 1997). The threshold live oocyst count of *Giardia* and *Cryptosporidium* needed to infect horses is unknown.

Algae

Cyanophyceae (blue-green) and other algae are being increasingly reported as contaminants of water in association with the eutrophication of worldwide water supplies (de Figueiredo et al., 2004). More importantly, the genera *Microcystis, Aphanizomenon, Planktothrix/Oscillatoria, Nostoc,* and *Anabaena* produce highly toxic hepatotoxins called microcystins that can affect humans and livestock (Romanowska-Duda et al., 2002; de Figueiredo et al., 2004). Cyanophytes can cause taste and odor adulteration of water described as moldy, musty, grassy, or with a septic-tank odor. Microcystin-producing algae in the U.S. Midwest favored growth in surface waters contaminated with high total suspended solids, chlorophyll, phosphorus, and nitrogen compounds, although these conditions were not invariable (Graham et al., 2004). The calculated trigger value for microcystin-LR in water for horses is 2.3 μg/L or

11,500 cells/mL (ANZECC, 2000). These values were based on maximal water intakes and incorporate several safety factors, including lowest observed adverse effects level and inter- and intraspecies variation, but were not based on studies in horses.

Bacteria

Total coliform bacteria and total fecal coliforms are used as sentinels of water contamination by fecal pollutants. Total coliforms are a generic group of gram-negative bacteria that are distinguished from thermotolerant coliforms (fecal coliforms) by a lower tolerance of high temperatures (45°C). Thermotolerant bacteria used to be considered more indicative of fecal contamination by warm-blooded animals, but some thermotolerant coliforms are now known to arise from environmental contaminants. Thermotolerant coliforms are more specifically related to *Escherichia coli*, but can also include the enterobacteria *Klebsiella*, *Citrobacter*, and others. Both methods of bacterial assessment indicate potential contamination of water and can be a gauge of the effectiveness of water treatment procedures. Increased colony counts of bacteria and, specifically, fecal streptococci and *Clostridium perfringens* were observed in runoff after extensive rainfall and after floods of forested or agricultural communities (Kistemann et al., 2002).

The median threshold guideline for thermotolerant coliforms for livestock has been given at 100 thermotolerant coliforms/100 mL (ANZECC, 2000). Canadian livestock water guidelines do not give a stated threshold coliform number for livestock because of the variation in pathogenicity of enterobacteria. The coliform bacteria in water most commonly associated with enteric disease in humans, *E. coli*, do not appear to affect horses similarly.

REFERENCES

Agabriel, J., W. Martin-Rosset, and J. Robelin. 1984. Croissance et besoins du poulain. Pp. 371–384 in Le Cheval, R. Jarrige and W. Martin-Rosset, eds. Paris: INRA.

Andrews, F. M., J. A. Nadeau, L. Saabye, and A. M. Saxton. 1997. Measurement of total body water content in horses, using deuterium oxide dilution. Am. J. Vet. Res. 58:1060–1064.

ANZECC (Australian and New Zealand Environment and Conservation Council). 2000. Livestock drinking water guidelines. Pp. 1–32 in Guidelines for Fresh and Marine Water Quality, vol. 3.

Backstrom, M., S. Karlsson, L. Backman, L. Folkeson, and B. Lind. 2004. Mobilisation of heavy metals by deicing salts in a roadside environment. Water Res. 38:720–732.

Betcher, R., G. Grove and C. Pupp. 1995. Groundwater in Manitoba. Hydrogeology, quality concerns, and management. NHRI Contribution No. CS-93017. Pp 53.

Bodley-Tickell, A. T., S. E. Kitchen, and A. P. Sturdee. 2002. Occurrence of Cryptosporidium in agricultural surface waters during an annual farming cycle in lowland UK. Water Res. 36:1880–1886.

Burwash, L., B. Ralston, and M. Olson. 2005. Effect of high nitrate feed on mature idle horses. Pp. 174–179 in Proc. 19th Equine Nutr. Physiol. Soc. Symp., Tucson, AZ.

Butudom, P., D. J. Barnes, M. W. Davis, B. D. Nielsen, S. W. Eberhart, and H. C. Schott II. 2004. Rehydration fluid temperature affects voluntary drinking in horses dehydrated by furosemide administration and endurance exercise. Vet. J. 167:72–80.

CCME (Canadian Council of Ministers of the Environment). 2002 (update). Canadian Environmental Quality Guidelines. Canadian Water Quality Guidelines for the Protection of Agricultural Water Uses. Chapter 5.

Collastos, C. 1999. Fluid therapy: when and where? Proc. Am. Assoc. Equine Pract. 45:271–272.

Crowell-Davis, S. L., K. A. Houpt, and J. Carnevale. 1985. Feeding and drinking behavior of mares and foals with free access to pasture and water. J. Anim. Sci. 60:883–889.

Cymbaluk, N. F. 1989. Water balance of horses fed various diets. Equine Pract. 11:19–24.

Cymbaluk, N. F. 1990a. Comparison of forage digestion by cattle and horses. Can. J. Anim. Sci. 70:601–610.

Cymbaluk N. F. 1990b. Cold housing effects on growth and nutrient demand of young horses. J. Anim. Sci. 68:3152–3162.

Cymbaluk, N. F., M. E. Smart, F. Bristol, and V. A. Pouteaux. 1993. Importance of milk replacer intake and composition in rearing orphan foals. Can. Vet. J. 34:479–486.

Danielsen, K., L. M. Lawrence, P. Siciliano, D. Powell, and K. Thompson. 1995. Effect of diet on weight and plasma variables in endurance exercised horses. Equine Vet. J. Suppl. 18:372–377.

de Figueiredo, D. R., U. M. Azeiteiro, S. M. Esteves, F. J. Goncalves, and M. J. Pereira. 2004. Microcystin-producing blooms—a serious global public health issue. Ecotoxicol. Environ. Safety 59:151–153.

Doreau, M., S. Boulot, W. Martin-Rosset, and J. Robelin. 1986. Relationship between nutrient intake, growth and body composition of the nursing foal. Reprod. Nutr. Develop. 26:683–690.

Doreau, M., S. Boulot, and W. Martin-Rosset 1991. Effect of parity and physiological state on intake, milk production and blood parameters in lactating mares differing in body size. Anim. Prod. 53:111–118.

Doreau, M., S. Boulot, D. Bauchart, J.-P. Barlet, and W. Martin-Rosset. 1992. Voluntary intake, milk production and plasma metabolites in nursing mares fed two different diets. J. Nutr. 122:992–999.

Dulphy, J. P., W. Martin-Rosset, H. Dubroeucq, J. M. Ballet, A. Detour, and M. Jailler. 1997. Compared feeding patterns in ad libitum intake of dry forages by horses and sheep. Livest. Prod. Sci. 52:49–56.

Ecke, P., D. R. Hodgson, and R. J. Rose. 1998. Induced diarrhoea in horses. Part I. Fluid and electrolyte balance. Vet. J. 155:149–159.

Ecker, G. L., and M. I. Lindinger. 1995. Water and ion losses during the cross-country phase of eventing. Equine Vet. J. Suppl. 20:111–119.

Fan, A.M. and V.E. Steinberg. 1996. Health implications of nitrate and nitrite in drinking water: an update on methemoglobinemia occurrence and reproductive and developmental toxicity. Regul. Toxicol. Pharmacol. 23:35–43.

Fielding, C. L., K. G. Magdesian, D. A. Elliott, L. D. Cowgill, and G. P. Carlson. 2004. Use of multifrequency bioelectrical impedance analysis for estimation of total body water and extracellular and intracellular fluid volumes in horses. Am. J. Vet. Res. 65:320–326.

Flannigan, G. 2001. Survey of stereotypies and time budgets of pregnant mares' urine (PMU) ranching industry production mares. M.Sc. Univ. Sask. 118 pp.

Forro, M., S. Cieslar, G. L. Ecker, A. Walzak, J. Hahn, and M. I. Lindinger. 2000. Total body water and ECFV measured using bioelectrical impedance analysis and indicator dilution in horses. J. Appl. Physiol. 89:663–671.

Freeman, D. A., N. F. Cymbaluk, H. C. Schott, K. Hinchcliff, S. M. McDonnell, and B. Kyle. 1999. Clinical, biochemical and hygiene assessment of stabled horses provided continuous or intermittent access to drinking water. Am. J. Vet. Res. 60:1445–1450.

Friend, T. H. 2000. Dehydration, stress and water consumption of horses during long-distance commercial transport. J. Anim. Sci. 78:2568–2580.

Gelberg, K. H., L. Church, G. Casey, M. London, D. S. Roerig, J. Boyd, and M. Hill. 1999. Nitrate levels in drinking water in rural New York state. Environ. Res. 80:34–40.

Geor, R. J., and L. J. McCutcheon. 1998. Hydration effects on physiological strain of horses during exercise-heat stress. J. Appl. Physiol. 84:2042–2051.

Geor, R. J., L. J. McCutcheon, and M. I. Lindinger. 1996. Adaptations to daily exercise in hot and humid conditions in trained Thoroughbred horses. Equine Vet. J. Suppl. 22:63–68.

Geor, R. J., L. J. McCutcheon, G. L. Ecker, and M. I. Lindinger. 2000. Heat storage in horses during submaximal exercise before and after humid heat acclimation. J. Appl. Physiol. 89:2283–2293.

Gibbs, A. E., and T. H. Friend. 2000. Effect of animal density and trough placement on drinking behavior and dehydration in slaughter horses. J. Equine Vet. Sci. 20:643–650.

Gibbs, P. G., G. D. Potter, R. W. Blake, and W. C. McMullan. 1982. Milk production of Quarter horse mares during 150 days of lactation. J. Anim. Sci. 54:496–499.

Graham, J. L., J. R. Jones, S. B. Jones, J. A. Downing, and T. E. Clevenger. 2004. Environmental factors influencing microcystin distribution and concentration in the midwestern United States. Water Res. 38:4395–4404.

Groenendyk, S., P. B. English, and I. Abetz. 1988. External balance of water and electrolytes in the horse. Equine Vet. J. 20:189–193.

Hargesheimer, E. E., and S. B. Watson. 1996. Drinking water treatment options for taste and odor control. Water Res. 30:1423–1430.

Hinchcliff, K. W., K. H. McKeever, L. M. Schmall, C. W. Kohn, and W. W. Muir. 1990. Renal and systemic hemodynamic responses to sustained submaximal exertion in horses. J. Appl. Physiol. 258:R1177–R1183.

Hodgson, D. S., L. J. McCutcheon, S. K. Byrd, W. S. Brown, W. M. Bayly, G. L. Brengelmann, and P. D. Gollnick. 1993. Dissipation of metabolic heat during exercise. J. Appl. Physiol. 74:1161–1170.

Houpt, K. A., K. Eggleston, K. Kunkle, and T. R. Houpt. 2000. Effect of water restriction on equine behavior and physiology. Equine Vet. J. 32:341–344.

Izraely, H., I. Chosniak, C. E. Stevens, M. W. Demment, and A. Shkolnik. 1989. Factors determining the digestive efficiency of the domesticated donkey (Equus asinus asinus). Quart. J. Exp. Physiol. 74:1–6.

Jansson, A. 1999. Sodium and potassium regulation with special reference to the athletic horse. Ph.D. thesis. Swed. Univ. Agric. Sci., Uppsala.

Jansson, A., and K. Dahlborn. 1999. Effects of feeding frequency and voluntary salt intake on fluid and electrolyte regulation in athletic horses. J. Appl. Physiol. 86:1610–1616.

Jansson, A., A. Lindholm, J. E. Lindberg, and K. Dahlborn. 1999. Effects of potassium intake on potassium, sodium and fluid balance in exercising horses. Equine Vet. J. Suppl. 30:412–417.

Kaneene, J. B., R. A. Miller, W. A. Ross, K. Gallagher, J. Marteniuk, and J. Rook. 1997. Risk factors for colic in the Michigan (USA) equine population. Prev. Vet. Med. 20:23–36.

Kingston, J., R. J. Geor, and L. J. McCutcheon. 1997. Use of dew-point hygrometry, direct sweat collection and measurements of body water losses to determine sweating rates in exercising horses. Am. J. Vet. Res. 58:175–181.

Kistemann, T., T. Classen, C. Koch, F. Dangendorf, R. Fischeder, J. Gebel, V. Vacata, and M. Exner. 2002. Microbial load of drinking water reservoir tributaries during extreme rainfall and runoff. Appl. Environ. Microbiol. 68:2188–2197.

Kristula, M. A., and S. M. McDonnell. 1994. Drinking water temperature affects consumption of water during cold weather in ponies. Appl. Anim. Behav. Sci. 41:155–160.

Marlow, C. H., E. M. van Tonder, F. C. Hayward, S. S. van der Merwe, and L. E. Price. 1983. A report on the consumption, composition and nutritional adequacy of a mixture of lush green perennial ryegrass (Lolium perenne) and cocksfoot (Dactylis glomerata) fed ad libitum to Thoroughbred mares. J. S. Afr. Vet Assoc. 54:155–157.

Martin, R. G., N. P. McMeniman, and K. F. Dowsett. 1992. Milk and water intakes of foals sucking grazing mares. Equine Vet. J. 24:295–299.

McCutcheon, L. J., and R. J. Geor 1999. Equine sweating responses to submaximal exercise during 21 days of heat acclimation. J. Appl. Physiol. 87:1843–1851.

McCutcheon, L. J., and R. J. Geor. 2000. Influence of training on sweating responses during submaximal exercise in horses. J. Appl. Physiol. 89:2463–2471.

McDonnell, S. M., D. A. Freeman, N. F. Cymbaluk, H. C. Schott, K. Hinchcliff, and B. Kyle. 1999. Behavior of stabled horses provided continuous or intermittent access to drinking water. Am. J. Vet. Res. 60:1451–1456.

McDonnell, S. M., and M. A. Kristula. 1996. No effect of drinking water temperature (ambient vs chilled) on consumption of water during hot summer weather in ponies. Appl. Anim. Behav. Sci. 49:159–163.

McKenzie, E. C., S. J. Valberg, S. M. Godden, J. D. Pagan, G. P. Carlson, J. M. Macleay, and F. D. DeLaCorte. 2003. Comparison of volumetric urine collection versus single-sample collection in horses consuming diets varying in cation-anion balance. Am. J. Vet. Res. 64:284–291.

McLeese, J. M., J. F. Patience, M. S. Wolynetz, and G. I. Christison. 1991. Evaluation of the quality of the ground water supplies used on Saskatchewan swine farms. Can. J. Anim. Sci. 71:191–203.

Morgan, K., A. Ehrlemark, and K. Sallvik. 1997. Dissipation of heat from standing horses exposed to ambient temperature between –3 and 37°C. J. Thermal Biol. 22:177–186.

Mueller, P. J., and K. A. Houpt. 1991. A comparison of the responses of donkeys (Equus asinus) and ponies (Equus caballus) to 36 hrs water deprivation. Pp. 86–95 in Donkey, Mules and Horses in Tropical Agricultural Development, D. Fielding and R. A. Pearson, eds. Univ. Edinburgh.

Nolan, B. T., K. J. Hitt, and B. C. Ruddy. 2002. Probability of nitrate contamination of recently recharged groundwaters in the conterminous United States. Environ. Sci. Technol. 36:2138–2145.

NRC (National Research Council). 1974. Nutrients and Toxic Substances in Water for Livestock and Poultry. Washington, DC: National Academy Press. 93 pp.

NRC. 1989. Nutrient Requirements of Horses. 5th rev. ed. Washington, DC: National Academy Press.

NRC. 2005. Water. Chapter 35 in Mineral Tolerance of Domestic Animals. Washington, DC: The National Academies Press.

Nyman, S., and K. Dahlborn. 2001. Effects of water supply method and flow rate on drinking behavior and fluid balance in horses. Physiol. Behav. 73:1–8.

Nyman, S., A. Jansson, A. Lindholm, and K. Dahlorn. 2002. Water intake and fluid shifts in horses: effects of hydration status during two exercise tests. Equine Vet. J. Suppl. 34:133–142.

Olson, M. E., C. L. Thorlakson, L. Deselliers, D. W. Morck, and T. A. McAllister. 1997. Giardia and Cryptosporidium in Canadian farm animals. Vet. Parasitol. 68:375–381.

Pagan, J. D., and P. Harris. 1999. The effects of timing and amount of forage and grain on exercise response in Thoroughbred horses. Equine Vet. J. Suppl. 30:451–457.

Pagan, J. D., P. Harris, T. Brewster-Barnes, S. E. Duren, and S. G. Jackson. 1998. Exercise affects digestibility and rate of passage of all-forage and mixed diets in Thoroughbred horses. J. Nutr. 128:2704S–2708S.

Petry, J., C. Soulsby, I. A. Malcolm, and A. F. Youngson. 2002. Hydrological controls on nutrient concentrations and fluxes in agricultural catchments. Sci. Total Environ. 294:95–110.

Pool-Anderson, K., R. H. Raub, and J. A. Warren. 1994. Maternal influences on growth and development of full-sibling foals. J. Anim. Sci. 72:1661–1666.

Ridder, W. E., F. W. Oehme, and D. C. Kelley. 1974. Nitrates in Kansas groundwaters as related to animal and human health. Toxicology 2:397–405.

Romanowska-Duda, Z., J. Mankiewicz, M. Tacznynska, Z. Walter, and M. Zalewski. 2002. The effect of toxic cyanobacteria (blue-green algae) on water plants and animal cells. Pol. J. Environ. Studies 11:561–566.

Rose, J. B. 1997. Environmental ecology of *Cryptosporidium* and public health implications. Annu. Rev. Public Health. 18:135–161.

Rumbaugh, G. E., G. P. Carlson, and D. Harrold. 1982. Urinary production in the healthy horse and in horses deprived of feed and water. Am. J. Vet Res. 43:735–737.

Schott, H. C., C. A. Ragle, and W. M. Bayly. 1995. Effects of phenylbutazone and frusemide on urinary excretory responses to high intensity exercise. Equine Vet. J. Suppl. 18:426–431.

Schott, H. C., K. S. McGlade, H. A. Molander, A. J. Leroux, and M. T. Hines. 1997. Body weight, fluid, electrolyte, and hormonal changes in horses competing in 50- and 100-mile endurance rides. Am. J. Vet. Res. 58:303–309.

Schott, H. C., S. M Axiak, K. A. Woody, and S. W. Eberhard. 2002. Effect of oral administration of electrolyte pastes on rehydration of horses. Am. J. Vet. Res. 63:19–27.

Schryver, H. F., M. T. Parker, P. D. Daniluk, K. I. Pagan, J. Williams, L. V. Soderholm, and H. F. Hintz. 1987. Salt consumption and the effect of salt on mineral metabolism in horses. Cornell Vet. 77:122–131.

Smith, B. L., J. H. Jones, W. J. Hornof, J. A. Miles, K. E. Longworth, and N. H. Willits. 1996. Effects of road transport on indices of stress in horses. Equine Vet. J. 28:446–454.

Sneddon, J. C., J. van der Walt, and G. Mitchell. 1993a. Effect of dehydration on the volumes of body fluid compartments in horses. J. Arid Environ. 24:397–408.

Sneddon, J. C., J. van der Walt, G. Mitchell, S. Hammer, and J. J. F. Taljaard. 1993b. Effects of dehydration and rehydration on plasma vasopressin and aldosterone in horses. Physiol. Behav. 54:223–228.

Spears, J.W. 2003. Trace mineral bioavailability in ruminants. J. Nutr. 133:1506S–1509S.

Sturdee, A. P., A. T. Bodley-Tickell, A. Archer, and R. M. Chalmers. 2003. Long-term study of *Cryptosporidium* prevalence on a lowland farm in the United Kingdom. Vet. Parasitol. 116:97–113.

Sufit, E., K. A. Houpt, and M. Sweeting. 1985. Physiological stimuli of thirst and drinking patterns in ponies. Equine Vet. J. 17:12–16.

Sweeting, M. P., and K. Houpt. 1987. Water consumption and time budgets of stabled pony geldings. New York: Elsevier.

Tasker, J. B. 1967a. Fluid and electrolyte studies in the horse. III. Intake and output of water, sodium, and potassium. Cornell Vet. 57:649–657.

Tasker, J. B. 1967b. Fluid and electrolyte studies in the horse. IV. The effects of fasting and thirsting. Cornell Vet. 57:658–667.

Tasker, J. B. 1967c. Fluid and electrolyte studies in the horse. V. The effects of diarrhea. Cornell Vet. 57:668–677.

Van den Berg, J. S., A. J. Guthrie, R. A. Meintjes, J. P. Nurton, D. A. Adamson, C. W. Travers, R. J. Lund, and H. J. Mostert. 1998. Water and electrolyte intake and output in conditioned Thoroughbred horses transported by road. Equine Vet. J. 30:316–323.

Warren, L. K., L. M. Lawrence, T. Brewster-Barnes, and D. M. Powell. 1999. The effect of dietary fiber on hydration status after dehydration with frusemide. Equine Vet. J. Suppl. 30:508–513.

Yarows, S. A., W. E. Fusilier, and A. B. Weder. 1997. Sodium concentrations of water from softeners. Arch. Int. Med. 157:218–222.

Zeyner, A., C. Geibler, and A. Dittrich. 2004. Effects of hay intake and feeding sequence on variables in feces and fecal water (dry matter, pH value, organic acids, ammonia, buffering capacity) of horses. J. Anim. Physiol. Anim. Nutr. 88:7–19.

8

Feeds and Feed Processing

FORAGES

Forages for horses are largely represented by the aerial portions of pasture grasses, legumes, and forbs. Forage grasses are divided into two main categories: cool-season species that are adapted to temperate conditions and warm-season grasses that are adapted to subtropical or tropical environments. Forages may either be grazed directly or conserved for use when fresh forage is scarce or when pasturing is not possible. Forages represent a significant portion of the diet for all classes of post-weaned horses and indeed may constitute the entire diet for equids in the wild and large numbers of domesticated horses.

Chemical Composition

Forages consist of the leaf, sheath, and stem of the plant and, depending on the stage of growth, may also include flowers and seed-heads. Each of these different plant parts differs in its chemical composition, and their relative proportions may change substantially during a growing season. Thus, young plants have a high proportion of leaf; are high in protein, water, and minerals; and are low in fiber and lignin. As the season progresses, leaf growth slows, stems elongate, reproductive structures develop, photosynthate accumulates, and the cell content:cell wall ratio decreases, all of which serve to change the overall chemical composition and hence nutritive value of the plant.

Forages are typically characterized by their high dietary fiber content, which is largely composed of the structural carbohydrates (SC) of the plant cell wall and varying amounts of lignin. Forages also contain nonstructural carbohydrates (NSC) originating from the cell contents and include the simple sugars, glucose fructose, sucrose, and storage carbohydrates such as starch or fructan (see Figure 10-1, Chapter 10). Together, the SC and NSC constitute the main energy-yielding fractions of forage. Starch can be digested to glucose by endogenous enzymes in the small intestine and, together with the free sugars, be absorbed across the small intestine of the horse and metabolized to yield adenosine triphosphate (ATP). However, the amount of starch digested in the foregut depends upon a number of factors, including the quantity and botanical origin of the starch, quantity of amylolytic enzymes present, other feeds fed, and interhorse variation. The cell wall carbohydrates and fructans cannot be digested by mammalian enzymes in the foregut (Nilsson, 1988; Åman and Graham, 1990), but are converted via fermentation by the gut microflora to volatile fatty acids (VFAs), which are then metabolized to yield ATP. The efficiency of energy yield via VFAs is lower than that from glucose absorbed in the small intestine. Furthermore, the degree to which SC and NSC are degraded depends upon factors such as their chemical composition, physical conformation, and association with poorly degraded noncarbohydrate compounds. As a consequence, the energy value of forage is governed to a large degree by the types and relative proportions of digestible and fermentable carbohydrate that it contains.

Dietary Fiber–Cell Wall Carbohydrates

Plant cell wall carbohydrates are traditionally divided into three fractions: cellulose (β-linked polymers of glucose), hemicelluloses (polymers of arabinose, xylose, glucose, fucose, mannose, and galactose), and pectins (containing β-D 1-4-linked galacturonic acid residues, arabinose, and galactose) (Butler and Bailey, 1973; Åman and Graham, 1990). The sum of these carbohydrates represents the nonstarch polysaccharide (NSP) fraction of the plant cell wall (see Figure 10-1, Chapter 10). The pectins and polymers of arabinose, galactose, and mannose are frequently readily degraded by the hindgut microflora of nonruminants, whereas those of cellulose and particularly xylan (composed of xylose residues) are more resistant to breakdown (Graham et al., 1986; Moore-Colyer and Longland, 2000). As the plant matures, these fractions, particularly cellulose, may become lignified to varying degrees. Lignin is not a carbohydrate, but is a generic term applied to a group of heterogeneous compounds derived from the phenylpropanoid pathway. Lignin can become intimately associated with cell wall carbohydrates, rendering them recalcitrant to degradation and thereby reducing the nutritive value of the forage (Hartley and Jones, 1977).

Cell Wall Content of Pasture Species

On average over the growing season, cool-season grasses may typically contain 350–650 g cell wall carbohydrates/kg dry matter (DM), of which approximately 50–60 percent may be cellulose, 30–50 percent hemicellulose (most of which is xylan), and 2–4 percent pectin (Longland et al., 1995). Cool-season grasses typically contain around 5 percent lignin (MAFF, 1992). Legumes, however, often contain 295–550 g cell wall carbohydrates/kg DM, of which 30–50 percent is cellulose, 25–30 percent hemicellulose (of which less than half is xylan), and up to 30 percent pectin (Nordkvist and Åman, 1986). Thus, in legumes the proportions of hemicellulose and pectins are lower and higher, respectively, compared with grasses. Lignin may account for 40–150 g/kg legume DM (Nordkvist, 1987). For routine feed analysis, the residue remaining after treatment with neutral detergent (termed neutral detergent fiber or NDF) is regarded as being representative of the cell wall content of gramminaceous feeds, being the sum of the lignin, cellulose, and most of the hemicellulose fractions. Acid detergent insoluble residues (acid detergent fiber or ADF) comprise the cellulose and lignin fractions (see Chapter 10 for further detail). Warm-season grasses mature more rapidly and tend to have a greater proportion of cell wall and be more highly lignified than their cool-season counterparts, and may exceed 800 g NDF/kg DM (Buxton et al., 1995) and 150 g lignin/kg DM (Woolfolk et al., 1975). Cell wall composition changes as the plant matures, with young vegetative growth being relatively high in readily degradable hemicelluloses, with comparatively little cellulose and lignin (Dulphy et al., 1997b). As the plant matures and produces more stem, the proportions of cellulose and lignin increase and those of hemicellulose decrease, with concomitant reductions in ruminal in vitro degradability as the season progresses (Givens et al., 1992). Various environmental factors affect cell wall content: high temperatures tend to increase cell wall content (Deinum et al., 1968) and lignification in legumes and in cool- and warm-season grasses (Wilson et al., 1991; Buxton et al., 1995). As a consequence, forages grown at high temperatures tend to be of reduced feeding value compared to those grown at lower temperatures. For example, ruminal NDF digestion was reduced by 13 and 19 percent, respectively, for leaf and stems of Bermudagrass grown at 32°C vs. 22°C (Buxton et al., 1995).

Cell Contents

The cell contents comprise the NSC (nonstructural carbohydrate fraction, which is the the sum of simple sugars, fructan, and starch), most of the plant protein, minerals, and lipids. In immature vegetative tissues, the cell contents may represent some 66 percent of the total DM; however, with increasing forage maturity, the proportion of cell contents decreases and in the mature plant may represent less than 40 percent of the forage DM. Declines in proportions of cell contents are associated with concomitant reductions in digestibility, the rate of the decline tending to be greater in legumes than cool-season grasses (Beever et al., 2000).

Carbohydrates

Starch is the major storage carbohydrate in most grass and legume seeds, and the vegetative (i.e., nonreproductive) tissues of legumes and warm-season grasses (Chatterton et al., 1989). Starch production and storage in vegetative tissues occurs within the chloroplasts, and is a self-limiting process as the chloroplasts become saturated with starch. However, the storage carbohydrates in the vegetative structures of many cool-season pasture grasses are fructans, composed of polymers of fructose and glucose (Ojima and Isawa, 1968; Smith, 1968; Bender and Smith, 1973), with starch as a relatively minor component (Cairns et al., 2002a,b; Turner et al., 2002). Photosynthate in excess of immediate plant requirements for growth and metabolism is converted to fructan and translocated from the leaf to stem. Thus, fructan production is not self-limiting, allowing high levels of fructan to accumulate. As a consequence, the average NSC content of warm-season grasses tends to be substantially lower than that of fructan-accumulating cool-season grasses when grown under the same conditions, with 129 and 209 g NSC/kg DM, respectively, observed by Chatterton et al. (1989) when studying more than 180 accessions of warm- and cool-season grasses grown under laboratory conditions.

The highest total NSC contents reported were 654 and 771 g/kg DM for *Phalaris aquatica* and *Bromus carinatus* spp., respectively, both of which contained 450 g fructan/kg DM (Chatterton et al., 1989). However, levels of fructan measured in 10 mixed grass and legume horse pastures in Germany varied from 10–74 g/kg DM (Vervuert et al., 2005), whereas orchardgrass in the Mediterranean accumulated up to 400 g fructan/kg DM in the stem bases (Volaire and Lelieve, 1997). In a study of total water-soluble carbohydrate (WSC, the sum of simple sugars and fructan) and fructan contents of various ryegrass species and varieties in fertilized field plots over three growing seasons in the United Kingdom, WSC contents of vegetative tissues ranged from less than 100 g/kg DM to more than 385 g/kg DM with fructan contents of 75–279 g/kg DM; the remainder of the WSC fraction was largely composed of sucrose, fructose, and glucose (Longland et al., 2006). Thus, levels of WSC and fructan in pasture grasses can vary widely. Although high levels of NSC may render a forage high in digestible energy (DE), there is evidence to suggest that overconsumption of starch (Potter et al., 1992a) or fructan (Pollit et al., 2003) may elicit the onset of metabolic disorders in horses, such as colic and laminitis, and high intakes of simple sugars may be involved in the development of insulin resistance in horses (Hoffman et al., 2003). Pastures sown with forage species that accumulate reduced concentrations of NSC should be used for equids susceptible to these conditions.

In addition to plant species, various other factors affect the amounts of NSC that accumulate in forage. Plant tissues differentially accumulate fructan, with bases of plant parts accumulating more fructans than the apices, (Williams et al., 1993), and stems more than leaves (Waite and Boyd, 1953a). Thus, stems of ryegrass, timothy, fescue, and orchardgrass contained 1.5- to 10-fold the amount of fructan found in the leaves of the same plant (Waite and Boyd, 1953b), and, as a consequence, the NSC content of a plant is influenced by the leaf:stem ratio. Environmental effects also influence herbage NSC content. Under conditions of reduced light, either through shading or cloud cover (Ciavarella et al., 2000) or with application of fertilizer nitrogen (Jacobs et al., 1989; O'Keily et al., 2002), NSC accumulation decreased, whereas drought resulted in an increase in NSC and fructan (Volaire and Lelievre, 1997). Furthermore, cool temperatures had a profound effect on NSC accumulation, resulting in 2- to 3-fold higher levels of total NSC in both warm- (166 vs. 92 g/kg DM) and cool-season (312 vs. 107 g/kg DM) grasses, respectively, when grown at night/day temperatures of 10/15°C as opposed to 15/25°C (Chatterton et al., 1989).

The NSC levels in plants are in constant flux, being a function of photosynthetic activity on the one hand and utilization, translocation, and storage for growth and development on the other. Thus, due to the combined effects of light and temperature on NSC accumulation, there are diurnal variations in NSC content, such that levels of NSC tend to rise during the morning to reach maxima in the afternoon, with levels declining overnight until the following daylight (Bowden et al., 1968; Holt and Hilst, 1969). Similar diurnal patterns of NSC accumulation have also been reported for legumes, with starch increasing 2-fold to 200 g/kg DM from 9 am–3 pm in alfalfa (Lechtenberg et al., 1971). There are also seasonal variations in NSC of grasses and legumes. Waite and Boyd (1953b), studying perennial ryegrass, timothy, orchardgrass, and fescue, reported that NSC was highest in late spring, declining mid-season and rising to intermediate levels in early autumn. Decreases in storage carbohydrates in legumes also occur with increasing maturity (Demarquilly, 1981). Although these generalized patterns of diurnal and seasonal variation largely hold true under standardized conditions, they are subject to considerable change in the field, as the effects of varying light intensity, temperature, fertilizer, water status, and other factors on NSC accumulation are superimposed upon these generalized profiles. Furthermore, where fluctuations in temperature and/or light intensity are minimal, e.g., under tropical conditions or mid-season in more temperate regions, the above generalized profiles of NSC accumulation may be less apparent or may not emerge (Van Soest et al., 1978). However, in general, environmental influences that both reduce photosynthetic activity (e.g., cloud cover) and enhance plant growth (e.g., warm, moist, fertile soils) result in lowered accumulation of NSC in vegetative tissues, whereas conditions that enhance photosynthesis but reduce growth (e.g., high light intensity coupled with cool temperatures) allow elevated levels of NSC, particularly fructan, to accumulate. It is of note that high levels of pasture NSC (starch, fructan, or total WSC) have been linked with the onset of disorders such as laminitis.

Protein

Protein in the vegetative tissues of forages is largely concentrated in the leaf, with much lower levels being found in the stem; thus, alfalfa and timothy leaves contained some 2- to 3-fold as much protein as the corresponding stem tissue (Collins, 1988). In addition to plant part, the protein content of forages also varies greatly with species and differing environments. However, when averaged across a growing season, legumes are higher in protein than grasses, with cool-season grasses generally higher in protein than warm-season grasses (Whitman et al., 1951). Stage of growth also had a profound influence on forage protein content; protein level declined with plant maturity (Green et al., 1971). In North Dakota, the average crude protein (CP) content of a number of cool-season grasses, was 220 g CP/kg DM in April, but declined to less than 70 g/kg by October. The corresponding values for a range of warm-season grasses were 150 and < 50 g CP (Whitman et al., 1951). Likewise, the CP content of alfalfa at the bud stage can be in the region of 250 g CP/kg DM, whereas at the mid-bloom stage, it may be 150 g CP/kg DM (Hunt, 1995). Ear emergence (heading) has been identified as a critical point after which there is a rapid decline in protein content and a concomitant increase in that of fiber. Although the timing of 50 percent heading is relatively constant within a species, the rate of protein decline varies considerably between plant species at a given growth stage (Harkess and Alexander, 1969). Management practices also affect the protein content of pastures. Frequent defoliation through clipping or grazing results in higher protein contents, because the herbage is maintained at a younger stage of growth. Clipping Coastal Bermudagrass once every 2 weeks resulted in swards that contained 88 percent leaf, 210 g CP/kg DM, and 90 g lignin/kg DM. The corresponding values for the swards clipped every 8 weeks were 51, 120, and 120, respectively (Burton et al., 1995). Fertilizer application also affects the CP content of grass. The average CP content of cool-season pastures managed for various DM yields rose from approximately 250 g CP/kg to 300 g/kg when fertilized with 100 or 400 kg nitrogen/hectare (Humphreys et al., 2001), and the protein content of Coastal Bermudagrass averaged over a season was reported to rise from 98 to 155 g CP/kg when receiving no fertilizer or 400 lbs/acre, respectively (Evers, 1998). Likewise, application of fertilizer increased the concentration of all protein fractions in Bermudagrass, stargrass, and bahiagrass (Johnson et al., 2001).

Lipid

The lipid content of fresh grass, alfalfa, and clovers is usually low, in the range of 10–50 g/kg DM (MAFF, 1992).

Minerals

There are wide interspecific variations in forage mineral contents. Thus, when grown on the same soil, legumes are generally higher in calcium, potassium, magnesium, copper, zinc, iron, and cobalt than grasses, whereas grasses tend to be higher in manganese and molybdenum. In a study of 17 North American grass species grown on the same soil and sampled at similar growth stages, copper ranged from 4.5–21.1 ppm and manganese from 96–815 ppm (Beeson et al., 1947). In addition to interspecies differences in forage mineral content, a number of environmental influences, such as season, plant maturity, geographical location, soil type, pH, and fertilizer history, can result in broad intraspecific variations in plant mineral status (Stout et al., 1977). There is often a rapid uptake of minerals during early growth that is reduced by the end of the season. The most common elements affected by plant growth stage are copper, zinc, iron, cobalt, and molybdenum (Underwood, 1981). During overwintering of forages, leaves, which are often higher in trace elements than the stem, are lost, with a concomitant reduction in minerals with a decrease in the leaf:stem ratio. Soil pH can have a profound effect on forage mineral status, with zinc, copper, cobalt, and manganese concentrations in clover and ryegrass decreasing with increasing soil pH (Mitchell, 1957). However, expected average mineral contents of forage foliage have been suggested to be approximately (in g/kg DM): calcium (5–20), phosphorus (2–5), sodium (0.1–0.3), magnesium (1.2–8), potassium (15–40), and sulfur (2–3.5) (McDonald et al., 1996; Barker and Collins, 2003). Average values for forage micromineral content (ppm) have been given as: iron (50–1,000), manganese (30–300), boron (10–50), copper (5–15), zinc (10–100), molybdenum (1–100), and nickel (0.2–2) (Barker and Collins, 2003).

Vitamins

Forages vary widely in vitamin content. However, immature, leafy forage should normally provide sufficient carotene and B vitamins for horses (Evans, 1973).

Summary

Clearly, overall forage quality is affected by plant species, maturity, and environmental effects. In general, factors that reduce plant growth and maintain swards at an immature growth stage will enhance forage digestibility through elevated cell content:cell wall ratios. Conversely, those factors (e.g., warm temperatures, strong light) that increase rates of growth and development will result in a decline in quality through decreased leaf:stem ratios and associated declines in cell contents and increased cell wall content and lignification. Thus, the quality of warm-season forages is generally lower than that of cool-season species. A mean difference of around 15 units of total digestible nutrients (TDN) for ruminants between warm-season and cool-season grasses was recorded (McDowell, 1972, in Van Soest et al., 1978).

Fresh Pastures for Horses

The feed value of pastures for horses is a function of pasture intake and forage nutrient composition, digestibility, and bioavailability. Although horses are preferential grazers, it has been found that some wild ponies in the United Kingdom and feral horses in the United States will ingest up to 20 percent of their daily intake from browse species, even at times of peak grass growth (Hansen, 1976; Putman et al., 1987). However, such access to browse species is often limited for pastured domestic equids: these animals rely on grass and legume swards, which will be the focus in the rest of this section.

Pasture Intakes

There is scant information on the voluntary dry matter intake (VDMI) of fresh forage by horses, largely due to the difficulties in measuring intakes by grazing animals. Methods used include subtraction of harvested residual herbage from calculated herbage mass allowance (Duren et al., 1989), marker studies such as use of n-alkanes (Nash, 2001; Grace and Brody, 2001), measurement of fecal outputs and known organic matter (OM) or DM digestibilities (Meschonia et al., 1998; Grace et al., 2002a), "cut and carry" techniques to housed animals (Chenost and Martin-Rosset, 1985), change in body weight (BW) after accounting for insensible weight loss and excretory outputs (Ince et al., 2005), or through determination of bite size, number, and duration of feedings (Duren et al., 1989).

Estimates of VDMI for grazing horses generally range from 1.5–3.1 percent of BW (Table 8-1). Average daily DM intakes were highest for lactating mares, which on average consumed 2.8 percent of BW whereas the remaining categories of horse ingested approximately 2 percent of their BW. This concurs with Dulphy et al. (1997b), who concluded that average DM intakes of fresh forage were in the region of 2 percent of BW.

TABLE 8-1 Estimated Voluntary Fresh Matter Intake (VFMI) and Voluntary Dry Matter Intake (VDMI) of Fresh Herbage[a]

Type of Horse	Type of Forage	VFMI (g FM/ kg BW)	VDMI (g DM/ kg BW)	VDMI (g DM/ kg BW$^{0.75}$)	Source
Mature trotters	Fresh cut grass (4 species) and alfalfa			98.6 (DM) 51.4 (DOM)	Chenost and Martin-Rosset (1985)
Mature light horses	Fresh pasture (first cut)		18		Dulphy et al. (1997a)
Mature light horses	Fresh pasture (second cut)		20		Dulphy et al. (1997a)
Nonlactating, heavy breed mares	Natural grassland			175.2 (DM) 166 (OM)	Fleurance et al. (2001)
Thoroughbred yearlings	Perennial ryegrass/white clover mix		20	85	Grace et al. (2002a)
Lactating Thoroughbred mares			24	118	Grace et al. (2002b)
Weanling Thoroughbreds			18	76.3	Grace et al. (2003)
Lactating Thoroughbred mares	Orchardgrass and perennial ryegrass early vegetative stage	117–122	24–26		Marlow et al. (1983)
Lactating Thoroughbred mares	Orchardgrass and perennial ryegrass mid bloom	84–100	26–31		Marlow et al. (1983)
Nonlactating Thoroughbred mares (n = 2)	Orchardgrass/perennial ryegrass	73–77	15–22		Marlow et al. (1983)
Weanling stock horses			20–30		McMeniman (2003)
1–2-year-old selle Francais				82 (OM)	Meschonia et al. (2000)
Draught breed mares	Semi-natural, medium-quality grassland			101–215	Menard et al. (2002)

[a]DOM = digestible organic matter, OM = organic matter, DM = dry matter

A number of authors have reported that increased herbage DM intakes are coincident with increased herbage quality, in terms of digestibility (Moffitt et al., 1987), high sugar content (Rogalski, 1984), or inferred increased CP and reduced cell wall contents arising from fertilizer nitrogen application (Benyovsky et al., 1998). However, other studies reported decreased intake of higher-quality pastures. For example, young Thoroughbred fillies on improved pastures were more active and spent less time grazing than those grazing less nutritious swards (Nash and Thompson, 2001). Thus, the VDMI response of growing horses to increasing pasture quality may be positive or negative. This has led to the suggestion that control of VDMI may be a function of DE intake in these animals (Hoskin and Gee, 2004). Thus, animals with previously insufficient or marginal DE intakes may show enhanced VDMI of high-quality pastures, whereas those with previously adequate DE intakes may reduce their VDMI to maintain constant DE intakes.

Pasture Digestibility

Digestibility of fresh pasture varies with plant species and type. In general, cool-season grasses are more digestible than warm-season grasses. This is purported to be due to the higher proportions of easily degraded mesophyll cells in cool-season grasses compared with their warm-season counterparts, which have higher proportions of more recalcitrant lignified vascular and schlerenchyma tissues (Akin and Burdick, 1975). Furthermore, plant maturity is an important determinant of forage digestibility, with digestibility declining with reductions in protein content, and of increases in fiber associated with the decreases in leaf:stem ratios that occur during reproductive development and stem elongation. Warm-season species tend to mature more rapidly than their cool-season counterparts, with concomitant declines in digestibility. Nutrient digestibilities of various forages at different growth stages are summarized in Table 8-2. Thus, the DM digestibility of bluegrass/alfalfa swards by horses was 73 percent for young pasture 11 cm tall and 52 percent for older, more mature swards 47 cm high with a higher proportion of stem than the younger material (McMeniman, 2003). The DM digestibilities of semi-natural grassland of medium quality were 61 percent in May and 53 percent in July (Menard et al., 2002). The energy value of pastures at different seasons has been determined by a number of researchers—the DE of leafy spring ryegrass/white clover swards and spring/summer pastures were respectively 2.88 (Hunt, 1995) and 2.82 Mcal/kg DM (Gallagher and McMeniman, 1988; Martin, 1993), declining to 1.9 and 1.8 Mcal/kg DM, when the pasture had a reduced leaf:stem ratio with the advancing seasons. Similarly the DE of alfalfa declined from 2.87 for immature material to 2.4 Mcal/kg DM when in full bloom (Hunt, 1995). Digestibility of forage protein is associated with protein content (Evans, 1973),

TABLE 8-2 Contents of Digestible Energy and Protein and Apparent Dry Matter and Protein Digestibilities[a] of Various Fresh Forages by Horses

Type of Forage	DE (Mcal/kg DM)	CP Content (g/kg DM)	DMD[b]	CPD[c]	Source[d]
Semi-natural medium-quality grassland					
–May			61		Menard et al. (2002)
–June			57		
–July			53		
–September			55		
–October			56		
Pasture spring/summer	2.3–2.82	103–130			Gallagher and McMeniman
Pasture/winter	1.8–2.5	121–151			(1988); Martin (1993)
Ryegrass				60	Hussein et al. (2001)
Tall fescue				66	
Orchardgrass				71	
Spring ryegrass/white clover	2.6–2.83	148–220			Martin (1993)
Spring ryegrass/white clover (leafy)	2.88	220			
Summer ryegrass/white clover (leafy)	2.5	150			Hunt (1995)
Late summer, stemmy ryegrass/white clover	1.9	100			
Ryegrass/white clover/autumn	2.6	250			
Ryegrass/white clover/winter (leafy)	2.7	250			
Pre-bloom red clover	2.64	230			
Full-bloom red clover	2.4	180			Hunt (1995)
Immature alfalfa	2.87	250			
Pre-bloom alfalfa	2.75	220			
Early-bloom alfalfa	2.64	200			
Mid-bloom alfalfa	2.51	160			
Young pitted bluegrass and alfalfa, 11 cm high			73		McMeniman (2003)
Mid-season pitted bluegrass and alfalfa, 23 cm high			68		
Late-season pitted bluegrass and alfalfa, 47 cm high			52		

[a]Digestibilities are expressed as percentages.
[b]DMD = dry matter digestibility.
[c]CPD = crude protein digestibility.
[d]All studies used mature horses except McMeniman (2003), which used young horses.

with CP digestibility declining with increased plant maturity and reduced protein levels.

Feeding Value of Pastures

Ad libitum access to pasture can support nonproductive adult horses. At certain times of year, this access can cause them to exceed their requirement for energy and protein, resulting in obesity (Elphinstone, 1981; Hughes and Gallacher, 1993; Marlow et al., 1983).

In a 2-year study on pregnant mares at pasture, it was found that although pasture nutrient content fluctuated throughout the seasons to well above and somewhat below the calculated requirements of the mares, their protein and energy requirements were met, as they gained weight in two successive seasons during lactation (Gallagher and McMeniman, 1988; Martin, 1993). A number of authors have concluded that providing that there is sufficient pasture of a DE no less than 2.4 Mcal/kg DM and 105 g CP/kg DM, lactating mares consuming pasture DM at a level equivalent to 2.4 percent of their BW per day would not require diet supplementation for these nutrients (Martin-Rosset et al., 1986; Doreau et al., 1988; Martin, 1993). However, high-quality, lush pastures of cocksfoot orchardgrass and perennial ryegrass, although able to support nonproductive mares, were unable to sustain lactating Thoroughbred mares. The high moisture content of the pastures was thought to prevent the lactating mares from ingesting sufficient dry matter, and they avidly ate all high-DM forages offered to them. It is of note that these mares were able to maintain body condition when the same pastures were of lower moisture content (Marlow et al., 1983). Keenan (1986) also reported on the need to provide high-fiber supplements to horses consuming irrigated, low-DM, low-fiber pastures to prevent bark-chewing and other undesirable behaviors.

In two separate studies, Bigot et al. (1987) and Staun et al. (1989) independently fed groups of young horses either a high or low plane of nutrition during the winter, then grazed the two groups of horses together each summer, for 3–3.5 years. Although growth was slower in the animals fed less intensively in winter, they exhibited compensatory growth such that there was no difference in body weight between the different groups by the time the animals were 3 years old, demonstrating that pasture was not only able to support growth, but also was able to redress deficits arising from suboptimal feeding. However, it is of note that compensatory growth may be associated with an increased risk of developmental orthopedic disease (DOD). In areas with an extended growing season, young horses can maintain steadier growth rates on pasture. For example, the growth rates of young Thoroughbreds raised entirely on ryegrass-based pastures in New Zealand (Brown-Douglas, 2003) were similar to those reported elsewhere for this type of horse fed cereal concentrates and hay in addition to pasture (Hintz, 1979; Pagan, 1996).

Pastures can only supply the nutrient requirements of horses if they are stocked appropriately, where due account is taken of (1) the quality and yields of the forages, and (2) the size, workload, and physiological status of the animal. Annual DM yields from natural unimproved pastures can be less than 1 ton/hectare (t/ha), whereas those from well-managed improved pastures can be 15 t/ha or more (Morrison et al., 1980; Hopkins et al., 1990). Blue couch, white clover, and lotononsis (*Lotononsis bainessi*) pastures that provided 2.15 Mcal/kg DM and 145 g CP/kg DM met the energy and protein requirements of breeding, lactating, and re-breeding Thoroughbred mares when stocked at density of 1.6 ha per animal (Gallagher and McMeniman, 1988). Grace et al. (2002a,b, 2003) estimated that 0.2, 0.25, and 0.5 ha per animal was sufficient for weanlings, yearlings, and lactating mares, respectively, grazing ryegrass pastures yielding approximately 2 t DM/ha, but no allowance was made for herbage wastage in these calculations. However, Hunt (1995) regarded 1 ha as sufficient to support one-and-a-half 500-kg mares plus foals in New Zealand. Elphinstone (1981) concluded that 1-ha pastures of kikuyu, blue couch, and Rhodes grass met the nutritional requirements for a mature horse at maintenance or a working horse in spring and autumn. If pasture is the sole feed for horses, then knowledge of annual DM yield is desirable to enable efficient stocking and utilization of the pastures.

Many well-managed pastures can yield at least 5 t DM/ha per year. Coupled with conservation of grass in times of plenty, if well managed, an area of 1 ha of such pasture should be able to provide sufficient annual forage DM for a 500-kg horse requiring 10 kg DM/d, after accounting for pasture wastage due to treading and defecation and for losses during herbage conservation.

Pasture can meet or often exceed the overall energy and protein needs of many types of horses. However, intensively exercised horses or those working for long hours may not be able to meet their nutritional needs entirely from pasture, due to increased nutrient demands and reduced time available for grazing. Furthermore, diets high in indigestible fiber increase gut fill and, as a consequence, may increase BW, which may be a disadvantage in certain disciplines such as racing (Caroll and Huntingdon, 1988) or may be regarded as unsightly in the show horse. Although appropriate gut fill is regarded as beneficial for the endurance horse, as large amounts of forage in the hindgut may act as a reservoir for water and electrolytes (Duren, 1998), the presence of a visibly distended "hay-belly" is not desirable.

Pastures for Horses

Pasture species do not grow throughout the year. Their growth depends on soil temperature, moisture, and fertility. Growth is also affected by management practice; overgrazing will reduce yields and encourage growth of unpalatable species and weeds. Ideally, horse pastures should contain a mix of grasses and legume species that are adapted to the prevailing soil and climatic conditions and that can also withstand close grazing and wear. It is outside the scope of this text to provide a comprehensive review of all forage species used for horse pastures, soonly some of the more commonly used forage species are described here. Suitable cool-season species (those that start to grow when temperatures reach 7°C, with optimal growth between 16–24°C) include orchardgrass (*Dactylis glomerata*), toxin or endophyte-free tall fescue (*Festuca arundinacea*), and Kentucky bluegrass (*Poa pratensis*), which can all resist tight grazing and treading. Other suitable, perennial cool-season species include endophyte-free perennial ryegrass (*Lolium perenne*) varieties, which are palatable, high yielding, and of high nutritive value. Timothy (*Phleum pretense*) is also useful. It is a traditional species for horses and is late flowering, producing leafy herbage mid-summer when such forage may be scarce. However, timothy does not tolerate very close grazing, and late summer and autumn production may be low. Meadow fescue (*Festuca pratensis*), smooth bromegrass (*Bromus inermis*), Matua prairiegrass (*Bromus wildenowii*), and low-alkaloid varieties of reed canary grass (*Phalaris arundinaceae*) are also used for horse pastures. Fine-leaved fescues such as creeping red fescue (*Festuca rubra*) are good for production of a wear-resistant turf and useful in areas of high traffic, such as exercise areas or around water sources or gateways, but are of mediocre grazing value. Inclusion of legumes in horse pastures as minority species provides a good source of dietary protein and calcium. Furthermore, through their ability to "fix" atmospheric nitrogen, legumes enhance the nitrogen status of the soil, reducing the need for additional nitrogen fertilizer. Legume species that proliferate by rhizomes and stolons are suitable for horse pastures as they are less susceptible to aggressive defoliation and wear. White clover (*Trifolium repens*) is commonly found in pastures grazed by horses, being generally tolerant of close grazing and mixing well with most grasses. With proper management, white clover can persist in swards for many years. Alfalfa (*Medicago sativa* L.) is often recommended for horse pastures because of its high quality, yield, and compatibility with grasses; varieties that have their crowns beneath the soil are better able to tolerate damage by horses than standard cultivars (Jordan et al., 1995). Red clover (*Trifolium pratense*) is less tolerant of close grazing than white clover and generally requires reseeding every 2–3 years. Other legumes for horse pastures include bird's-foot trefoil (*Lotus corniculatus*) and sainfoin (*Onobrychis viciifolia*), although these often need careful establishment and grazing management if they are to persist in the sward. Both annual or perennial species of lespedeza (*Kummerowia* spp.) may also be used in horse pasture seed mixtures.

In hot, dry environments when most cool-season forages lie dormant, warm-season grasses (which start growth at 15°C with temperature optima of 32–35°C) can grow, providing a good source of forage in the summer months. Warm-season perennial grasses suitable for horses include Bermudagrass (*Cynodon dactylon*), which tolerates tight grazing and wear as does bahiagrass (*Paspalum notatum*), which will also grow in soils of low to mediocre fertility. Dallisgrass (*Paspalum dilatatum*) is also suitable, but requires more fertile soils with higher water content than bahiagrass. Various bluestem species (*Andropogon* spp.), such as Caucasian or big bluestem, may also be used. The warm-season annual species are generally of higher nutritive value than the warm-season perennials. Species used for horse pastures include pearl millet (*Pennisetum glaucum*) and crabgrass (*Digitaria* spp.). During cool periods, warm-season grasses are dormant. In areas that will allow their growth, use of both cool- and warm-season species can greatly extend the grazing season, as the majority of the cool-season grass production occurs in spring and autumn, whereas that of warm season species occurs in the summer. In suitable areas, this strategy allows grazing for much of the year, and annual herbage production can be further extended by seeding dormant warm-season perennial pastures with cool-season annual species such as annual ryegrass or small-grain species, e.g., wheat, rye, or oats.

Horses are spot grazers. They overgraze some areas of a pasture and defecate in others, which, if left unmanaged, results in overgrazed "lawns" and rank overgrowth of herbage in latrine areas, termed "roughs" (Odberg and Francis-Smith, 1976). Long-term rotational or co-grazing of large horse pastures with sheep or cattle is beneficial, as the ruminants will remove the roughs and may help break the lifecycle of equine parasites. This practice helps prevent the pasture from becoming "horse sick," where overgrazed lawns become subject to ingress of weed species, some of which may be toxic (e.g., *Seneccio* spp.) and the roughs grow unchecked, eventually producing overgrown herbage unpalatable even to ruminants. In the absence of other species of grazing livestock, strip grazing or division of grazing into three or four smaller paddocks will allow short-term rotation (often either 2 weeks grazing and 4 weeks rest, or 1 week grazing and 3 weeks rest) (Matches, 1992; Emmick and Fox, 1993; Henning, 1994). Coupled with daily removal of manure, this practice will help to prevent the development of roughs and lawns, and it can do much to increase the yield and quality of available grazing (Odberg and Francis-Smith, 1977). To prevent pasture deterioration, soils should be analyzed to enable appropriate maintenance levels of fertilizer to be applied. If lawns have developed, they can be preferentially fertilized to maintain the nutrient status of the sward.

Where growth of grass is excess to immediate requirements, the grass can be either stockpiled for winter feed or conserved. Stockpiling is the practice of allowing pastures to grow from mid-late summer onwards to produce stands of fairly mature sward. When autumn pastures have become depleted, animals can be strip-grazed on stockpiled pastures. Strip-grazing is necessary to maximize the use of the stockpiled fodder and to prevent excessive wastage via trampling and defecation on fresh sward, rendering it unpalatable. Stockpiling of permanent pastures can only be considered for free-draining soils or in areas subject to only moderate winter rainfall. Where these conditions are not met, the pasture may become irrecoverably damaged, necessitating complete reseeding. Stockpiling can be an economical alternative to forage preservation, but most domesticated equines receive some form of conserved forage for at least a portion of the year.

Conserved Forage for Horses

Forages may be conserved for use when there is little fresh forage available or when animals are confined to stalls. Such conservation is achieved by drying, ensiling, or applying preservatives. After drying, the forage may be chopped, ground and pelleted, cubed, or wafered, whereas ensiled forages are either bulk-stored in bunkers (clamps) or silos, or baled and wrapped in plastic film. The feed quality of conserved forage can be no greater than the original sward, and thus stage of plant maturity at time of harvest is an important factor influencing the feeding value of the final product. Young leafy swards have the highest feed quality but low yields. As plants mature, their DM increases. The leaf:stem ratio decreases with concomitant increases and decreases in fiber and protein, respectively. Preservation of high-moisture, young, leafy herbage as hay can be problematical in areas where good haymaking weather is uncertain; under those circumstances, such herbage is often ensiled.

Hay

The ultimate aim of haymaking is to produce a palatable, hygienic product that retains much of the nutrient quality of the original sward. This is achieved by minimizing nutrient losses in the field and curing the herbage to a stage that prevents molding and reduces nutrient losses and deterioration during storage.

There are inevitable biological and physical losses of DM and nutrients during haymaking, associated with drying, baling, and subsequent storage and usage. Drying of forage begins immediately after it is cut, but the rate of drying depends upon the differential in water vapor pressure between the surrounding air and in the surface tissues of the plant. When plant and air vapor pressure are equal, no further drying occurs (Technical Committee, 1964). Vapor pressure is affected by temperature, air movement, solute concentration, and water movement within the plant tissues. Hays made and stored in humid environments cannot achieve a DM as high as those made and stored under more arid conditions.

Different plant parts dry at different rates, with leaves tending to dry more rapidly than the thicker stem. This can lead to leaf shatter during mechanical handling and loss of the more nutritious leaf material (Shepherd et al., 1954; Rotz and Muck, 1994). Leaf shatter may account for DM losses from grass and legume hays of 2–5 and 3–35 percent, respectively. Use of mower/conditioners in which the stems are crushed and cuticular wax is scarified during cutting can help reduce losses due to leaf shatter by reducing the disparity in drying rates by various plant parts (Rotz and Muck, 1994; Rotz, 1995).

Plant respiration continues post-cutting and is responsible for loss of nutrients, particularly the NSC fractions (Wylam, 1953; Raguse and Smith, 1965), which account for the majority of respiratory DM losses during field curing of hay. Thus, the average WSC content of fresh, cool-season pasture grasses was 16 percent, whereas that of sun-cured hay was 10 percent (MAFF, 1992), and the NSC contents of fresh forage legume pasture vs. legume hays were 15 and 11 percent, respectively (Dairy One, 2003). In a summary of literature, Shephard et al. (1954) reported that such DM losses ranged from 4–16 percent, higher losses being associated with slower drying rates. Losses of CP and changes in constituent nitrogen fractions can occur during haymaking. Proteolysis during drying causes a rise in nonprotein nitrogen (NPN) and changes in amino-acid profiles (Brady, 1960), whereas the nitrate content is largely unaffected (Butler and Bailey, 1973). Other nutrient losses include some organic acids (James, 1953) and vitamins. Upward of 80 percent of carotene (the precursor of vitamin A) may be lost (Butler and Bailey, 1973), and vitamin E (alpha tocopherol) content also declines during haymaking (Miller, 1958). As the fiber fractions are relatively unaffected by plant respiration, their proportions increase during herbage drying. Once herbage moisture has been reduced to 400 g moisture/kg, plant respiration ceases, and further nutrient losses in the field are largely due to weathering and handling.

Hay yield and quality are reduced if exposed to rain during curing, through leaching of soluble components, with the amount of loss increasing with numbers of showers, amounts of rain, and the DM of the crop. Leaching has been reported to remove 20–40 percent of the DM, 20 percent of CP, 35 percent of NFC, and 30 and 65 percent, respectively, of phosphorus and potash (Shepherd et al., 1954). The average WSC contents of hays made from four cool-season species, which had received a light rain shower during drying, averaged half those of the original swards and losses of CP were up to 27 percent (Ince et al., 2006). Losses of NSC leached from alfalfa and red-clover hays exposed to heavy rain during curing resulted in a 45 percent increase in the proportion of fiber relative to hays protected from rain (Collins, 1983). Rain not only leaches nutrients, but also increases leaf shatter due to the extra mechanical operations required to dry the hay.

High-moisture hays may be effectively preserved through artificial drying in barns. Nutrient losses from hays dried in barns without added heat are usually lower than for hays dried in the field; addition of heat to 60°C to accelerate the drying process reduces DM losses still further through rapid inhibition of enzyme activity (Butler and Bailey, 1973). However, such heating can result in the formation of Maillard products (protein/carbohydrate complexes), which are resistant to proteases, thus reducing protein digestibility (Goering and Van Soest, 1967).

High-moisture (250 g/kg) hays can also be preserved via application of microbial inhibitors such as organic acids, buffered acids, or ammonia. Propionic acid or acid mixtures applied to hay at rates of 1–2:100 (volume:weight) generally reduce mold growth and heating. Short-term (30-day) studies with growing horses fed hay preserved with a propionate/acetic acid mixture showed no difference in acceptance or growth rate compared with those fed untreated hay, with no apparent ill effects, whereas in another study, horses preferred untreated alfalfa hay to that which had been treated with a similar propionate/acetic acid preparation (Lawrence et al., 1987, 2000). However, the expense incurred with barn drying and the corrosiveness and difficulties in working with acid or alkaline preservatives have limited their use in hay preservation (Collins and Owens, 2003).

Forages conserved as hay by desiccation should contain no more than 200 g moisture/kg, to prevent proliferation of microorganisms, heating (due to microbial respiration), and subsequent reduction of nutritive quality (Collins and Owens, 2003). However, under conditions of high (90–100 percent) relative humidity that favor microbial growth, hay stored at 200 g moisture/kg can become moldy. Under these circumstances, baling at lower moisture contents is necessary. For low-density bales, recommended moisture contents are around 180 g/kg; for more densely packed bales, drier hay of 120–140 g moisture/kg is suggested to improve preservation (Rotz and Muck, 1994; Rotz, 1995). There are usually minimal losses of DM or nutrients in hays stored at less than 150 g moisture/kg (Czerkawski, 1967). However, in hays of greater moisture content, varying losses occur during storage, mainly associated with microbial respiration (and heating), which, in turn, is affected by ambient conditions. It has been estimated that on average, during storage, hay of 150 g moisture/kg will lose 5 percent of DM, and this loss increases by 1 percent for every further 10 g/kg increase in moisture up to 200 g moisture/kg (Collins and Owens, 2003). Thus, DM losses were small for hays of 880–930 g DM/kg stored at temperatures of 7°C or less, but losses of 8 percent were recorded for hays of 820 g DM/kg stored at 36°C for 9 months, largely accounted for by losses in NSC (Czerkawski, 1967). Mineral content, lignin, and fiber fractions remained relatively stable during bale storage. DM losses during storage of large round bales of alfalfa hay (average DM 810 g/kg), which were either stored in a barn or outside with or without a cover, were 2.5, 6, and 15 percent, respectively (Belyea et al., 1985). Losses (biological and mechanical) of ryegrass hay stored on the ground over 7 months were 27 percent, whereas those for hays stored in a barn were 2.3 percent (Nelson et al., 1983). Total DM field and storage losses of conserved grass-legume mixes have been reported to range from 15–30 percent (Hoglund, 1964).

Large reductions in DM and quality occur during storage of hays containing more than 200 g moisture/kg, with excessive heating (due to microbial respiration) playing a significant role in the deterioration of high-moisture hays. Thus, hays of 840 g DM/kg heated little during storage and microbial contamination was low, whereas hays of 750 g DM/kg heated to more than 45°C and became obviously moldy with *Aspergillus* spp. Hays with DM contents of less than 600 g/kg reached temperatures of 60–65°C and contained thermophilic fungi (Gregory et al., 1963). Storage of hays of less than 700 g DM/kg may result in a charred product of lowered nutritive value, and extreme heating can result in spontaneous combustion (Browne, 1933). Studies on alfalfa hay baled at either 700 or 800 g DM/kg indicated that forage quality deterioration (increased NDF and unavailable nitrogen content) was greater for the higher moisture hays, deterioration being highly correlated with accumulated days of heating to > 30°C. The greatest changes in forage quality occurred between days 4 and 11 post-baling, but in the higher moisture hays, microbial activity was prolonged and caused further deterioration between days 11 and 22. Thereafter, there was little change in nutritive value (Coblentz et al., 1996). Likewise, in Bermudagrass hays baled at moistures ranging from 208–325 g/kg, there was a positive linear relationship between hay moisture content and spontaneous heating that, in turn, was significantly correlated with increased deterioration of nitrogen fractions (Coblentz et al., 2000). Hays visibly contaminated with molds should not be fed to horses. In addition to the reduction in feeding value, such hays may contain mycotoxins, and inhalation of fungal spores from molded forage can lead to respiratory compromise in both horses and their human attendants.

There is a paucity of information on comparisons of the nutritive value of hay and the sward of origin in equines. However, studies with ruminants have reported OM digestibilities of 73 and 65 percent for the original sward and hay, respectively (Shepperson, 1960), and well-cured alfalfa hay was reported to contain 15 percent less CP and be 10 percent less digestible than the original standing crop (Collins, 1990). Field losses of TDN in well-cured hays and those exposed to rain were, respectively, 26 and 42 percent (Shepherd et al., 1954.). Similarly, alfalfa and red-clover hays exposed to rain were 12 percent less digestible relative to hays protected from rain (Collins, 1983). Furthermore, ruminant digestibility of Bermudagrass hays was little affected by heating up to 48°C, but declined by 14 percent when internal bale temperatures exceeded 60°C (Coblentz et al., 1998). It is likely that reductions in the feeding value of such hays would also be seen in horses.

There may also be further DM losses of hay at feed-out. Weathered or otherwise unpalatable hay may be rejected, resulting in considerable wastage. When fed to heifers, losses from large round bales of alfalfa hay stored indoors or outside with or without cover were 12, 14, and 25 percent, respectively, resulting in total losses of 15, 20, and 40 percent of the original DM (Belyea et al., 1985). In the uncovered bales stored outside, rain weathered the outer portions equating to approximately 40 percent of the original hay DM. At feed-out, the animals wasted much of this material in their search for more palatable fodder in the center of the bale (Belyea et al., 1985). Likewise, feed refusals of ryegrass hay stored on the ground were 22 percent, compared with 1.2 percent of barn-stored hay; the sum of storage losses and animal wastage of these ryegrass hays equated to 49 and 3.5 percent of the original harvested DM for the ground and barn-stored hays, respectively (Nelson et al., 1983).

Hays of high nutritive value are characterized by a large proportion of leaf, and high protein and low NDF contents. DM yields of such "prime" quality hay are low, and a compromise between the nutritive value of the hay and DM yield is usually made to produce hays of various feed value or "grades." With the possible exception of lactating mares and growing youngstock, many horses are unlikely to require the very high CP contents of "prime" hay. If such high-protein forage is fed in conjunction with sufficient energy, the protein excess to requirements will be excreted, contributing to the environmental burden of excretory nitrogen. Furthermore, excess protein intakes may have detrimental acidogenic effects in sports horses (Graham-Thiers et al., 1991). Horses can be fed well-preserved hays with lower nutrient value, which can be supplemented as necessary during times of increased nutrient demand. Threshed mature hay, in which the seed has been removed, may also be fed to horses, but it is of low nutritional value (Schurg et al., 1978; Hyslop et al., 1998b).

It is of note, however, that the visual appearance of conserved forages is an imprecise indicator of their potential nu-

Hay Intakes

Contrary to fresh pasture intakes, higher voluntary dry matter intakes (VDMI) generally occur with alfalfa hay compared with long-grass hays (Cymbaluk, 1990a; Dulphy et al., 1997b; Crozier et al., 1997; LaCasha et al., 1999). The range of VDMI of long hays reported by a number of studies is detailed in Table 8-3. Intakes typically averaged between 2 and 2.4 percent of BW for grass and alfalfa hays, respectively. The mechanisms that control VDMI of hay in horses are unclear: it has been proposed that VDMI of hay is governed by energy requirement (Aiken et al., 1989), dry matter digestibility (Crozier et al., 1997), and cell wall content (St. Lawrence et al., 2001). However, Martin-Rosset and Vermorel (1991) found no consistent relationship between VDMI and energy requirement, and Dulphy et al. (1997a) failed to find a relationship between NDF, CF or CP, and VDMI of hay. Nevertheless, St. Lawrence et al. (2001) reported a significant relationship between the NDF content of four cool-season grass hays and VDMI ($p < 0.001$), and they were able to use this relationship to predict intakes of different hays by horses. Similarly, Reinowski and Coleman (2003) found a significant correlation between warm-season grass hay NDF content and VDMI. However, the reported relationships between NDF content and intakes did not account for all of the variation, and it is likely that VDMI of hay is controlled by a number of interacting factors.

Effect of Particle Size

Grass hay is normally fed to horses in the long form, and there was no difference in intakes of the same hay when chopped (Hyslop et al., 1998a; Morrow et al., 1999). However, when hays are presented in a dense form such as wafers or pellets, intakes have been reported to be greater than when hay of similar composition was fed loose, such that horses ate 0.17 and 0.24 more wafered and pelleted alfalfa hay, respectively, than when it was fed in the loose form (Haenlein et al., 1966). Likewise, the VDMI of horses fed long-stem, threshed ryegrass hay was significantly increased when the same material was pelleted, cubed, or briquetted (Schurg et al., 1978). Reported daily VDMI of horses fed loose alfalfa hays range from 73–122 g DM/kg $BW^{0.75}$ (Haenlein et al., 1966; Cymbaluk and Christiensen, 1986; Cymbaluk, 1990a; Crozier et al., 1997; Dulphy et al., 1997a,b), compared to 88.3–139 g DM/kg $BW^{0.75}$ for wafers, cubes, or pellets (Haenlein et al., 1966; Cymbaluk and Christiensen, 1986; Cymbaluk, 1990a; Todd et al., 1995). Furthermore, VDMI of horses fed pelleted high-fiber complete diets was some 2.6-fold that of the same complete feed offered as a chaff, when pellets were fed as the first

TABLE 8-3 Estimated Voluntary Dry Matter Intake (VDMI) of Various Hays by Horses and Ponies

Type of Horse	Type of Hay	VDMI (g DM/kg BW)	VDMI (g DM/kg $BW^{0.75}$)	Source
Yearling	Bermudagrass	21–25	111	Aiken et al. (1989); La Casha et al. (1999)
	Matua	28	128	LaCasha et al. (1999)
	Alfalfa	31	142	LaCasha et al. (1999)
Mature horses	Alfalfa	17.2–31	73–142	Crozier et al. (1997); Dulphy et al. (1997a,b); Haenlein et al. (1966); LaCasha et al. (1999)
	Altai wildrye		81.2	Cymbaluk (1990a)
	Bermudagrass		95.6	Aiken et al. (1989)
	Bluestem	22	115	Reinowski and Coleman (2003)
	Bromegrass		114	Cymbaluk (1990a)
	Crested wheatgrass		85	Cymbaluk (1990a)
	Eastern gammagrass	19		Reinowski and Coleman (2003)
	India grass	22		Reinowski and Coleman (2003)
	Kentucky bluegrass		82.3	Cymbaluk (1990a)
	Oat hay		81.2	Cymbaluk (1990a)
	Reed canarygrass		99.4	Cymbaluk (1990a)
	Tall fescue		111	Crozier et al. (1997)
	Timothy	29.2		Reinowski and Coleman (2003)
	Early cut grass	18.2	87	Dulphy et al. (1997a, 1997b)
	Re-growth grass	20	96	Dulphy et al. (1997a, 1997b)
Mature ponies	High-quality grass hay		110	Hyslop et al. (1998a)
	Poor-quality grass hay		113	Hyslop et al. (1998a)
	Mature threshed grass hay		95.6	Hyslop et al. (1998b)
	Meadow hay	26	153	Pearson and Merrit (1991)
	Mature meadow hay	14.7	63	Moore-Colyer and Longland (2000)

feed in a crossover design experiment. The pellets were more rapidly consumed than the chaff, largely due to faster bite rates and decreased chewing, and thus the chaff-fed animals spent more time feeding (Argo et al., 2002). It is of note that rapid intakes of pelleted diets may elicit the onset of undesirable behaviors such as wood-chewing (Haenlein et al., 1966), and it is a common perception that addition of chopped conserved forage to sweet feeds, grains, or pelleted feeds will reduce the rate of meal intake. However, although Ellis et al. (2005) recorded a 120 percent increase in feed intake time by horses when chopped Lucerne straw was added to pelleted feeds, there was no effect on speed of consumption when similar types of chaff were fed with oats (Harris et al., 2005; Brussow et al., 2005).

Digestibility of Hay

The digestibility of hay depends upon the plant species, maturity at harvest, leaf:stem ratio, speed of drying, and conditions under which it has been stored. Nutrient digestibilities of several long-grass and legume hays by horses reported in the literature are shown in Table 8-4. It is of note that artificially, rapidly dehydrated grass had higher digestibilities of DM, CP, NDF, and gross energy (GE) than when the same crop was field-cured as hay (Hyslop et al., 1998a). The DE of grass hays averaged 1.79 Mcal/kg DM, the range being 1.40–2.13 Mcal/kg DM, with the DE of alfalfa hay averaging 2.42. The digestibility of CP in grass hays averaged 53 percent (range 20–74), whereas that for alfalfa was 74 (range 64–83 percent). In a survey of the literature of the digestibility of grass hays by horses, Chenost and Martin-Rosset (1985) found digestibilities of OM, CP, and crude fiber (CF) to average 56, 72, and 38 percent, respectively, for hays with a CP content of greater than 120 g/kg. These authors found corresponding values for hays containing 80–120 g CP/kg to be 49, 55, and 44. For low-protein hays of less than 80 g CP/kg, the digestibilities for OM, CP, and CF were 44, 27, and 47 percent, respectively. Although densification of forages appears to increase intakes, total tract nutrient digestibility does not usually appear to be affected. Thus, processing alfalfa hay into pellets, cubes, or by chopping had little effect on total tract digestibility of DM, CF, CP, or minerals (Jackson et al., 1985; Pagan and Jackson, 1991a; Todd et al., 1995). Likewise, similar apparent digestibilities of DM, GE, and NDF of a chaffed or pelleted high-fiber diet fed to ponies were observed by Argo et al., (2002) and the nutritive value (digestibility and mean retention time) of long hay or long silage was similar to that of the corresponding short chopped feed (Morrow et al., 1999). No differences in digestibility of OM, NDF, or CP were observed by Drogoul et al. (2000a) when pelleted or chopped hay was fed at similar intakes to ponies. The pelleted hay rations were retained in the large intestine longer, which when combining evidence of similar digestibility, suggests pelleting slowed the rate of fiber degradation in the hindgut. Certainly, grinding and pelleting hay caused a significant decrease in both the rate and extent of in situ NDF degradation (Drougoul et al., 2000a,b). However, the apparent DM, CP, ADF, and cell wall constituent digestibilities of long-stem threshed ryegrass hay were reported to be 58, 60, 34, and 40 percent, respectively, when fed to horses at 1.5 percent of BW (Schurg et al., 1978). However, when the same material was cubed, briquetted, or pelleted, DMD was significantly reduced ($P < 0.05$). Furthermore, the ADF digestibility of the pellets was 25 percent, being significantly lower ($P < 0.05$) than for the long-stem (34 percent), cubed (34 percent), or briquetted (31 percent) material.

Cereal Straw

Voluntary dry matter intakes of horses fed cereal straws ad libitum are generally reported as being lower than for grass or legume hays (see Chapter 11). Thus, pooled data from a number of studies showed that VDMI of cereal straw averaged 54 and 64 percent of the intakes of alfalfa and grass hays, respectively (Dulphy et al., 1997b). However, if oat (Hyslop and Calder, 2001) or wheat (Hansen et al., 1992) straw was fed with alfalfa (1:1), VDMI was similar to a 100 percent alfalfa diet.

The calculated DE value of wheat straw was low, at only 43 and 57 percent of alfalfa and Midwest prairie hays, respectively, with DMD and fiber digestibilities of 23 and 11 percent (Hansen et al., 1992). The DM, CP, and fiber digestibilities of oat straw calculated by difference were 32–50 percent with a DE of 1.97 Mcal/kg DM (Hyslop and Calder, 2001). Treatment can improve the nutrient digestibility of straw. When wheat straw was ammoniated, there was a significant ($P < 0.05$) increase in both the digestibility of DM (23 percent untreated vs. 44 percent ammoniated) and NDF (11 vs. 36 percent) (Hansen et al., 1992). Low intakes of straw may be related to an increased mean gastrointestinal particle retention time (Pearson and Merrit, 1991; Pearson et al., 2001) and are associated with extended feeding and chewing times, presumably due, at least in part, to the recalcitrant nature of the lignified cell walls of the stem.

Problems with Feeding Hay and Straw

Alfalfa hay is high in minerals, especially calcium and magnesium, and their possible role in the formation of enteroliths is discussed in Chapter 12. Furthermore, some alfalfa hay harvests can be contaminated with blister beetles that produce cantharidin, a highly toxic chemical that can be fatal to horses (Schoeb and Panciera, 1978). The generally low intake of cereal straws precludes their use as the sole diet unless they are being fed to occupy animals undergoing a weight reduction program. Some cereal straws contain high levels of silica, which has been implicated in the formation of urinary calculi (Nash, 1999). Forages high in sil-

FEEDS AND FEED PROCESSING

TABLE 8-4 Apparent Dry Matter, Organic Matter, Energy, Protein, and Fiber Digestibilities[a] of Various Hays in Horses

Type of Horse	Type of Hay	DMD[b]	DE (Mcal/kg DM)	OMD[c]	CPD[d]	GED[e]	NDFD/(ADFD)[f]	Source
Mature mares	Elephant grass	43		45	25	41	40	Almeida et al. (1999)
	Alfalfa	55		57	71	53	36	
	Coastgrass	50		51	56	48	63	
Yearling Quarter horse	Matua bromegrass	51		64	74		47	LaCasha et al. (1999)
	Coastal Bermudagrass	46		60	64		52	
	Alfalfa	63		74	83		24	
Mature cross-bred geldings	Altai wildrye	47	2.03		54	44	50	Cymbaluk (1990a)
	Bromegrass	48	2.12		51	45	44	
	Crested wheatgrass	42	1.82		29	40	41	
	Kentucky bluegrass	45	1.95		59	44	51	
	Oat hay	48	2.08		60	47	44	
	Reed canarygrass	38	1.58		52	38	34	
Mature Arabians	Alfalfa	58			73		47	Crozier et al. (1997)
	Tall fescue	48			67		44	
	Caucasian bluestem	44			43		41	
Mature ponies	Alfalfa	62	2.58		77		41[a]	Cymbaluk and Christiensen (1986)
	Oat	55	2.33		68		37[a]	
	Bromegrass	51	2.13		67		39[a]	
	Slough	43	1.75		57		42[a]	
Mature ponies	Chopped alfalfa	53	2.25	51	64	49	29	Hyslop and Calder (2001)
	Meadow hay	36–44	1.4	36–40	20–29	33–33	40–41[g]	Moore-Colyer and Longland (2000) McClean et al. (2000); Hale and Moore-Colyer (2001)
Mature ponies	Dehydrated grass	47	2.3	50	62	50	51	Hyslop et al. (1998a)
	Mature meadow hay	0.41	2.17	44	48	45	40	
Mature ponies	Mature threshed grass hay	30	1.49	30	31	33	28	Hyslop et al. (1998b)
Mature horses	Alfalfa			56	75			Van der Noot and Gilbreath (1970)
	Timothy orchardgrass			49	54			
	Bromegrass			49	60			
Mature horses	Hay > 120 g CP/kg			56	68–75			Hintz (1969); Van der Noot and Gilbreath (1970) in Chenost and Martin-Rosset (1985)
	Hay 81–119 g CP/kg			49	54			
	Hay < 80 g CP/kg			38–49	10–43			

[a] Digestibilities are expressed as percentages.
[b] DMD = dry matter digestibility.
[c] OMD = organic matter digestibility.
[d] CPD = crude protein digestibility.
[e] GED = gross energy digestibility.
[f] NDFD/ADFD = NDF or ADF digestibility.
[g] Total nonstarch polysaccharides (NSP) digestibility.

ica are known to be of reduced digestibility for a number of livestock species (Laca et al., 2001).

Although there have been a number of studies on the role of dried forage in the elicitation of colic, the evidence is contradictory. Thus, in a study in the United States of 21,800 horses across 28 states on 1,026 premises, no association was found between development of colic and either type of dried forage or frequency of feeding (Traub-Dargatz et al., 2001). However, other studies have reported forage type, form, or a change in dietary forage to influence colic risk (Tinker et al., 1997; Cohen et al., 1999; Hudson et al., 2001; Hillyer et al., 2002; Little and Blickslager, 2002). Bearing in mind such equivocal findings, it may be prudent to introduce new feeding regimens, forage types, or batches gradually over time.

Other problems associated with feeding hay include the elicitation of respiratory compromise. Even well-made and stored hay, which to the naked eye appears "clean," contains considerable numbers of respirable particles (such as dust and fungal spores), which can lead to the onset of allergic respiratory disease in horses (Clarke, 1992; Robinson et al., 1995; Robinson, 2001). In an effort to prevent such problems, it is common practice to soak hay in water to reduce the number of respirable particles; however, if soaked for more than 10 minutes, this operation results in the loss of considerable amounts of minerals, particularly sodium, potassium, and phosphorus, and extended periods of soaking reduces WSC content (Moore-Colyer, 1996; Blackman and Moore-Colyer, 1998), substantially reducing the nutrient content of the hay. Hay contaminated with nonforage plant species can also present a hazard to equine health. During forage harvesting, poisonous weeds, which may normally be avoided in the fresh state by grazing equids, can become incorporated into the swath. In some cases, drying or wilting of such weeds renders them palatable to horses without affecting their toxicity. One such example is the hepatotoxic weed, ragwort (*Sennecio* spp.); the repeated ingestion of even small amounts of ragwort can prove fatal (Knottenbelt, 2000). It is therefore essential that fields destined for conservation as hay or silage are free of such weeds.

Ensiled Forages

Forages may be conserved as silage when weather conditions are not sufficiently reliable for hay production. During ensiling, forage is preserved by anaerobic fermentation of the NSC fraction to organic acids, resulting in a decline in pH usually from about pH 6 to 4.5. The acidity prevents the growth of spoilage microorganisms. As a consequence of fermentation of NSC fractions during ensilage, ensiled forages are low in NSC compared to the original sward. Silage is classified according to DM content: low-DM silages are approximately 30 percent DM, wilted silages are commonly 30–40 percent DM, and high-DM silages (often referred to as haylage) are usually between 40–65 percent DM.

There are few reports on feeding ensiled forages to horses, as they have historically been regarded as unsuitable for horses due to (1) their acidity and perceived laxative effects (Pillner, 1992) and (2) questionable hygienic quality, as silage can occasionally contain *Listeria* spp. or *Clostridium botulinum* (the causal agent of botulism), to which horses are highly susceptible (Ricketts et al., 1984). However, with the advent of high-DM-baled silage, there is often insufficient moisture for the proliferation of *Clostridia* spp. and feeding haylage to horses is becoming increasingly popular. Especially as compared to hay, well-preserved silage is relatively low in aeroallergens (Vandenput et al., 1997). In a survey of 99 silages (mean DM 631g/kg ± 137) and 53 hays fed to a total of 323 horses, Coenen et al. (2003) did not detect any problems of intake or nutrient digestibility associated with feeding silage, and although average fecal DM was significantly ($P < 0.05$) lower in the silage-fed horses compared to those given hay, the differences were small (188 vs. 203 g/kg, respectively). Furthermore fecal pH was significantly ($P < 0.05$) higher in the horses fed the silage diets compared with those fed hay (pH 6.78 vs. 6.62). The authors concluded that grass silage was suitable forage for horses, although silages can be relatively high in nonprotein nitrogen, which is of little nutritional value to horses (see Chapter 4).

Silage Intakes

High-DM grass silage (haylage) was well accepted by ponies. Daily VDMI ranged from 61–98 g DM/kg $BW^{0.75}$, equivalent to 1.47–2.2 percent of BW (Morrow et al., 1999; Moore-Colyer and Longland, 2000; Bergero et al., 2002), as shown in Table 8-5. It is of note that the highest haylage intakes were by ponies in medium work compared with those at maintenance or in light work (Bergero et al., 2002), which may suggest that nutrient requirements were influencing intakes. However, comparatively low-DM clamp (bunker) silage was not so palatable, and VDMI was 38.8 g DM/kg $BW^{0.75}$ d (0.92 percent BW/d) (Moore-Colyer and Longland, 2000). McLean et al. (1995) reported that intakes of low-DM clamp grass silage were less than 50 percent of intakes of hay, as were intakes of 32 percent DM maize (corn) silage (Martin-Rosset and Dulphy, 1987; Martin-Rosset et al., 1987). However, low-DM cannot be the sole determinant for reduced intakes of ensiled forages by horses, as intakes of red-clover silage were 31 and 20 percent higher than for hay and haylage, respectively, despite the red-clover silage having a DM content of 268 g/kg vs. 852 and 371 g DM/kg for hay and haylage, respectively (Hale and Moore-Colyer, 2001). High-DM alfalfa silage was also found to be highly palatable for ponies at 76.8 g DM/kg $BW^{0.75}$ d (1.9 percent of BW/d) (Murray, 2004). With the exception of the low-DM grass and maize silages, it was concluded that ad libitum access to grass and legume haylage could lead to obesity in ponies, and therefore intakes of such forages should be restricted.

Digestibility of Ensiled Forages

The digestibility of ensiled grass were substantially higher than grass hays (Table 8-6). Thus, percentage digestibilities of DM, CP, and fiber for haylage and clamp silage (in parenthesis) averaged 58 (66), 61 (67), and 60 (76), respectively, with the corresponding values for the grass hay being 37, 25, and 41 (Morrow et al., 1999; Moore-Colyer and Longland, 2000; Bergero et al., 2002). Thus the

FEEDS AND FEED PROCESSING

TABLE 8-5 Voluntary Dry Matter Intakes (VDMI) of Ensiled Forages by Ponies and Horses

Type of Horse	Type of Forage	DM %	VDMI (kg/d)	VDMI (g DM/kg BW/d)	VDMI (g DM/kg BW$^{0.75}$ d)	Source
Ponies	Meadow hay	92	4.95	14.7	62.9	Moore-Colyer and Longland (2000)
	Haylage	67	6.3	18.4	79.2	
	Big bale silage	50	5.96	17.3	74.6	
	Clamp silage	34	2.95	9.17	38.8	
	Meadow hay	85	5.5			Hale and Moore-Colyer (2001)
Ponies	Big bale grass silage	37	6.1			
	Big bale red-clover silage	27	7.2			
Ponies	Long or short chop grass silage	36	4.4	14.6	61	Morrow et al. (1999)
Ponies at maintenance	Grass haylage	55	6.5		85	Bergero et al. (2002)
Ponies in light work^a	Grass haylage	63	6.7	20.5	87	
Ponies in medium work^b	Grass haylage	65	7.6	22.3	98	
Horses	Maize silage	31			40.6	Martin-Rosset and Dulphy (1987)
Ponies	Alfalfa silage	30		19.3	76.8	Murray (2004)

^{a}10-min walk, 20-min trot, and 5-min gallop per day.
^{b}40-min walk, 80-min trot, and 20-min gallop per day.

DE and digestible crude protein (DCP) values of the hay were 1.38 Mcal/kg DM and DCP 6 g/kg DM, respectively, while the corresponding average values for the haylages were 2.28 Mcal/kg DM and 54 g DCP/kg DM (Moore-Colyer and Longland, 2000). These authors reported that the theoretical DE and DCP maintenance requirements of ponies fed the haylages were exceeded by up to 1.7- and 2.2-fold for DE and DCP, respectively, but the DE and DCP intakes of ponies fed a poor-quality hay were only 0.9 and 0.2 of their requirements. Although the clamp silage was of high

TABLE 8-6 Apparent Dry Matter, Organic Matter, Protein, and Energy Digestibility of Ensiled Forages by Ponies

Horse Type	Type of Forage	DMD^a	OMD^b	CPD^c	GED^d	CFD^e	TNSPD/ NDFD^f	Source
Welsh ponies	Grass hay	39	40	20	33		41	Moore-Colyer and Longland (2000)
Welsh ponies	Grass haylage	57	57	48	52		45	
Welsh ponies	Big bale silage	61	62	66	55		67	
Welsh ponies	Clamp silage	67	67	68	55		76	
					65			
Ponies at maintenance	Haylage	58	57	77	52	48		Bergero et al. (2002)
Ponies in light work^g	Haylage 63% DM	55	55	57	50	45		
Ponies in medium work^h	Haylage 65% DM	49	49	60	50	33		
					44			
Ponies	Hay	36	36	29				Hale and Moore-Colyer (2001)
Ponies	Big bale grass silage	69	70	68				
Ponies	Big bale red-clover silage	74	74	80				
Ponies	Long or short chop grass silage	67		74			62	Morrow et al. (1999)
Ponies	Alfalfa silage	62	60	76	59		55/49	Murray (2004)

NOTE: Digestibilities are expressed as percentages.
^{a}DMD = dry matter digestibility.
^{b}OMD = organic matter digestibility.
^{c}CPD = crude protein digestibility.
^{d}GED = gross energy digestibility.
^{e}CFD = crude fiber digestibility.
^{f}TNSPD/NDFD = total nonstarch polysaccharides (NSP) digestibility or neutral detergent fiber (NDF) digestibility.
^{g}10-min walk, 20-min trot, and 5-min gallop per day.
^{h}40-min walk, 80-min trot, and 20-min gallop per day.

nutritive value with a DE of 2.87 Mcal/kg DM and 104 g DCP/kg DM, intakes were only just sufficient to meet the maintenance energy requirement of the ponies. The digestibility of red-clover silage was significantly greater than either grass silage or hay with a DE value of approximately 3 Mcal/kg DM and 154 g DCP/kg DM. Intakes of red-clover silage by ponies exceeded their theoretical energy and protein maintenance requirements by 2.7- and 5.5-fold, respectively (Hale and Moore-Colyer, 2001). There is clearly a need to restrict intakes of such highly nutritious forms of conserved forage. In a survey of 239 horses fed high-DM (average 63 percent DM, 12.4 percent CP) grass haylage and 147 fed hay (85 percent DM, 10 percent CP), Coenen et al. (2003) reported that grass silage yielded sufficient nutrients to meet the requirements of most classes of horses except lactating mares.

Potential Problems of Feeding Ensiled Forage

The hygienic quality of ensiled products for horses is paramount, as horses do not possess the ability of ruminants to metabolize certain toxins. Care should be exercised to ensure that no soil or animal carcasses are ensiled with the forage as this can lead to proliferation of the bacterium *Clostridium botulinum*, the causal agent of botulism that can be fatal in horses (Ricketts et al., 1984). Furthermore, ensiled products that have been subject to aerobic spoilage (molding) should not be fed.

Anti-Quality Factors in Forages

Although all of the pasture species described in Chapter 11 have been fed to horses, some may contain substances that are injurious to health and performance. These anti-quality factors may be inherent to the forage, or they may be the result of microbial or insect contamination of fresh or conserved forages. In many cases, only very small amounts of anti-quality factors are required to exert an unfavorable effect on horse health. Some of these anti-quality factors are described below.

Inherent Plant Anti-Nutrients

High oxalate and phytate levels in some warm-season grasses including kikuyu grass or setaria may cause calcium and phosphorus deficiency in horses, leading to osteodystrophia fibrosa (ODF) (Elphinstone, 1981; Williams, 1987), and calcium and phosphorus supplements should be provided for growing or lactating mares grazing such pastures (McKenzie et al., 1981), as detailed more fully in Chapter 14. Sorghum, Sudan grass, hybrid Johnson grass, and sorghum-Sudan grass hybrids are not recommended for horses as they contain varying levels of cyanogenic glycosides, with particularly high levels observed in young rapidly growing plants. When the plant tissues are stressed, such as through frost, drought, or mechanical injury, free cyanide can be released.

Some varieties of white clover are also cyanogenic, and these varieties should be avoided in horse pastures (Clark et al., 1990). Acute ingestion of significant amounts of cyanide can lead to rapid death due to respiratory paralysis, and consumption of low levels over a prolonged period can cause abortion in mares, a staggering gait, cystitis, and weight loss (Adams et al., 1969; Turner and Szczawinski, 1991). Alsike clover (*Trifolium hybridum*) contains hepatotoxic alkaloids. Consumption by horses may result in photosensitization of unpigmented skin, loss of condition, neurological disturbance, and eventual hepatic failure (Cooper and Johnson, 1984; Cheeke and Schull, 1985). There is a widely held belief that horses ingesting fresh or conserved forages containing high levels of nitrates can suffer from nitrate poisoning. High levels of herbage nitrate can be caused by excessive application of nitrogen fertilizer or when plants have been subject to cool temperatures, low light intensity, or water stress (Allison, 1998). Pasture species known to accumulate nitrates include barley, bromegrass, corn, Johnson grass, oat hay, orchardgrass, rape, sorghum, sweet clover, and wheat. Nitrates remain stable in well-cured hay, but in moist hay, microbial action can convert nitrate to the more toxic nitrite. Nitrates, however, are substantially reduced in ensiled forages. As nitrates tend to accumulate in plant bases, harvesting herbage with a raised cutting height may help reduce the nitrate content of conserved forages. Alfalfa hay grown in soils high in selenium may accrue selenium levels up to 50 ppm (Davies et al., 2004). Ingestion of such hay in horses can lead to selenium toxicosis.

Contamination by Insects

Alfalfa hay can contain blister beetles (*Epicauta vittat* and *E. pennsylvanica*), which produce cantharidin that is highly toxic to horses and can be fatal (Schoeb and Panciera, 1978).

Microbial Contamination

Bacteria

The bacterium *Clostridium botulinum*, the casual agent of botulism, can be found in ensiled forages that are contaminated with soil or small animal carcasses. Botulism in horses is frequently fatal (Ricketts et al., 1984; Hunter et al., 2002). *Listeria monocytogenes*, the causal agent of listeriosis in horses, may also be found in poorly preserved silages and was associated with listeriosis in a number of Icelandic ponies that had consumed spoiled grass silage contaminated with the bacterium (Gudmundsdottir et al., 2004).

Fungi

Contamination of forages by fungi depends upon a number of factors, including the health and physiological status of the plant, harvesting methods, weather conditions during harvest, speed of stabilizing the conserved forage, and ambient conditions during transport and storage. Fungi may be surface contaminants of herbage or may invade plant tissues and cause disease (plant pathogens) or reside within the plant without causing any immediate, overt negative effects (endophytes) (Bacon and White, 2000). Contamination of forages with any of the above classes of fungi can reduce both their palatability and intake. It may result in some form of mycotoxicosis, the degree of which depends upon the amount and duration of mycotoxin ingestion. The cumulative effects of ingestion of low levels of mycotoxins may possibly contribute to a gradual deterioration of equine health and performance. As a general rule, feeding forages contaminated with fungi should be avoided.

Fresh pastures in Europe have been found contaminated with *Claviceps*, *Pythomyces*, *Neotyphodium*, and *Rhizoctonia* spp. (Le Bars and Le Bars, 1996). *Claviceps* spp. produce sclerotia, termed ergots, and infect a number of gramminaceous forages, including species of ryegrass, canarygrass, dallisgrass, and various native species. Ergots produce a range of toxic alkaloids, such as ergotamine, which may result in death within hours of ingestion (Wilcox, 1899). Ergots are found on seed heads, and thus ingestion can be avoided by ensuring pastures are regularly clipped or tightly grazed to prevent seed-head formation. *Fusarium* spp. are frequently associated with fresh pastures and, under appropriate environmental conditions, may produce tricothecenes zearolone and/or fumonisins (Scudamore and Livesey, 1998; Yiannikouris and Jouany, 2002), the latter being known to cause blind staggers (equine leucoencephalomalacia) and death in horses. Red clover or alfalfa infected with *Rhizoctonia leguminicola* may contain slaframine, resulting in excessive salivation and increased water consumption by horses. Slaframine breaks down with storage; levels were reported to decline from 100 mg/kg to 7 mg/kg after 10 months (Hagler and Behlow, 1981).

Hay produced and stored under humid conditions may contain a wide range of fungal contaminants in addition to *Fusarium* spp. Thus, *Asperigillus*, *Stachybotrys*, and *Penicillium* spp. may all be found in insufficiently dried hay or straw, and, as a result, these conserved forages may contain an array of mycotoxins including aflatoxins and patulin, in addition to those produced by *Fusarium* spp. (Le Bars, 1976; Clevstroem et al., 1981; Scudamore and Livesey, 1998). Aflatoxins cause reduced feed intakes, weight loss, hepatic disease, and brain, kidney, and heart damage in horses (Hintz, 1990). Patulin has been shown to be carcinogenic in laboratory animals and symptoms may include neurological disorders (Riley, 1998), but there is little information pertaining to effects in horses. Certain strains of *Stachybotrys* spp. that are common saprophytes of improperly dried hay and straw produce trichothecene satratoxins, which cause stachybotrytoxicosis, a fatal hemorrhagic disorder in horses (Forgacs, 1965, 1972). Cereal straws may be contaminated with the tricothecene deoxynivalenol (DON), known to cause a range of severe disorders in many livestock species, although the reported effects of this mycotoxin on horses is an area of debate. Reports range from no apparent effect on barren mares or geldings when fed over 40 days (Johnson et al., 1997) through reduced intake (Raymond et al., 2003) to being implicated in colic cases in a retrospective study by North Carolina State University. However, the presence of other mycotoxins in the feed of the latter two studies make it difficult to ascribe a strict cause-and-effect relationship between DON and unfavourable effects on horses.

Properly ensiled forages (whereby near-anaerobic conditions have been achieved coupled with a rapid decline in pH) should be relatively free of fungal contaminants. However, where conditions are aerobic and pH reduction is compromised, fungal contamination may occur, with the resultant production of a number of mycotoxins (Dutton et al., 1984). Patulin was found in the majority of corn silages tested in a study in France (Escoula, 1977) and ochratoxin A and citrinin (nephrotoxic in many species) have been found in corn silages and hays (Carlton and Tuite, 1977). *Penicillium roqueforti* varieties that can produce patulin, botryodiploidin, and penitrem A were the main contaminant of European grass, sugar-beet, and corn silages (Nout et al., 1993). Although no reference to the activity of such mycotoxins in horses has been found, they have been reported to be injurious to cattle. *Aspergillus*, *Penicillium*, and *Fusarium* spp. have all been found present in silage 2–3 months old, whereas *Byssochlamys nivea*, a patulin producer, appeared after 6 months of silage storage (Le Bars and Le Bars, 1996). Improperly conserved yellow sweet-clover (*Melilotus officinalis*) or white sweet-clover (*Melilotus alba*) hay, haylage, or silage may be contaminated with *Penicillium* spp., which can convert nontoxic coumarin to the toxin dicoumarol. Symptoms of dicoumarol poisoning include nasal bleeding, joint swelling, lameness, and respiratory difficulties (Hendrix, 2003). Dicoumarol levels are often higher in large round bales where the hay tends to be of lower dry matter than in small, rectangular bales. Forages may harbor a number of fungal contaminants at any one time, and mycotoxins have been reported to act in synergy in some species. Thus, fusaric acid enhanced fumonisin activity in poultry (D'Mello and MacDonald, 1997), and diacetoxyscirpenol acted in synergy with trichothecenes in pigs (Smith et al., 1997). It is conceivable that similar synergistic mechanisms between mycotoxins may also occur in horses.

Endophyte Contamination

The toxic endophyte *Neotyphodium coenophialum* (formerly *Acremonium coenophialum*), an inhabitant of tall fescue in U.S. pastures, is a common problem, due to production of the alkaloid ergovaline, causing late abortion, prolonged gestation, dystocia, and agalactia in broodmares and reduced growth in young horses (Hoveland, 1992; Aiken et al., 1993). In the United States, the threshold levels of ergovaline in horse feeds are 0.3–0.5 mg/kg. Varieties of tall fescue are now available that are inhabited by nontoxic strains of endophyte; however, tall fescue containing the toxic form of the endophytes may be more hardy and can reestablish in pastures. Perennial ryegrass infected with the endophyte *Neotyphodium lolii* produces the toxic alkaloid lolitrem B, which causes ryegrass staggers (Stynes and Bird, 1983). Although there is no threshold set for lolitrem B concentrations in horse fodder, two groups of horses were observed to suffer ataxia, tremors, and paralysis when fed ryegrass hay containing 5–6 mg lolitrem B/kg (Sloet van Oldruitenborgh-Oosterbaan et al., 1999), and ponies fed a sole diet of ryegrass seed cleanings containing 5.3 mg lolitrem B/kg were symptomatic of ryegrass staggers.

Good-quality hay should be free of mold, dust, and weeds. Contamination of hay and straw by fungi can be reduced by drying to at least 85 percent DM. Where such conditions cannot be achieved, the use of antifungal agents such as propionic acid to reduce the pH to levels below that tolerated by most contaminating fungi can be employed. During ensilage, ensuring anaerobic conditions and enhancing a rapid decline in pH immediately post-harvest by the use of various biological inoculants and/or enzyme preparations can help reduce levels of fungal contaminants. Other biological strategies for reducing the effects of mycotoxins include use of bacterial strains that limit mycotoxin bioavailability (El-Nezami et al., 1988; Yoon and Baeck, 1999) or those that metabolize or biotransform them (Nakazato et al., 1990). These latter methods are as yet somewhat slow and inefficient, and methods for inoculating feedstuffs with non-mycotoxin-producing strains to outcompete those that produce toxins have been areas of investigation (Cotty and Bhatnagar, 1994). Use of forage varieties bred for resistance to fungal contaminants is a more direct and potentially efficient approach to reducing the incidence of mycotoxicosis from forages (Yiannikouris and Jouany, 2002).

Forage/Fiber Requirement

There are no reports of trials that prove a direct requirement for forage/fiber in horse diets. Nevertheless, fibrous forages clearly form the basis of the diet of wild equids, and there is a large body of circumstantial evidence that suggests that insufficient dietary fiber in equid diets can lead to hindgut acidosis (Medina et al., 2002), colic (Tinker et al., 1997), gastric ulcers (Murray and Schusser, 1989), increased risk of crib-biting and wood-chewing (Keenan, 1986; McGreevy et al., 1995; Redbo et al., 1998), and behavioral problems (Gillham et al., 1994). It is known that oversupply of starch or other rapidly fermentable carbohydrates can result in lactate acidosis, hindgut dysfunction, colic, and laminitis in horses (Garner et al., 1977; Pollit et al., 2003). Potter et al. (1992a) recommended a maximum of 4.0 g starch/kg BW/meal to prevent such disorders, whereas Meyer et al. (1993) were more conservative in their recommendation of a maximum of 2 g starch/kg BW/meal to prevent hindgut dysfunction. Even the latter recommendation for maximum amounts of starch to be fed per meal may be somewhat high for some equids, as even 2.1 g starch/kg BW/meal from a hay-cube:rolled-barley diet (50:50) was sufficient to elicit unfavorable changes in intracecal fermentation in ponies (McClean et al., 2000). However, the undesirable effects of high starch intakes (3.4 g starch/kg BW/meal) on hindgut function were reduced when the diet contained an NDF:starch ratio of 1:1 (Medina et al., 2002). Keenan (1986) reported that young horses that grazed on lush, low-fiber pastures indulged in substantial bark-stripping. Lactating mares grazing low-DM, low-fiber pastures avidly consumed supplemental high-fiber feedstuffs (Marlow et al., 1983). The incidence of horses performing oral stereotypies, such as wood-chewing, was reduced when long hay, as opposed to a pelleted diet, was fed (Willard et al., 1977) and increasing the amount of hay and decreasing the amount of sweet feed resulted in decreased incidence of crib-biting (Gillham et al., 1994). Extended feeding time and greater buffering of gastric contents (due to increased saliva production) have been implicated in the reduction of undesirable oral behaviors through increased provision of long forage. Certainly, surveys have shown that the risk of crib-biting is increased by low-forage or high-starch diets (McGreevy et al., 1995; Redbo et al., 1998), and foals fed concentrates at weaning were four times more likely to crib-bite than those that were not (Waters et al., 2002; Bachmann et al., 2003). Bachmann et al. (2003) concluded that management strategies to prevent development of stereotypic behaviours in horses included providing diets high in fiber with minimal amounts of concentrates. Reduced gastric pH, elicited by a combination of high-concentrate/low-forage diets and long periods of fasting between feeds, may be related to the incidence of gastric ulcers in horses. Endoscopic examination of racehorses in training receiving high levels of cereals indicated that more than 80 percent of the animals had significant gastric ulceration (Hammond et al., 1986). However, when such racehorses were turned out to pasture for 1 month or more, the incidence of ulcers decreased to 52 percent (Murray et al., 1989). Gastric ulcers are rare in horses maintained solely on pasture, and the gastric pH of horses with ad libitum access to timothy hay was significantly higher than in horses that had been fasted (Murray and Schusser, 1989). Such evidence, although not conclusive, strongly suggests that diets high in dietary fiber are beneficial to horses. The NRC (1989) recommended that equid diets should contain no less than 1 percent of BW as forage (DM) per day. Indeed, the necessity for feeding fibrous forages is implicit in redressing the energy deficit in diets of less than 2 g starch/kg BW/meal, as exclusive use of oil and/or protein in this regard would be unpalatable on the one hand and impractical, energetically inefficient, and environmentally unsound on the other.

GRAINS AND GRAIN BYPRODUCTS

A wide variety of grains and grain byproducts may be used as feeds for horses, usually to increase the energy density of horse diets. Grains and their byproducts vary in protein content and quality, but are usually low in sodium and calcium. The calcium:phosphorus ratio of grains and grain byproducts may be 1:3 or wider. Approximately 60 percent of the phosphorus in oats, corn, and barley is contained in phytate (Ravindran, 1996). These characteristics do not relate directly to the value of grains as energy supplements, but they affect the quantity and type of other feeds that must be included in the diet to provide a balanced ration. Variation in the nutrient content of grains can arise from differences in soil fertility and growing conditions. In general, the composition of grains is less variable than the composition of forages. However, because processing methods can vary from mill to mill, the nutrient composition of a byproduct feed is subject to much greater variation than the composition of a whole grain. Nevertheless, byproduct feeds are often economically priced, and they can have many nutritional characteristics that make them effective as horse feeds.

In the United States, grains may be marketed on the basis of grade. The grading criteria vary for each grain, but characteristics such as bushel weight, percentage of damaged kernels, and the presence of foreign material are considered. A higher grade is associated with higher bushel weight, fewer damaged kernels, and less foreign material.

Common Grains and Grain Byproducts Fed to Horses

Corn (maize) is often an economical energy source for horse feeds. Dent corn is the most common type of corn used in animal feeds, whereas sweet corn and popcorn are usually grown for human consumption. Corn is frequently fed cracked, rolled, or flaked, and is highly palatable. Corn is lower in CP and lysine, but higher in DE, than oats or barley (Table 16-6). Corn has a high bushel weight, and it is higher in starch and lower in fiber than barley or oats (Table 2-2). The small intestinal digestibility of the starch in whole corn is lower than for the starch in whole oats (Radicke et al., 1991), although some types of processing will improve the small intestinal availability of corn starch. The effects of starch source and grain processing on starch digestibility are discussed in detail later in this chapter.

Corn is often processed to produce ingredients used in the manufacture of food for human consumption, such as corn oil, corn starch, and corn syrup. Many of the residues (byproducts or co-products) of these processes may be incorporated into feeds for horses as energy sources. Hominy feed is produced during the manufacture of corn grits or corn meal for human use and is sometimes called corn grits byproduct. Hominy feed usually contains at least 4 percent fat and is relatively low in fiber. Protein quantity and quality are relatively low, but the energy value is at least comparable to barley or oats. Corn gluten feed, corn gluten meal, and corn distillers' dried grains are the residues from processing or distilling. These products are much higher in protein and fiber than corn, and much lower in starch. Distillers' dried grains have been shown to be palatable to horses (Pagan and Jackson, 1991b).

On a volume basis and on a weight basis, oats are much less energy-dense than corn. The bushel (bu) weight of corn will be greater than 50 lb/bu, whereas the bushel weight of oats will often be less than 40 lb/bu. Bushel weight can be affected by the variation in the ratio of hull to kernel. When the proportion of hull increases, the bushel weight decreases. In addition, the oat hull contains high levels of cellulose and xylan, which are much less digestible than the starch in the kernel. Therefore, as the proportion of hull increases, the energy value of the oats decreases. Oats contain more fiber and less starch than corn. However, oat starch has been reported to be more readily digested than corn starch in the small intestine (Radicke et al., 1991). Therefore, if grains are fed at high intakes, the use of oats may result in less overflow of starch to the large intestine. Oats also tend to be higher in protein, lysine, and fat than corn, but like corn, oats have an inverted calcium:phosphorus ratio. Oats are palatable to horses, but the rate of consumption of oats is often much less than for textured sweet feed or pelleted feed (Harbor et al., 2003). White oats are the most common type grown in the United States, but red oats and gray oats are also available. High fat (12–15 percent oil) varieties of oats have been produced, termed "naked oats," which thresh free of the hull and are higher in energy than traditional oats (Valentine, 1999). Oats are often fed whole, crimped, or rolled. Oats may be cleaned to remove loose hulls and contaminating material. When the hull is removed from the oat, the remaining product is referred to as the groat. Oat groats are used primarily in the production of human foods, but some may be incorporated into horse feeds. They are higher in starch, fat, and energy than whole oats. Byproducts of oat milling that are available for animal feeds include feeding oat meal, oat mill byproduct (oat mill feed), and oat hulls. Oat hulls are high in NDF and ADF and can be used to increase the fiber content of a diet, but are only marginally digestible, so they provide little energy to horses. Feeding oat meal is relatively low in fiber and contains pieces of oat groats and some oat flour. Oat mill feed is a byproduct intermediate to feeding oat meal and oat hulls in fiber content and contains some pieces of oat groats as well as some oat hulls.

Barley is an important energy feed worldwide. It is the basic unit of energy for the French horse feeding standards.

The DE, CP, starch, and lysine content of barley is intermediate to oats and corn (Table 16-6 and Table 2-2). Using ileally fistulated animals, Meyer et al. (1993) reported that the preileal digestibility of starch in rolled barley was approximately 21.4 percent, compared to 85.2 percent for oats. In addition, de Fombelle et al. (2004) reported that small intestinal digestion of barley starch was lower than oat starch (87.4 percent vs. 99.8 percent, respectively, in horses fed a high-starch diet). De Fombelle et al. (2004) used a mobile nylon bag technique and the substrates were ground, which may have resulted in the high small intestinal starch digestibilities. Barley is the primary grain used in the brewing industry and brewers' dried grains are often incorporated into animal feeds. As with distillers' dried grains, brewers' dried grains tend to be higher in protein, higher in fiber, and lower in starch than whole grains. Hordenine (N,N-dimethyltyramine) may be found in some barley ingredients, particularly in barley sprouts (Schubert et al., 1988). Hordenine originating from reed canarygrass or barley sprouts has been found in urine samples collected for drug-testing purposes in horses (Irvine, 1988; Sams, 1997).

Most wheat grown in the United States is used for human consumption, so the inclusion of wheat grain in horse diets is somewhat uncommon. However, wheat byproduct feeds are often used in horse feeds, wheat middlings (midds) being one of the most common. Because most of the flour has been removed, wheat midds are higher in fiber and protein, but lower in energy than wheat grain (Table 16-6). Wheat midds may contain more than 1 percent phosphorus (Table 16-6). Approximately 80 percent of the phosphorus in wheat midds is found as phytate (Ravindran, 1996). Because of the high phosphorus content, calcium supplementation is usually necessary when wheat midds constitute a significant portion of the diet. Due to their fine texture, wheat middlings are not easily fed alone; however, they are commonly used in pelleted feeds. Wheat bran is higher in ADF and NDF than wheat midds, and it is also high in phosphorus. Other wheat byproducts that may be incorporated in horse feeds include wheat mill run, wheat shorts, and red dog. Wheat mill run is a combination of bran and midds. Wheat shorts and red dog contain slightly more flour than wheat midds.

Other grains that can be fed to horses include rye and sorghum grain. Sorghum grain is very small in size, and it is commonly processed prior to incorporation in horse diets. The nutrient composition of sorghum is similar to corn, although it may be slightly lower in energy value. Rye is lower in palatability than most other cereal grains, but the chemical composition is similar to oats. Rye may be contaminated with ergot (see section Mycotoxins in Grains).

Other Byproduct Feeds

Molasses is a byproduct of sugar manufacturing and is usually produced from sugar cane or sugar beets. Molasses is usually incorporated into horse feeds because it is palatable, helps to reduce dust, and may also aid in preventing sifting of ingredients in a mixed feed. Typical inclusion rates of molasses vary, but are usually less than 10 percent of a concentrate. On a DM basis, molasses contains 4 to 6 percent potassium (Table 16-6) and 62–90 percent NFC (Table 2-2). Under some circumstances molasses may be blended with other liquids; for example, a low level of fat may be added to molasses that will be incorporated in textured feeds (sweet feeds) to enhance the appearance of the feed and decrease caking in cold weather.

Another byproduct of the sugar industry is beet pulp. Dried beet pulp is available with or without added molasses. The addition of molasses increases the sugar and potassium content of beet pulp. Beet pulp has a higher water holding capacity than hay cubes or soy hulls (Moore-Colyer et al., 2002) and may be fed moistened. Several research studies have fed diets containing sugar-beet pulp to horses (Harris and Rodiek, 1993; Crandell et al., 1999; Warren et al., 1999; Palmgren-Karlsson, 2002). Beet pulp is usually used as a component of mixed concentrate feeds; however, Harris and Rodiek (1993) fed diets consisting of 45 percent beet pulp and 55 percent alfalfa pellets without negative effects, and Warren et al. (1999) fed horses a diet containing 55 percent beet pulp.

Moore-Colyer et al. (2002) reported a total tract disappearance of 85 percent for unmolassed sugar-beet pulp using a mobile nylon bag technique in ponies. This estimate of dry matter digestibility for beet pulp compares well with the results of Harris and Rodiek (1993). In their study, dry matter digestibility of a beet pulp/alfalfa pellet diet was 72 percent compared to 63 percent for the alfalfa pellets alone. Palmgren-Karlsson (2002) found that replacing 40 percent of the oats in a hay-oat diet with a combination of molassed beet pulp and dried brewers' grains (86:14 ratio) did not affect the energy digestibility of the diet. These studies suggest that the energy value of beet pulp is higher than alfalfa pellets and possibly as high as oats. Pagan (1998) reported a DE value of 2.8 Mcal/kg for beet pulp on an as-fed basis. However, the beet pulp used in nutrition studies with horses has been very diverse. For example, Moore and Colyer et al. (2002) studied the digestibility of sugar-beet pulp containing 54.7 percent NDF and 7.8 percent CP (DM basis), while Palmgren-Karlsson (2002) fed beet pulp containing 23.6 percent NDF and 11.5 percent CP. In Table 16-6 the DE content (2.8 Mcal DE/kg DM) of beet pulp was calculated using an equation that was derived from feeding experiments that primarily evaluated forages and grains. It is possible that this equation underestimates the DE content of beet pulp. The nonstarch polysaccharide and NDF fractions of beet pulp appear to be more digestible than those found in hay (Moore-Colyer et al., 2002).

Citrus pulp has also been fed to horses (Ott et al., 1979b). Palatability was low when citrus pulp was incorporated at a rate of 30 percent of a coarse concentrate but was considered adequate when the citrus pulp constituted 15 percent of a pelleted concentrate. Citrus pulp is somewhat more readily fermented in vitro than beet pulp (Sunvold et al., 1995). Ott et al. (1979b) suggested that the DE content of citrus pulp was slightly higher than the DE content of pulverized oats.

Soybean hulls (soyhulls) are a byproduct of the soybean processing industry. Soyhulls contain 53–70 percent NDF and less than 3 percent starch (Table 2-2). Coverdale et al. (2004) used soyhulls to replace up to 75 percent of the diet of mature horses receiving alfalfa/bromegrass hay and found no effect on apparent total-tract dry matter digestibility. The NDF and ADF concentration in the soyhulls (60.6 and 43.7 percent, respectively) was similar to the NDF and ADF concentration in the hay (58.1 and 39.1 percent, respectively). Soyhulls containing 59.1 percent NDF and 43.8 percent ADF had a higher total-tract dry matter digestibility than hay cubes containing 62.3 percent NDF and 35.5 percent ADF (Moore-Colyer et al., 2002). Using cecal inocula, Bush et al. (2001) reported that the in vitro dry matter disappearance of soyhulls was higher than for low-quality alfalfa, but lower than oats (Bush et al., 2001). Pagan (1998) reported a DE value for soyhulls of 2.6 Mcal/kg (as-fed basis), which would be similar to immature legume hay. As with beet pulp, the equation for estimating DE may underestimate the DE content of soyhulls. The feeding value of almond hulls has also been investigated (Clutter and Rodiek, 1991). Almond hulls (22 percent ADF) were well accepted by mature horses and increased dry matter digestibility of an alfalfa and oat hay ration.

Although rice is not commonly incorporated into horse diets in the United States, rice bran may be used. Rice bran contains approximately the same amount of NDF as oats, but it is relatively high in crude fat (19–28 percent: DePeters et al., 2000). Rice bran contains a moderate amount of nonfiber carbohydrates, including starch (DePeters et al., 2000). Unless it has been combined with other ingredients, rice bran may have an inverted calcium:phosphorus ratio. Rice bran can contain a naturally occurring lipase that can be inactivated by some types of processing. Rice bran that is processed soon after milling in order to inactivate this lipase is referred to as stabilized rice bran. Stabilization reduces the potential for rancidification. According to AAFCO (2005), the free fatty acid content of crude fat in rice bran must be less than 4 percent. Like rice bran, whole soybeans are a high-fat feed ingredient that may be incorporated into horse feeds. Whole soybeans may be roasted or extruded prior to incorporation to inactivate naturally occurring trypsin inhibitors.

Mycotoxins in Grains

Under some conditions, cereal grains or cereal grain byproducts may contain mycotoxins. The concentrations and types of mycotoxins found in grains can vary greatly. An interaction between environmental temperature and moisture is an important determinant of preharvest mycotoxin contamination of grains (CAST, 2003), although no single combination of conditions can define mycotoxin production potential. It is possible that the concentration of some mycotoxins in grains may increase during storage (Bacon and Nelson, 1994). Temperature and moisture conditions during harvesting and storage can promote mycotoxin production along with insect infestation and mechanical damage to grain kernels. Mycotoxins may depress feed intake, impair growth, or cause disease in animals; however, the signs are not consistent among species. Many factors may influence the susceptibility of an animal to a specific mycotoxin, including animal species, age, general health, and immune status (Hollinger and Ekperigin, 1999).

The *Fusarium* spp. produce a variety of mycotoxins including zearalenone, deoxynivalenol (vomitoxin), T-2 toxin, and fumonisin B1, B2, and B3. *Fusarium* spp. can affect the plant during growth, causing stalk and ear rot in corn, and scab or head blight in other plants (Whitlow and Hagler, 2002). Zearalenone, deoxynivalenol, and T-2 toxin can be found in a variety of feedstuffs, whereas the fumonisins are usually associated with corn or corn byproducts. There is great variation in the susceptibility of different animal species to the *Fusarium* spp. mycotoxins. Swine are affected by concentrations of deoxynivalenol and zearalenone as low as 1 ppm and 0.1 ppm, respectively (Whitlow and Hagler, 2002). By comparison, feed consumption was not affected when horses were fed barley containing more than 36 ppm deoxynivalenol (Johnson et al., 1997). Other studies have reported that grain intake by horses was affected when the grain contained a mix of mycotoxins (15 ppm deoxynivalenol and 2 ppm zearalenone, or 11 ppm deoxynivalenol and 0.8 ppm zearalenone), but no effects on animal health were noted (Raymond et al., 2003, 2005).

Equine leucoencephalomalacia, often referred to as blind staggers, or moldy corn poisoning has been reported to occur in horses fed diets containing corn or corn byproducts contaminated with *Fusarium verticilliodes* (syn. *moniliforme*) (Vesonder et al., 1989; Wilson et al., 1990a.). Toxicosis is believed to result from the consumption of high levels of fumonisin B_1 (Wilson et al., 1990b; Ross et al., 1991), although fumonisin B_2 and B_3 occur in close association with fumonisin B_1 (Murphy et al., 1993). Horses affected by leucoencephalomalacia may exhibit facial paralysis and ataxia. Morbidity and mortality are high (Ross et al., 1991). Equine leucoencephalomalacia has been produced experimentally by feeding corn screenings known to be contaminated with fumonisin B_1 and B_2 (Wilson et al., 1992; Ross et al., 1993). Ross et al. (1993) found that susceptibility to toxicosis was variable among ponies and suggested that animals with impaired liver function had increased susceptibility. The Food and Drug Administration recommends 5 ppm as the upper limit for fumonisin in corn and corn byproducts intended for equine consumption, with the stipulation that the contaminated feed will not constitute more than 20 percent of the diet (FDA, 2001a).

Fumonisin contamination of corn is variable and may be influenced by growing conditions. Surveys in 1995 and 1996 found that 6.9 and 3.9 percent, respectively, of samples from the preharvest U.S. corn crop contained more than 5 ppm fumonisin (APHIS, 1995, 1996). Fumonisin contamination of corn is more likely to occur when the crop has been subjected to stress from weather or insect damage. The fumonisin-producing molds may proliferate during storage if moisture content is favorable (Bacon and Nelson, 1994). Corn screenings have been reported to be higher in fumonisin than whole corn grain (Murphy et al., 1993). The FDA Center for Veterinary Medicine does not recommend that corn screenings be used in feeds for horses (FDA, 2001b). In 1998, the National Animal Health Monitoring System of the U.S. Department of Agriculture collected samples from more than 900 equine operations to assess the incidence of fumonisin contamination of equine feeds. Approximately 95 percent of all samples contained less than 2 ppm fumonisin, and slightly less than 1 percent contained more than 5 ppm fumonisin. Samples that were obtained from horse operations that used homegrown grain had a greater incidence of high concentrations of fumonisin than samples obtained from operations that used grain obtained from a retail supplier.

The mycotoxins produced by *Aspergillus* spp. include aflatoxin B1, B2, G1, and G2. Aflatoxins are not unique to cereal grains and may be found in peanuts, cottonseed, and other feeds. Aflatoxins are considered to be carcinogenic (FDA, 1994). In horses, aflatoxins have been associated with liver disease and death (Angsubhakorn et al., 1981; Vesonder et al., 1991). The toxic level of aflatoxin in horse feeds has not been clearly established. Angsubhakorn et al. (1981) reported that horses consuming feed containing more than 200 ppb aflatoxin B1 became ill soon after the feed was introduced to the diet, and that several horses died. Vesonder et al. (1991) reported that three horses that died had consumed corn containing more than 100 ppb aflatoxin. Hasso (2003) attributed a bout of soft feces observed in Arabian horses in Iraq to aflatoxin contamination of the barley in the diet. The barley contained 12.5 ppb aflatoxin, and horses received 5–6 kg/d. No effects on feed or water intake were noted. The FDA has suggested action levels for aflatoxin concentration in specific feeds used in certain circumstances for cattle, swine, and poultry, but not for horses (FDA, 1994). An action level of 20 ppb has been given for animal feeds and feed ingredients used for animal species and uses not specifically designated by other guidelines. An action level is not a formal tolerance level but has been described as a level that a qualified expert witness would consider injurious to health during testimony in a federal court (Price et al., 1993).

Mycotoxins associated with *Penicillium* spp. include ochratoxins and citrinin. Ochratoxins are believed to negatively affect other species, but little documentation of effects on horses can be found.

Another contaminant that may be found in some cereal grains is ergot. An ergot is a small brown mass (sclerotium) that is produced by molds in the *Claviceps* genus. Ergots contain ergot alkaloids that may cause neurological, behavioral, vascular, and reproductive effects in animals. In horses, agalactia, dystocia, and placental abnormalities have been reported in mares consuming oats contaminated with ergot (Riet-Correa et al., 1998; Copetti et al., 2002).

FATS AND OILS

The digestion and metabolism of fats by horses have been discussed at length in Chapter 3. In general, fats and oils do not contain any appreciable amounts of protein or minerals and are usually included in horse diets for their energy value and associated metabolic benefits. Depending upon the extent of processing, some vegetable oils may contain some natural antioxidants.

Many different types of fats and oils are available for incorporation into equine diets. Animal fats include tallow, lard, and rendered fat. Vegetable fats include corn oil, soybean (soya) oil, sunflower oil, canola oil, and rice oil. Blends of animal and vegetable fats have also been fed to horses (Bowman et al., 1979; McCann et al., 1987). Animal fats are typically higher in saturated fatty acids than vegetable oils, which are predominantly unsaturated fatty acids. An exception would be coconut oil, which is low in unsaturated fats but high in medium-chain saturated fatty acids. Corn oil is typically high in linoleic acid and low in linolenic acid, whereas linseed oil is comparatively lower in linoleic acid and higher in linolenic acid. The fatty acid composition of various fats and oils is shown in Table 8-7.

Fats and oils are usually incorporated into horse feeds for their nutritional characteristics, but they are also used to affect the physical characteristics of the feed. Addition of fats and oils may decrease the dustiness of a feed and decrease caking in sweet feeds. Addition of fat may also enhance mixing qualities. However, inclusion of high levels of fat in pelleted feeds may negatively affect pellet quality. In addition, fats may be susceptible to oxidation, resulting in rancidity. Unsaturated fats are usually more susceptible to oxidation than saturated fats. To minimize oxidation and increase shelf life, antioxidants may be added to feeds containing high levels of fat. The use of antioxidants in horse diets is reviewed in Chapter 9.

Different fat sources vary in their palatability to horses. In a study conducted on the acceptance of various plant and animal lipid sources when incorporated at 15 percent of the concentrate ration, corn oil was found to be most palatable, followed by corn oil blended with other oils of plant or animal origin. Compared to corn oil, peanut and safflower oils were moderately palatable, whereas cottonseed oil and tallow were largely unpalatable (Holland et al., 1998). In further studies, 10 percent coconut and soya oils percent were well accepted by horses (Pagan et al., 1993).

FEEDS AND FEED PROCESSING

TABLE 8-7 Fatty Acid Composition of Some Fats and Oils Available for Use in Equine Feeds

Type of Oil	International Feed Number	Selected Fatty Acids (% of total fatty acids)[a]							Other Fatty Acids[b]
		C14:0	C16:0	C16:1	C18:0	C18:1	C18:2	C18:3	
Animal Fats and Fish Oils									
Tallow	4-08-127	3.0	24.5	3.7	19.3	40.9	3.2	0.7	4.9
Lard	4-04-790	1.3	23.8	2.7	13.5	41.2	10.2	1.0	6.3
Herring	7-08-048	7.2	11.7	9.6	0.8	12.0	1.1	0.8	56.8
Menhaden	7-08-049	8.0	15.1	10.5	3.8	14.5	2.2	1.5	44.5
Vegetable Oils									
Canola (rapeseed)	4-06-144	—	4.8	0.5	1.6	53.8	22.1	11.1	6.1
Corn	4-07-882	0	10.9	—	1.8	24.2	58.0	0.7	4.4
Cottonseed	4-20-836	0.8	22.7	0.8	2.3	17.0	51.5	0.2	4.7
Linseed	—	—	5.3	—	4.1	20.2	12.7	53.3	4.4
Olive	—	0	11.0	0.8	2.2	72.5	7.9	0.6	5.0
Palm	—	1.0	43.5	0.3	4.3	36.6	9.1	0.2	5.0
Peanut	4-03-658	0.1	9.5	0.1	2.2	44.8	32.0	—	11.3
Safflower	4-20-256	0.1	6.2	0.4	2.2	11.7	74.1	0.4	4.9
Sesame	—	—	8.9	0.2	4.8	39.3	41.3	0.3	5.2
Soybean	4-07-983	0.1	10.3	0.2	3.8	22.8	51.0	6.8	5.0
Sunflower	4-20-833	—	5.4	0.2	3.5	45.3	39.8	0.2	5.6

[a]Values from the U.S. Department of Agriculture *Food Composition Standard Release 12* (1998) and Pearl (1995) of the Fats and Protein Research Foundation.
[b]Other fatty acids are predominantly polyunsaturated fatty acids greater than 18 carbons long.

PROTEIN SUPPLEMENTS

The quality of protein supplements fed to horses is a function of both the amino acid profile and digestibility of the protein source. Protein supplements are either from plant or animal sources. Those of animal origin are superior in terms of their amino acid profile to those of plant origin. However, animal protein sources are more expensive and often unpalatable compared to protein supplements of plant origin. It is of note that in some countries, such as the United Kingdom, feeding animal protein products to horses is banned (DEFRA, 2006).

Many protein supplements such as canola meal, soybean meal, brewers' dried grains, fishmeal, linseed meal, and cottonseed meal, have been fed to adult horses with no ill effects (Slade et al., 1970; Hintz and Schryver, 1972; Reitnour and Salsbury, 1976; Gibbs et al., 1996; Martin et al., 1996). However, protein sources such as milk byproducts and soybean meal, as well as canola meal, have proved superior to other protein sources for growing horses based on greater ADG (Borton et al., 1973; Prior et al., 1974; Ott et al., 1979a; Cymbaluk, 1990b). This is probably due to a better amino acid profile in these protein sources, as well as a potentially superior digestibility in the foregut of the horse. Soybeans and some varieties of peas contain a trypsin inhibitor that can interfere with protein digestion, and cottonseed meal contains gossypol, which has been suggested to bind iron and interfere with protein digestion. During processing, heating can destroy the trypsin inhibitors in soybeans and peas and inactivate the toxins from gossypol in cottonseed meal, making them acceptable for inclusion in horse feeds. Others protein supplements used in horse feeds include sunflower meal, peanut meal, lupin seed meal, beans, linseed meal, brewers' dried grains, and distillers' grains (Frape, 1998).

Particular attention should be paid to the lysine level in the protein source especially for growing horses and lactating mares. Deficient lysine levels will limit growth in young horses (Ott et al., 1979a) and may affect milk protein quality thereby, ultimately affecting the growth and development of the nursing foal (Glade and Luba, 1990). Table 8-8 gives amino acid profiles of some common feedstuffs for horses.

Dietary supplement with urea has been shown to increase blood and urine concentrations of urea but has improved nitrogen balance when protein in the diet was deficient (Slade et al., 1970; Godbee and Slade, 1981; Martin et al., 1991, 1996). However, it should be noted that large quantities of urea in the diet can result in death. Feeding 450 g of urea resulted in ammonia toxicity (Hintz et al., 1970) and death of the horses in the study. Inclusion of urea in the diet does not improve the quality (i.e., the amino acid profile) of the diet and should be avoided in the diets of growing horses and lactating mares.

MINERAL AND VITAMIN SUPPLEMENTS

Mineral Supplements

Supplemental minerals differ in chemical form, concentration, and bioavailability. Supplemental minerals are gen-

TABLE 8-8 Amino Acid Contents of Some Horse Feed Ingredients and Forages (percentage DM basis)

Feed Name	Feed Description	IFN[a]	DM %	CP %	Arg (%)	His (%)	Ile (%)	Leu (%)	Lys (%)	Met (%)	Cys (%)	Phe (%)	Tyr (%)	Thr (%)
Alfalfa														
	meal dehydrated, 17% CP	1-00-023	92	17	0.77	0.41	0.74	1.32	0.77	0.27	0.22	0.92	0.60	0.77
	meal dehydrated, 20% CP	1-00-024	92	19.6	1.0	0.98	0.98	1.54	0.99	0.37	0.33	1.02	0.66	0.90
Bakery waste														
	dried bakery product	4-00-466	91	10.8	0.52	0.26	0.46	0.88	0.33	0.20	0.22	0.55	0.42	0.36
Barley														
	grain, two row	4-00-572	89	11.3	0.61	0.30	0.43	0.88	0.44	0.22	0.33	0.62	0.32	0.39
	grain, six row	4-00-574	89	10.5	0.53	0.24	0.40	0.77	0.44	0.19	0.22	0.54	0.35	0.37
	grain, hulless	4-00-552	88	14.9	0.61	0.25	0.45	0.88	0.44	0.18	0.22	0.67	0.44	0.44
Beet, sugar														
	pulp, dried	4-00-669	91	8.6	0.35	0.25	0.4	0.55	0.55	0.08	0.11	0.33	0.44	0.41
Brewers' grains														
	dried	5-02-141	92	26.5	1.68	0.58	1.12	2.31	1.31	0.49	0.55	1.42	0.97	1.04
Buckwheat, common														
	grain	4-00-994	88	11.1	1.10	0.28	0.44	0.66	0.66	0.21	0.22	0.51	0.34	0.45
Canola (rapeseed)														
	meal, sol. extr.	5-06-145	90	35.6	2.42	1.06	1.57	2.86	2.31	0.81	0.99	1.47	1.24	1.74
Casein														
	dried	5-01-162	91	88.7	3.59	3.10	5.13	9.68	8.14	3.00	0.44	4.84	5.25	4.38
Cassava (tapioca or manioc)														
	meal	4-01-152	88	3.3	0.20	0.09	0.21	0.22	0.11	0.04	0.11	0.16	0.04	0.12
Citrus														
	pulp dried	4-01-237	85	6.9	0.23	0.12	0.19	0.34	0.18	0.07	0.01	0.23	—	0.26
Coconut (copra)														
	meal, sol. extr.	5-01-573	92	21.9	2.40	0.43	0.83	1.54	0.66	0.38	0.33	0.92	0.63	0.73
Corn, yellow														
	distillers' grain	5-02-842	94	24.8	0.99	0.69	1.00	2.86	0.77	0.47	0.33	1.09	0.90	0.68
	distillers' grain with solubles	5-02-843	93	27.7	1.24	0.77	1.13	2.86	0.66	0.55	0.55	1.47	0.91	1.03
	distillers' solubles	5-02-844	92	26.7	0.99	0.73	1.33	2.53	0.88	0.56	0.55	1.33	0.88	1.13
	gluten feed	5-02-903	90	21.5	1.14	0.74	0.73	2.20	0.66	0.39	0.55	0.78	0.63	0.81
	gluten meal, 60% CP	5-28-242	90	60.2	2.12	1.41	2.73	11.0	1.10	1.57	1.31	3.88	3.56	2.29
	grain	4-02-935	89	8.3	0.41	0.25	0.31	1.10	0.33	0.19	0.22	0.43	0.27	0.38
	grits byproduct (hominy feed)	4-03-011	90	10.3	0.61	0.31	0.40	1.10	0.44	0.19	0.22	0.47	0.44	0.44
	grain, steam-flaked	4-02-854	88	9.4	0.44	0.29	0.31	1.04	0.30	0.19	0.22	0.43	—	0.34
Cottonseed														
	meal, mech. extr. 41% CP	5-01-617	92	42.4	4.68	1.22	1.42	2.75	1.87	0.74	0.77	2.17	1.35	1.47
	meal, sol. extr. 41% CP	5-07-872	90	41.4	5.01	1.29	1.43	2.75	1.87	0.74	0.77	2.32	1.34	1.49
Fababean (broadbean)														
	seeds	5-09-262	87	25.4	2.51	0.74	1.43	2.10	1.76	0.22	0.33	1.13	0.96	0.98
Flax (linseed)														
	meal, sol. extr.	5-02-048	90	33.6	3.26	0.75	1.72	2.31	1.32	0.65	0.66	1.73	1.13	1.27
Lentil														
	seeds	5-02-506	89	24.4	2.26	0.86	1.10	1.98	1.87	0.20	0.33	1.42	0.77	0.92
Lupin (sweet white)														
	seeds	5-27-717	89	34.9	3.71	0.85	1.54	2.64	1.65	0.30	0.55	1.34	1.48	1.32
Milk (cattle)														
	dried	5-01-175	96	34.6	1.28	1.15	2.06	4.07	3.19	1.01	0.33	1.96	2.06	1.78
Millet (proso)														
	grain	4-03-120	90	11.1	0.45	0.22	0.51	1.32	0.22	0.34	0.22	0.62	0.34	0.44
Molasses														
	beet-sugar	4-00-668	77.9	8.5	0.42	0.14	0.38	0.31	0.09	0.02	0.07	0.23	—	0.14
	sugarcane	4-00-696	74.3	5.8	0.28	0.09	0.26	0.21	0.06	0.01	0.05	0.16	—	0.09
Oat														
	grain	4-03-309	89	11.5	0.96	0.34	0.53	0.99	0.44	0.24	0.44	0.72	0.45	0.48
	grain, naked	4-25-101	86	17.1	0.85	0.31	0.53	0.99	0.55	0.22	0.33	0.66	0.46	0.44
	groat	4-03-331	90	13.9	0.94	0.26	0.61	1.10	0.55	0.22	022	0.72	0.56	0.48
Pea														
	seeds	5-03-600	89	22.8	2.06	0.59	0.95	1.65	1.65	0.23	0.33	1.09	0.78	0.85
Peanut (groundnut)														
	meal, mech. extr.	5-03-649	92	43.2	5.27	1.11	1.55	3.08	1.65	0.55	0.66	2.22	1.91	1.28
	meal, sol. extr.	5-03-650	92	49.1	5.60	1.17	1.96	3.10	1.87	0.57	0.77	2.58	1.98	1.39

TABLE 8-8 continued

Feed Name	Feed Description	IFN[a]	DM %	CP %	Arg (%)	His (%)	Ile (%)	Leu (%)	Lys (%)	Met (%)	Cys (%)	Phe (%)	Tyr (%)	Thr (%)
Potato	protein concentrate	5-25-392	91	73.8	4.18	1.88	4.49	8.36	6.38	1.85	1.32	5.48	4.69	4.73
Rice	bran	4-03-928	90	13.3	1.10	0.37	0.48	0.99	0.66	0.29	0.33	0.61	0.44	0.52
Safflower	meal, sol. extr.	5-04-110	92	23.4	2.24	0.65	0.73	1.65	0.77	0.37	0.44	1.17	0.84	0.71
	meal without hulls, sol. extr.	5-07-959	92	42.5	3.95	1.17	1.86	2.86	1.32	0.72	0.77	2.20	1.19	1.41
Sesame	meal, mech. extr.	5-04-220	93	42.6	5.35	1.08	1.61	2.97	1.10	1.26	0.88	1.95	1.67	1.58
Sorghum	grain	4-20-893	88	9.2	0.42	0.25	0.41	1.32	0.22	0.19	0.22	0.54	0.38	0.34
Soybean	meal, sol. extr.	5-04-604	89	43.8	3.55	1.29	2.20	3.74	3.08	0.67	0.77	2.40	1.86	1.90
	meal without hulls	5-04-612	90	47.5	3.83	1.41	2.38	4.07	3.30	0.74	0.77	2.63	2.00	2.04
	protein concentrate	—	90	64.0	6.37	1.98	3.63	5.83	4.62	0.99	1.10	3.74	2.75	3.08
	protein isolate	5-08-038	92	85.8	7.56	2.48	4.68	7.26	5.83	1.11	1.32	4.77	3.41	3.47
	seeds, heat processed	5-04-597	90	35.2	2.86	1.06	1.78	3.08	2.42	0.58	0.66	2.01	1.45	1.55
Sunflower	meal, sol. extr.	5-09-340	90	26.8	2.62	0.73	1.42	2.09	1.10	0.65	0.55	1.35	0.84	1.14
	meal without hulls, sol. extr.	5-04-739	93	42.2	3.22	1.01	1.58	2.53	1.32	0.90	0.77	1.83	1.13	1.46
Triticale	grain	4-20-362	90	12.5	0.63	0.28	0.43	0.88	0.44	0.22	0.33	0.54	0.35	0.39
Wheat	bran	4-05-190	89	15.7	1.18	0.48	0.54	1.10	0.66	0.27	0.33	0.68	0.47	0.57
	grain, hard red spring	4-05-258	88	14.1	0.74	0.37	0.52	0.99	0.44	0.25	0.33	0.73	0.44	0.45
	grain, hard red winter	4-05-268	88	13.5	0.66	0.35	0.44	0.99	0.33	0.22	0.33	0.66	0.41	0.40
	grain, soft red winter	4-05-294	88	11.5	0.55	0.22	0.50	0.99	0.44	0.24	0.33	0.69	0.40	0.42
	grain, soft white winter	4-05-337	89	11.8	0.61	0.30	0.48	0.88	0.33	0.22	0.33	0.60	0.39	0.38
	middlings, 9.5% fiber	4-05-205	89	15.9	1.07	0.48	0.58	1.21	0.66	0.28	0.33	0.77	0.31	0.56
	red dog, 4% fiber	4-05-203	88	15.3	1.06	0.45	0.60	1.21	0.66	0.25	0.44	0.72	0.50	0.55
	shorts, 7% fiber	4-05-201	88	16.0	1.12	0.47	0.64	1.10	0.77	0.27	0.33	0.77	0.56	0.62
Whey	dried	4-01-182	96	12.1	0.29	0.25	0.68	1.21	0.99	0.18	0.33	0.42	0.27	0.79
	low lactose, dried	4-01-186	96	17.6	0.58	0.36	1.28	1.76	1.65	0.42	0.55	0.69	0.57	1.28
	permeate, dried	—	96	3.8	0.07	0.06	0.18	0.22	0.22	0.03	0.00	0.06	—	0.15
Yeast, brewers'	dehydrated	7-05-527	93	45.9	2.42	1.20	2.37	3.41	3.52	0.81	0.55	1.91	1.71	2.42
Forages														
Cool-season grasses	pasture intensively managed	2-02-260	20	26.5	0.30	0.13	0.23	0.43	0.24	0.09	0.07	0.32	—	0.24
	hay, all samples	1-02-250	88	10.6	0.04	0.01	0.03	0.06	0.03	0.01	0.01	0.04	—	0.04
	hay, immature	1-02-212	84	18.0	0.12	0.05	0.10	0.20	0.11	0.04	0.041	0.12	—	0.12
	hay, mid maturity	1-02-243	84	13.3	0.07	0.03	0.06	0.11	0.06	0.03	0.02	0.07	—	0.06
	hay, mature	1-02-244	84	10.8	0.04	0.01	0.03	0.07	0.04	0.01	0.01	0.04	—	0.04
	silage, all samples	3-02-222	37	12.8	0.05	0.03	0.06	0.10	0.05	0.02	0.01	0.08	—	0.06
	silage, immature	3-02-217	36	16.8	0.09	0.05	0.10	0.17	0.09	0.03	0.02	0.12	—	0.09
	silage, mid-maturity	3-02-218	42	16.8	0.09	0.05	0.10	0.17	0.09	0.03	0.02	0.12	—	0.09
	silage, mature	3-02-219	39	12.7	0.05	0.03	0.06	0.10	0.06	0.02	0.01	0.07	—	0.06
Grass-legume mixtures predominantly grass (17–22% hemicellulose)	hay, immature	1-02-275	84	18.4	0.14	0.06	0.12	0.22	0.132	0.05	0.04	0.14	—	0.12
	hay, mid-maturity	1-02-277	87	17.4	0.12	0.05	0.11	0.19	0.12	0.04	0.04	0.12	—	0.11
	hay, mature	1-02-280	85	13.3	0.07	0.03	0.06	0.11	0.07	0.02	0.02	0.07	—	0.06
	silage, immature	3-02-302	47	18.0	0.10	0.05	0.11	0.19	0.11	0.04	0.03	0.14	—	0.11
	silage, mid-maturity	3-02-265	45	17.6	0.10	0.05	0.11	0.19	0.11	0.04	0.03	0.14	—	0.11
	silage, mature	3-02-266	39	15.4	0.08	0.04	0.09	0.09	0.09	0.03	0.02	0.10	—	0.08
Mixed grass and legume (12–15% hemicellulose)	hay, immature	1-02-275	83	19.7	0.18	0.07	0.15	0.28	0.18	0.06	0.06	0.17	—	0.16
	hay, mid-maturity	1-02-277	85	18.4	0.15	0.06	0.12	0.23	0.08	0.05	0.04	0.14	—	0.80
	hay, mature	1-02-280	90	18.2	0.14	0.06	0.12	0.22	0.14	0.05	0.04	0.14	—	0.79

TABLE 8-8 continued

Feed Name	Feed Description	IFN[a]	DM %	CP %	Arg (%)	His (%)	Ile (%)	Leu (%)	Lys (%)	Met (%)	Cys (%)	Phe (%)	Tyr (%)	Thr (%)
	silage, immature	3-02-302	46	20.3	0.14	0.06	0.16	0.26	0.16	0.06	0.04	0.18	—	0.77
	silage, mid-maturity	3-02-265	44	19.1	0.13	0.06	0.14	0.24	0.15	0.05	0.03	0.16	—	0.76
	silage, mature	3-02-266	43	17.4	0.10	0.05	0.11	0.19	0.12	0.04	0.02	0.13	—	0.63
Predominantly legume (10–13.5% hemicellulose)	hay, immature	1-02-275	84	20.5	0.21	0.08	0.18	0.32	0.21	0.06	0.06	0.20	—	0.20
	hay, mid-maturity	1-02-277	84	19.1	0.18	0.07	0.15	0.26	0.17	0.06	0.05	0.17	—	0.15
	hay, mature	1-02-280	84	17.2	0.14	0.06	0.12	0.21	0.14	0.04	0.04	0.13	—	0.12
	silage, immature	3-02-302	43	20.0	0.15	0.07	0.15	0.24	0.17	0.05	0.03	0.17	—	0.15
	silage, mid-maturity	3-02-265	43	19.0	0.14	0.06	0.15	0.24	0.16	0.05	0.03	0.16	—	0.14
	silage, mature	3-02-266	43	18.3	0.12	0.06	0.13	0.21	0.13	0.04	0.03	0.14	—	0.12
Legumes, forage	pasture intensively managed	2-29-431	21	26.5	0.38	0.14	0.30	0.52	0.34	0.11	0.10	0.08	—	0.31
	hay, all samples	1-20-648	88	20.2	0.20	0.08	0.17	0.30	0.21	0.06	0.06	0.19	—	0.18
	hay immature	1-07-792	84	22.8	0.27	0.10	0.10	0.38	0.27	0.08	0.07	0.24	—	0.22
	hay, mid-maturity	1-07-788	84	20.8	0.21	0.08	0.18	0.31	0.21	0.07	0.06	0.20	—	0.18
	hay, mature	1-07-789	84	17.8	0.16	0.06	0.13	0.23	0.16	0.05	0.05	0.16	—	0.14
	silage, all samples	3-07-796	39	20.1	0.16	0.07	0.16	0.25	0.18	0.06	0.03	0.17	—	0.15
	silage, immature	3-07-795	41	23.2	0.21	0.09	0.20	0.32	0.24	0.07	0.04	0.22	—	0.18
	silage mid-maturity	3-07-797	43	21.9	0.185	0.08	0.18	0.30	0.21	0.06	0.04	0.20	—	0.19
	silage, mature	3-07-798	43	20.3	0.16	0.07	0.16	0.26	0.19	0.06	0.03	0.16	—	0.16
Bermudagrass (Cynodon dactylon)	coastal hay, early heading	1-20-900	87	10.4	0.04	0.02	0.03	0.07	0.04	0.01	0.01	0.04	—	0.04
Oat	silage, headed	3-21-843	35	13.0	0.04	0.03	0.09	0.11	0.06	0.03	0.01	0.08	—	0.02
	hay	1-09-099	92	9.1	0.20	0.18	0.50	0.61	0.32	0.17	0.07	0.42	—	0.38
Wheat	straw	1-05-175	93	4.8	0.05	0.08	0.08	0.16	0.16	0.06	0.05	0.09	—	0.15
	silage, early head	3-21-865	33	12.0	0.25	0.45	0.50	0.83	0.53	0.22	0.08	0.53	—	0.52
Corn, yellow	silage, normal	3-28-248	35	8.8	0.17	0.15	0.29	0.76	0.22	0.13	0.12	0.34	—	0.28

[a]NOTE: IFN = International Feed Number
First digit is class of feed: 1, dry forages and roughages; 2, pasture, range plants, and forages fed green; 3, silages; 4, energy feeds; 5, protein supplements; 6, minerals; 7, vitamins; 8, additives; the other five digits are the International Feed Number.

erally in the form of salts (e.g., carbonates, oxides, sulfates) or in a complex with a chelating agent (e.g., polysaccharides, proteinates, amino acids). Mineral chelates are defined as metal complexes in which the metal is held in the complex through more than one point of attachment to the ligand (chelating agent), with the metal atom occupying a central position in the complex (McDowell, 2003). The concentration of a mineral for any given form depends upon the relative mass of the element, compared to the compound in which it is bound. For example the molecular weight of cupric oxide (CuO) is 79.5454 (i.e., Cu = 63.546 + O = 15.9994). Therefore, copper oxide contains 80 percent Cu (i.e., 63.546/79.5454). In comparison, cupric sulfate ($CuSO_4 \cdot 5\ H_2O$) only contains 25 percent Cu (63.546/249.68). Mineral concentrations of supplemental mineral forms commonly used in feeding horses are shown in the Table 16-7.

Bioavailability, defined as the degree to which an ingested nutrient in a particular source is absorbed in a form that can be utilized in metabolism by the animal (Ammerman et al., 1995), varies between different chemical forms of mineral. Unfortunately, information regarding bioavailability of different forms of minerals specific to horses is lacking. However, it is a commonly held view that chelated minerals are more bioavailable to horses than nonchelated forms. Chelated minerals are chemically altered and bound to proteins or amino acids and do not have to compete for ligands in the stomach to be absorbed; thus, in theory they should be more bioavailable than those that are not chelated (Baker et al., 2005). However, the limited studies on the relative bioavailability of chelated minerals in horses have produced equivocal results, thus making it difficult to generalize on the merits or otherwise of using chelated mineral supplements in horse feeds. Wagner et al. (2005) reported no difference in absorption and retention of copper, manganese, and zinc when fed as the oxide, sulfate, or organic-chelate form. Likewise, Highfill et al. (2005) reported calcium from a calcium-amino acid proteinate was no more available than the calcium from calcium carbonate. Baker et al. (2005) reported mature horses did not appear to digest and retain organically chelated copper and zinc sources as efficiently as inorganic sources. In comparison, Baker et al. (2003) reported yearling geldings fed a supplemental organic copper and zinc source had a greater apparent copper digestibility, higher daily copper balance, and higher daily zinc balance as compared to those fed a diet supplemented with an inorganic source. Wagner et al. (2005) suggested that growing horses may find more benefit from chelated sources than mature, idle horses.

In the absence of further information on mineral bioavailability specific to horses, estimates for some nonruminant (e.g., swine) and ruminant species have been summarized (McDowell, 2003) and may provide a rough estimate of bioavailability differences between mineral sources.

Vitamin Supplements

Supplemental vitamins differ in chemical form, vitamin activity, and stability. Several vitamins (A, D, E, and K) are susceptible to destruction by various factors associated with feed manufacturing (e.g., heat, moisture, pH, light, pro-oxidants). Vitamin stability of supplemental forms is often improved by synthesis of stable derivatives (e.g., esterification of retinol to retinyl-palmitate), addition of antioxidants (e.g., ethoxyquin, butylated hydroxytoluene), fat coating, incorporation into gelatin-carbohydrate matrix (e.g., beadlets, spray-dried powder), and absorbance and adsorbance of vitamins to various carrier substances (e.g., adsorbance to silica) (McDowell, 2003). Several detailed reviews on vitamin stability and factors influencing stability have been published (Roche Vitamins Inc., 2000; BASF Corp., 2001). Table 8-9 lists different forms of vitamins, vitamin activity of each form, physical form, applications, and information regarding vitamin stability. More specific information regarding numerous factors and the magnitude of their effect on stability is available (Roche Vitamins Inc., 2000; BASF Corp., 2001).

FEED PROCESSING AND MANUFACTURING

Rations fed to horses routinely contain feed ingredients that are processed post-harvesting. Processing can affect the physical, chemical, and microbiological properties of the feedstuff to be processed and may improve animal performance, feed manufacturing and storage, ease of feed handling, and consumer acceptance (Fahrenholz, 1994; Van Der Poel et al., 1995; Behnke, 1996; Hancock and Behnke, 2001). Processing alters the size, density, and texture of feed, which can positively influence animal utilization and purchaser acceptance. Processing may improve the intake and digestibility of rations, and deleterious compounds may be denatured or inactivated. Hygienic specifications may be improved by reducing bacterial and/or fungal infestations. In addition, processing allows more varieties of feedstuffs to be incorporated into rations, and reduces the level of dust. Diet uniformity, feed handling, and storage may be enhanced.

Animal feed processing systems use equipment that shapes and thermally treats feed. Processing methods that are common to horse rations include chopping, cubing, wafering, and pelleting of forages and complete feeds. Grains, grain byproducts, and complete feeds are routinely pelleted; extruded; compressed by rolling, flaking, or crimping; or treated with steam and high temperatures that alter their physical and chemical properties. Feeds may be cleaned, screened, or sifted to remove various sized particles. Supplements and additives are commonly processed to produce finely ground powders, crumbles, bricks, blocks, gels, or emulsified liquids. There are other processing methods inherent to the preparation of individual feedstuffs prior to mixing such as culturing of biological materials, curing forages for preservation, extracting oils or other compounds intended for other uses, or removing or denaturing undesirable compounds that might affect the health or performance of a horse.

The Official Publication of the Association of American Feed Control Officials (AAFCO, 2005) serves as one source of information and recognized standard in the United States for feed manufacturing regulations, guidelines, and feed terms and ingredients. Some of the terminology more commonly used in formulation of horse diets is defined in Appendix 8-1.

There are many reported advantages for processing feeds intended for animal consumption. A review of research conducted by Hancock and Behnke (2001) identified several benefits with processing swine feeds. Pelleting can increase rates of gain, increase palatability, decrease feed wastage, and decrease environmental wastes as compared with meal feeding. Grinding complete diets can increase feed utilization. Differences in the particle size of ground feed can influence gain efficiency, digestibility, and feed intake. However, the review also pointed out the complexity of diet processing technology and the need for evaluating the conditions under which each trial was conducted. Animal response can be significantly influenced by differences in feed ingredients, intakes, and processing technologies.

The effect of processing feed in ruminant diets also has received considerable attention. Research areas include the influence of ration particle size on ruminal function, ruminally protected amino acids, and a significant amount of interest with processing and carbohydrate utilization (NRC, 2000,

TABLE 8-9 Supplemental Vitamin Sources: Chemical Form, Vitamin Activity, Physical Form, and Applications[a]

Vitamin	Chemical Form	Vitamin Activity/	Physical Form	Applications
A				
	retinyl-acetate	2.9 IU/μg	beadlets	dry feeds
			spray- or drum-dried powders	dry feeds and water-dispersible vitamin products
	retinyl-palmitate	1.82 IU/μg	liquid water-soluble emulsions	liquid feed supplements
D				
	cholecalciferol	40 IU/μg	beadlets with vitamin A	dry feeds
			spray- or drum-dried powders	dry feeds, water-dispersible vitamin products
			liquid concentrates	liquid feed supplements
E				
	dl-α-tocopheryl acetate (all-rac)	1 IU/mg	adsorbate powders, dry dilutions, oils	dry feeds
			spray-dried coated powders	dry feeds, water-dispersible vitamin products
	d-α-tocopheryl acetate (RRR)	1.36 IU/mg	liquid concentrates	liquid feed supplements
K				
	menadione sodium bisulfite	500 g/kg	dry dilutions	dry feeds
	menadione dimethyl-pyrimidinol bisulfite	454 g/kg	water-dispersible powders	water-dispersible vitamin products
	menadione sodium bisulfite complex	330 g/kg		
Thiamin				
	thiamin mononitrate	920 g/kg	crystalline; fine powder	dry feeds
	thiamin hydrochloride	890 g/kg	crystalline; dry dilution	dry feeds and water-dispersible vitamin products
Riboflavin				
	crystalline riboflavin	1 g/g	spray-dried powder	dry feeds
Niacin				
	crystalline nicotinic acid	1 g/g	crystalline and dried dilutions	dry feeds
	crystalline nicotinamide	1 g/g		
Folic acid				
	crystalline folic acid	1 g/g	crystalline and dried dilutions	dry feeds
Biotin				
	crystalline d-biotin	1 g/g	crystalline and dried dilutions	dry feeds
Vitamin C				
	L-ascorbic acid (100% crystalline)	1 g/g	crystalline	water-dispersible vitamin products
	L-ascorbic acid (50%; fat coated)	500 g/kg	fat coated	dry feeds
	L-ascorbic acid (97.5%; ethylcellulose-coated)	975 g/kg	ethylcellulose-coated	dry feeds
	ascorbyl palmitate	400 g/kg	ascorbic acid ester	dry feeds
	calcium ascorbyl-2-monophosphate	350 g/kg	ascorbic acid ester	dry feeds

[a]Adapted from Roche Vitamins Inc. (2000); McDowell (2000).

2001). In a review of research with feedlot cattle, Owens et al. (1997) stressed the need to carefully analyze the conditions under which specific trials were conducted. The effects of processing on animal performance differed among trials, probably due to differences in the grain processing methods, grain choices, and characteristics of additional ingredients.

Reviewing research in other species is beneficial to develop a more comprehensive knowledge of how processing affects different production parameters, as results can be extrapolated in areas where specific research in the equine is lacking. However, the level of accuracy of predicting responses may be low because of differences in physiology and management of horses.

There are fewer research trials reported and there is less depth of information available, about the effects of feed processing of horse feeds compared to the effects of processing of feedstuffs for other species of livestock.

Most of the investigations and reports have centered on comparative utilization of feeds processed by different methods or on the effect of processing on ingestive behavior.

Total Tract Digestibility

The past NRC committee reported that processing increased the total tract digestibility of oats and barley by only a small percentage (2–5 percent) with increased benefits for grains with harder seed coats (NRC, 1989). The suggestion that processing of softer seed-coated grains, such as oats, has little effect on total tract digestibility has been confirmed by several trials.

Coleman et al. (1985) reported similar dry matter and energy digestibility for oats fed whole, rolled, or pelleted when mature horses were fed the grains at two different intake levels with an alfalfa cube forage. Lopez et al. (1988) found no differences in digestibility of energy, CP, ether extract, ADF, or NDF for rations containing alfalfa hay cubes with whole, cut and vacuum-cleaned, or cut and recombined oats.

Similar to the results with processed oats, Coleman et al. (1985) found no improvement in total tract digestibility of DM or energy when whole barley was rolled and fed to mature horses. McLean et al. (1999) found no differences in total tract apparent digestibility of DM, OM, GE, starch, CP, ADF, or NDF when ponies were fed rolled, micronized, or extruded barley.

Pelleting a diet of rolled barley, alfalfa hay, and wheat bran did not affect CF, CP, and nitrogen-free extract (NFE) digestibility of growing-horse rations (Hintz and Loy, 1966). Pipkin et al. (1991) noted similar digestibility of rations fed as a complete, wafered form or as a textured grain mix and long-stem forage. Raina and Raghavan (1985) reported decreased DM and CF digestibility of a ground concentrate fed with chopped hay as compared to the same grain mix in pelleted or unprocessed form. They postulated the decrease in digestibility might be due to an increased rate of flow in the hindgut associated with the smaller particle size of the ground mix.

There are reported increases in the total tract digestibility of ether extract. Hintz and Loy (1966) reported a 6 percent increase in the total tract digestibility of ether extract when a complete ration was fed in a pelleted vs. a nonpelleted form. Pagan and Jackson (1991a) noted that pelleting alfalfa hay decreased total tract digestibility of fat. Diets in both studies contained low amounts of fat with values reported between 2.8 to 4 percent ether extract.

Even though most of these reports suggest little benefit of processing oats, barley, or alfalfa forage on total tract digestibility, these methods may have more significance if feeding horses with poor dentition or horses with limited digestive capacities, such as young horses that are meal-fed large amounts of grains. It is reasonable also to assume that coarsely processing hard-seed coat grains such as corn has more benefit.

The unique arrangement of the horse's digestive tract may limit the significance of measurements such as total tract digestion. As the digestive processes of the stomach and small intestine are significantly different than digestion in the hindgut, site of digestion may be of more importance when addressing the relative benefit of processing. Most notably, recent research interests have focused on site of digestion of starch.

Starch Digestibility

Many horses are fed meals containing significant amounts of starch in combination with hay or green forage. Starch is highly digestible, with total tract digestibility ranging from 87 percent to nearly 100 percent (Potter et al., 1992a). Starch not digested in the small intestine is readily digested by microbial digestion in the hindgut. Large amounts of starch bypassing the small intestine is thought to increase digestive upset because of adverse changes in the microbial population and dysfunction of the hindgut.

The rate and site of digestion of starch is influenced by many factors, including intake level, morphology and processing of starch, intake of the total ration, forage intake, rate of passage through the small intestine, level of amylase, and individual differences between horses (Potter et al., 1992a; Kienzle et al., 1992, 1997; Meyer et al., 1993; Kienzle, 1994; Cuddeford, 1999; Hussein and Vogedes, 2003; Jose-Cunilleras et al., 2004).

Processing is but one of the potential influences on the site of starch digestion, and the interaction of associated factors increases the difficulty of independently assessing the effect of processing. Regardless, processing can affect the site of starch digestion. Comparisons of whole, crushed, ground, or popped corn suggest that grinding increases small intestinal starch digestibility about 15 percent over digestibility of whole or cracked corn (Table 8-10) (Meyer et al., 1993). In addition, the percent preileal starch digestibility was higher for popped corn than for whole, crushed, or ground corn. Digestibility estimates were obtained from five ponies fitted with permanent fistulas at the end of the jejunum. Chromic oxide was used as a marker. The ponies were fed at 12-hour intervals, and the grains were fed with green meal. Starch intake per meal and digestibility are provided in Table 8-10.

The increase in preileal starch digestibility of processed corn may parallel the degree of molecular disruption of the starch molecule. Popping is thought to destroy the structure of starch in corn to a greater level than grinding or crushing, and this greater level of destruction enhances solubility of starch molecules and absorption in the small intestine of the horse (Potter et al., 1992a; Meyer et al., 1993; Kienzle, 1994). The disruption of the structure of starch is more extensive with heat- and steam-processed corn than with

TABLE 8-10 Comparison of Small Intestinal Starch Digestibility of Processed Corn[a,b]

	Whole Corn	Crushed Corn	Ground Corn	Popped Corn
Starch intake (g/kg BW/meal) morning:evening	1.9:1.0	1.9:1.1	2.1:2.0	1.3:1.5
Preileal starch digestibility (%)	28.9[c]	29.9[c]	45.6[d]	90.1[e]

[a]Adapted from Meyer et al. (1993).
[b]Digestibility reflective of total ration of grain fed with green meal.
[c,d,e]Values with different superscripts reported different at $P < 0.05$.

ground corn and more extensive with ground corn than whole or broken corn (Kienzle et al., 1997). The proposed relationship between processing methods, disruption of the structure of starch, and the potential effects on digestibility and animal performance receives considerable support with research conducted on other species (Gray, 1992; NRC, 2001; Zinn et al., 2002; Zarkadas and Wiseman, 2002).

Gelatinization refers to the irreversible swelling and the destruction of the internal crystalline structure of starch granules brought about by thermal processing (Selmi et al., 2000; Zinn et al., 2002; Vervuert et al., 2004). The ability of thermal, high-pressure processing methods to gelatinize starch in cereal grains has been well established (Selmi et al., 2000). Processing methods, such as steam flaking of corn and micronizing of barley and wheat, can increase the degree of gelatinization of starch in cereal grains. Increases in solubility and availability of starch to enzymatic and microbial digestion should increase feed value; however, research findings in other species provide differing results with diet digestibility and animal performance.

Work with growing-finishing beef cattle suggests that steam flaking sorghum improves the feeding value by 12–15 percent above dry rolling (Swingle et al., 1999). Similarly, Zinn et al. (2002) suggested steam flaking corn increases the net energy for maintenance and gain in growing cattle by 14 percent and 17 percent, respectively, over dry rolling. Studies with mature dairy cows suggest less consistent improvements in feed utilization (NRC, 2001), as does research with growing swine (Hongtrakul et al., 1998; Zarkadas and Wiseman, 2001, 2002).

Associative interactions such as intake level, degree of retrogradation, differences in starch morphology between grain species and varieties, animal differences, and processing methods will influence the results of research relating processing, starch morphology, and animal performance. The degree of structural breakdown of a starch molecule may vary with different sources of a specific grain processed similarly because of differences in equipment and conditions at mills, and differences in nutrient content and harvesting methods of the grain (Kienzle et al., 1997; Zinn et al., 2002). Meyer et al. (1993) reported that ground corn milled at different locations to similar maximally allowed size (maximum particle size < 2 mm) had enough differences in the degree of starch alteration to influence trial results.

Similar to corn, grinding can increase preileal starch digestibility of oats over values obtained with whole or rolled oats (Table 8-11) (Kienzle et al., 1992). Estimates in Table 8-11 were obtained from six horses with cannulas in the terminal jejunum. Chromic oxide was used as a marker. The horses were fed at 12-hour intervals. Grass meal was added to both meals when ground oats were fed, and to the evening meal only when the whole and rolled oats were fed.

The degree of small intestinal digestibility of whole or coarsely processed oats appears to be greater than corn (Kienzle et al., 1992; Meyer et al., 1993). The relatively high small intestinal starch digestibility of oats, whether processed or not, is supported by examination of oat starch granules retrieved from intestinal chyme. The structure of the starch granules in both whole and rolled oats appears to be greatly altered by enzymatic digestion, possibly a result of the normal morphology of the starch molecule in oats and the effect of normal chewing on the disruption of the oat seed coat (Kienzle et al., 1997).

Studies have been conducted to compare digestibility of different grains that are similarly processed. Preileal starch digestibility of rolled oats has been reported to be over three times that of rolled barley (Table 8-12) (Meyer, 1993). Observations of the morphology of starch granules suggest that the susceptibility to enzymatic digestion of starch molecules in rolled barley is somewhat intermediate between starch in processed corn and rolled oats (Kienzle et al., 1997).

Potter et al. (1992a) reported little difference in the prececal starch digestibility of rolled corn, oats, barley, or sorghum when fed in low amounts to ponies (Table 8-13). Four ileally cannulated ponies were fed at 12-hour intervals, and rations included chopped Bermudagrass hay with the grains. The prececal starch digestibility of rolled barley was numerically higher; however, this value may have been influenced by an abnormally high digestibility of rolled barley by one of the ponies used in the experiment (Potter, 1992a).

When combining results with oats and sorghum, Potter et al. (1992a) reported higher prececal starch digestion with micronizing as compared with crimping (61 percent vs. 42

TABLE 8-11 Comparison of Small Intestinal Starch Digestibility of Processed Oats[a,b]

	Whole Oats	Rolled Oats	Ground Oats
Starch intake (g/kg BW/meal) morning:evening	2.0:1.0	1.8:0.9	1.8:1.8
Preileal starch digestibility (%)	83.50[c]	85.23[c]	98.05[d]

[a]Adapted from Kienzle et al. (1992).
[b]Digestibility reflective of total ration of grain fed with grass meal.
[c,d]Values with different superscripts were reported to be significantly different (P < 0.05).

TABLE 8-12 Comparison of Small Intestinal Starch Digestibility of Processed Oats and Barley[a,b]

	Rolled Oats	Rolled Barley
Starch intake (g/kg BW/meal) morning:evening	1.8:0.9	2.0:2.0
Preileal starch digestibility (%)	85.2[c]	21.4[d]

[a]Adapted from Meyer et al. (1993).
[b]Digestibility reflective of total ration of grain fed with green meal.
[c,d]Values with different superscripts were reported to be significantly different (P < 0.05).

TABLE 8-13 Comparison of Small Intestinal Starch Digestibility of Grains[a,b,c]

	Rolled Corn	Rolled Oats	Rolled Barley	Rolled Sorghum	Mean
Starch intake (g/kg BW/meal[d])	1.3	1.2	1.5	1.2	1.3
Prececal starch digestibility (%)	80.9	81.0	95.9	80.3	85.1
Total tract starch digestibility (%)	98.9	98.9	98.9	97.6	98.6

[a]Adapted from Arnold (1982) as reported in Potter et al. (1992a).
[b]Digestibility reflective of total ration of grain fed with chopped Bermudagrass hay.
[c]No significant differences observed between grains.
[d]Meals fed twice daily.

percent). Four ileally cannulated horses were fed at 12-hour intervals, and rations consisted of a 50:50 ratio of grain and Bermudagrass hay. An interaction between grain type and processing method was noted (Table 8-14), with micronized oats having higher prececal starch digestibility than crimped sorghum.

Small intestinal starch absorption is not only energetically efficient compared with microbial digestion in the cecum and large intestine, but also it guards against digestive disorders resulting from soluble carbohydrate digestion by microbes in the cecum and large intestine (Lewis, 1995; Longland, 2001). It is apparent that processing grains can significantly influence the relative amounts of starch digested in the small intestine. However, as influencing factors such as differences in the degree of starch disruption of similarly processed grains, differences in intake, and differences between horses affect results, application of results from single trials should be guarded, and differences in animal response should be expected.

TABLE 8-14 Comparison of Small Intestinal Starch Digestibility of Grains Fed at Moderate Intakes[a,b]

	Crimped Oats	Micronized Oats	Crimped Sorghum	Micronized Sorghum	Mean
Starch intake (g/kg BW/meal)	2.6	2.4	2.9	2.8	2.7
Prececal starch digestibility (%)	48.0	62.3[c]	36.0[d]	59.0	51.3
Total tract starch digestibility	94.4	93.8	94.0	94.5	94.1

[a]Adapted from Householder (1978) as reported in Potter et al. (1992a).
[b]Digestibility reflective of total ration of grain fed with Bermudagrass hay.
[c,d]Values with different superscripts reported different at $P < 0.1$.

Even though results appear to be specific to intake levels, types of processing, and types of grains, digestibility trials show that processing can influence the degree of small intestinal starch digestibility. Indirect measures of prececal starch digestibility support results identified in digestion trials. Intracecal lactate concentrations following meals of rolled, micronized, or extruded barley have been reported to be higher when ponies were fed rolled barley as compared to the other two processed barley meals (McLean et al., 2000). Steam flaked corn fed to mature horses produced a greater glycemic response and higher peak plasma glucose concentration than did ground or cracked corn (Hoekstra et al., 1999). Other research conducted to evaluate the effect of processing on glycemic and insulinemic responses in horses has not elicited as clear a response. Horses fed finely ground, steamed, micronized, steam flaked, or popped corn had similar responses in post-prandial blood glucose and insulin concentrations regardless of processing treatment (Vervuert et al., 2004).

Similarly, Vervuert et al. (2003) found little effect on post-prandial plasma glucose or insulin response when oats were processed by grinding, steam flaking, or popping. Associative interactions such as individual horse responses, differences in the degree of starch gelatinization of similar grains processed similarly, and intake levels may partially explain the differences in results from various researchers. Additionally, Kronfeld et al. (2004) reinforced the need to use glycemic indices cautiously as large errors in their mean values and the nonlinearity of glucose-insulin regulatory system limited glycemic indices' use.

Processing also influences the rate of starch digestion. McLean et al. (1998) compared the rate of starch degradation of whole, micronized, and extruded barley by placing incubation bags in situ of cecally fistulated ponies. Little differences in degradation of dry matter or starch were evident after 40 hours of incubation. However, there was a reported increased rate of degradation of micronized barley as compared with whole barley during the first 20 hours of incubation.

Protein Digestibility

The lack of research relating processing to protein digestibility in horses makes recommendations difficult. As mentioned in the previous section on total tract nutrient digestibility, most reports suggest little to no influence of processing on protein digestibility. Horses are capable of both enzymatic digestion of protein leading to absorption of amino acids in the small intestine and fermentative digestion of protein leading to absorption of ammonia in the large intestine. This capability, with the differences in the absorbed products of digestion, limits the usefulness of total tract protein digestibility as a measurement to determine the relative value of different processing methods.

In a summary of several trials conducted in their laboratory, Potter et al. (1992b) identified compensatory digestion of protein similar to that found with digestion of energy. They concluded that large intestine true digestibility of protein from several different feedstuffs was 80–90 percent, while small intestine true digestibility of protein varied from 45–80 percent. Prececal digestibility differed with inclusions of different feedstuffs and levels of intake.

One of the trials compared mixed diets of grass hay and either oats or sorghum where the grains were fed crimped or micronized (Table 8-15). Four ileally cannulated horses were fed at 12-hour intervals, and rations consisted of a 50:50 ratio of grain and Bermudagrass hay. Total tract apparent digestibility of nitrogen of crimped sorghum was lower than either of the two sources of oats. Prececal digestibility of micronized oats appeared to be lower than crimped oats or either source of sorghum, although other sources of variation apparently were so large that there were no significant differences due to grain type or processing method.

The effect of processing on amino acid absorption in the small intestine requires further investigation, especially in horses fed large amounts of protein in meal feeding. By calculating expected absorption of amino acids from results of several different trials, Gibbs and Potter (2002) emphasized the potential for deficiencies of amino acids in diets fed to growing horses, even when rations met protein requirements based on total tract digestion.

Underprocessing may leave a deleterious level of anti-nutritional factors, such as trypsin in soybean meal, which has been shown to affect performance and growth in other species. Excessive heating may reduce the availability of essential amino acids (Dale, 1996). Research on the utilization of feedstuffs by other species shows that some processing methods can decrease the availability of amino acids because of the Maillard reaction, in which protein combines with other nutrients to form large compounds with differing volatility and solubility (Hardy et al., 1999; Mavromichalis and Baker, 2000).

SUMMARY

Specific horse diets vary greatly in form, ranging from rations consisting solely of nonharvested forages to those containing feeds processed by a variety of methods. Feed processing provides many potential advantages to the feed milling industry. Formulations may include a greater variety of ingredients, feed handling may be eased, storage time lengthened, and consumer acceptance increased. Some processing methods may have a small effect on total tract digestibility for some feeds. In addition, some processing methods may influence the site of digestion for specific feed components, such as starch. Therefore, improvements in the utilization of energetic nutrients may be more related to site of digestion rather than observable differences in total tract digestibility. As energetic efficiency is higher with small intestinal starch digestion, shifting the percentage of starch digested prececally should also increase the energy value of grains. Benefits appear to be related to differences in the structure of starch molecules of different grains, and with processing methods that combine sufficient heat and steam to affect the chemical structure of starch. Research is limited, and results have varied between trials. However, processing has had the most dramatic effect on the small intestinal starch digestibility of corn. Effects have also been observed from the micronizing of barley and oats. Estimates from the previous version of the NRC (1989) of 2–5 percent increase in the digestibility of barley, with more benefits to processing hard-seed coat grains such as corn and milo, are supported with recently reported research on the site of starch digestion. Improvements with energy utilization are expected to be largest with processes that significantly disrupt the structure of the starch molecule, such as micronizing, steam flaking, and popping.

Quantifying expected benefits of processing for all feeding plans and horses is difficult. The relative benefit of processing will depend on many influencing factors including grain type, horse differences, processing method, and level of starch and dry matter intake. Processing has a significant potential for reducing digestive upset of horses that are fed meals containing high amounts of starch that is resistant to small intestinal digestion. Horses with limited ability to chew rations because of poor dentition should respond more favorably to processed feeds than those horses able to break up feed prior to swallowing.

Behavioral and intake differences observed with differently processed feeds could be large enough to alter other management routines (see Chapter 11). Slower intakes may be desirable to reduce boredom with confined horses. However, the relative behavioral and physiological importance of processing appears to be specific to intake, feedstuffs, processing method, and horses.

TABLE 8-15 Comparison of Small Intestinal Nitrogen Digestibility of Diets Containing Micronized and Crimped Oats and Sorghum[a,b]

	Crimped Oats	Micronized Oats	Crimped Sorghum	Micronized Sorghum	Mean
Nitrogen intake (mg/kg BW/meal)	130	132	138	130	132
Prececal apparent digestibility (%)	45.4	35.9	51.5	52.0	46.2
Total tract apparent digestibility	68.6[d,e]	70.9[e]	62.2[c]	65.1[c,d]	66.7

[a]Adapted from Klendshoj (1979) as reported in Potter et al. (1992b).
[b]Digestibility reflective of total ration of grain fed with a soybean meal based supplement in a 50:50 ratio with Bermudagrass hay.
[c,d,e]Values with different superscripts reported different at P < 0.05.

APPENDIX 8-1 SELECTED TERMINOLOGY RELATED TO FEED IDENTIFICATION AND PROCESSING

SOURCE: Adapted from AAFCO (2005).

Additive. An ingredient or combination of ingredients added to the basic feed mix or parts thereof to fulfill a specific need. Usually used in micro quantities and requires careful handling and mixing.

Balanced. A term that may be applied to a diet, ration, or feed having all the known required nutrients in proper amount and proportion based upon recommendations of recognized authorities in the field of animal nutrition, such as the National Research Council, for a given set of physiological animal requirements.

Blocks. Agglomerated feed compressed into a solid mass cohesive enough to hold its form and weighing over 2 pounds, and generally weighing 14 to 22 kg.

Bricks. Agglomerated feed, other than pellets, compressed into a solid mass cohesive enough to hold its form and weighing less than 0.91 kg.

Byproduct. Secondary products produced in addition to the principal product.

Carriers. An edible material to which ingredients are added to facilitate uniform incorporation of the latter into feeds. The active particles are absorbed, impregnated, or coated into or onto the edible material in such a way as to physically carry the active ingredient.

Chopped, chopping. Reduced in particle size by cutting with knives or other edged instruments.

Cleaned, cleaning. Removal of material by such methods as scalping, aspirating, magnetic separation, or by any other method.

Commercial feed. As defined in the Uniform State Feed Bill, all materials except unmixed whole seeds or physically altered entire unmixed seeds, when not adulterated, which are distributed for use as feed or for mixing in feed.

Complete feed. A nutritionally adequate feed for animals other than humans; by specific formula is compounded to be fed as the sole ration and is capable of maintaining life and/or promoting production without any additional substance being consumed except water. *Note: Other regulatory agencies also include those feeds that provide all of the nutritional requirements necessary for maintenance of life or for promoting production except water* **and** *roughage within the definition of complete feeds.*

Concentrate. A feed used with another to improve the nutritive balance of the total and intended to be further diluted and mixed to produce a supplement or complete feed.

Conditioning. Having achieved predetermined moisture characteristics and/or temperature of ingredients or a mixture of ingredients prior to further processing.

Cooked, cooking. Heated in the presence of moisture to alter chemical and/or physical characteristics or to sterilize.

Cracked, cracking. Particle size reduced by a combined breaking or crushing action.

Crimped, crimping. Rolled by use of corrugated rollers, which may curtail tempering or conditioning and cooling.

Crumbled, crumbling. Pellets reduced to a granular form.

Customer-formula feed. Consists of a mixture of commercial feeds and/or feed ingredients each batch of which is manufactured according to the specific instructions of the final purchaser.

Dehulled, dehulling. Having removed the outer covering of grains or other seeds.

Dehydrating, dehydrated. Having been freed of moisture by thermal means.

Diet. Feed ingredients or mixture of ingredients including water, which is consumed by animals.

Expanded. Subjected to moisture, pressure, and temperature to gelatinize the starch portion.

Extracted, mechanical. Having removed fat or oil from materials by heat and mechanical pressure. Similar terms: expeller extracted, hydraulic extracted, "old process."

Extracted, solvent. Having removed fat or oil from materials by organic solvents. Similar term: "new process."

Extruded. A process by which feed has been pressed, pushed, or protruded through orifices under pressure. Feed is fed through the extruder from a holding bin, through a mixing cylinder and into the extruder barrel. The feed is subjected to increased pressure, friction, and attrition as it passes through the barrel. As the feed is released from the extruder barrel, it expands violently as steam is released because of the sudden drop in pressure.

Feed(s). Edible material(s) that are consumed by animals and contribute energy and/or nutrients to the animal's diet. (Usually refers to animals rather than humans.)

Fines. Any materials that will pass through a screen whose openings are immediately smaller than the specified minimum crumble size or pellet diameter.

Flakes. An ingredient rolled or cut into flat pieces with or without prior steam conditioning.

Fodder. The green or cured plant, containing all the ears or seed heads, if any, grown primarily for forage.

Formula feed. Two or more ingredients proportioned, mixed, and processed according to specifications.

Gelatinized, gelatinizing. Having had the starch granules completely ruptured by a combination of moisture, heat, and pressure, and, in some instances, by mechanical shear.

Germ. (Part) The embryo found in seeds and frequently separated from bran and starch endosperm during the milling.

Gluten. The tough, viscid nitrogenous substance remaining when the flour or wheat or other grain is washed to remove the starch.

Grain. Seed from cereal plants.

Ground, grinding. Reduced in particle size by impact, shearing, or attrition.

Hay. The aerial portion of grass or herbage especially cut and cured for animal feeding.

Hulls. Outer covering of grain or other seed.

Ingredient, feed ingredient. A component part or constituent of any combination or mixture making up a commercial feed.

Kibbled, kibbling. Cracked or crushed baked dough, or extruded feed that has been cooked before the extrusion process.

Meal. An ingredient that has been ground or otherwise reduced in particle size.

Middlings. A byproduct of flour milling comprising several grades of granular particles containing different proportions of endosperm, bran, and germ, each of which contains different amounts of crude fiber.

Nutrient. A feed constituent in a form and a level that will help support the life of an animal. The chief classes of feed nutrients are proteins, fats, carbohydrates, minerals, and vitamins.

Pellets. Agglomerated feed formed by compacting and forcing through die openings by a mechanical process.

Premix. A uniform mixture of one or more microingredients with diluents and/or carrier. Premixes are used to facilitate uniform dispersion of the microingredients in a large mix.

Ration. The amount of total feed that is provided to one animal over a 24-hour period.

Rolled, rolling. Changing the shape and/or size of particles by compressing between rollers. It may entail tempering or conditioning.

Seed. The fertilized and ripened ovule of a plant.

Self fed. A feeding system where animals have continuous free access to some or all component(s) of a ration either individually or as mixtures.

Steamed, steaming. Treating ingredients with steam to alter physical and/or chemical properties.

Supplement. A feed used with another to improve nutritive balance or performance of the total and intended to be:

(1) Fed undiluted as a supplement to other feeds;
(2) Offered free choice with other parts of the ration separately available; or
(3) Further diluted and mixed to produce a complete feed.

Trace minerals. Mineral nutrients required by animals in micro amounts only (measured in milligrams per pound or smaller units).

Wafered, wafering. Having agglomerated a feed of a fibrous nature by compressing into a form usually having a diameter or cross-section measurement greater than its length.

Whole. Complete, entire.

REFERENCES

AAFCO (Association of American Feed Control Officials, Inc.). 2005. Official Publication. Oxford, IN: Association of American Feed Control Officials.

Adams, L. G., J. W. Dollahite, W. M. Romane, T. L. Bullard, and C. H. Bridges. 1969. Cystitis and ataxia associated with sorghum ingestion in horses. J. Am. Vet. Med. Assoc. 155:518–524.

Aiken, G. E., G. D. Potter, B. E. Conrad, and J. W. Evans. 1989. Voluntary intake and digestion of coastal Bermuda grass hay by yearling and mature horses. J. Equine Vet. Sci. 9:262–264.

Aiken, G. E., D. I. Bransby, and C. A. McCall. 1993. Growth of yearling horses compared to steers on high endophyte and low endophyte infected tall fescue. J. Equine Vet. Sci. 13:26–28.

Akin, D. E., and D. Burdick. 1975. Percentage of tissue types in tropical and temperate leaf blades and degradation of tissues by rumen microorganisms. Crop Sci. 15:661–668.

Allison, C. D. 1998. Nitrate poisoning of livestock. New Mexico State University Guide B-802.

Almeida, M. I. V., W. M. Ferreira, F. Q. Almeida, C. A. S. Just, L. C. Goncalves, and A. S. C. Rezende. 1999. Nutritive value of elephant grass (*Pennisetum purpureum,* Schum), alfalfa hay (*Medicago sativa*) and coast-grass cross hay (*Cynodon dactylon* L.) for horses. Zootech. Doutorando Zootecnica, DZO, UFV, 36571-000. Vicosa, MG, Brazil.

Åman, P., and H. Graham. 1990. Chemical evaluation of polysaccharides in animal feeds. Pp. 161–178 in Feedstuff Evaluation, J. Wiseman and D. J. A. Cole, eds. London: Butterworths.

Ammerman, C. B., D. H. Baker, and A. J. Lewis. 1995. Bio-availability of nutrients for animals: amino acids, minerals and vitamins. San Diego, CA: Academic Press.

Angsubhakorn, S., P. Poomvises, K. Romruen, and P. M. Newberne. 1981. Aflatoxicosis in horses. J. Am. Vet. Med. Assoc. 1778:274–278.

APHIS (Animal and Plant Health Inspection Service). 1995. Factsheet: mycotoxin levels in the 1995 Midwest corn crop. USDA-APHIS, Publication N195.1295.

APHIS. 1996. Infosheet: mycotoxin levels in the 1996 Midwest corn crop. USDA-APHIS, Publication N222.1296.

Argo, C. M. G., Z. Fuller, C. Lockyer, and J. E. Cox. 2002. Adaptive changes in appetite, growth and feeding behaviour of pony mares offered *ad libitum* access to a complete diet in either a pelleted or chaff-based form. Anim. Sci. 74:517–528.

Bachmann, I., L. Audige, and M. Stauffacher. 2003. Risk factors associated with behavioural disorders of crib-biting, weaving and box-walking in Swiss horses. Equine Vet. J. 35:158–163.

Bacon, C. W., and P. E. Nelson. 1994. Fumonisin production in corn by toxigenic strains of Fusarium moniliforme and Fusarium proliferatum. J. Food Protect. 57:514–521.

Bacon, C. W., and J. F. White. 2000. Microbial Endophytes. New York: Marcel Dekker.

Baker, L. A., T. Kearney-Moss, J. L. Pipkin, R. C. Bachman, J. T. Haliburton, and G. O. Veneklasen. 2003. The effect of supplemental inorganic and organic sources of copper and zinc on bone metabolism in exercised yearling geldings. Pp. 100–105 in Proc. 18th Equine Nutr. Physiol. Symp., East Lansing, MI.

Baker, L. A., M. R. Wrigley, J. L. Pipkin, J. T. Haliburton, and R. C. Bachman. 2005. Digestibility and retention of inorganic and organic sources of copper and zinc in mature horses. Pp. 162–167 in Proc. 19th Equine Sci. Soc., Tucson, AZ.

Barker, D. J., and M. Collins. 2003. Forage fertilisation and nutrient management. In Forages, vol. 11. The Science of Grassland Agriculture, 6th ed., R. F. Barnes, C. J. Nelson, M. Collins, and K. J. Moore, eds. Ames: Iowa State University Press.

BASF Corp. 2001. Vitamin Stability in Premixes and Feeds: A Practical Approach. Available at http://www.basf.com/animalnutrition/pdfs/kc_9138.pdf.

Beeson, K. K., L. Gray, and M. B. Adams. 1947. The absorption of mineral elements by plants. 1. the phosphorous, cobalt, magnesium and copper content of some common grasses. J. Am. Soc. Agron. 39:356.

Beever, D. E., N. Offer, and M. Gill. 2000. The feeding value of grass and grass products. Chapter 7 in Grass: Its Production and Utilisation, 3rd ed., A. Hopkins, ed. Oxford, UK: British Grassland Society, Blackwell Science Publications.

Behnke, K. C. 1996. Feed manufacturing technology: current issues and challenges. Anim. Feed Sci. Technol. 62:49–57.

Belyea, L., F. A. Martz, and S. Bell. 1985. Storage and feeding losses of large round bales. J. Dairy Sci. 68:3371–3375.

Bender, M., and D. Smith. 1973. Classification of starch and fructosan—accumulating grasses as C3 or C4 species by carbon-isotope analysis. J. Br. Grassland Soc. 28:97–100.

Benyovsky, B. M., K. Penksza, and J. Hausenblasz. 1998. Quality requirements of pasture for horses (pp. 216–223). Zavod za Pomurje, Murska Sobota, Slovenia.

Bergero, D., P. G. Peiretti, and E. Cola. 2002. Intake and apparent digestibility of perennial ryegrass haylages fed to ponies either at maintenance or at work. Livest. Prod. Sci. 77:325–329.

Bigot, G., C. Trilland-Geyl, M. Jussiaux, and W. Martin-Rosset. 1987. Elevage du cheval de selle du severage an debourrage: alimentation hivonale croissance et development. Bulletin Technicale Centre de Recherche Zootechniques et Veterinaires de Thiex 69:45–53.

Blackman, H., and M. J. S. Moore-Colyer. 1998. Hay for horses: the effects of three different wetting treatments on dust and mineral content. Anim. Sci. 66:745–750.

Borton, A., D. R. Anderson, and S. Lyford. 1973. Studies of protein quality and quantity in the early weaned foal. P. 19 in Proc. 3rd Equine Nutr. Phys. Soc. Symp., Gainesville, FL.

Bowden, D. M., D. K. Taylor, and W. E. P. Davis. 1968. Water-soluble carbohydrates in orchardgrass and mixed forages. Can. J. Plant Sci. 48:9–15.

Bowman, V. A., J. P. Fontenot, T. N. Meacham, and K. E. Webb, Jr. 1979. Acceptability and digestibility of animal, vegetable and blended fats by equines. Pp. 74–75 in Proc. 6th Equine Nutr. Physiol. Symp., College Station, TX.

Brady, C. J. 1960. Redistribution of nitrogen in grass and leguminous fodder during wilting and ensilage. J. Sci. Food Agric. 11:276–284.

Brown-Douglas, G. C. 2003. Aspects of puberty and growth in pasture-raised New Zealand Thouroughbreds born in spring and autumn. Ph.D. Thesis. Massey University, Palmerston North, New Zealand.

Browne, C. A. 1933. The spontaneous heating and ignition of hay and other agricultural products. Science 77:223–232.

Brussow, N., K.Voigt, I.Vervuert, T. Hollands, D. Cuddeford, and M. Coenen. 2005. The effect of order of feeding oats and chopped alfalfa to horses on the rate of feed intake and chewing activity. Pp 37–38, ENUCO conference, Pferdeheilkunde, Stuttgart, Germany.

Burton, G. W., and W. W. Hanna. 1995. Bermudagrass. In Forages, vol. 1. An Introduction to Grassland Agriculture, R. F. Barnes, D. A. Miller, and C. J. Nelson, eds. Ames: Iowa State University Press.

Bush, J. A., D. E. Freeman, K. H. Kline, N. R. Merchen, and G. C. Fahey, Jr. 2001. Dietary fat supplementation effects on *in vitro* nutrient disappearance and *in vivo* nutrient intake and total tract digestibility by horses. J. Anim. Sci. 79:232–239.

Butler, G. W., and R. W. Bailey. 1973. Chemistry and Biochemistry of Herbage. New York: Academic Press.

Buxton, D. R., D. R. Mertens, and K. J. Moore. 1995. Forage quality for ruminants: plant and animal considerations. Prof. Anim. Scientist 11:121.

Cairns, A. J., P. Begley, and I. M. Sims. 2002a. The structure of starch from seeds and leaves of the fructan-accumulating ryegrass, *Lolium temulentum* L. J. Plant Physiol. 159:221–230.

Cairns A. J., A. Cookson, and B. J. Thomas. 2002b. Starch metabolism in the fructan-grasses: Patterns of starch accumulation in excised leaves of *Lolium temulentum* L. J. Plant Physiol. 159:293–305.

Carlton, W. W., and J. Tuite. 1977. Metabolites of P. viridicatum toxicology. Pp. 525–555 in Mycotoxins in Human and Animal Health, J. V. Rodricks, C. W. Hesseltine, and M. A. Mehlman, eds. Park Forest South, IL: Pathotox Publications.

Caroll, C. L., and P. J. Huntingdon. 1988. Body condition scoring and weight estimation of horses. Equine Vet. J. 20:41–104.

CAST (Council on Agricultural Science and Technology). 2003. Mycotoxins: Risks in Plant, Animal, and Human Systems. Ames, IA: Council on Agricultural Science and Technology.

Chatterton, N. J., P. A. Harrison, J. H. Bennett, and K. H. Asay. 1989. Carbohydrate partitioning in 185 accessions of graminae grown under warm and cool temperatures. J. Plant Physiol. 143:169–179.

Cheeke, P. R., and L. R Schull. 1985. Natural toxicants in feeds and poisonous plants. Westport, CT: AVI Publishing.

Chenost, M., and W. Martin-Rosset. 1985. Comparison between species (sheep, horses, cattle) on intake and digestibility of fresh herbage. Ann. Zootech. 34:291–312.

Ciavarella, T. A., H. Dove, B. J. Leury, and R. J. Simpson. 2000. Diet selection by sheep grazing *Phalaris aquatica*. L. pastures differing in water-soluble carbohydrate content. Aust. J. Ag. Res. 51:757–764.

Clark, S., J. Taylor, and K. Smith. 1990. Winter growth, seed production and cyanogenic potential of white clovers under irrigation at Neuapur, Victoria. Report No. 2, Department of Agriculture and Rural Affairs, Victoria, Australia.

Clarke, A. 1992. Environmental monitoring in relation to equine respiratory disease. Pp. 310–315 in Current Therapy in Equine Respiratory Medicine, 3rd ed., N. E. Robinson, ed. Philadelphia: W. B. Saunders.

Clevstroem, G., B. Goransson, R. Hodverson, and H. Pettersson. 1981. Aflatoxin formation in hay treated with formic acid and in isolated strains of *Aspergillus flavus*. J. Stored Prod. Res. 17:151–161.

Clutter, S. H., and A. V. Rodiek. 1991. Feeding value of diets containing almond hulls. Pp. 37–42 in Proc. 12th Equine Nutr. Phys. Symp., University of Calgary, Alberta.

Coblentz, W. K., J. O. Fritz, K. K. Bolsen, and R. C. Cochran. 1996. Quality changes in alfalfa hay during storage in bales. J. Dairy Sci. 79:873–885.

Coblentz, W. K., J. O. Fritz, K. K. Bolsen, C. W. King, and R. C. Cochran. 1998. The effects of moisture concentration, moisture type, and bale density on quality characteristics of alfalfa hay in a model system. Anim. Feed Sci. Technol. 72:53–69.

Coblentz, W. K., J. E. Turner, D. A. Scarbrough, K. E. Lesmeister, Z. B. Johnson, D. W. Kellogg, K. P. Coffey, L. J. McBeth, and J. S. Weyers. 2000. Storage characteristics and nutritive value changes in Bermudagrass hay as affected by moisture content and density of rectangular bales. Crop Sci. 40:1375–1383.

Coenen, M., G. Muller, and H. Enbergs. 2003. Grass silages vs. hay in feeding horses. Pp. 140–141 in Proc. 18th Equine Nutr. Physiol. Soc. Symp., East Lansing, MI.

Cohen, N. D., P. G. Gibbs, and A. M. Woods. 1999. Dietary and other management factors associated with colic in horses. J. Am. Vet. Med. Assoc. 215:53–60.

Coleman, R. J., J. D. Milligan, and R. J. Christopherson. 1985. Energy and dry matter digestibility of processed grain for horses. Pp. 162–167 in Proc. 9th Equine Nutr. Physiol. Symp., East Lansing, MI.

Collins, M. 1983. Wetting and maturity effects on the yield and quality of legume hay. Agron. J. 75:523–527.

Collins, M. 1988. Composition and fiber digestion in morphological components of an alfalfa/timothy hay. Anim. Feed Sci. Technol. 19:135–143.

Collins, M. 1990. Composition of alfalfa forage, field-cured hay and pressed forage. Agron. J. 82:91–95.

Collins, M., and V. N. Owens. 2003. Preservation of forage as hay and silage. Pp. 443–447 in Disorders in Forages, vol. 11. The Science of Grassland Agriculture, 6th ed., R. F. Barnes, C. J. Nelson, M. Collins, and K. J. Moore, eds. Ames: Iowa State University Press.

Cooper, M. R., and A. W. Johnson. 1984. Poisonous Plants in Britain and Their Effects on Animals and Man. London: Her Majesty's Stationery Office.

Copetti, M. V., J. M. Santurio, A. A. P. Boeck, R. B. Silva, L. A. Bergermaier, I. Lubeck, A. B. M. Leal, A. T. Leal, S. H. Alves, and L. Ferreiro. 2002. Agalactia in mares fed grain contaminated with *Claviceps purpura*. Mycopathalogia 154:199–200.

Cotty, P. J., and D. Bhatnagar. 1994. Variability among atoxigenic Aspergillus flavus strains to prevent aflatoxin contamination and production of aflatoxin biosynthetic pathway enzymes. Appl. Environ. Microbiol. 60:2248–2251.

Coverdale, J. A., J. A. Moore, H. D. Tyler, and P. A. Miller-Auwerda. 2004. Soybean hulls as an alternative feed for horses. J. Anim. Sci. 82:1663–1668.

Crandell, K. G., J. D. Pagan, and S. E. Duren. 1999. A comparison of grain, oil and beet pulp as energy sources for the exercised horse. Equine Vet. J. Suppl. 30:485–489.

Crozier, J. A., V. G. Allen, N. E. Jack, J. P. Fontenot, and M. A. Cochran. 1997. Digestibility, apparent mineral absorption and voluntary intake by horses fed alfalfa, tall fescue and Caucasian bluestem. J. Anim. Sci. 75:1651–1658.

Cuddeford, D. 1999. Starch digestion in the horse. Pp. 129–139 in Advances in Equine Nutrition, Proc. 1998 Equine Nutr. Conf. Feed Manufacturers, Kentucky Equine Research, Inc.

Cymbaluk, N. F. 1990a. Comparison of forage digestion by cattle and horses. Can. J. Anim. Sci. 70:601–610.

Cymbaluk, N. F. 1990b. Using canola meal in growing horse diets. Equine Pract. 12:13–19.

Cymbaluk, N., and D. A. Christiensen. 1986. Nutrient utilization of pelleted and unpelleted forages by ponies. Can. J. Anim. Sci. 66:237–244.

Czerkawski, J. W. 1967. The effects of storage on fatty acids of dried grass. Br. J. Nutr. 21:599–608.

D'Mello, J. P. F., and A. M. C. MacDonald. 1997. Mycotoxins. Anim. Feed Sci. Tech. 69:155–166.

Dairy One. 2003. Available at http://www.dairyone.com/Forage/Feed Comp. Accessed March 12, 2006.

Dale, N. 1996. Variation in feed ingredient quality: oilseed meals. Anim. Feed Sci. Technol. 59:129–135.

Davies, J. G, T. J. Steffens, T. E. Engle, K. L. Mallow, and S. E. Cotto. 2004. Preventing Selenium Toxicity. Colorado State University Extension Services, Publication No. 611.

De Fombelle, A., L. Veiga, C. Drogoul, and V. Julliand. 2004. Effect of diet composition and feeding pattern on the prececal digestibility of starches from diverse botanical origins measured with the mobile nylon bag technique in horses. J. Anim. Sci. 82:3625–3634.

DEFRA (UK Department for Environment, Food and Rural Affairs). 2006. Guidance Note on Feed Controls in the TSE Regulations. Available at http://www.defra.gov.uk/animalh/bse/animal-health/feedbanguide. Accessed April 1, 2006.

Deinum, B., A. J. H. Van Es, and P. J. Van Soest. 1968. Climate, nitrogen and grass. II. The influence of light intensity, temperature and nitrogen on in vivo digestibility of grass and the prediction of these effects from some chemical procedures. Neth. J. Agr. Sci. 16:217–223.

Demarquilly, C. 1981. Prevision de la Valeur Nutritive de Aliments des Ruminants. Thieux, France: INRA.

DePeters, E. J., J. G. Fadel, M. J. Arana, N. Ohanesian, M. A. Etchebarne, C. A. Hamilton, R. G. Hinders, M. D. Maloney, C. A. Old, T. J. Riordan, H. Perez-Monti, and J. W. Pareas. 2000. Variability in the chemical composition of seventeen selected byproduct feedstuffs used by the California dairy industry. Prof. Anim. Scientist 16:69–99.

Doreau, M., W. Martin-Rosset, and S. Boulot. 1988. Energy requirements and the feeding of mares during lactation. A. Review Livest. Prod. Sci. 20:53–68.

Drogoul, C., C. Poncet, and J. L. Tisserand. 2000a. Feeding ground and pelleted hay rather than chopped hay to ponies 1. Consequences for in vivo digestibility and rate of passage of digesta. Anim. Feed Sci. Technol. 87:117–130.

Drogoul, C., J. L. Tisserand, and C. Poncet. 2000b. Feeding ground and pelleted hay rather than chopped hay to ponies. 2. Consequences on fiber degradation in the cecum and colon. Anim. Feed Sci. Technol. 87:131–145.

Dulphy, J. P., W. Martin-Rosset, H. Dubroeucq, J. M. Ballet, A. Detour, and M. Jailler. 1997a. Compared feeding patterns in *ad libitum* intakes of dry forages by horses and sheep. Livest. Prod. Sci. 52:49–56.

Dulphy, J. P., W. Martin-Rosset, H. Dubroeucq, and M. Jailler. 1997b. Evaluation of voluntary intake of forage trough-fed to light horses. Comparison with sheep. Factors of variation and prediction. Livest. Prod. Sci. 52:97–104.

Duren, S. E. 1998. Feeding the endurance horse. Pp. 351–364 in Advances in Equine Nutrition, J. Pagan, ed. Nottingham, UK: Nottingham University Press.

Duren, S. E., C. T. Dougherty, S. G. Jackson, and J. P. Baker. 1989. Modification of ingestive behaviour due to exercise in yearling horses grazing orchard grass. Appl. Anim. Behav. Sci. 22:335–345.

Dutton, M. F., K. Westlake, and M. S. Anderson. 1984. The interaction between additives, yeasts and patulin production in silage. Mycopathologia 87:20–33.

El-Nezami, H., P. Kankaanpaa, S. Salinen, H. Mykkanen, and J. Abokas. 1998. Use of probiotic bacteria to reduce aflatoxin uptake. Rev. Med. Vet. 149:570.

Ellis, A. D., S. Thomas, K. Arkell, and P. A. Harris. 2005. Adding chopped straw to concentrate feed: the effect of inclusion rate and particle length on intake behaviour of horses. Pp. 53–37, ENUCO conference, Pferdeheilkunde, Stuttgart, Germany.

Elphinstone, G. D. 1981. Pastures and fodder crops for horses in southern coastal Queensland. Queensland Ag. J. 107:122–126.

Emmick D. L., and D. G. Fox. 1993. Prescribed grazing management to improve pasture productivity in NY. USDA Soil Cons. Serv. and Cornell Dept. An. Sci.

Escoula, L. 1977. Moissures des ensilages et consequences toxicologique. Fourrages 69:97–114.

Evans, J. L. 1973. Forages for horses. Pp. 723–732 in Forages: The Science of Grassland Agriculture, 3rd ed., M. E. Heath, D. S. Metcalfe, and R. F. Barnes, eds. Ames: Iowa State University Press.

Evers, G. W. 1998. Comparison of broiler poultry litter and commercial fertilizer for coastal Bermudagrass production in the southeastern U.S. J. Sustainable Agric. 12:55–77.

Fahrenholz, C. 1994. Cereal grains and byproducts: What's in them and how are they processed? Pp. 23–42 in Proc. for the 1994 Short Course: Feeding the Performance Horse, Kentucky Equine Research, Inc.

FDA (Food and Drug Administration). 1994. Action Levels for Aflatoxins in Animal Feeds (CPG 7126.33). Available at http://www.fda.gov/ora/compliance_ref/cpg/cpgvet/cpg683-100.html. Accessed August 25, 2005.

FDA. 2001a. Guidance for Industry. Fumonisin levels in human foods and animal feeds. Available at http://www.cfsan.fda.gov/~dms/fumongu2.html. Accessed September 23, 2005.

FDA. 2001b. Background Paper In Support of Fumonisin Levels in Animal Feed: Executive Summary of This Scientific Support Document. Available at http://www.cfsan.fda.gov/~dms/fumongu4.html. Accessed September 23, 2005.

Fleurance, G., P. Duncan, and B. Mallevaud. 2001. Daily intake and selection of feeding sites by horses in heterogeneous wet grasslands. Anim. Res. 50:149–156.

Forgacs, J. 1965. Stachybotrytoxicosis and moldy corn toxicosis. Pp. 87–104 in Mycotoxins in Foodstuffs, G. N. Wogan, ed. Cambridge, MA: MIT Press.

Forgacs, J. 1972. Stachybotrytoxicosis. Pp. 294–298 in Microbial Toxins VIII, S. Kadis et al., eds. New York: Academic Press.

Frape, D. 1998. Equine Nutrition and Feeding, 2nd ed. Malden, MA: Blackwell Science.

Gallagher, R., and N. P. McMeniman. 1988. The nutritional status of pregnant and non-pregnant mares grazing South East Queensland pastures. Equine Vet. J. 20:414–419.

Garner, H. E., D. P. Hutcheson, J. R. Coffman, and A. W. Hahn. 1977. Lactic acidosis. A factor associated with equine laminitis. J. Anim. Sci. 45:1037–1041.

Gibbs, P. G., and G. D. Potter. 2002. Review: concepts in protein digestion and amino acid requirements of young horses. Prof. Anim. Scientist 18:295–301.

Gibbs, P. G., G. D. Potter, G. T. Schelling, J. L. Kreider, and C. J. Boyd. 1996. The significance of small vs large intestinal digestion of cereal grain and oilseed protein in the equine. J. Equine Vet. Sci. 16:60–65.

Gillham, S. B., N. H. Dodman, L. Shuster, R. Kream, and W. Rand. 1994. The effect of diet on cribbing behaviour and plasma beta-endorphin in horses. Appl. Anim. Behav. Sci. 41:147–153.

Givens, D. I., A. R. Moss, and A. H. Adamson. 1992. The chemical composition and energy value of high temperature dried grass produced in England. Anim. Feed. Sci. Technol. 36:215–228.

Glade, M. J., and N. K. Luba. 1990. Benefits to foals of feeding soybean meal to lactating broodmares. J. Equine Vet. Sci. 10:422–428.

Godbee, R. G., and L. M. Slade. 1981. The effect of urea or soybean meal on the growth and protein status of young horses. J. Anim. Sci. 53:670–676.

Goering, H. K., and P. J. Van Soest. 1967. Effect of moisture, temperature and pH on the relative susceptibility of forages to non-enzymatic browning. J. Dairy Sci. 50:989–990.

Grace, N. D., and D. R. Brody. 2001. The possible use of long chain (C_{19}–C_{32}) fatty acids in herbage as an indigestible fecal marker. J. Agric. Sci. Camb. 126:743–745.

Grace, N. D., E. K. Gee, E. C. Firth, and H. I. Shaw. 2002a. Digestible energy intake, dry matter digestibility and mineral status of grazing thoroughbred yearlings in New Zealand. N. Z. Vet. J. 50:63–69.

Grace, N. D., E. K. Gee, E. C. Firth, and H. I. Shaw. 2002b. Determination of the digestible energy intake and apparent absorption of macro elements in pasture-fed lactating Thoroughbred mares. N. Z. Vet. J. 50:182–185.

Grace, N. D., C. W. Rogers, E. C. Firth, T. L. Faram, and H. I. Shaw. 2003. Digestible energy intake, dry matter digestibility and effect of increased calcium intake on bone parameters of thoroughbred weanlings grazing in New Zealand. N. Z. Vet. J. 51:165–173.

Graham, H., K. Hesselman, and P. Åman. 1986. The influence of wheat bran and sugar beet pulp on the digestibility of dietary components in a cereal-based pig diet. Br. J. Nutr. 54:719–726.

Graham-Thiers, P. M., D. S. Kronfeld, K. A. Kline, and D. J. Sklan. 1991. Dietary protein restriction and fat supplementation diminish the acidogenic effects of exercise during repeated sprints in horses. J. Nutr. 131:1959–1964.

Gray, G. 1992. Starch digestion and absorption in nonruminants. J. Nutr. 122:172–177.

Green, J. O., A. J. Corrall, and R. A. Terry. 1971. Grass species and varieties: relationships between stage of growth, yield and forage quality. GRI Technical Report No. 8. Hurley, UK: Grassland Research Institute.

Gregory, P. H., M. E. Lacey, G. W. Festenstein, and F. A. Skinner. 1963. Microbial and biochemical changes during moulding of hay. J. Gen. Microbiol. 33:147–174.

Gudmundsdottir, K. B., V. Svansson, B. Aalbaek, E. Gunnarsson, and S. Sigurdarson. 2004. Listeria monocytogenes in horses in Iceland. Vet. Rec. 155:456–459.

Haenlein, G. F., R. D. Holdren, and Y. M. Yoon. 1966. Comparative responses of horses and sheep to different physical forms of alfalfa. J. Anim. Sci. 25:740–743.

Hagler, W. M., and R. F. Behlow. 1981. Salivary syndrome in horses: identification of slaframine in red clover hay. Appl. Environ. Microbiol. 42:1067–1073.

Hale, C., and M. J. S. Moore-Colyer. 2001. Voluntary feed intakes and apparent digestibilities of hay, big bale grass silage and red clover silage by ponies. Pp. 468–469 in Proc. 17th Equine Nutr. Physiol. Soc. Symp., Lexington, KY.

Hammond, C. J., D. K. Mason, and K. L. Watkins. 1986. Gastric ulceration in mature Thouroughbred horses. Equine Vet. J. 18:284–287.

Hancock, J. D., and K. C. Behnke. 2001. Use of ingredient and diet processing technologies (Grinding, mixing, pelleting, and extruding) to produce quality feeds for pigs. Pp. 469–497 in Swine Nutrition, 2nd ed., A. J. Lewis and L. L. Southern, eds. Boca Raton, FL: CRC Press LLC.

Hansen, D. K., G. W. Webb, and S. P. Webb. 1992. Digestibility of wheat straw or ammoniated wheat straw in equine diets. J. Equine Vet. Sci. 12:223–226.

Hansen, R. M. 1976. Foods of free-roaming horses in southern New Mexico. J. Range Manage. 29:347.

Harbor, L. E., L. M. Lawrence, S. H. Hayes, C. J. Stine, and D. M. Powell. 2003. Concentrate composition, form and glycemic response in horses. Pp. 329–330 in Proc. 18th Equine Nutr. Physiol. Symp., East Lansing, MI.

Hardy, J., M. Parmentier, and J. Fanni. 1999. Functionality of nutrients and thermal treatments of food. Proc. Nutr. Soc. 58:579–585.

Harkess, R. D., and R. A. Alexander. 1969. The digestibility and productivity of selected herbage varieties. J. Br. Grassland Soc. 24:282–289.

Harris, D. M., and A. V. Rodiek. 1993. Dry matter digestibility of diets containing beet pulp fed to horses. Pp. 100–101 in Proc. 13th Equine Nutr. Physiol. Symp., Gainesville, FL.

Harris, P. A., M. Sillence, R. Inglis, C. Siever-Kelly, M. Friend, K. Munn, and H. Davidson. 2005. Effect of short Lucerne chaff on the rate of intake and glycaemic response to an oat meal. Pp. 151–152 in Proc. 19th Equine Sci. Soc., Tucson, AZ.

Hartley, R. D., and E. C. Jones. 1977. Phenolic compounds and degradability of cell walls of grass and legume species. Phytochem. 16:1531.

Hasso, S. A. 2003. Non-fatal aflatoxicosis in Arabian horses in Iraq. Vet. Rec. 152:657–658.

Hendrix, W. F. 2003. Pasture management and problems while grazing. Central Washington Agricultural Team Fact Sheet 1004.

Henning, J. C. 1994. The establishment and management of horse pastures. In Proc. Kentucky Forage and Grassl. Council Ann. Mtng., November 1–2, Lexington, KY. Available at http://www.neosoft.com/~iaep/pages/protected/jissues/j1909/j1909p540.html. Accessed December 20, 2005.

Highfill, J. L., G. D. Potter, E. M. Eller, P. G. Gibbs, B. D. Scott, and D. M. Hood. 2005. Comparative absorption of calcium fed in varying chemical forms and effects on absorption of phosphorus and magnesium. Pp. 37–42 in Proc. 19th Equine Sci. Soc., Tucson, AZ.

Hillyer, M. H., F. G. Taylor, C. J. Proudman, G. B. Edwards, J. E. Smith, and N. P. French. 2002. Case control study to identify risk factors for simple colonic obstruction and distension colic in horses. Equine Vet. J. 34:455–463.

Hintz, H. 1969. Review article. Equine nutrition. Comparison of digestion coefficients obtained with cattle sheep, rabbits and horses. The Veterinarian 6:45–51.

Hintz, H. 1979. Factors affecting growth in the horse. Pp. 210–226 in Proc. Cornell Nutr. Conf. Feed Manufacturers. Ithaca, NY: Cornell University.

Hintz, H. F. 1990. Molds, mycotoxins, and mycotoxicosis. Vet. Clinic No. Am. Equine Pract. 6:419–431.

Hintz, H. F., and R. G. Loy. 1966. Effects of pelleting on the nutritive value of horse rations. J. Anim. Sci. 25:1059–1062.

Hintz, H. F., and H. F. Schryver. 1972. Nitrogen utilization in ponies. J. Anim. Sci. 34:592–595.

Hintz, H. F., J. E. Lowe, A. J. Clifford, and W. J. Visek. 1970. Ammonia intoxication resulting from urea ingestion by ponies. J. Am. Vet. Med. Assoc. 157:963–966.

Hoekstra, K. E., K. Newman, M. A. P. Kennedy, and J. D. Pagan. 1999. Effect of corn processing on glycemic response in horses. Pp. 144–148 in Proc. 16th Equine Nutr. Physiol. Symp., Raleigh, N.C.

Hoffman, R. M., R. C. Boston, D. Stefanovski, D. S. Kronfeld, and P. A. Harris. 2003. Obesity and diet affect glucose dynamics and insulin sensitivity in Thoroughbred geldings. J. Anim. Sci. 81:2333–2342.

Hoglund, C. R. 1964. Comparative losses and feeding values of alfalfa and corn silage crops when harvested at different moisture levels and stored in gas tight and conventional tower silos. An appraisal of research results. Agricultural Economics Publication No. 947, Michigan State University, East Lansing.

Holland, J. L., D. S. Kronfeld, G. A. Rich, K. A. Kilne, J. P. Fontenot, T. N. Meachen, and P. A. Harris, P A. 1998. Acceptance of fat and lecithin containing diets by horses. Appl. Anim. Behav. Sci. 56:91–96.

Hollinger, K., and H. E. Ekperigin. 1999. Mycotoxicosis in food producing animals. Vet. Clinics N. Am. 15:133–165.

Holt, D. A., and A. R. Hilst. 1969. Daily variation in carbohydrate content of selected forage crops. Agron. J. 61:239–242.

Hongtrakul, K., J. R. Bergstrom, W. B. Nessmith, I. H. Kim, M. D. Tokach, R. D. Goodband, K. C. Behnke, and J. L. Nelssen. 1998. The effects of extrusion processing of carbohydrate sources on weanling pig performance. J. Anim. Sci. 76:3034–3042.

Hopkins, A., J. Gilbey, C. Dibb, P. J. Bowling, and P. J. Murray. 1990. Response of permanent and reseeded grassland to fertiliser nitrogen. 1. Herbage production and herbage quality. Grass Forage Sci. 45:43–55.

Hoskin, S. O., and E. K. Gee. 2004. Feeding value of pastures for horses. N. Z. Vet. J. 52:332–341.

Householder, D. D. 1978. Pre-cecal, postileal and total tract digestion and growth performance in horses fed concentrate rations containing oats or sorghum grain processed by crimping or micronizing. Ph.D. Dissertation. Texas A&M University.

Hoveland, C. S. 1992. Grazing systems for humid regions. J. Prod. Agric. 5:23–27.

Hudson, J. M., N. D. Cohen, P. G. Gibbs, and J. A. Thompson. 2001. Feeding practices associated with colic in horses. J. Am. Vet. Med Assoc. 219:1419–1425.

Hughes, T. P., and J. R. Gallacher. 1993. Influence of sward height on the mechanics of grazing and intake by racehorses. Pp. 1325–1326 in Proc. XVII Inter. Grassland Congress, Palmerston North, NZ.

Humphreys, J., E. G. O'Riordan, and P. O'Kiely. 2001. Maximizing annual intake of grazed grass for beef production. Beef Production Series No. 29, Teagasc Grange Research Centre.

Hunt, W. F. 1995. Pastures for horses: a New Zealand perspective. Pp. 17–24 in Proceedings of the Equine Nutrition and Pastures for Horses Workshop, February 14–16, Richmond, NSW.

Hunter J. M., B. W. Rohrbach, F. M. Andrews, and R. H. Whitlock. 2002. Round bale grass hay: a risk factor for botulism in horses. Comp. Cont. Educ. Prac. Vet. 24:166–169.

Hussein, H. S., and L. A. Vogedes. 2003. Review: forage nutritional value for equine as affected by forage species and cereal grain supplementation. Prof. Anim. Scientist 19:388–397.

Hussein, H. S., H. Han, L. A. Vogedes, and J. P. Tanner. 2001. Utilisation of grasses by grazing horses. Available at http://www.ag.un.edu/AG/extension/cattleman/cattleman2001/2001-012.pdf. Accessed November 12, 2005.

Hyslop, J. J., A. Bayley, A. L. Tomlinson, and D. Cuddeford. 1998a. Voluntary feed intake and apparent digestibility *in vivo* in ponies given *ad libitum* access to dehydrated grass or hay harvested from the same crop. P. 131 in Proc. Br. Soc. Anim. Sci.

Hyslop, J. J., A. L. Tomlinson, A. Bayley, and D. Cuddeford. 1998b. Voluntary feed intake and apparent digestibility *in vivo* in ponies offered mature threshed grass hay *ad libitum*. P. 131 in Proc. Br. Soc. Anim. Sci.

Hyslop, J. J., and S. Calder. 2001. Voluntary intake and apparent digestibility in ponies offered alfalfa-based forages. P. 90 in Proc. Br. Soc. Anim. Sci.

Ince, J. C., A. C. Longland, M. J. S. Moore-Colyer, C. J. Newbold, and P. A. Harris. 2005. A pilot study to estimate the intake of grass by ponies with restricted access to pasture. P. 109 in Proc. Br. Soc. Anim. Sci.

Ince, J. C., A. C. Longland, and M. J. S. Moore-Colyer. 2006. Preservation of Timothy, meadow fescue and two varieties of perennial ryegrass as hay: effect on water soluble carbohydrate content. Proc. App. Equine Sci. Symp., Royal Agricultural College, Cirencester, UK (in press).

Irvine, C. H. G. 1988. Responses of horses to hordenine and related substances. Pp. 47–50 in Proc. 7th Inter. Conf. of Racing Analysts and Veterinarians, T. Tobin, J. Blake, M. Potter, and T. Wood, eds., Louisville, KY.

Jackson, S. A., V. A. Rich, S. L. Ralston, and E. W. Anderson. 1985. Feeding behavior and feed efficiency of horses as affected by feeding frequency and physical form of hay. Pp. 78–83 in Proc. 9th Equine Nutr. Physiol. Soc. Symp., East Lansing, MI.

Jacobs, J., S. Rigby, F. McKenzie, M. Ryan, G. Ward, and S. Burch. 1989. Effect of nitrogen on pasture yield and quality for silage in western Victoria. Pp. 29–32 in Proc. Australian Agronomy Conf., Australian Society of Agronomy.

James, W. O. 1953. Plant Respiration. Oxford, UK: Oxford University Press.

Johnson, C. R., B. A. Reiling, P. Mislevy, and M. B. Hall. 2001. Effects of nitrogen fertilization and harvest date on yield, digestibility, fiber, and protein fractions of tropical grasses. J. Anim. Sci. 79:2439–2448.

Johnson, P. J., S. W. Casteel, and N. T. Messer. 1997. Effect of feeding deoxynivalenol contaminated barley to horses. J. Vet. Diag. Invest. 9:219–221.

Jordan, S. A., K. R. Pond, J. C. Burns, D. S. Fisher, D. T. Barnets, and P. A. Evans. 1995. Controlled grazing of horses with electric fences. Pp. 238–239 in Proc. Am. Forage and Grassl. Counc., Lexington, KY.

Jose-Cunilleras, E., L. E. Taylor, and K. W. Hinchcliff. 2004. Glycemic index of cracked corn, oat groats and rolled barley in horses. J. Anim. Sci. 82:2623–2629.

Keenan, D. M. 1986. Bark chewing by horses grazed on irrigated pastures. Austral. Vet. J. 63:234–235.

Kienzle, E. 1994. Small intestinal digestion of starch in the horse. Revue Med. Vet. 145:199–204.

Kienzle, E., S. Radicke, S. Wilke, E. Landes, and H. Meyer. 1992. Preileal starch digestion in relation to source and preparation of starch. Pp. 103–107 in Eur. Conf. on Nutrition for the Horse, Hannover, Germany.

Kienzle, E., J. Pohlenz, and S. Radicke. 1997. Morphology of starch digestion in the horse. J. Am. Vet. Med. Assoc. 44:207–221.

Knottenbelt, D. C. 2000. Ragwort—a killer in disguise. Pp. 29–35 in 3rd International Conference on Feeding Horses, Perth, UK.

Kronfeld, D., A. Rodiek, and C. Stull. 2004. Glycemic indices, glycemic levels, and glycemic dietetics. J. Equine Vet. Sci. 24:399–404.

Laca, E. A, L. A. Shipley, and E. D. Reid. 2001. Structural anti-quality characteristics of range and pasture plants. J. Range Mgmt. 54:413–419.

LaCasha, P. A., H. A. Brady, B. G. Allen, C. R. Richardson, and K. R. Pond. 1999. Voluntary intake, digestibility and subsequent selection of matua bromegrass, coastal Bermuda grass and alfalfa hays by yearling horses. J. Anim. Sci. 77:2766–2773.

Lawrence, L. M., K. J. Moore, H. F. Hintz, E. H. Jaster, and L. Wischow. 1987. Acceptability of alfalfa hay treated with an organic acid preservative. Can. J. Anim. Sci. 67:217–220.

Lawrence, L. M., R. Coleman, and J. C. Henning. 2000. Choosing hay for horses. University of Kentucky College of Agriculture, Co-operative Extension Service Sheet ID-146.

Le Bars, J. 1976. Mycoflore des fourrages secs: croissance et development des especes selon les conditions hydrothermique de conservation. Rev. Mycol. 40:347–360.

Le Bars, J., and P. Le Bars. 1996. Recent acute and sub-acute mycotoxicoses recognised in France. Vet. Res. 27:383–394.

Lechtenberg, V. L., D. A. Holt, and H. W. Youngberg. 1971. Diurnal variation in nonstructural carbohydrates, *in vitro* digestibility, and leaf to stem ratio of alfalfa. Agron. J. 63:719.

Lewis, L. D. 1995. Equine Clinical Nutrition: Feeding and Care. Media, PA: Williams & Wilkins.

Little, D., and A. T. Blickslager. 2002. Factors associated with development of ileal impaction in horses with surgical colic: 78 cases (1968–2000). Equine Vet. J. 34:464–468.

Longland, A. C. 2001. Plant carbohydrates: analytical methods and nutritional implications for equines. Pp. 173–175 in Proc. 17th Equine Nutr. Physiol. Soc. Symp., Lexington, KY.

Longland, A. C., R. Pilgrim, and I. J. Jones. 1995. Comparison of oven drying vs. freeze drying on the analysis of non-starch polysaccharides in gramminaceous and leguminous forages. P. 60 in Proc. Br. Soc. Anim. Sci.

Longland, A. C., M. Halling, S. Thomas, M. Scott, and M. K. Theodorou. 2006. Effect of grazing or conservation management on seasonal variation of WSC content and composition in eight varieties of ryegrass over two growing seasons. In Final Report to the EU-funded Framework V project (QLK-2001-0498).

Lopez, N. E., J. P. Baker, and S. G. Jackson. 1988. Effect of culling and vacuum cleaning on the digestibility of oats by horses. J. Equine Vet. Sci. 8:375–378.

MAFF (UK Ministry of Agriculture, Fisheries and Food). 1992. Feed Composition. UK Tables of Feed Composition and Nutritive Value for Ruminants, 2nd ed. Canterbury, UK: Chalcombe Publications.

Marlow, C. H. B., E. M. van Tonder, F. C. Hayward, S. S. van der Merwe, and L. E. G. Price. 1983. A report on the consumption, composition and nutritional adequacy of a mixture of lush green perennial ryegrass (*Lolium perenne*) and cocksfoot (*Dactylis glomerata*) fed *ad libitum* to thoroughbred mares. J. S. Afr. Vet. Assoc. 54:155–157.

Martin, R. G. 1993. Effects of nitrogen and energy supplementation on grazing broodmares and aspects of nitrogen metabolism in horses. Ph.D. Thesis. University of Queensland, Brisbane.

Martin, R. G., N. P. McMeniman, and K. F. Dowsett. 1991. Effects of protein deficient diet and urea supplementation on lactating mares. J. Reprod. Fert. Suppl. 44:543–550.

Martin, R. G., N. P. McMeniman, B. W. Norton, and K. F. Dowsett. 1996. Utilization of endogenous and dietary urea in the large intestine of the mature horse. Br. J. Nutr. 76:373–386.

Martin-Rosset, W., and J. P. Dulphy. 1987. Digestibility. Interactions between concentrates and forages in horses; influence of feeding level. Comparison with sheep. Livestock Prod. Sci. 17:263–276.

Martin-Rosset, W., and M. Vermorel. 1991. Maintenance energy requirements determined by indirect colorimetry and feeding trials in light horses. Equine Vet. Sci. 11:42–45.

Martin-Rosset, W., M. Doreau, and J. Espinasse. 1986. Alimentation de la jument lourde allaitante. Evolution du poids uif des jumants et croissance des polains. Ann. Zootech. 35:21–36.

Martin-Rosset, W. M., M. Vermorel, P. Doreau, and P. Thivend. 1987. Digestion de regimes a base de foin ou ensilages de mais chez le cheval en croissance. Reprod. Nutr. Develop. 27:291–292.

Matches, A. G. 1992. Plant response to grazing: a review. J. Prod. Agric. 5:1–7.

Mavromichalis, I., and D. H. Baker. 2000. Effects of pelleting and storage of a complex nursery pig diet on lysine bio-availability. J. Anim. Sci. 78:341–347.

McCann, J. S., T. N. Meacham, and J. P. Fontenot. 1987. Energy utilization and blood traits of ponies fed fat-supplemented diets. J. Anim. Sci. 65:1019–1026.

McDonald, M., R. A. Edwards, J. F. D. Greenhalgh, and C. Morgan. 1996. Animal Nutrition, 5th ed. Harlow, UK: Longman Scientific and Technical.

McDowell, L. R. 2000. Vitamins in Animal and Human Nutrition, 2nd ed. Ames: Iowa State University Press.

McDowell, L. R. 2003. Minerals in Animal and Human Nutrition, 2nd ed. Amsterdam: Elsevier.

McDowell, R. E. 1972. Improvement of livestock production in warm climates. San Francisco, CA: Freeman.

McGreevy, P. D., P. J. Cripps, N. P. French, L. E. Green, and C. J. Nicol. 1995. Management factors associated with stereotypic and redirected behavior in the Thoroughbred horse. Equine Vet. J. 27:86–91.

McKenzie, R. A., B. J. Blaney, and R. J. W. Gartner. 1981. The effect of dietary oxalate on calcium, phosphorus and magnesium balances in horses. J. Agr. Sci. 97:69–74.

McLean, B. M. L. 2000. Methodologies to determine digestion of starch in ponies. Ph.D. Thesis. University of Edinburgh, UK.

McLean, B. M. L., A. Afzalzadeh, L. Bates, R. W. Mayes, and F. D. Hovell. 1995. Voluntary intake, digestibility and rate of passage of hay and silage fed to horses and to cattle. Anim. Sci. 60:555.

McLean, B. M. L., J. J. Hyslop, A. C. Longland, and D. Cuddeford. 1998. Effect of physical processing on *in situ* degradation of barley in the cecum of ponies. P. 127 in Proc. Br. Soc. Anim. Sci.

McLean, B. M. L., J. J. Hyslop, A. C. Longland, D. Cuddeford, and T. Hollands. 1999. Apparent digestibility in ponies given rolled, micronised or extruded barley. P. 133 in Proc. Br. Soc. Anim. Sci.

McLean, B. M. L., J. J. Hyslop, A. C. Longland, D. Cuddeford, and T. Hollands. 2000. Physical processing of barley and its effects on intra-caecal fermentation parameters in ponies. Anim. Feed Sci. Tech. 85:79–87.

McMeniman, N. P. 2003. Pasture intake by young horses. A report for the Rural Industries Research and Development Corporation, RIDRC Publication No. 00W03/005.

Medina, B., I. D. Girard, E. Jacotot, and V. Julliand. 2002. Effect of a preparation of *Saccharomyces cerevisiae* on microbial profiles and fermentation patterns in the large intestine of horses fed a high fiber or a high starch diet. J. Anim. Sci. 80:2600–2609.

Menard, C., P. Duncan, G. Fleurance, J. Y. Georges, and M. Lila. 2002. Comparative foraging nutrition of horses and cattle in European wetlands. J. Appl. Ecol. 39:120–133.

Meschonia, P., M. W. Martin-Rosset, J. L. Peyraud, P. Duncan, D. Micol, and S. Boulot. 1998. Prediction of digestibility of the diet of horses: evaluation of faecal indices. Grass Forage Sci. 53:159–196.

Meschonia, P., J. L. Peyraud, P. Duncan, D. Micol, and C. Tillaud-Geyl. 2000. Grass intake by growing horses at pasture: a test on the effect of the horse's age and sward biomass. Ann. Zootech. 49:505–515.

Meyer, H., S. Radicke, E. Kienzle, S. Wilke, and D. Kleffken. 1993. Investigations on preileal digestion of oats, corn and barley starch in relation to grain processing. Pp. 92–97 in Proc. 13th Equine Nutr. Physiol. Soc. Symp., Gainesville, FL.

Miller, D. F., ed. 1958. Composition of cereal grains and forages. NRC Publication No. 585. Washington, DC: NAS.

Mitchell, R. L. 1957. The trace element content of plants. UK Research 10:357.

Moffitt, D. L., T. N. Meacham, J. P. Fontenot, and V. G. Allen. 1987. Seasonal differences in apparent digestibilities of fescue and orchard grass/clover pastures in horses. P. 79 in Proc. 10th Equine Nutr. Physiol. Soc. Symp., Fort Collins, CO.

Moore-Colyer, M. J. S. 1996. Effects of soaking hay fodder for horses on dust and mineral content. Anim. Sci. 63:337–342.

Moore-Colyer, M. J. S., and A. C. Longland. 2000. Intakes and *in vivo* apparent digestibilities of four types of conserved grass forage by ponies. Anim. Sci. 71:527–534.

Moore-Colyer, M. J. S., J. J. Hyslop, A. C. Longland, and D. Cuddeford. 2002. The mobile bag technique as a method for determining the degradation of four botanically diverse fibrous feedstuffs in the small intestine and total digestive tract of ponies. Br. J. Nutr. 88:729–740.

Morrison, J., M. V. Jackson, and P. E. Sparrow. 1980. The response of perennial ryegrass to fertiliser nitrogen in relation to climate and soil. GRI Technical Report No. 27. Hurley, UK: Grassland Research Institute.

Morrow, H. J., M. J. S. Moore-Colyer, and A. C. Longland. 1999. The apparent digestibilities and rates of passage of two chop-lengths of big-bale silage and hay in ponies. P. 142 in Proc. Br. Soc. Anim. Sci.

Murphy, P. A., L. G. Rice, and P. F. Ross. 1993. Fumonisin B1, B2 and B3 content of Iowa, Wisconsin and Illinois corn and corn screenings. J. Agric. Food Chem. 41:263–266.

Murray, J. M. D. 2004. The effect of enzyme treatment and supplementary feedstuffs on the degradation of conserved forages by ponies. Ph.D. Thesis. University of Wales, Aberystwyth.

Murray, M. J., and G. Shusser. 1989. Application of gastric pH-metry in horses: measurement of 24 h gastric pH in horses fed, fasted and treated with ranitidine. J. Vet. Internal Med. 6:133.

Murray, M. J., C. Grodinsky, C. W. Anderson, P. F. Radue, and G. R. Schmidt. 1989. Gastric ulcers in horses: a comparison of endoscopic findings in horses with and without clinical signs. Equine Vet. J. Suppl. 7:68–72.

Nakazato, M., S. Morozumi, K. Saito, K. Fujinuma, T. Nishima, and N. Kasai. 1990. Interconversion of aflatoxin B1 and antiflatoxicol by several fungi. Appl. Envir. Microbiol. 56:1465–1470.

Nash, D. 1999. Drought feeding and management of horses. RIRDC publication No. 99/98.

Nash, D. 2001. Estimation of intake in pastured horses. Pp. 161–167 in Proc. 17th Equine Nutr. Physiol. Soc. Symp., Lexington, KY.

Nash, D. G., and Thompson. 2001. Grazing behaviour of Thoroughbred weanlings on temperate pastures. Pp. 326–327 in Proc. 17th Equine Nutr. Physiol. Soc. Symp. Lexington, KY.

Nelson, B. D., L. R. Verma, and C. R. Montgomery. 1983. Effects of storage method on losses and quality changes in round bales of ryegrass and alfalfa hay. LA Agric. Exp. Sta. Bull. 750.

Nilsson, U. 1988. Cereal fructans—preparation, fermentation and bioavailability. Ph.D. Thesis. Department of Applied Nutrition, University of Lund, Sweden.

Nordkvist, E. 1987. Composition and degradation of cell walls in red clover, Lucerne and cereal straw. Ph.D. Thesis. Swedish University of Agricultural Sciences, Uppsala.

Nordkvist, E., and P. Åman. 1986. Changes during growth in anatomical and chemical composition of in vitro degradability. J. Sci. Feed Agric. 31:1–7.

Nout, M. J. R., H. M. Boumeester, J. Haaksma, and H. van Dijk. 1993. Fungal growth in silages of sugar beet press pulp and maize. J. Agric. Sci. 121:323–326.

NRC (National Research Council). 1989. Nutrient Requirements of Horses, 5th ed. Washington, DC: National Academy Press.

NRC. 2000. Nutrient Requirements of Beef Cattle, 7th ed. Washington, DC: National Academy Press.

NRC. 2001. Nutrient Requirements of Dairy Cattle, 7th ed. Washington, DC: National Academy Press.

Odberg, F. O., and K. Francis-Smith. 1976. A study on eliminative and grazing behaviour—the use of the field by captive horses. Equine Vet. J. 8:147–149.

Odberg, F. O., and K. Francis-Smith. 1977. Studies on the formation of ungrazed eliminative areas in fields used by horses. Appl. Anim. Ethology 3:27–34.

O'Keily, P., A. Moloney, and E. G. Riordan. 2002. Reducing the cost of beef production by increasing silage intakes. Teagasc Beef Production Series No. 51.

Ojima, K., and T. Isawa. 1968. The variation of carbohydrate in various species of grasses and legumes. Can. J. Bot. 46:1507–1511.

Ott, E. A., R. L. Asquith, J. P. Feaster, and F. G. Martin. 1979a. Influence of protein level and quality on growth and development of yearling foals. J. Anim. Sci. 49:620–626.

Ott, E. A., J. P. Feaster, and S. Lieb. 1979b. Acceptability and digestibility of dried citrus pulp by horses. J. Anim. Sci. 49:983–987.

Owens, F. N., D. S. Secrist, W. J. Hill, and D. R. Gill. 1997. The effect of grain source and grain processing on performance of feedlot cattle: a review. J. Anim. Sci. 75:868–879.

Pagan, J. 1996. A survey of growth rates of Thoroughbreds in Kentucky. Pferdheilkunde 12:285–289.

Pagan, J. D. 1998. Measuring the digestible energy content of horse feeds. Pp. 71–76 in Advances in Equine Nutrition, J. D. Pagan, ed. Nottingham, UK: Nottingham University Press.

Pagan, J. D., and S. G. Jackson. 1991a. Digestibility of pelleted verses long stem alfalfa hay in horses. Pp. 29–32 in Proc. 12th Equine Nutr. Physiol. Soc. Symp., University of Calgary, Alberta.

Pagan, J. D., and S. G. Jackson. 1991b. Distillers dried grains as a feed ingredient for horse rations: A palatability and digestibility study. Pp. 49–54 in Proc. 12th Equine Nutr. Physiol. Soc. Symp., University of Calgary, Alberta.

Pagan, J. D., W. Tiegs, S. G. Jackson, and H. O. W. Murphy. 1993. The effect of different fat sources on exercise performance in Thoroughbred racehorses. Pp. 125–129 in Proc. 13th Equine Nutr. and Physiol. Soc., Gainesville, FL.

Palmgren-Karlsson, C., A. Jansson, B. Essen-Gustavsson, and J. E. Lindberg. 2002. Effect of molassed sugar beet pulp on nutrient utilisation and metabolic parameters during exercise. Equine Vet. J. Suppl. 34:44–49.

Pearl, G. G. 1995. Fatty Acid Composition of Fats and Oils. Alexandria, VA: Fats and Proteins Research Foundation.

Pearson, R. A., and J. B. Merrit. 1991. Intake, digestion and gastrointestinal transit time in resting donkeys and ponies and exercised donkeys given ad libitum hay and straw diets. Equine Vet. J. 23:339–343.

Pearson, R. A., R. F. Archibald, and R. H. Muirhead. 2001. The effect of forage quality and level of feeding on digestibility and gastrointestinal transit time of oat straw and alfalfa given to ponies and donkeys. Br. J. Nutr. 85:599–606.

Pillner, S. 1992. Horse Nutrition and Feeding. London: Blackwell Scientific Publications.

Pipkin, J. L., L. J. Yoss, C. R. Richardson, C. F. Triplitt, D. E. Parr, and J. V. Pipkin. 1991. Total mixed ration for horses. Pp. 55–56 in Proc. 12th Equine Nutr. Physiol. Soc. Symp., University of Calgary, Alberta.

Pollitt, C. C., M. Kyaw-Tanner, K. R. French, A. W. Van Eps, J. K. Hendrikz, and M. Daradka. 2003. Equine Laminitis. Pp. 103–115 in 49th Annual Convention of the American Association of Equine Practitioners, New Orleans, LA: American Association of Equine Practitioners..

Potter, G. D., F. F. Arnold, D. D. Householder, D. H. Hansen, and K. M. Brown. 1992a. Digestion of starch in the small or large intestine of the equine. Pp. 107–111 in European Conference on Nutrition for the Horse, Hannover, Germany.

Potter, G. D., P. G. Gibbs, R. G. Haley, and C. Klendshoj. 1992b. Digestion of protein in the small and large intestines of equines fed mixed diets. Pp. 140–143 in European Conference on Nutrition for the Horse, Hannover, Germany.

Price, W. D., R. A. Lovell, and D. G. McChesney. 1993. Naturally occurring toxins in feedstuffs: Center for Veterinary Medicine perspective. J. Anim. Sci. 71:2556–2562.

Prior, R. L., H. F. Hintz, J. E. Lowe, and W. J. Visek. 1974. Urea recycling and metabolism of ponies. J. Anim. Sci. 38:565–571.

Putman, R. J., R. M. Pratt, J. R. Ekins, and P. J. Edwards. 1987. Food and feeding-behavior of cattle and ponies in the New Forest, Hampshire. J. Appl. Ecol. 24:369–380.

Radicke, S., E. Kienzle, and H. Meyer. 1991. Preileal apparent digestibility of oats and corn starch and consequences for cecal metabolism. Pp. 43–48 in Proc. 12th Equine Nutr. Physiol. Soc. Symp., University of Calgary, Alberta.

Raguse, C. A., and D. Smith. 1965. Carbohydrate content in alfalfa herbage as influenced by methods of drying. J. Agric. Feed. Chem. 13:306–309.

Raina, R. N., and G. V. Raghavan. 1985. Processing of complete feeds and availability of nutrients to horses. Indian J. Anim. Sci. 55:282–287.

Ravindran, V. 1996. Occurrence of phytic acid in plant feed ingredients. Pp. 85–92 in Phytase in Animal Nutrition and Waste Management, M. B. Coelho and E. T. Kornegay, eds. BASF Reference Manual DC9601. Mount Olive, NJ: BASF Corporation.

Raymond, S. L, T. K. Smith, H. V. L. N. Swamy. 2003. Effects of feeding of grains naturally contaminated with Fusarium mycotoxins on feed intake, serum chemistry, and hematology of horses, and the efficacy of a polymeric glucomannan mycotoxin adsorbent. J. Anim. Sci. 81: 2123–2130.

Raymond, S. L., T. K. Smith, and H. V. L. N. Swamy. 2005. Effects of feeding a blend of grains naturally contaminated with Fusarium mycotoxins on feed intake, metabolism, and indices of athletic performance of exercised horses. J. Anim. Sci. 83:1267–1273.

Redbo, I., P. Redbo-Torstensson, F. O. Odberg, A. Hedendahl, and J. Holm. 1998. Factors affecting behavioural disturbances in race-horses. Anim. Sci. 66:475–481.

Reinowski, A. R., and R. J. Coleman. 2003. Voluntary intake of big bluestem, eastern gamagrass, indiangrass and timothy grass hays by mature horses. Pp. 3–4 in Proc. 18th Equine Nutr. Physiol. Soc. Symp., East Lansing, MI.

Reitnour, C. M., and R. L. Salsbury. 1976. Utilization of proteins by the equine species. Am. J. Vet. Res. 37:1065–1067.

Ricketts, S. W., T. R. Greet, P. J. Glyn, C. D. R. Ginnet, E. P. McAllister, J. McCaig, P. H. Skinner, P. M. Webbon, D. L. Frape, G. R. Smith, and L. G. Murray. 1984. Thirteen cases of botulism in horses fed big bale silage. Equine Vet. J. 16:515–518.

Riet-Correa, F., M. C. Mendez, A. L. Shild, P. N. Bergamo, and W. N. Flores. 1988. Aglactia, reproductive problems and neonatal mortality in horses associated with the ingestion of *Claviceps purpurea*. Austral. Vet. J. 65:192–193.

Riley, R. T. 1998. Mechanistic interactions of mycotoxins: theoretical considerations Pp. 227–253 in S. K. K. Sinha, and D. Bhatnagar, eds. Mycotoxins in Agriculture and Food Safety, S. K. K. Sinha and D. Bhatnagar, eds. New York: Marcel Dekker.

Robinson, N. E. 2001. Recurrent airway obstruction (Heaves). Pp. 1–14 in Equine Respiratory Diseases, P. Lekeuk, ed. Ithaca, NY: IVIS.

Robinson, N. E., F. J. Derksen, and M. A. Olszewski. 1995. The pathogenesis of chronic obstructive disease of horses. Br. Vet. J. 152:283–306.

Roche Vitamins Inc. 2000. Vitamin Nutrition Compendium. Parsippany, NJ: Roche Vitamins.

Rogalski, M. 1984. Effect of carbohydrates or lignin on preferences for and intakes of pasture plants by mares. Roczniki Akademii Rolniczej Poznaniu 27:183–193.

Ross, P. F., L. G. Rice, J. C. Reagor, G. D. Osweiler, T. M. Wilson, H. A. Nelson, D. L. Owens, R. D. Plattner, K. A. Harlin, and J. L. Richard. 1991. Fumonisin B1 concentrations in feeds from 45 confirmed equine leukoencephalomalacia cases. J. Vet. Diagn. Invest. 3:238–241.

Ross, P. F., A. E. Ledet, D. L. Owens, L. G. Rice, H. A. Nelson, G. D. Osweiler, and T. M. Wilson. 1993. Experimental equine leukoencephalomalacia, toxic hepatosis and encephalopathy caused by corn naturally contaminated with fumonisins. J. Vet. Diagn. Invest. 5:69–74.

Rotz, C. A. 1995. Field Curing of Forages. Pp. 39–65 in Post-Harvest Physiology and Preservation of Forages. CSSA Special Publication No. 22. Madison, WI: Crop Sci. Soc. Agron. and Am. Soc. Agron.

Rotz, C. A., and R. E. Muck. 1994. Changes in forage quality during harvest and storage. Pp. 828–868 in Forage Quality, Evaluation, and Utilization, G. C. Fahey, Jr. et al., eds. Madison, WI: Am. Soc. Agron.

Sams, R. A. 1997. Review of possible sources of exposure of horses to natural products and environmental contaminants resulting in regulatory action. AAEP Proceedings 43:220–223.

Schoeb, T. R., and R. J. Panciera. 1978. Blister beetle poisoning in horses. J. Am. Vet. Med. Assoc. 173:75–77.

Schubert, B., P. Kallings, M. Johannsson, A. Ryttman, and U. Bondesson. 1988. Hordenine- N,N,-Dimethyltyramine—Studies of occurrence in animal feeds, disposition and effects on cardiorespiratory and blood lactate responses to exercise in the horse. Pp. 51–63 in Proc. 7th Inter. Conf. of Racing Analysts and Veterinarians, T. Tobin, J. Blake, M. Potter, and T. Wood, eds., Louisville, KY.

Schurg, W. A., R. E. Pulse, D. W. Holtan, and J. E. Oldfield. 1978. Use of various quantities and forms of ryegrass straw in horse diets. J. Anim. Sci. 47:1287–1291.

Scudamore, K. A., and C. T. Livesey. 1998. Occurrences and significance of mycotoxins in forage crops and silage: a review. J. Sci. Food Agric. 77:1–17.

Selmi, B., D. Marion, J. M. Perrier Cornet, J. P. Douzals, and P. Gervais. 2000. Amyloglucosidase hydrolysis of high pressure and thermally gelatinized corn and wheat starches. J. Agric. Food Chem. 48:2629–2633.

Shepherd, J. B., H. G. Wiseman, R. E. Ely, C. G. Melin, W. J. Sweetman, C. H. Gordon, L. G. Scheonleber, R. E. Wagner, L. E. Campbell, and G. D. Roane. 1954. USDA Tech. Bull. 1079:1–147.

Shepperson, G. 1960. Effect of time of cutting and method of making on the feed value of hay. Pp. 704–708 in Proc. 8th Inter. Grassland Congress, Reading, UK.

Slade, L. M., D. W. Robinson, and K. E. Casey. 1970. Nitrogen metabolism in nonruminant herbivores. I. The influence of nonprotein nitrogen and protein quality on the nitrogen retention of adult mares. J. Anim. Sci. 30:753–760.

Sloet Van Oldruitenborgh-Oosterbaan, M. M., F. C. M. Schipper, L. S. Goehring, and J. F. Gremmels. 1999. Pleasure horses with neurological signs: EHV1-infection or mycotoxin intoxication? Tijdschrift voor Diergeneeskunde 124:679–681.

Smith, D. 1968. Classification of several North American grasses as starch or fructosan accumulators in relation to taxonomy. J. Br. Grassland Soc. 23:306–309.

Smith, T. A., E. G. McMillan, and J. B. Castillo. 1997. Effects of feeding blends of mycotoxins-contaminated grains containing deoxynivalenol and fusaric acid on growth and feed consumption of immature swine. J. Anim. Sci. 75:2194–2191.

Staun, H., F. Linneman, L. Erikson, K. Mielsen, H. V. Sonnicksen, J. Valk-Ronne, P. Schamleye, P. Henkel, and E. Fachr. 1989. The influence of feeding intensity on the development of the young growing horse until three years of age. Beretning fra Statens Husdyrbrugsforsog No. 657.

St. Lawrence, A. C., L. M. Lawrence, and R. J. Coleman. 2001. Using an empirical equation to predict the voluntary intake of grass hays by mature equids. Pp. 99–100 in Proc. 17th Equine Nutr. Physiol. Soc. Symp., Lexington, KY.

Stout, W. L., D. P. Belesky, G. A. Jung, R. S. Adams, and B. L. Moser. 1977. A survey of Pennsylvania forage mineral levels with respect to dairy and beef nutrition. Prog. Rep. No. 364. Pennsylvania Agric. Exp. Stn., University Park.

Stynes, B. A., and A. F. Bird. 1983. Development of annual ryegrass toxicity. Aust. J. Ag. Res. 34:653–660.

Sunvold, G. D., H. S. Hussein, G. C. Fahey, Jr., N. R. Merchen, and G. A. Reinhart. 1995. *In vitro* fermentation of cellulose, beet pulp, citrus pulp and citrus pectin using fecal inoculum from cats, dogs, horses, humans and pigs and ruminal fluid from cattle. J. Anim. Sci. 73:3639–3648.

Swingle, R. S., T. P. Eck, C. B. Theurer, M. De la Llata, M. H. Poore, and J. A. Moore. 1999. Flake density of steam-processed sorghum grain alters performance and sites of digestibility by growing-finishing steers. J. Anim. Sci. 77:1055–1065.

Technical Committee. 1964. Delaware Agr. Exp. Sta. Tech. Bull. 349:1–17.

Tinker, M. K., N. A. White, P. Lessard, C. D. Thatcher, K. D. Pelzer, B. Davis, and D. K. Carmel. 1997. A prospective study of equine colic risk factors. Equine Vet. J. 29: 454–458.

Todd, L. K., W. C. Sauer, R. J. Christopherson, R. J. Coleman, and W. R. Caine. 1995. The effect of feeding different forms of alfalfa on nutrient digestibility and voluntary intake in horses. J. Anim. Physiol. 73:1–8.

Traub-Dargatz, J. L., C. A. Kopral, A. H. Seitzinger, L. P. Garber, K. Forde, and N. A. White. 2001. Estimate of the national incidence of and operation-level risk factors for colic among horses in the United States spring 1998-spring 1999. J. Am. Vet. Med. Assoc. 219:67–71.

Turner, L. B., M. O. Humphreys, and A. J. Cairns. 2002. Carbon assimilation and partitioning into non-structural carbohydrate in contrasting varieties of *Lolium perenne*. J. Plant Physiol. 159:257–263.

Turner, N. J., and N. F. Szczawinski. 1991. Common poisonous plants and mushrooms of North America. Portland, OR: Timber Press.

Underwood, E. J. 1981. Mineral Nutrition of Livestock. Slough, UK: Commonwealth Agricultural Bureau.

USDA (United States Department of Agriculture). 1998. National Nutrient Database for Standard Reference Release 12. Accessible at http://www.nal.usda.gov/fnic/foodcomp. Accessed August 15, 2006.

Valentine, J. 1999. Oats—the way forward. Pp. 24–29 in IGER Innovations.

Van der Noot, G. W., and E. B. Gilbreath. 1970. Comparative digestibility of components of forages by geldings and steers. J. Anim. Sci. 31:351–355.

Van Der Poel, A. F. B., M. W. A. Verstegen, and S. Tamminga. 1995. Chemical, physical and nutritional effects of feed processing technology. Pp. 70–86 in Proc. 16th Western Nutrition Conference, Saskatoon, Saskatchewan.

Van Soest, P., D. R. Mertens, and B. Deinum. 1978. Pre-harvest factors influencing quality of conserved forage. J. Anim. Sci. 47:713–720.

Vandenput S., L. Istasse, and B. Nicks. 1997. Airborne dust and aeroallergen concentration in a horse stable under two different management systems. Vet. Quarterly 19:154–158.

Vervuert, I., M. Coenen, and C. Bothe. 2003. Effects of oat processing on the glycaemic and insulin responses in horses. J. Anim. Physiol. Anim. Nutr. 87:96–104.

Vervuert, I., M. Coenen, and C. Bothe. 2004. Effects of corn processing on the glycaemic and insulin responses in horses. J. Anim. Physiol. Anim. Nutr. 88:348–355.

Vervuert, I., M. Coenen, S. Dahlhoff, and W. Sommer. 2005. Fructan content in roughage for horses. Proc. Waltham–Virginia Tech Symp.: Innovative, Nutritional, Metabolic, and Genetic Countermeasures to Equine Laminitis, September 14, Washington, DC.

Vesonder, R., J. Haliburton, and P. Golinski. 1989. Toxicity of field samples and Fusarium moniliforme from feed associated with equine-leucoencephalomalacia. Arch. Environ. Contam. Toxicol. 18:439–442.

Vesonder, R., J. Haliburton, R. Stubblefield, W. Gilmore, and S. Peterson. 1991. Aspergillus flavus and aflatoxins B1, B2 and M1 in corn associated with equine death. Arch. Environ. Contam. Tox. 20:151–153.

Volaire, F., and F. Lelievre. 1997. Production, persistence, and water-soluble carbohydrate accumulation in 21 contrasting populations of *Dactylis glomerata*. L. subjected to severe drought in the South of France. Aust. J. Agric. Res. 48:933–944.

Wagner, E. L., G. D. Potter, E. M. Eller, P. G. Gibbs, and D. M. Hood. 2005. Absorption and retention of trace minerals in adult horses. Prof. Anim. Scientist 21:207–211.

Waite, R., and J. Boyd. 1953a. The water-soluble carbohydrates in grasses. I. Changes occurring during the normal life cycle. J. Sci. Food Agric. 4:197–204.

Waite, R., and J. Boyd. 1953b. The water-soluble carbohydrates of grasses. II. Grasses cut at grazing height several times in the grazing season. J. Sci. Food Agric. 4:257–261.

Warren, L. K., L. M. Lawrence, T. Brewster-Barnes, and D. M. Powell. 1999. The effect of dietary fibre on hydration status after dehydration with frusemide. Equine Vet. J. Suppl. 30:508–513.

Waters A. J., C. J. Nicol, and N. P. French. 2002. Factors influencing the development of stereotypic and redirected behaviours in young horses: findings of a four year prospective epidemiological study. Equine Vet. J. 34:572–579.

Whitlow, L. W., and W. M. Hagler. 2002. Mycotoxins in feeds. Feedstuffs 74(28):66–74.

Whitman, W. C., D. W. Bolin, E. W. Klosterman, H. J. Klostermann, K. D. Ford, L. Moomaw, D. G. Hoag, and M. L. Buchanan. 1951. Carotene, protein, and phosphorus in range and tame grasses of western North Dakota. North Dakota Agric. Exp. Sta. Bull. 370. Fargo, ND.

Wilcox, E. C. 1899. Ergotism in horses. Montana Agri. Exp. Sta. Bull. 22:49.

Willard, J. G., J. C. Willard, S. A. Wolfram, and J. P. Baker. 1977. Effect of diet on cecal pH and feeding behaviour of horses. J. Anim. Sci. 45:87–93.

Williams, J. H. H., B. E. Collis, C. J. Pollock, M. Williams, and J. F. Farrar. 1993. Variability in the distribution of photoassimilates along leaves of temperate Gramineae. New Phytologist 123:699–703.

Williams, M. C. 1987. Nitrate and soluble oxalate accumulation in Kikuyugrass (*Pennisetum clandestinum*). Proc. Western Soc. Weed Sci. 40:78–79.

Wilson, J. R., B. Deinum, and F. M. Engels. 1991. Temperature effect on anatomy and digestibility of leaf and stem of tropical and temperate forage species. Neth. J. Agric. Sci. 39:31–48.

Wilson, T. M., P. E. Nelson, W. F. O. Marasas, P. G. Thiel, G. S. Shephard, E. W. Sydenham, H. A. Nelson, and P. F. Ross. 1990a. A mycological evaluation and in vivo toxicity evaluation of feed from 41 farms with equine leukoencephalomalacia. J. Vet. Diagn. Invest. 2:352–354.

Wilson, T. M., P. F. Ross, L. G. Rice, G. D. Osweiler, H. A. Nelson, D. L. Owens, R. D. Plattner, C. Reggiardo, T. H. Noon, and J. W. Pickrell. 1990b. Fumonisin B1 levels associated with an epizootic of equine leukoencephalomalacia. J. Vet. Diagn. Invest. 2:213–216.

Wilson, T. M., P. F. Ross, D. L. Owens, L. G. Rice, S. A. Green, S. J. Jenkins, and H. A. Nelson. 1992. Experimental reproduction of ELEM. Mycopathalogia 117:115–120.

Woolfolk, J. S., E. F. Smith, R. R. Schalles, B. E. Brent, L. H. Harbers, and C. E. Owensby. 1975. Effects of nitrogen fertilization and late-spring burning of bluestem range on diet and performance of steers. J. Range Manage. 28:190–193.

Wylam, C. B. 1953. Analytical studies on the carbohydrates of grasses and clovers. 111. Carbohydrate breakdown during ensilage. J. Sci. Food Agric. 4:527–531.

Yiannikouris, A., and J. P. Jouany. 2002. Mycotoxins in feed and their fate in animals: a review. Anim. Res. 51:81–99.

Yoon, Y., and Y. J. Baeck. 1999. Aflatoxin binding and antimutagenic activities of *Bifidiobacterium bifidum* HY strains and their genotypes. Korean J. Dairy Sci. 21:291–298.

Zarkadas, L. N., and J. Wiseman. 2001. Influence of processing variables during micronization of wheat on starch structure and subsequent performance and digestibility in weaned piglets fed wheat-based diets. Anim. Feed Sci. Technol. 93:93–107.

Zarkadas, L. N., and J. Wiseman. 2002. Influence of micronization temperature and pre-conditioning on performance and digestibility in piglets fed barley-based diets. Anim. Feed Sci. Techol. 95:73–82.

Zinn, R. A., F. N. Owens, and R. A. Ware. 2002. Flaking corn: processing mechanics, quality standards and impacts on energy availability and performance of feedlot cattle. J. Anim. Sci. 80:1145–1156.

9

Feed Additives

Foods are defined by the Federal Food, Drug, and Cosmetic Act (Title 21 Code of Federal Regulations (CFR) §321 (f)) as "articles used for food or drink for man or other animals and articles used for components of any other such article." Inherently, food and feed (used in reference to animals) articles provide taste, aroma, nutritive value, or some combination. Natural and commercially prepared feeds intended for horses include substances that do not directly provide essential nutrients, but may influence animal intake, health, and performance or feed characteristics. Food additives, as described within Title 21 CFR (§321 (s)), include any substance intended or reasonably expected to become, either directly or indirectly, a component of food or alters the characteristics of any food and including any substance intended for use in the manufacturing, processing, packaging, and storing of food. No distinction is made between feeds or food additives for food-producing or nonfood-producing animals. Concerns about animal safety and potential for residues in human foods derived from animal sources have resulted in feed additives being regulated by the U.S. Food and Drug Administration (FDA).

A more conventional description of animal diet feed additives suggests nonnutritive ingredients that stimulate growth or other types of production, improve the efficiency of feed utilization, or benefit the health or metabolism of the animal (Church and Kellems, 1998). The focus here is on medications and therapeutic agents in livestock feeds. This perception of feed additives is consistent with the legal definition of a drug. Besides medicinal agents recognized by various official pharmacopoeia agencies, the CFR additionally defines a drug (21 CFR §321 (g)) as any "article intended for use in the diagnosis, cure, mitigation, treatment, or prevention of disease in man or other animals and articles (other than food) intended to affect the structure or any function of the body of man or other animals." Substances fitting the legal definition of a drug must undergo stringent and extensive evaluation to document safety and efficacy before being approved by the FDA for use in medicated feeds. A distinction is made where dietary substances providing one or more defined nutrients that affect body structure or function are not considered a drug (Hoestenbach, 2004). In contrast, feed products not containing recognized nutrients and claiming health, structure, or performance responses are potentially subject to regulatory scrutiny. Additionally, feed additives used for something other than their intended purpose as defined in the CFR can result in regulatory action by the FDA.

The Association of American Feed Control Officials (AAFCO) writes and revises model bills. A model bill encompasses food and drug regulations set forth in the CFR and often is the basis of individual state feed regulations (AAFCO, 2005). A publication published by AAFCO contains a listing of approved animal feed additives and guidelines for their intended use and is updated yearly as approved uses of feed additives are subject to change. Other countries have similar regulatory bodies that define acceptable uses for various nonnutrient feed components. Given the complexity of regulations, potential for change, and differences across countries, the scope of this chapter will be limited to current feed additive regulations within the United States.

ADDITIVES AFFECTING FEED CHARACTERISTICS

As previously defined, feeds provide nutrients required to sustain normal body structure, metabolism, and productivity. Physical characteristics of feed that affect sight, smell, taste, and texture impact feed intake (Dulphy et al., 1997; Goodwin et al., 2005a), thereby influencing the animal's ability to consume sufficient amounts to meet nutrient needs. Additionally, chemical or microbiological alteration or degradation of the feed and its components during the manufacturing and storage process can adversely affect intake, animal health, or both (Raymond et al., 2003). Nonnutritive food additives can provide a number of technologic functions to enhance physical characteristics, suitability, and stability of feed during manufacturing, processing, and storage (FDA, 1992; Kantor, 1996; Sumner and Eifert, 2002). Technical food additives are used in foods to promote product consistency, improve or maintain nutritional value, maintain palatability, retard spoilage, and provide characteristics to influence taste and color (FDA, 1992).

Food additives used for technical effects on feeds are all defined and approved for their intended use within specific guidelines for rate of incorporation within Title 21 CFR and the current AAFCO publication, or by similar regulatory bodies in other countries. These substances are categorized either as generally recognized as safe (GRAS; 21 CFR §582) or permitted (21 CFR §573) food additives. An additive with GRAS status (21 CFR §570.30) is established by either recognizing the substance has been used for many years with public knowledge of its use and safety or has been scientifically evaluated to be without documented health, residue, or toxicity concerns. Most food additives used prior to 1958 were classified as GRAS as a result of their prolonged use without safety concerns under good manufacturing or feeding practices. Most nutrients, except selenium, are considered GRAS. Specific selenium sources have been approved as food additives for animals following extensive scientific documentation (21 CFR §573.920). It should be noted that GRAS substances, although recognized as safe, are not without potential hazard if not used within the defined guidelines of good manufacturing or feeding practices. Any nutrient if fed in amounts greatly exceeding a defined requirement can induce toxicosis.

Following the food additives amendment to the Federal Food, Drug, and Cosmetic Act in 1958, food additives not considered GRAS and all new food additive requests were and are required to provide substantial documentation of safety and utility before being approved. Though no differentiation is made in defining food additives for humans or animals, food additives approved for humans are not necessarily approved for use in animal feeds. To date, no exceptions or qualifications exist for the inclusion of GRAS or permitted food additives in horse feeds.

Antioxidants and Preservatives

Antioxidant preservative compounds are added to dietary ingredients for the purpose of inhibiting oxidation reactions to polyunsaturated fats and vitamins. Reactions from exposure to oxidizing agents induce formation of highly reactive, unstable, and self-replicating peroxides and free radicals (unpaired electron species) within fatty acid structures. Fat oxidation results in feed discoloration, deterioration, and fat rancidity and ultimately reduces feed palatability and quality. Feed vitamin activity can be markedly reduced by oxidation.

Ethoxyquin (21 CFR §573.380) is a commonly used synthetic antioxidant approved for use in animal feeds, although some concerns regarding its safety for use in dog foods have been raised (Dzanis, 1991) and subsequently a lower inclusion rate was recommended (FDA, 1997). However, no adverse effects have been reported with its use in horse feeds. Other synthetic feed-based antioxidants include butylated hydroxyanisole (BHA; 21 CFR §582.3169), butylated hydroxytoluene (BHT; 21 CFR §582.3173), and tertiary butyl hydroquinone (TBHQ). Both BHA and BHT compounds are considered GRAS. As of 2005, TBHQ is considered an acceptable feed ingredient by AAFCO as it is undergoing informal review by FDA (AAFCO, 2005). Inclusion of BHT, BHA, and TBHQ is limited to a total preservative content not more than 0.02 percent (200 mg/kg) of fat or oil (including volatile oils) content (AAFCO, 2005).

Mixed tocopherols (21 CFR §582.3890) are combined forms of vitamin E isomers with similar antioxidant activity to synthetic compounds, though greater quantities are needed compared to synthetic antioxidants (Gross et al., 1994; Ohshima et al., 1998). Being derived from plants and not chemically altered, mixed tocopherols are often marketed as "natural" antioxidants. The antioxidant properties of tocopherols are complex and vary by isomer, concentration, and combination interactions (Huang et al., 1994, 1995). Stabilization of tocopherol isomers by esterification to acetate or succinate limits their food preservation activity.

A number of additional GRAS substances are used as chemical preservatives (21 CFR §582 Subpart D) to maintain feed value and inhibit microbial colonization and growth in feeds. Propionic acid (21 CFR §582.3081) incorporated at 0.3 and 1 percent (weight/weight) has been shown to be an effective mold-inhibiting agent for dried grains (Kiessling and Pettersson, 1991). A number of other organic acids and their combinations are used as chemical preservatives (Kiessling and Pettersson, 1991; AAFCO, 2005). Feed labels must indicate the inclusion of preservative agents by identifying the compound as "a preservative," using a statement "preserved with," "added to inhibit mold growth," or similar designation (AAFCO, 2005).

Colors

Color additives may be added to feeds to replace, enhance, or accentuate inherent colors of feed. Allowed substances used for color in feeds are either certified synthetic compounds (21 CFR §74.101 through §74.706) or noncertified natural or synthetic sources (21 CFR §73.1 through §73.615). Certified colors not only require premarket approval, but each manufactured batch must be certified to ensure safety. Inclusion of certified color additives must be identified on product labels by color and number ("Green 3" or "Yellow 5") (21 CFR §70.25). Natural color sources include certain spices, vegetables, fruits, caramel, and others. Color additives have little to no impact on feed acceptability, but may play an important role in product marketing and consumer appeal.

Flavors

A wide variety of spices, seasonings, flavorings, natural oils, and extracts are considered GRAS (21 CFR §582.10 through §582.50) and could be used to add natural flavors to horse feeds. Additionally, synthetic GRAS compounds (21 CFR §582.60) mimicking various fruit, mint, and other flavors can be added to horse feeds. Beyond the intended purpose of providing flavor, a number of herbs and spices have been attributed effects often associated with health or disease mitigation. Inclusion rate for these flavor ingredients using good manufacturing practices are unlikely to have potential for other beneficial effects. Additionally, any product claim to this effect is contrary to recognized intended purpose of the additive and could prompt regulatory action.

Flavors are often used to improve feed palatability and acceptability directly or indirectly by masking off-taste or off-odor constituents in feed. Anorectic or sick horses may potentially benefit from flavors if intake is increased, but use in feeds for healthy horses is questionable and potentially is more for marketing aimed at the horse owner. Randall et al. (1978) assessed taste response of weanlings (202 kg bodyweight [BW]) to salty (sodium chloride), sweet (sucrose), sour (acetic acid), and bitter (quinine hydrochloride) tasting solutions using a two-choice preference test procedure (water as the control solution). Foals showed weak to moderate preference for sweet solutions between 1.25 and 10 g sucrose per 100 ml (Randall et al., 1978). Sucrose solutions were not discriminated against compared to water, which is in agreement with observed feeding preferences of horses for sweetened concentrates (Houpt, 1990). Foals discriminated against salty, sour, and bitter solutions compared to water above 0.63 g NaCl, 0.16 ml acetic acid (3.1 pH), and 20 mg quinine per 100 ml water (Randall et al., 1978). Other studies have addressed flavor preferences in feeds for horses (Burton et al., 1983; Hintz et al., 1989; Pollack and Burton, 1991; Goodwin et al., 2005b).

Peppermint-, carrot-, and wheat syrup-flavored feeds had lower consumption rate compared to apple- or orange-flavored feeds or a control feed containing molasses (Pollack and Burton, 1991). Using flavorings at incorporation rates of 500 or 2,500 g/ton, within-flavor comparisons showed apple and peppermint flavors were preferred at the higher and lower inclusion rates, respectively (Pollack and Burton, 1991). There also was a reported tendency for preference of the lower inclusion rate for orange flavor compared to the higher incorporation rate (Pollack and Burton, 1991). Another study found peppermint flavor, added at the manufacturer's recommended level, to have no effect on intake (Hintz et al., 1989). Time to consume 2 kg of a mixed cereal grain sweet feed was increased 45, 57, and 213 percent when flavored with apple, caramel, and anise, respectively (Burton et al., 1983). Paired preference testing with 15 different flavors added to 100 g cereal byproduct meal (1 g/100 g) fed to eight mature horses showed nutmeg, coriander, and echinacea to be selected against (Goodwin et al., 2005b). Apple, banana, carrot, cherry, cumin, fenugreek, garlic, ginger, oregano, peppermint, rosemary, and turmeric were all universally accepted, but mean consumption rates varied, with apple, garlic, ginger, and turmeric having the slower consumption times (Goodwin et al., 2005b). In the same study, using paired flavor-testing comparisons, fenugreek and banana flavors were highest ranked. Consumption time of a mineral pellet was lower ($P < 0.01$) for banana- and fenugreek-flavored compared to unflavored pellets with no difference between flavored pellets (Goodwin et al., 2005b). Studies evaluating flavor preferences of horses are limited, and feed intake response to flavor additives is influenced by individual preference, concentration, and feed characteristics.

Pellet Binders and Anticaking Agents

Pellet binders are compounds added to feed ingredients to be compressed through a pellet mold that promote cohesiveness and inhibit pellet crumbling or breakdown prior to feeding. Bentonite (21 CFR §582.1155) and attapulgite (21 CFR §582.1) clays and kaolin (21 CFR §582.1) can be added to a maximum of 2 percent of total ration as pelleting aids. Both clays and kaolin have restricted use in medicated feeds as they potentially interfere in analysis of certain drugs. Lignin sulfonate (21 CFR §573.600) can be incorporated up to 4 percent of the finished pellet as a binding aid. Ball clay is no longer approved as a feed ingredient (AAFCO, 2005).

Anticaking agents are substances included in finely powdered or crystalline feeds to prevent caking, lumping, or agglomeration. Iron ammonium citrate (21 CFR §573.560) and yellow prussiate of soda (21 CFR §573.1020) are used as anticaking agents in granular salt and are limited to 25 and 13 ppm in finished product, respectively. Various silicate compounds are either GRAS (21 CFR §582.2122 through §582.2906) or permitted (calcium silicate, 21 CFR §573.260; diatomaceous earth, 21 CFR §573.340; pyrophyllite, 21 CFR §573.900) food additives as anticaking or pellet-binding aids. Good manufacturing practices limit the incorporation of silicate agents to a maximum of 2 percent of the finished product.

Hydrated sodium calcium aluminosilicate (HSCAS, 21 CFR §582.2729), as well as other aluminosilicate compounds (zeolites), have been purported as potential mycotoxin sorbent in animal feeds (CAST, 2003). Bentonite clays have also been suggested to bind mycotoxins in feeds making them less available for absorption. Philips et al. (1987, 1988) showed a protective effect of feeding HSCAS to growing chicks fed a diet containing 7.5 ppm aflatoxin B_1. In the CAST (2003) report on mycotoxins, 25 studies were cited as having shown enterosorbent effects of HSCAS or other bentonite clays in protecting against aflatoxins in a wide variety of young animals. None of the cited studies had used horses as an animal model. Although data are supportive of a sorbent effect of clays, primarily HSCAS, evidence suggests the response is limited to aflatoxins and does not carry over to other mycotoxins. Inclusion of HSCAS in diets did not ameliorate effects of zearalenone (Bursian et al., 1992), deoxynivalenol (DON; Patterson and Young, 1993), or ergotamine (Chestnut et al., 1992). Additionally, zeolites are potential binders of cations and could reduce availability of calcium, magnesium, and zinc if fed in excess of the approved rate of 2 percent of total feed (Chung et al., 1990; Chestnut et al., 1992). Any product labeling claim relative to mycotoxin binding ability for these compounds is contrary to the specified purpose of these ingredients as defined in current regulations and could prompt regulatory action.

Other Additives

A number of other nonnutritive substances are potentially added to horse feeds to alter form and uniformity. Mineral oil (21 CFR §573.680), paraffin, petrolatum (21 CFR §573.720), and petroleum jelly (21 CFR §573.720) can be included in mineral mixes to reduce dust (AAFCO, 2005). The inclusion rate of any dust reducer must be less than 3 or 0.06 percent of the mineral mix or total ration, respectively. Talc and mineral oil can be used as die lubricants in the feed manufacturing process. Emulsifying agents (21 CFR §582.4101 through §582.4666) are used to maintain uniform dispersion of fats and oils in aqueous components of a product. Stabilizers (21 CFR §582.7115 through §582.7724), primarily gums and alginate substances, maintain final product uniformity or consistency over various conditions of manufacturing, processing, and storage. Sequestrants (21 CFR §582.6033 through §582.6851) are polyvalent metal ion binders that form soluble metal complexes to minimize oxidation from free metal ions and improve final product stability.

ADDITIVES AFFECTING ANIMAL HEALTH AND PERFORMANCE

In addition to substances added to enhance the technical or nonnutritive characteristics of food, a wide variety of nutritive and nonnutritive substances are potentially added to enhance animal health. Most recognized of these substances are medicinal compounds (e.g., antibiotics, anthelmintics) used to prevent or treat disease conditions. Medicinal compounds require extensive premarket study and documentation of safety and efficacy for their intended purpose. Medicinal compound documentation is completed by the manufacturer, at considerable expense, prior to consideration for FDA approval as a new animal drug. Beyond medicinal compounds, much interest has been focused on the potential role of food or food components in promoting health and well-being, performance, and disease mitigation or prevention. These foods or food components may include essential nutrients provided in amounts above those suggested to prevent a deficiency state. Or they can be other food components known to have vital role(s) in metabolism that are not currently recognized as an essential nutrient. Other substances may include those for which no function in metabolism is known, yet their inclusion in the diet is purported to augment production or facilitate body function.

With emphasis on human health, fitness, and good nutrition, inclusion of dietary substances for purposes of improving health and performance has spawned an expanding market of products and generated new terminology of "nutraceutical," "functional foods," "designer foods," and similar descriptors. There are similar interests within horse nutrition. The term "nutraceutical" was coined to encompass perceived dual roles of providing nutritive value (e.g., food) and pharmaceutical activity; however, there is little agreement on a precise definition (Boothe, 1997). Concerns have been raised relative to safety and efficacy of such products as well as the role of regulatory oversight (Boothe, 1998). In 1994 the U.S. Congress passed the Dietary Supplement Health and Education Act (DSHEA), which permitted the inclusion of such substances in dietary supplements without prior documentation of safety and utility. Citing safety concerns for the human food supply, the FDA determined that DSHEA does not apply to animal feeds (FDA, 1996). This determination was made because a distinction between animal feeds intended for food-producing or nonfood species is not considered. Thus, from a regulatory viewpoint, nutraceutical products for use in animal feeds do not exist. Dietary supplements included in animal feeds are classified legally as either drug, food, or both and regulated as either drug or food according to a written policy matrix (FDA, 1998). Legal status as a food or drug is determined by the intended use of the substance. Under current regulations, manufacturers may be restricted in terms of statements regarding substance functions within foods, including some of the functions described below.

In feeding horses, as with any species, emphasis should be on feeding a complete and balanced diet. Interest in additional dietary supplements to maintain or improve health and performance is warranted, but safety to the animal should take precedence. The following discussion provides documentation from the scientific literature on the efficacy of a number of commonly used dietary supplements in horses. Discussion of such supplements does not imply essentiality, but only serves to provide information on which to base an informed decision as whether or not to use such substances in diets provided to horses.

Antioxidants

Production of reactive oxygen species (ROS) is a normal consequence of cellular metabolism, leukocyte-induced inflammatory response (respiratory burst), and exposure to environmental oxidizing agents (UV radiation, pollution, chemical agents, tobacco smoke). Generated ROS molecules include free radicals (molecules containing an unpaired electron) and various peroxides (e.g., hydrogen peroxide, lipid hydroperoxides, singlet oxygen). These molecules once generated by pro-oxidative reactions are self-perpetuating and are capable of damaging DNA, lipids, proteins, and carbohydrates (Evans and Halliwell, 2001). Production and continued propagation of ROS is believed integral to the pathogenesis of carcinogenesis, aging osteoarthritis, cardiovascular, and other degenerative diseases (Clark, 2002). In the horse, oxidative stress from ROS propagation has been associated in the pathogenesis of joint disease (Dimock et al., 2000) and recurrent airway obstruction (RAO) (Art et al., 1999; Kirschvink et al., 2002a; Deaton et al., 2004a).

A number of essential nutrients perform all or part of their biological role as a metabolic antioxidant protecting against environmental or metabolic oxidizing agents (Frei, 1994; Clark, 2002). A number of trace minerals are constituents of enzymes having antioxidant activities, namely glutathione peroxidases (selenium), superoxide dismutases (copper, zinc, manganese), and catalases (iron). Other nonenzymatic mineral-dependent antioxidants include ceruloplasmin (copper) and ferritin (iron). Additionally, the essential fat-soluble vitamins A and E perform part or all of their biologic functions as cellular antioxidants (Frei, 1994). Antioxidants acting individually or collectively are capable of chemically converting ROS to less reactive or inactive molecules, thus reducing potential cellular damage. Specific discussions on biologic activities of these essential trace minerals and vitamins and their requirements are covered in their respective chapters elsewhere in this report.

Other Antioxidants

Other compounds have also been characterized as having cellular or extracellular antioxidant properties. These compounds are currently considered nonessential in the diet of the horse as they can either be sufficiently synthesized by the body to meet needs (vitamin C, lipoic acid) or there is insufficient evidence suggesting a dietary requirement (β-carotene, lutein, lycopene). Beyond being a precursor for vitamin A, β-carotene and other carotenoids (lutein, lycopene) have been suggested to possess antioxidant properties (Frei, 1994). There is a paucity of data supporting any benefit of adding these compounds (carotenoids and lipoic acid) as antioxidants to equine diets. Beta-carotene is addressed in more detail elsewhere in this report (see Chapter 6, Vitamins).

Vitamin C functions as a water-soluble intra- and extracellular antioxidant and interacts with vitamin E as a co-antioxidant to restore the antioxidant form of vitamin E (Bowery et al., 1995). However in vivo relevance of this interaction is uncertain (Carr and Frei, 1999). Supplementation and availability of dietary ascorbic acid is complex, influenced by chemical form, dose, dosing frequency, and dose response, and is extremely variable among individuals (Snow and Frigg, 1990). Oral bioavailability of crystalline L-ascorbic acid in the horse is low, using dosages ranging from 5–20 g/d to either single (Löscher et al., 1984; Snow et al., 1987; Snow and Frigg, 1989) or continuous (Snow and Frigg, 1990) dosing. Horses supplemented with crystalline ascorbic acid at either 4.5 or 20 g/d had an approximate doubling of plasma ascorbic acid concentration compared to unsupplemented control horses, but the response was not different between 4.5- or 20-g dosages (Snow et al., 1987). Ascorbyl palmitate, but not ascorbyl stearate, showed greater bioavailability compared to crystalline ascorbic acid with a single oral dose (Snow and Frigg, 1989). Deaton et al. (2003) supplemented ponies with 20 mg/kg BW ascorbic acid equivalent weight from ascorbyl palmitate or calcium ascorbyl monophosphate. Plasma and bronchoalveolar lavage fluid (BALF) ascorbic acid concentrations were 61 and 68 percent greater with ascorbyl palmitate supplementation compared to control. Calcium ascorbyl monophosphate supplementation increased BALF, but not plasma, ascorbic acid concentration 39 percent above unsupplemented controls (Deaton et al., 2003). Snow and Frigg (1990) using seven horses in a cross-over study design did not see any significant increases in mean plasma ascorbic acid concentration with daily crystalline ascorbic acid (20 g/d; 3.2 ± 0.6 mg/l) or ascorbyl palmitate (47 g/d; 4.2 ± 0.9 mg/l) compared to control and unsupplemented periods (2.8 ± 1.1 mg/l).

Thoroughbred horses (n = 14) treated intravenously with 5 g ascorbic acid prior to racing had no change in thiobarbiturate reactive substances (TBAR) compared to a 29 percent increase (P < 0.01) in untreated cohorts (n = 30), but treated horses experienced a greater increase (212 vs. 97 percent, P < 0.01) in creatine kinase activity (White et al., 2001). No influence on physical performance was determined. Though plasma ascorbic acid concentrations were greatly increased with supplementation (75.9 mg/l) and greatly exceeded observed plasma concentrations with oral ascorbate supplementation, there was no effect of racing on plasma concentration in treated or untreated horses.

Supplementing ascorbic acid may have adverse consequences. Snow and Frigg (1990) observed significant declines in plasma ascorbic acid concentration below that of unsupplemented controls following periods of supplementation (20 g/d ascorbic acid). A decline in endogenous synthesis was hypothesized, but a mechanism was not elucidated. Tsao and Young (1989) determined that endogenous synthesis of ascorbic acid can be down regulated by feeding between 0.5 and 5 percent ascorbic acid in the total diet to mice. Ascorbic acid toxicity was not recognized in horses administered up to 20 g/d for 1 day (NRC, 1987), but potential long-term administration has not been evaluated. Ascorbic acid can act as a pro-oxidant with copper and iron potentially generating lipid radicals and requiring antioxidants to return ascorbic acid to its antioxidant form (Clark,

2002). Excess ascorbic acid intake could overwhelm the body's capacity to recycle ascorbic acid back to its antioxidant state.

Reported differences in ascorbic acid in RAO-affected horses with and without inflammation compared to healthy horses and the implied protective effect of ascorbic acid in RAO pathogenesis is enticing (Kirschvink et al., 2002a; Deaton et al., 2004a); however, data substantiating an independent ascorbic acid effect on disease amelioration are unavailable. Based on the limited data, variable response to oral ascorbic acid dosing and clinical trials (White et al., 2001; Deaton et al., 2002) with equivocal responses to supplementation, recommendations for additional supplementation of ascorbic acid to promote antioxidant function cannot be determined.

Alpha-lipoic acid has been reported to perform antioxidant function in humans and laboratory animals (Packer et al., 1995). A similar function was suggested for horses evidenced by reduced total plasma lipid hydroperoxide concentration in Thoroughbred geldings (687 kg BW, n = 10) supplemented once daily with 10 mg/kg BW d,l-α-lipoic acid compared to unsupplemented control horses (Williams et al., 2002). In this study, supplemented geldings had an unexplained greater plasma concentration of total lipid hydroperoxidases compared to control geldings at initiation of the study. Other than red and white blood cell total glutathione and glutathione peroxidase, no other antioxidants that may have impacted overall antioxidant status were measured; thus, the implied role of lipoic acid in observed response may be questioned. No adverse health effects were observed in lipoic acid-supplemented horses over the duration of the study (14 days), but long-term safety in horses is unknown and must be evaluated before a recommendation for use made.

In a second study using 12 mature Arabian horses (450 kg BW), antioxidant supplementation with 10 g/kg BW lipoic acid or 5,000 IU/d α-tocopheryl acetate was compared to unsupplemented horses completing a treadmill-based endurance (55 km) exercise (Williams et al., 2004a). Supplementation with either lipoic acid or α-tocopherol improved a number of parameters measured to assess antioxidant status. Plasma lipid hydroperoxide concentration was not different across treatments. However, only white blood cell apoptosis (programmed cell death) showed significant interaction between supplementation and stage (time points during exercise). White blood cell apoptosis was lower (P = 0.05) and tended (P = 0.06) to be lower in vitamin E and lipoic acid supplemented horses, respectively, compared to unsupplemented horses (Williams et al., 2004a). Results from this study suggest potential antioxidant effects with lipoic acid; however, animal numbers were limited to make any broad-based interpretation. Vitamin E status of experimental horses was adequate based on initial plasma α-tocopherol concentrations of control horses (> 4.0 μg/ml). Ability for lipoic acid to provide antioxidant protection when the horse is vitamin E-deficient has not been tested. Without further studies, supplementation of α-lipoic acid as an antioxidant is not warranted.

Dietary Application of Antioxidants

Exercise or other activity increasing oxygen consumption will increase the generation of ROS and potentially tip the balance away from the body's antioxidant defense ability in favor of oxidative reactions and resulting cellular damage (Hargreaves et al., 2002; Deaton and Marlin, 2003; Williams, 2004). Antioxidants have been advocated for dietary inclusion in exercising horses to minimize oxidative stress associated with physical activity, especially for horses with RAO (Deaton and Marlin, 2003; Williams, 2004). Healthy horses supplemented with a commercial dietary antioxidant mixture (vitamins E and C, and selenium) or a placebo for 4 weeks and subjected to an intermittent, moderate-intensity exercise test (2 minutes at 70, 80, and 90 percent individual oxygen maximum) showed no benefit or detriment of additional antioxidant supplementation (Deaton et al., 2002). A lack of response may be attributed to exercise intensity not being sufficient to induce oxidative stress. However, antioxidant supplementation increased plasma ascorbic acid (P = 0.007) and α-tocopherol (P = 0.02) concentrations compared to placebo-treated horses (Deaton et al., 2002). Antioxidant effects on pulmonary epithelial lining fluid (ELF) ascorbic acid and α-tocopherol concentrations were not significant (Deaton et al., 2002).

Recurrent airway obstruction-affected horses in acute crisis (exposed to bedding and hay allergens) have indicators of oxidative stress evidenced by increased oxidized glutathione concentration and glutathione redox ratio in ELF (Art et al., 1999; Kirschvink et al., 2002b). Reduced antioxidant status was correlated with measures of impaired pulmonary function and increased airway inflammation (Kirschvink et al., 2002b). Horses affected with RAO and having evidence of airway inflammation had lowest ELF ascorbic acid concentration compared to RAO-affected without airway inflammation and unaffected horses (Deaton et al., 2004a, 2005a). Collectively, these studies suggest RAO-affected horses have lower airway antioxidant status and might benefit from antioxidant supplementation. Dietary supplementation of an antioxidant mixture (vitamins E and C and selenium) for 4 weeks in RAO-affected horses showed improvement in exercise ability and inflammatory score (Kirschvink et al., 2002c) or no effect (Deaton et al., 2004b); however, neither study had healthy control horses for comparison. Nonneutrophilic airway inflammation induced by ozone exposure resulted in oxidation of glutathione, but not ascorbic acid in both RAO-affected and healthy horses (Deaton et al., 2005b). Response to ozone-induced inflammation was not greater in RAO-affected horses, in spite of their lower ELF ascorbic acid concentration compared to healthy horses.

Supplementation of exercising horses with vitamin E (Siciliano et al., 1997) or vitamins E and C (Hoffman et al., 2001; Williams et al., 2004b), though significantly increasing plasma vitamin E and ascorbic acid concentrations compared to unsupplemented horses, failed to show significant reduction in exercise-induced muscle damage as evaluated by plasma muscle enzyme activities. Racing Thoroughbreds provided an antioxidant mixture supplement (containing 11.5 g ascorbic acid; 7 g d,l-α-tocopheryl acetate; 7 mg selenium; 769 mg zinc; 187 gm copper; and 500 mg β-carotene) over a 3-month period had lower creatine phosphokinase activity at 6, but not 12, weeks, compared to unsupplemented controls (de Moffarts et al., 2005). The basal hay and oats diet consumed by all horses provided less than NRC (1989) recommended daily amounts of vitamin E (120 IU), selenium (0.4 mg), zinc (48 mg), and copper (75 mg).

A lack of consistent markers of oxidative stressors or responses to antioxidants in exercising horses may be attributed to differences in level of training, duration, and intensity of exercise; ambient conditions; and nutrition (Marlin et al., 2002; Williams et al., 2003; de Moffarts et al., 2004). Additionally, interpretation of oxidative stress response may be influenced by the analytic marker used (Balogh et al., 2001), source of oxidative stress (Deaton et al., 2005a,b), and the form of antioxidant. At present, there is a lack of data on which to base specific recommendations beyond those for the essential vitamins and minerals that are components of antioxidants. Recent research using antioxidant mixtures is encouraging, but specific recommendations are not available.

Direct Fed Microbials (Probiotics)

Direct fed microbials (DFM, also termed "probiotics") are products intended to be consumed and provide live colonies of lactic acid bacteria, namely *Lactobacilli*, *Bifidobacteria*, and entercoli, typically present in the intestinal lumen of healthy animals. Provision of live bacteria is believed to exclude or reduce growth of potential pathogenic bacteria by competitive inhibition, production of inhibitory substances, promotion of localized immune responses, or alteration of the luminal environment (Weese, 2002a). These bacteria may also provide benefit to the host animal through production of vitamins, enzymes, and volatile fatty acids (VFAs), which may provide nutritional value, aid digestion, and benefit gastrointestinal health. Microbial viability and concentration within commercial human and veterinary products has been questioned (Canganella et al., 1997; Weese, 2002b), as well as the applicability of cultured bacterial organisms to specific host animals (Weese et al., 2004).

Attempts to determine colonization capacity of a human strain organism (*Lactobacillus rhamnosus* strain GG) in horses found low colonization in adults, even at a very high dose, and consistent colonization in foals with administration over 5 days (Weese et al., 2003). An equine-specific organism, *Lactobacillus pentosus* WE7, was identified as having good inhibitory activity against enteric pathogens and colonization ability (Weese et al., 2004). However, it induced clinical disease and diarrhea when specifically used as a probiotic agent in neonatal foals (Weese and Rousseau, 2005).

Administration of *Lactobacillus acidophilus* to cecally cannulated geldings had minimal effects on pH, bacterial populations, and volatile fatty acids with the exception of reduced butyrate production (Booth et al., 2001). Although fecal lactate concentrations were higher in treated foals, supplementing a commercial product of mixed lactobacillus bacteria had no effect on foals fed either a starch- or fiber-based diet at weaning (Swanson et al., 2003). In a double-blind study using two commercial probiotic products administered for 7 days following colic surgery, no effect was seen on *Salmonella* shedding, prevalence of diarrhea, duration of antibiotic therapy, or length of hospitalization (Parraga et al., 1997). In contrast, Ward et al. (2004) found a marked reduction in *Salmonella* shedding in hospitalized horses without gastrointestinal disease administered a probiotic agent compared to a placebo. Concerns about safety and utility and limited number of clinical studies in horses require further evaluation of probiotic products.

Enzymes

Enzymes of various sorts have been added to livestock diets to facilitate digestion of ingested feed (Officer, 2000). In ruminant animals, cellulases, hemicellulases, or other cell wall carbohydrate enzymes have been applied to improve dietary fiber digestibility. Similarly, various carbohydrases (pentosanases and β-gluconases) and proteases have been used in poultry to improve feed energy availability and animal performance. In poultry and pigs, phytase has been successfully used to improve dietary phosphorus availability from plant sources (NRC, 1998; Augspurger and Baker, 2004). Phytate phosphorus accounts for a significant amount of total phosphorus in cereal grains and wheat byproducts (Eeckhout and De Paepe, 1994). In horses, potential exists for the use of phytase and various cell wall carbohydrate enzymes in improving net availability of dietary phosphorus and fiber, respectively.

Fibrolytic enzymes in horse diets could improve energy availability from low-quality grass forages. Cellulase added to a concentrate (330 g/d) fed with ad libitum timothy hay forage resulted in no improvement in fiber digestibility in mature Arabian geldings (O'Connor et al., 2005). Microbial xylanase and cellulase were administered orally at the time of feeding to eight yearling geldings (341 kg mean BW) receiving Coastal Bermudagrass (fed at 1.5 percent of BW) and provided sufficient supplements to meet recommended energy and protein needs (Hainze et al., 2003). Four dietary supplements in this study consisted of alfalfa cubes, whole oats, sweet feed (corn, oats, molasses, soybean meal), or pelleted concentrate (wheat midds, corn, dehydrated alfalfa). All horses received all four dietary treatments with and without enzymes. Modest increases ($P < 0.1$) in dry matter (DM), neutral detergent fiber (NDF), acid detergent fiber (ADF), and hemicellulose digestibility were found in diets supplemented with oats or sweet feed and enzymes. In contrast, DM, NDF, and ADF digestibility slightly declined ($P < 0.1$) for diets supplemented with alfalfa and enzymes. Alfalfa contains minimal xylans compared to the other supplements and efficacy of dietary fibrolytic enzymes is dependent upon matching feedstuff carbohydrate content to the enzymes supplied (Officer, 2000). Additionally, applicability of acid insoluble ash methodology as an internal marker for estimating cell wall digestibility of alfalfa is questioned, as it does not contain significant amounts of silica compared to grass forages (Van Soest, 1994).

Four studies from different laboratories evaluated the application of phytase in equine diets and the impact on dietary phosphorus availability (Morris-Stoker et al., 2001; Patterson et al., 2002; van Doorn et al., 2004; Hainze et al., 2004). In all studies, true total tract dietary phosphorus digestibility was not improved, and only van Doorn et al. (2004) showed increased phytate phosphorus digestibility with added phytase (see discussion in Chapter 5). This is in contrast to results observed in pigs and poultry. Although phytase source and range of activity was similar across studies, variation in amount of phytate phosphorus supplied or dietary calcium content may account for observed poor responses of dietary phytase. Further research is required to adequately assess applicability of enzymes to facilitate nutrient availability from the equine diet.

Herbs and Botanicals

Many herbs are generally recognized as safe (GRAS) and are used in foods as seasoning and flavoring agents. Although in whole form, herbs and other botanicals contain some nutritive value (fiber, vitamins, minerals), their typical inclusion rate does not contribute appreciably to dietary nutrient content. However, a number of herbs and botanicals contain alkaloids and other phytochemicals that may or may not be safe when fed to the horse. Although many herbs and botanicals are used for various health or medicinal effects in humans, dietary use of herbs or botanicals with the intention of preventing or treating a disease or altering body structure, function, or performance defines the supplement as a drug, thus requiring regulatory evaluation. Data supporting such efficacy of use and safety in the horse are not available, and discussion of potential applications beyond nutritional value is not within the scope of this report. Given the paucity of research data about herbs pertaining directly to horses and the hazards of extrapolating from other species, any claims about the benefits of herbs must be viewed cautiously.

Of greater concern are safety issues for herbs and botanicals that might be incorporated into horse feed or supplemented by an owner. Acute and chronic toxicity data for various herbal compounds in horses are not well documented and extrapolation of data from other species may not be valid in many cases. Garlic is one of the most popular herbs used for medicinal purposes and perceived to be natural and safe. Garlic is considered GRAS as a flavoring agent in feed, but has potential to cause oxidative damage when consumed in greater quantities in a variety of species. Horses consuming freeze-dried garlic received greater than 0.2 mg/kg BW in two daily meals showed oxidative damage to red blood cells evidenced by increasing Heinz body anemia over time of exposure (Pearson et al., 2005). Horses showed improved hematologic parameters 4–5 weeks following removal of garlic supplementation. In this study horses voluntarily consumed a toxic dose (0.25 g/kg BW twice daily) of freeze-dried garlic for 71 days.

Additional concerns with phytochemicals in herbs and botanicals relate to potential interactions with administered pharmacologic agents and positive drug residue violations in show and performance horses. Herb compound interactions with conventional pharmacologic agents may potentially enhance, diminish, or induce a novel response to drug or herb. A number of human dietary supplements containing compounds with either sedative or stimulating effects on the central nervous system could result in residue violations (Short et al., 1998). Though few reports have been published documenting adverse effects of herbs and botanicals in horses, potential risks extrapolated from reports in other species have been reviewed for horses (Poppenga, 2001).

Joint Supplements

Products containing glucosamine, chondroitin sulfate, or a combination, and possibly including manganese ascorbate, are one of the most common feed additives fed to horses. Products may contain various forms of glucosamine (hydrochloride or sulfate) or substances that may provide a glucosamine source. The main impetus for use of these supplements is the perception that they are "chondroprotective," supplying "building blocks" for articular cartilage and potentially effective in delaying, stabilizing, or even repairing osteoarthritis lesions (Neil et al., 2005). Any such claim would fit the regulatory definition of a drug, thus requiring extensive documentation of safety and efficacy by the FDA. At present (2005), no dietary product containing these substances has received FDA approval for such intended purposes. However, an injectable drug product containing one form of a glycosaminoglycan is approved for use in horses to treat osteoarthritis (reviewed by McIlwraith, 2004).

Glucosamine is an amino monosaccharide that can be synthesized in the body from other dietary constituents and, thereby, not considered an essential nutrient in the diet. Further metabolic modification of glucosamine generates intermediate substrates for chondrocytes and synoviocytes to synthesize various glycosaminoglycan (GAG) compounds including hyaluronan, keratan sulfate, and chondroitin sulfate (Neil et al., 2005). Chondroitin sulfate is a GAG consisting of alternating disaccharide subunits of glucuronic acid and N-acetylgalactosamine. Chondroitin sulfate is a large polymer and has hydrophilic properties that impart compressive resistance to articular cartilage. Glycosaminoglycan components are structural components of synovial fluid (hyaluronan) and articular cartilage matrix (chondroitin sulfate) and provide protective and nutritive functions to the joints. The premise for the inclusion of glucosamine, chondroitin sulfate, or their combination in the diet is to augment endogenous synthesis and reduce catabolic joint degradation (reviewed by McIlwraith, 2004; Neil et al., 2005).

A number of in vitro studies have examined the effect of glucosamine and chondroitin sulfate, either individually or combined, on the catabolic response of cartilage explants for a number of species, including the horse. There is some in vitro evidence that glucosamine and chondroitin sulfate limit GAG degradation and enhance GAG synthesis in cartilage explants incubated with lipopolysaccharide (LPS) or preconditioned with interleukin-1, the end result being an increase in total GAG content when compared to placebo-treated explants (Fenton et al., 2000; Orth et al., 2002; Dechant et al., 2005). Using in vitro bovine articular cartilage explants, glucosamine also inhibited the release of nitric oxide and prostaglandin E2 from explants incubated with LPS, suggesting it may exert anti-inflammatory effects (Chan et al., 2005). Collectively, the results of these in vitro studies suggest that glucosamine and chondroitin sulfate could be beneficial to articular cartilage metabolism by preventing GAG degradation, enhancing GAG synthesis, or both. However, these data cannot be taken as proof of efficacy by oral supplementation in the treatment or prevention of osteoarthritis in horses.

Quantitative aspects of oral glucosamine and chondroitin sulfate administration bioavailability are debated. Of concern is whether target tissue (synovial fluid or articular cartilage) concentrations, consistent with in vitro studies, of such compounds can be achieved following oral dosing. Oral bioavailabilies of glucosamine and chondroitin sulfate have been determined in rats, dogs, and humans, but few studies have been completed in horses. Mean oral bioavailability of low molecular weight chondroitin sulfate (8-kDa and 16.9-kDa forms, 3 g each) in horses was 32 and 22 percent, respectively, and these values were not different (Du et al., 2004). However, oral bioavailability of glucosamine HCl (single dose of 125 mg/kg BW) was lower in horses at 2.5 percent, much lower than values reported for the dog (Du et al., 2004). Low bioavailability might be due to poor intestinal absorption, extensive first pass metabolism, or some combination. This single oral dose in horses was 5- to 10-fold higher than typical recommended levels (9 g) and needed to achieve concentrations within sensitivity of methods used. Glucosamine concentrations were not detectable when 9 g were administered orally (Du et al., 2004). In another horse study, after nasogastric administration of 20 mg/kg BW glucosamine HCl, bioavailability was determined to be 5.9 percent (Laverty et al., 2005). Maximum serum and synovial fluid glucosamine concentrations were 5.8 ± 1.7 µM and 0.3–0.7 µM, respectively, with glucosamine still detectable in synovial fluid up to 12 hours after dosing (Laverty et al., 2005). Corresponding peak serum and synovial fluid concentrations after intravenous administration of the same dose were 288 ± 53 µM and 250 µM. The glucosamine concentration achieved in synovial fluid after oral administration was markedly lower when compared to concentrations used in the previously described in vitro studies. Multiple dosing studies of glucosamine or chondroitin sulfate in horses have not been reported.

The number of in vivo studies performed in horses to examine efficacy of glucosamine, chondroitin sulfate, or their combination for the treatment of joint disease are limited. Two clinical studies evaluated utility of oral glucosamine and chondroitin sulfate supplementation using a population of horses diagnosed with degenerative joint (Hanson et al., 1997) or navicular (Hanson et al., 2001) disease. Both studies showed improvement in lameness evaluation, but neither study included negative controls (nonlame) horses for comparison, placebo group (1 study), nor blinding of investigators to treatment (1 study). An experimentally controlled study in healthy horses (n = 12) and healthy horses with chemically induced joint disease found no improvement in supplemented horses (White et al., 1994). A second study using healthy horses (n = 15) and healthy horses with chemically induced arthritis compared response of oral (2.5 g/d for 30 d) or intramuscular (600 mg/d for 5 days) chondroitin sulfate (25 kDa) to nonsupplemented horses (Videla and Guerrerro, 1998). Orally treated horses showed some improvements in measured lameness markers compared to untreated horses, but not for all parameters. Both of these studies also had flaws in experimental design (McIlwraith, 2004). Thus, there is a need for appropriately designed clinical trials to truly determine utility of oral joint supplements. Long-term studies also are needed to address the efficacy of these agents for the prevention of osteoarthritis, which appears to be the basis for widespread use of oral joint supplements in horses.

Beyond issues of oral availability, variability in product content and quality, as well as safety, are all potential problems with nutritional supplements that need to be considered. Studies of oral chondroprotective products intended for human or animal use have demonstrated that few consistently meet label claims of guaranteed analysis (Adebowale et al., 2000; Russell et al., 2002). In one study of equine products, actual composition in comparison to label claims ranged from 63–112 percent for five glucosamine products and 22–155 percent for five chondroitin sulfate products

(Ramey et al., 2002). Most of the published clinical studies have used a single product form of glucosamine and chondroitin sulfate, and extrapolation of these results to other products containing different chemical forms or concentrations of GAGs or chondroitin sulfate cannot be inferred. Short-term safety of glucosamine and chondroitin sulfate has been evaluated in horses (Kirker-Head and Kirker-Head, 2001). Healthy horses (n = 6) were administered a commercial product at 5 times its recommended dose (daily total: 18 g glucosamine HCl, 6 g chondroitin sulfate, and 160 mg manganese ascorbate) for 34 days. Although significant differences were found over the course of the study for some hematologic values, all hematologic, serum chemistry, and synovial fluid parameters remained within normal reference ranges. Definitive, long-term safety studies have not been reported for horses or other species.

Other compounds characterized to have "chondroprotective" effects include green-lipped mussel (*Perna canaliculus*) extract and methylsulfonylmethane (MSM). Extract of green-lipped mussel consists of various GAG compounds, omega-3 fatty acids, and other substances believed to provide anti-inflammatory activity and may show potential benefit in managing osteoarthritis, though clinical responses have been equivocal (Cobb and Ernst, 2005). Methylsulfonylmethane is intended as a source of bioavailable sulfur. Sulfur is a component of many compounds associated with joint structure and function. Studies evaluating a potential chondroprotective effect of MSM in horses have not been reported.

Medicinal Compounds

Antimicrobial agents, primarily antibacterial (antibiotic) compounds, can be naturally or synthetically derived. Antibiotics have been included in livestock feeds for three main purposes: disease treatment, disease prevention, or performance enhancers (CAST, 1981; NRC, 1999). In some species, low-level incorporation (subtherapeutic) has been shown to promote growth rate, improve feed utilization, reduce morbidity and mortality, and improve reproductive function. Higher antimicrobial levels (therapeutic) are administered to prevent or treat infectious disease conditions (NRC, 1999).

Regulatory control of medicinal compounds is maintained by the FDA to address concerns about animal safety, drug residues in foods, and microbial drug resistance. Extensive scientific evaluation and controlled studies must be completed to show safety (animal and residue concerns) and efficacy before a therapeutic drug can be included into feed. If approved, strict guidelines are defined for target species, drug incorporation rate into feed, and specific time periods for the drug to be removed from the feed before animals can enter the human food chain.

Horses can respond to feed-based antimicrobials similar to other livestock species. It must be emphasized that for most world jurisdictions, no antibiotic agent, including chlortetracycline, is approved for use as a growth promotant in horses. Quarter horse weanlings (n = 8) fed chlortetracycline (27.5 mg/kg total diet) over a 112-day feeding period showed greater ($P < 0.10$) average daily gain (0.97 vs. 0.87 kg/d) and height gain (11.2 vs. 9.1 cm) compared to non-supplemented controls (DuBose and Sigler, 1991). Currently (2005), no antibiotics and only two anthelmintics (dewormers) are approved for inclusion in horse feeds (21 CFR §558; AAFCO, 2005). Pyrantel tartrate (21 CFR §558.485) can be fed continuously as a top dress or mixed grain supplement to horses at 1.2 mg/kg BW for the prevention of intestinal helminthes (large and small stronglyes, pinworms, and ascarids). Febendazole (21 CFR §558.258) can be fed at either 5 or 10 mg/kg BW for one treatment to control large and small strongyles and pinworms or ascarids, respectively, with repeat dosing at 6- to 8-week intervals. Neither compound can be fed to horses intended for food. Specific feed regulations for any given country must be reviewed to ascertain legal status for food additive use.

Of greater concern with horses is the potential for feed-based toxicity from a number of antimicrobial agents approved for use in other livestock species, but errantly fed to horses (Hall, 2001). Colitis and diarrhea have been reported in horses fed feeds contaminated with lincomycin (Raisbeck and Osweiler, 1981) and tetracycline (Keir et al., 1999), as well as others (Hall, 2001; Larsen, 1997). Although the mechanism is unknown, antibiotics are believed to impart their toxic effect on horses by altering cecal and colonic microbial populations allowing proliferation of pathogenic bacteria (Larsen, 1997; Hall, 2001).

Ionophores are a special class of feed-based antibiotic agents commonly used in poultry and ruminant diets to control coccidia parasites and promote feed efficiency and growth (Russell and Strobel, 1989). Currently approved ionophore compounds for some livestock species (primarily ruminants) include lasalocid, maduramycin, monensin sodium, narasin, salinomycin, and virginiamycin (21 CFR §558; AAFCO, 2005). Potential for ionophore agents to induce toxicosis varies by compound and target species, with horses being more sensitive compared to other livestock species. Ionophore toxicity cases in horses have been reported for monensin (Matsuoka, 1976; Bila et al., 2001; Peek et al., 2004), lasalocid (Hanson et al., 1981), and salinomycin (Rollinson et al., 1987; Nel et al., 1988; Nicpon et al., 1997).

In contrast to other ionophore agents, virginiamycin has been administered at subtherapeutic levels to manipulate hindgut microbial populations in horses fed high-grain diets (Rowe et al., 1994; Johnson et al., 1998). Standardbred horses (496 kg BW) fed high-grain diets (8 kg/d) supplemented with 0, 4, or 8 g/kg grain of virginiamycin showed lower blood d-lactate concentration, higher ($P < 0.05$) fecal pH, and lower ($P < 0.001$) lameness incidence when consuming either dose of virginiamycin (Rowe et al., 1994). In an in vitro model using equine cecal contents, virginiamycin inhibited overgrowth of lactic acid-producing gram positive bacteria and production of vasoactive amine compounds associated with grain overload and altered colonic fermentation (Bailey et al., 2002). Although some positive effects might be realized, use of virginiamycin or any other ionophore agent in horses is not recommended because of their potential toxicity in horses. Virginiamycin is not available in most countries as a feed additive due to its antibiotic properties. In the limited jurisdictions where legally permitted, virginiamycin may only be fed when under the direct supervision of a veterinarian.

Oligosaccharides

Oligosaccharides are a diverse group of complex polysaccharides containing various sugar moieties resistant to hydrolysis by mammalian digestive enzymes, but are readily fermentable by enteric bacteria. Dietary supplementation of oligosaccharides in various species has been suggested to promote nonpathogenic colonic bacterial growth and maintain colonic health (Roberfroid, 1997; Flickinger et al., 2003). Since the intended purpose of dietary oligosaccharide supplementation is to stimulate bacterial growth, it had previously been characterized as "prebiotic" (Roberfroid, 1997). Specific mode of activity in promoting colonic health is dependent upon the constituent sugar moiety of the oligosaccharide. Fructooligosaccharides (FOS) are naturally occurring short to medium chains of fructose residues linked with β 2-1 glycosides bonds. Bacterial species such as *Bifidobacteria* are capable of hydrolyzing these β-glycosidic bonds, using FOS as a potential energy source to support bacterial growth (Campbell et al., 1997). Fermentation production of VFAs is believed to decrease intestinal pH adversely altering the environment for pathogenic bacteria. Alternatively, FOS-stimulated bacterial growth may lead to competitive exclusion of pathogenic bacteria. Fructooligosaccharide (T60.105) has tentative status as a feed ingredient (AAFCO, 2005).

Oligosaccharides of mannose are also believed to reduce adverse affects of pathogenic bacteria by inhibiting their adherence to enterocytes by mannose-specific lectins, as shown in human cell culture (Ofek and Beachey, 1978) and poultry models (Oyofo et al., 1989a,b). Saturating the gut environment with dietary mannose supplementation can reduce the probability of bacterial attachment to epithelial cell membrane mannose moieties. Glucomannans may also play a protective role in preventing absorption of mycotoxins in horses (Raymond et al., 2003, 2005).

Limited studies have addressed potential benefits of oligosaccharide supplements for horses. Yearling Quarter horses (n = 9; 401 kg mean BW) supplemented with FOS at three levels (0, 8, 24 g/d) in a 3 × 3 Latin square study design showed a linear dose effect of lower fecal pH and increased short-chain VFA concentrations, consistent with increased bacterial fermentation (Berg et al., 2005). Fecal *E. coli* population was reduced in the 8-g treatment, with no difference between 0- and 24-g treatment groups. Other bacteria were not different across treatment groups. Foals drenched with 10-g arabinogalatan, another fermentable oligosaccharide complex, for the first 14 days of life had less days with high fecal scores (diarrhea) and therapeutic treatments compared to placebo-drenched foals (Werner et al., 2001). No differences were seen between foal groups on serum immunoglobulin concentrations or hematology parameters over a 30-day period from birth.

Pregnant Thoroughbred and Quarter horse mares (n = 6 per group) were fed 0 or 10 g mannose oligosaccharide supplement from 56 days prior to foaling through 84 days of lactation (Ott, 2002). Supplementation had no effect on mare BW, body condition, or immunologic parameters measured. Foal blood immunoglobulin A, G, and M, concentrations were not influenced by supplementation, though foals from supplemented mares had higher blood immunoglobulin M concentration on the day of birth. Although unexplained, foals from supplemented mares had lower birth weights and maintained lower body weight throughout the duration of the study. Foals from unsupplemented mares experienced more cases of diarrhea requiring treatment (5/6 control vs. 0/5 supplemented, P = 0.02). Diarrhea cases were defined as only those severe enough to justify therapy, suggesting normal foal heat diarrhea was not confounding study results. It could not be ascertained whether the observed protective effect against foal diarrhea was a result of indirect (mare) or direct (foal) consumption of the supplement. Benage et al. (2005) did not find any effect of mannan oligosaccharide on immunity, measured as white blood cell counts or antibody titers, in young, mature, or aged horses. Based on these limited number, mostly preliminary studies, evidence is not supportive of a perceived role of immune system stimulation from feeding oligosaccharides; however, their role in reducing risk of intestinal disease in the horse should be further explored.

Omega-3 Fatty Acids

Linoleic acid (C18:2, n-6) and α-linolenic acid (C18:3, n-3) are considered essential fatty acids for most species. A minimum requirement for linoleic acid in horses was defined as 0.5 percent of DM (see Chapter 3); however, no specific requirement has been defined for α-linolenic acid. Potential health effects of supplementing omega-3 fatty acids are related to antagonistic biologic responses to eicosanoid mediators derived from cyclooxygenase or lipooxygenase from membrane-derived omega-3 fatty acids compared to similar metabolites from omega-6 fatty acids (Miles and Calder, 1998; Calder, 2001). In general, omega-3 derived eicosanoid mediators have antagonistic properties to omega-6 derived mediators. Collectively, data from studies where omega-3 fatty acid-enriched diets were fed to horses (see Chapter 3, Health Effects of Dietary (n-3) vs. (n-6) Fatty Acids) show promotion of anti-inflammatory mediators for various inflammatory cell types similar to what is observed in other species (Henry et al., 1991; Morris et al., 1991; Hansen et al., 2002; Hall et al., 2004a,b). Based on their anti-inflammatory properties, several potential health benefits from supplementing omega-3 fats to horses have been proposed (McCann and Carrick, 1998). Practical application suggests inflammatory mediated disease processes, such as recurrent airway obstruction (heaves) or fly-bite hypersensitivity, might possibly be mitigated with omega-3 fatty acid supplementation; however, few clinical trials have been completed to support this contention.

Two studies using a similar double-blinded, cross-over experimental design tested potential mediation of allergic skin reactions to *Culicoides* spp. with omega-3 fat supplementation in hypersensitive horses (Friberg and Logas, 1999; O'Neill et al., 2002). Calculated daily intake of α-linolenic acid in the two studies was between 108 and 110 g α-linolenic acid from linseed. This intake was consistent with a suggested dose extrapolated from human studies, but not substantiated for the horse (McCann and Carrick, 1998). Friberg and Logas (1999) found no quantifiable effect of oil source (linseed [n-3] vs. corn [n-6]) on improvement in dermatologic lesion size (quantified by digital imaging) or pruritic behavior (timed observations) exhibited by the horses. Interestingly, these findings are in contrast to participating horse owners' perceptions (study was double blind) where 12 of 16 owners believed supplementation with linseed oil reduced pruritis in their horse compared to 1 of 16 with corn oil supplementation.

In a separate study, mean skin reaction area (mm^2) to an intradermal injection of *Culicoides* spp. extract was smaller ($P = 0.02$) in horses supplemented with 0.45 kg flaxseed compared to 0.45 kg wheat bran after 42 days of supplementation (O'Neill et al., 2002). However, fatty acid profiles from skin biopsy samples did not show expected changes in omega-3 or omega-6 fatty acids reflective of supplementation. Neither of these studies included negative control horses (nonsensitized to *Culicoides* spp.) for comparison. Also, both studies used shorter supplementation periods (6 weeks) compared to other horse studies (8–12 weeks) monitoring fatty acid composition and inflammatory cell responses to different fat sources (Henry et al., 1991; Morris et al., 1991; Hansen et al., 2002; Hall et al., 2004a,b). Although measured changes in biochemical mediators of inflammation in response to dietary fatty sources (n-3 vs. n-6) are persuasive, further research is needed to determine if such changes have potential in mediating inflammatory disease processes in horses and an appropriate therapeutic dose.

Organic Trace Minerals

Inorganic trace mineral sources, principally oxide, sulfate, chloride, and carbonate forms of a specific mineral ion, have been primary sources of dietary mineral supplementation. Metal ion availability from these inorganic sources is variable. Generally, oxide and sulfate forms have the lowest and highest availability, respectively (Ammerman et al., 1995). Concerns about availability have prompted interest in use of organic trace mineral sources. On a relative availability scale, organic mineral forms are equal to or modestly greater in mineral bioavailability compared to inorganic sulfate sources across most species (Ammerman et al., 1995). Reviews of organic mineral supplementation studies in cattle (Spears, 1996) and swine (Jondreville and Revy, 2002) note the mechanism accounting for improved bioavailability of organic minerals is unknown and tremendous variability exists among sources.

Jondreville and Revy (2002) suggested a lack of clear evidence in swine feeding studies supporting greater mineral availability from organic sources compared to inorganic forms. In contrast, Spears (1996) noted improved animal performance in a number of ruminant studies, but whether the response was truly due to organic mineral source or additional dietary mineral intake was undetermined. Prevailing perceptions suggest greater metal absorptive efficiency via cotransportation across the intestinal mucosa, but evidence is lacking. A preponderance of data using rat intestinal loop models suggest no difference in absorptive efficiency between metals from inorganic or organic forms (Hill et al., 1987; Hempe and Cousins, 1989; Beutler et al., 1998). Organic mineral forms may protect the metal ion from microbial alteration in the rumen environment thus accounting for the differential response to organic mineral supplementation observed in swine and ruminant studies.

Organic mineral sources are not equivalent and encompass a wide spectrum of metal-ligand structures. Potential ligands include one or more amino acids, proteins of varying size, polysaccharides, or propionate. Feed ingredient definitions for various organic mineral products have been designated, as shown in Table 9-1 (AAFCO, 2005). Mineral availability from an organic source is dependent upon the type of bonding (ionic or covalent) between metal and ligand, ligand size, and how each are influenced by pH (Hynes and Kelly, 1995). Weaker metal-ligand bonds (ionic) and small ligand size result in a less stable molecule, whereas strong bonds (covalent) and large ligand size result in greater stability, but also create availability concerns (Hynes and Kelly, 1995).

Eight studies from five laboratories have compared organic and inorganic mineral sources supplemented to horses. Study designs varied in organic mineral source (proteinates, n = 5 vs. amino acid chelates, n = 3); partial (45–80 percent, n = 4) or complete (n = 4) replacement of inorganic mineral sources; animal age (weanlings, n = 1; yearlings, n = 3; adult, n = 4); and evaluation criteria. With the exception of the Ott and Asquith (1994) study, where mineral supplementation was at or slightly below (copper only) NRC (1989) recommendations, all other studies supplemented trace minerals in excess of NRC (1989) recommendations,

TABLE 9-1 AAFCO Feed Ingredient Definitions for Organic Mineral Products

Product	Feed Ingredient Number	Description
Metal amino acid complex	57.150	Product resulting from complexing of a soluble metal salt with amino acid(s). Declared as a specific metal amino acid complex ("Zinc, amino acid complex")
Metal (specific amino acid) complex	57.151	Product resulting from complexing a soluble metal salt with a specific amino acid. Declared as a specific metal, specific amino acid complex ("Zinc lysine complex")
Metal amino acid chelate	57.142	Product resulting from the reaction of a metal ion from a stable metal salt with amino acids with a mole ratio of one metal to one to three moles of amino acids to form coordinate covalent bonds and heterocyclic ring(s). Declared as a specific metal amino acid chelate ("Manganese amino acid chelate")
Metal polysaccharide complex	57.29	Product resulting from complexing of a soluble salt with a polysaccharide solution. Declared as specific metal complex ("Copper polysaccharide complex")
Metal proteinate	57.23	Product resulting from chelation of a soluble salt (mineral) with amino acids and/or partially hydrolyzed protein. Declared as specific metal proteinate ("Copper proteinate")
Metal propionate	57.160	Product resulting from a reaction of a metal salt with propionic acid. Declared as a specific metal propionate ("Zinc propionate")
Selenium yeast	T57.163	Dried nonviable yeast cultivated in a selenium-supplemented fermentation allowing selenium to be incorporated into cellular organic material

ranging from 30 to 80 percent increase to nearly four times the recommendations. Most studies stated the higher rate of supplementation was consistent with current industry feeding standards.

Using weanlings (n = 12) and 100 percent replacement of inorganic mineral sources with amino acid chelate sources, no effects of organic compared to inorganic minerals were found on hoof growth, hardness, or tensile strength (Siciliano et al., 2003a). However, improved ($P < 0.01$) immunologic response, measured as higher total immunoglobulin and mean IgM concentrations, to porcine red blood cell injection was observed in organic mineral supplemented weanlings (Siciliano et al., 2003b). In yearlings (n = 15), hoof growth, but not strength, was increased ($P = 0.02$) and hip height gain was greater ($P = 0.02$) when fed proteinated minerals compared to similar concentrations from inorganic mineral sources (Ott and Johnson, 2001). No effects of trace mineral source (inorganic vs. proteinated) on bone density or mineral content were observed (Ott and Johnson, 2001; Baker et al., 2003). Improved copper digestibility and availability and greater average daily copper and zinc balance were reported in yearlings fed proteinated mineral sources (45 percent replacement of inorganic amounts) compared to inorganic sources (Miller et al., 2003). These data are difficult to interpret as they are confounded by altered trace mineral regulation as a result of experimental animals experiencing an infectious disease during the study. Yearlings fed specific amino acid chelates (100 percent replacement) or inorganic trace mineral sources at similar levels (4 × NRC recommendations) showed no difference in growth or trace mineral digestibility and balance (Naile et al., 2005).

Studies were completed with mature and miniature horses fed either proteinate or specific amino acid chelate organic trace mineral sources. Organic sources were fed at either 45–50 or 100 percent of the inorganic supplementation rate and dietary mineral content ranged from slightly below to four times NRC (1989) recommendations. No effects of trace mineral source were found in hoof growth characteristics (Siciliano et al., 2001a), liver mineral content (Siciliano et al., 2001b), or trace mineral digestibility and retention (Wagner et al., 2005; Baker et al., 2005). Pregnant mares fed either proteinated (50–80 percent replacement) or inorganic trace mineral sources at or slightly below NRC (1989) recommendations showed no effects of mineral source on mare trace mineral status, weight gain, or subsequent reproductive efficiency (Ott and Asquith, 1994). Growth rate and bone mineral content were not different between foals born to organic or inorganic mineral-supplemented mares.

Collectively, all studies comparing organic to inorganic sources of trace minerals suggested minimal to no difference in biologic utilization or animal performance, consistent with results from swine studies. In fact, some studies reported improved responses to inorganic compared to organic mineral sources (Siciliano et al., 2003a; Baker et al., 2005). However, age and rate of supplementation effects on trace mineral metabolism need to be further evaluated. Results from studies using weanling and yearling horses tended to show more positive responses from organic mineral sources (Ott and Johnson, 2001; Siciliano et al., 2003b; Miller et al., 2003). Further study is needed to find a proper balance between sufficient dietary mineral supplementation in support of productive animals and minimizing manure mineral content and environmental load all within an economically viable system.

In 2004, the FDA permitted use of selenium (Se) yeast in horse feed at a rate not to exceed 0.3 ppm of added selenium in the total diet (21 CFR §573.920(h); FDA, 2004). Selenium yeast (T57.163) contains selenomethione and selenocysteine, organic forms of selenium quite different from those previously described. In contrast to organic chelates and complexes where the metal ion is bound to one or more ligands, selenium in seleno-amino acids has replaced the sulfur atom within methionine and cysteine amino acids. Seleno-amino acid absorption is believed to occur via amino acid transporters (Weiss, 2003), thus improving bioavailability over inorganic forms (selenite, selenate) as evidenced in ruminants by improved muscle, milk, and liver selenium content compared to inorganic sources (Ullrey et al., 1977; Ammerman et al., 1980; Pehrson et al., 1999; Gunter et al., 2003). Direct incorporation of seleno-amino acids into body and milk proteins accounts for these observations and may also account for a lesser response in selenium-dependent glutathione peroxidase activity in comparing inorganic selenium and selenium yeast sources (Weiss, 2003).

Few studies have addressed selenium yeast supplementation in the horse. Pagan et al. (1999) reported improved digestibility and retention comparing selenium yeast (2.75 mg/d Se) to sodium selenite (2.9 mg/d Se) sources. However, no differences in serum or whole blood selenium concentrations were observed. Similar to observations in cattle, late pregnant mares supplemented with selenium yeast (3 mg/d Se) compared to inorganic sources (selenite at 1 or 3 mg/d Se) had greater colostrum and milk selenium concentration and gave birth to foals with improved selenium status (Janicki, 2001). Further study is needed to determine the potential physiologic effects improved selenium status might have on animal health and performance.

Yeast Culture or Extract

A number of yeast products are defined as feed ingredients by AAFCO (2005), including dried yeast (active or nonfermentative), yeast culture, and yeast extract (tentative ingredient designation). Most yeast products are derived from *Saccharomyces* spp. cultures, primarily *S. cerevisiae*, or *Aspergillus oryzae*. Active dry yeast must contain a minimum of 15 billion live yeast cells per gram. Yeast culture is a dried product containing viable yeast cells and the culture media on which the yeast was grown. Yeast extract is a dried or concentrated product of cell contents from mechanically ruptured *Saccharomyces cerevisiae* cells. Dried yeast must contain a minimum of 40 percent crude protein, whereas yeast extract contains a minimum of 9 percent crude protein.

Various yeast products are used in ruminant diets. Yeast additives are believed to either directly facilitate fiber digestion and dry matter intake (active cultures) or contain metabolites or compounds having stimulatory properties on bacterial growth to facilitate fermentation and animal performance (active or nonfermentative). Robinson (2002) reviewed results from 71 published scientific reports on the use of yeast additives in ruminant diets. Modest changes were reported for measures of rumen fermentation, dry matter intake, growth, and feed efficiency with live yeast cultures. Most pronounced was the observed increase in rumen bacterial numbers, both cellulolytic (20 percent) and noncellulolytic (95 percent) bacteria. Across yeast products (active and nonfermentative culture), modest improvement (1–3 percent) in dry matter intake and milk production were observed. Consistency across studies on observed effects suggests the greatest impact of yeast products are through promotion of bacterial growth and independent of live yeast in the fermentation system (Robinson, 2002).

Similar to published ruminant studies with yeast additives, live yeast cultures were most studied in horses. A majority of these studies evaluated the potential of enhanced fermentation and fiber or nutrient digestibility in the horse. Unlike observed effects in ruminant studies, supplementation of yeast in horse diets tended to show some beneficial effects on fermentation, but results were equivocal across studies. Using an in vitro fermentation system with cecally fistulated inocula, time to reach 50 percent gas production was shortened with the addition of 10 mg live yeast culture added to hay, beet pulp, or 50:50 mix of hay and beet pulp as substrate, suggesting augmentation of fermentation (McLean et al., 1997). Yeast supplementation induced minimal (Moore et al., 1994) to no increase (Medina et al., 2002; Lattimer et al., 2005) in cecal or colonic bacterial colonies. Similarly, yeast supplementation effects on fermentation products were minimal to none (McDaniel et al., 1993; Krusic et al., 2001), though when feeding low-forage or high-starch diets, yeast supplementation altered fermentation to increase (9–14 percent) acetate (Medina et al., 2002; Lattimer et al., 2005) and lower (36 percent, high-starch diet) lactate (Medina et al., 2002). Studies measuring cecal and colonic pH found minimal effect of supplemental yeast (McDaniel et al., 1993; Krusic et al., 2001; Lattimer et al., 2005). In contrast, more alkaline cecal pH with yeast supplementation was observed when feeding higher concentrate diets (Moore and Newman, 1993). Yeast supplementation attenuated the decline in cecal pH at 4 hours post-feeding when low-forage (43 percent: Hall and Miller-Auwerda, 2005) or high-starch (3.4 g/kg BW: Medina et al., 2002) diets were fed to horses.

No improvement in nutrient apparent digestibility was reported for mature horses (Webb et al., 1985; Hall et al., 1990), but others have reported improved digestibility for one or more nutrients when horses were fed yeast cultures. Improvement in DM, NDF, and ADF digestibility with yeast supplementation was reported for mature (Pagan, 1990; Glade, 1991a) and yearling (Glade and Sist, 1988) horses, whereas another study using yearlings found only hemicellulose digestibility improved with yeast supplementation (Glade and Biesik, 1986). Improved nitrogen digestibility (5.1–8.8 percent) and retention with yeast supplementation was the most consistently reported response to yeast supplementation (Godbee, 1983; Glade and Biesik, 1986; Glade and Sist, 1988; Glade, 1991a,c; Switzer et al., 2003). Two studies reported improved digestibility with one or more minerals. Improved magnesium digestibility was reported by Pagan (1990) and Switzer et al. (2003) with yeast supplementation. Phosphorus digestibility, independent of source, was increased 22.3 percent across two different whole collection trials feeding forage (66 percent) and sweet feed (Pagan, 1990).

Studies evaluating the role of yeast on horse performance are limited. Improved weight gain, height, and feed efficiency were observed in weanling horses supplemented with live yeast culture (Mason, 1983; Glade and Sist, 1990). No growth advantage was observed with yearlings (Bennett et al., 1991). Pregnant mares fed 20 g live yeast 4 weeks prior to foaling had improved digestibility of dietary energy, protein, and fiber resulting in greater milk production and improved foal growth (Glade, 1991a,b,c). Administration of 10×10^9 live *Saccharomyces boulardii* every 12 hours for 14 days resulted in reduced severity and duration of clinical signs associated with enterocolitis compared to placebo-treated horses (Desrochers et al., 2005). In this study, supplemented yeast could be found in feces during supplementation, but there was no ability to determine colonization potential of the colon.

Variation in observed responses between studies may be attributed to differences in the amount of yeast supplement being fed, composition and treatment diet interaction, and diet adaptation time. Results across the studies would suggest some potential benefits to feeding yeast when high-starch or low-fiber diets are being fed (Medina et al., 2002; Hall and Miller-Auwerda, 2005). Improvements in nutrient digestibility, especially nitrogen, are suggested, but the exact mechanism for this response is not evident. Constant feeding of yeast may have greater potential for mediating an effect as compared to sporadic supplementation. Given most reported studies used live yeast cultures, application of non-fermentative yeast cultures requires further study in horses.

REFERENCES

AAFCO (Association of American Feed Control Officials, Inc.). 2005. Official Publication. Oxford, IN: Association of American Feed Control Officials.

Adebowale, A. O., D. S. Cox, Z. Liang, and N. D. Eddington. 2000. Analysis of glucosamine and chondroitin sulfate content in marketed products and the Caco-2 permeability of chondroitin sulfate raw materials. J. Am. Nutraceutical Assoc. 3:37–44.

Ammerman, C. B., H. L. Chapman, G. W. Bouwman, J. P. Fontenot, C. P. Bagley, and A. L. Moxon. 1980. Effect of supplemental selenium for beef cows on the performance and tissue selenium concentrations of cows and suckling calves. J. Anim. Sci. 51:1381–1386.

Ammerman, C. B., D. H. Baker, and A. J. Lewis. 1995. Bioavailability of Nutrients for Animals. San Diego: Academic Press.

Art, T., N. Kirschvink, N. Smith, and P. Lekeux. 1999. Indices of oxidative stress in blood and pulmonary epithelium lining fluid in horses suffering from recurrent airway obstruction. Equine Vet. J. 31:397–401.

Augspurger, N. R., and D. H. Baker. 2004. High dietary phytase levels maximize phytate phosphorus utilization but do not affect protein utilization in chicks fed phosphorus- or amino acid-deficient diets. J. Anim. Sci. 82:1100–1107.

Bailey, S. R., A. Rycroft, and J. Elliott. 2002. Production of amines in equine cecal contents in an in vitro model of carbohydrate overload. J. Anim. Sci. 80:2656–2662.

Baker, L. A., T. Kearney-Moss, J. L. Pipkin, R. C. Bachman, J. T. Haliburton, and G. O. Vneklasen. 2003. The effect of supplemental inorganic and organic sources of copper and zinc on bone metabolism in exercised yearling geldings. Pp. 100–105 in Proc. 18th Equine Nutr. Physiol. Soc. Symp., East Lansing, MI.

Baker, L. A., M. R. Wrigley, J. L. Pipkin, J. T. Haliburton, and R. C. Bachman. 2005. Digestibility and retention of inorganic and organic sources of copper and zinc in mature horses. Pp. 162–167 in Proc. 19th Equine Sci. Soc., Tucson, AZ.

Balogh, N., T. Gaal, P. S. Ribiczeyne, and A. Petri. 2001. Biochemical and antioxidant changes in plasma and erythrocytes of pentathlon horses before and after exercise. Vet. Clin. Path. 30:214–218.

Benage, M. C., L. A. Baker, G. H. Loneragan, J. L. Pipkin, and J. C. Haliburton. 2005. The effect of mannan oligosaccharide on horse herd health. Pp. 17–22 in Proc. 19th Equine Sci. Soc., Tucson, AZ.

Bennett, K., J. C. Loch, E. M. Lattimer, and E. M. Green. 1991. Effect of yeast culture supplementation on weight gains, skeletal growth and bone density of third metacarpal in yearling Quarter horses. J. Anim. Sci. 69(Suppl. 1):324 (Abstr.).

Berg, E. L., C. J. Fu, J. H. Porter, and M. S. Kerley. 2005. Fructooligosaccharide supplementation in the yearling horse: effects on fecal pH, microbial content, and volatile fatty acid concentrations. J. Anim. Sci. 83:1549–1553.

Beutler, K. T., O. Pankewycz, and D. L. Brautigan. 1998. Equivalent uptake of organic and inorganic zinc by monkey kidney fibroblasts, human intestinal epithelial cells, or perfused mouse intestine. Biol. Trace Elem. Res. 61:19–31.

Bila, C. G., C. L. Perreira, and E. Gruys. 2001. Accidental monensin toxicosis in horses in Mozambique. J. S. Afr. Vet Assoc. 72:163–164.

Booth, J. A., P. A. Miller-Auwerda, and M. A. Rasmussen. 2001. The effect of a microbial supplement (Horse-Bac) containing *Lactobacillus acidophilus* on the microbial and chemical composition of the cecum in the sedentary horse. Pp. 183–185 in Proc. 17th Equine Nutr. Physiol. Soc. Symp., Lexington, KY.

Boothe, D. M. 1997. Nutraceuticals in veterinary medicine. Part I. Definitions and regulations. Comp. Cont. Educ. Pract. Vet. 19:1248–1255.

Boothe, D. M. 1998. Nutraceuticals in veterinary medicine. Part II. Safety and efficacy. Comp. Cont. Educ. Pract. Vet. 20:15–21.

Bowery, V. W., D. Mohr, J. Cleary, and R. Stocker. 1995. Prevention of tocopherol-mediated peroxidation in ubiquinol-10-free human low density lipoprotein. J. Biol. Chem. 270:5756–5763.

Bursian, S. J., R. J. Aulerich, J. K. Cameron, N. K. Ames, and B. A. Steficek. 1992. Efficacy of hydrated sodium calcium aluminosilicate in reducing the toxicity of dietary zearalenone to mink. J. Appl. Toxicol. 12:85–90.

Burton, J. H., D. J. Price, and J. Aspinal. 1983. The effect of feed flavour and feed consumption in horses. P. 27 in Proc. 8th Equine Nutr. Physiol. Soc. Symp., Lexington, KY.

Calder P. C. 2001. Omega-3 polyunsaturated fatty acids, inflammation and immunity. World Rev. Nutr. Diet 88:109–116.

Campbell, J. M., G. C. Fahey, Jr., and B. W. Wolf. 1997. Selected indigestible oligosaccharides affect large bowel mass, cecal and fecal short-chain fatty acids, pH and microflora in rats. J. Nutr. 127:130–136.

Canganella, F., S. Paganini, M. Ovidi, A. M. Vettraino, L. Bevilacqua, S. Massa, and L. D. Trovatelli. 1997. A microbiological investigation on probiotic pharmaceutical products used for human health. Microbiol. Res. 152:171–179.

Carr, A. C., and B. Frei. 1999. Toward a new recommended dietary allowance for vitamin C based on antioxidant and health effects in humans. Am. J. Clin. Nutr. 69:1086–1107.

CAST (Council for Agricultural Science and Technology). 1981. Antibiotics in Animal Feeds. Report No. 88. Ames, IA.

CAST. 2003. Mycotoxins: Risks in Plants, Animal and Human Systems. Report No. 139. Ames, IA.

Chan, P. S., J. P. Caron, G. J. Rosa, and M. W. Orth. 2005. Glucosamine and chondroitin sulfate regulate gene expression and synthesis of nitric oxide and prostaglandin E(2) in articular cartilage explants. Osteoarth. Cart. 13:387–394.

Chestnut, A. B., P. D. Anderson, M. A. Cochran, H. A. Fribourg, and K. D. Gwinn. 1992. Effects of hydrated sodium calcium aluminosilicate on fescue toxicosis and mineral absorption. J. Anim. Sci. 70:2838–2846.

Chung, T. K., J. W. Erdman, Jr., and D. H. Baker. 1990. Hydrated sodium calcium aluminosilicate: effects on zinc, manganese, vitamin A and riboflavin utilization. Poult. Sci. 69:1364–1370.

Church, D. C., and R. O. Kellems. 1998. Feed additives. Pp. 177–190 in Livestock Feeds & Feeding, 4th ed. Upper Saddle River, NJ: Prentice Hall.

Clark, S. F. 2002. The biochemistry of antioxidants revisited. Nutr. Clin. Pract. 17:5–17.

Cobb, C. S., and E. Ernst. 2005. Systematic review of a marine nutraceutical supplement in clinical trials for arthritis: the effectiveness of the New Zealand green-lipped mussel Perna canaliculus. Clin. Rheumatol. 12:1–10.

Deaton, C. M., and D. J. Marlin. 2003. Exercise-associated oxidative stress. Clin. Techniques Equine Pract. 2(3):278–291.

Deaton, C. M., D. J. Marlin, C. A. Roberts, N. Smith, P. A. Harris, F. J. Kelly, and R. C. Schroter. 2002. Antioxidant supplementation and pulmonary function at rest and exercise. Equine Vet. J. Suppl. 34:58–65.

Deaton, C. M., D. J. Marlin, N. C. Smith, C. A. Roberts, P. A. Harris, F. J. Kelly, and R. C. Schroter. 2003. Pulmonary bioavailability of ascorbic acid in an ascorbate-synthesizing species, the horse. Free Radical Res. 37:461–467.

Deaton, C. M., D. J. Marlin, N. C. Smith, P. A. Harris, C. A. Roberts, R. C. Schroter, and F. J. Kelley. 2004a. Pulmonary epithelial lining fluid and plasma ascorbic acid concentrations in horses affected by recurrent airway obstruction. Am. J. Vet. Res. 65:80–87.

Deaton, C. M., D. J. Marlin, N. C. Smith, P. A. Harris, R. C. Schroter, and F. J. Kelly. 2004b. Antioxidant supplementation in horses affected by recurrent airway obstruction. J. Nutr. 134(8S):2065S–2067S.

Deaton, C. M., D. J. Marlin, N. C. Smith, P. A. Harris, M. P. Dagleigh, R. C. Schroter, and F. J. Kelly. 2005a. Effect of acute airway inflammation on the pulmonary antioxidant status. Exp. Lung Res. 31:653–670.

Deaton, C. M., D. J. Marlin, N. C. Smith, C. A. Roberts, P. A. Harris, R. C. Schroter, and F. J. Kelly. 2005b. Antioxidant and inflammatory responses of healthy horses and horses affected by recurrent airway obstruction to inhaled ozone. Equine Vet. J. 37:243–249.

Dechant, J. E., G. M. Baxter, D. D. Frisbie, G. W. Trotter, and C. W. McIlraith. 2005. Effects of glucosamine hydrochloride and chondroitin sulphate, alone or in combination, on normal and interleukin-1 conditioned equine articular cartilage explant metabolism. Equine Vet. J. 37:227–231.

de Moffarts, B., N. Kirshvink, T. Art, J. Pincemail, C. Michaux, K. Cayeux, and J. O. Defraigne. 2004. Impact of training and exercise intensity on blood antioxidant markers in healthy Standardbred horses. Equine Comp. Ex. Physiol. 1:211–220.

de Moffarts, B., N. Kirschvink, T. Art, J. Pincemail, and P. Lekeux. 2005. Effect of oral antioxidant supplementation on blood antioxidant status in trained Thoroughbred horses. Vet. J. 169:65–74.

Desrochers, A. M., B. A. Dolente, M. F. Roy, R. Boston, and S. Carlisle. 2005. Efficacy of Saccharomyces boulardii for treatment of horses with acute enterocolitis. J. Am. Vet. Med. Assoc. 227:954–959.

Dimock, A. N., P. D. Siciliano, and C. W. McIlwraith. 2000. Evidence supporting an increased presence of reactive oxygen species in the diseased equine joint. Equine Vet. J. 32:439–443.

Du, J., N. White, and N. D. Eddington. 2004. The bioavailability and pharmacokinetics of glucosamine hydrochloride and chondroitin sulfate after oral and intravenous single dose administration in the horse. Biopharm. Drug. Dispos. 25:109–116.

DuBose, L. E., and D. H. Sigler. 1991. Effect of antibiotic feed additive on growth of weanling horses. Pp. 65–66 in Proc. 12th Equine Nutr. Physiol. Soc. Symp., Calgary, Alberta.

Dulphy, J. P., W. Martin-Rosset, H. Dubroeucq, J. M. Ballet, A. Detour, and M. Jailler. 1997. Compared feeding patterns in ad libitum intake of dry forages by horses and sheep. Livest. Prod. Sci. 52:49–56.

Dzanis, D. A. 1991. Safety of ethoxyquin in dog foods. J. Nutr. 121(Suppl.):S163–S164.

Eeckhout, W., and M. De Paepe. 1994. Total phosphorus, phytate-phosphorus and phytase activity in plant feedstuffs. Anim. Feed Sci. Technol. 47:19–29.

Evans, P., and B. Halliwell. 2001. Micronutrients: oxidant/antioxidant status. Br. J. Nutr. 85:S67–S74.

FDA (U.S. Food and Drug Administration). 1992. Food additives. Food and Drug Administration/International Food Information Council brochure. Available at http://www.cfsan.fda.gov/~lrd/foodaddi.html. Accessed April 1, 2006.

FDA. 1996. Inapplicability of the Dietary Supplement Health and Education Act to animal products. Fed. Reg. 61:17706–17708.

FDA. 1997. FDA Requests That Ethoxyquin Levels Be Reduced in Dog Foods. Available at http://www.fda.gov/cvm/CVM_Updates/dogethox.html. Accessed August 9, 2006.

FDA. 1998. Regulating animal foods with drug claims. Guide 1240.3605, Center for Veterinary Medicine Program Policy and Procedures Manual. Available at http://www.fda.gov/cvm/Policy_Procedures/3605.pdf Accessed August 2, 2006.

FDA. 2004. FDA Permits the Use of Selenium Yeast in Horse Feed. CVM Update on U.S. Food and Drug Administration website (October 14, 2004). Available at http://www.fda.gov/cvm/CVM_Updates/selenium horse.htm. Accessed September 29, 2005.

Fenton J. I., K. A. Chlebek-Brown, T. A. Peters, J. P. Caron, and M. W. Orth. 2000. Effects of glucosamine derivatives on equine articular degradation in explant culture. Osteoarth. Cart. 8:444–451.

Flickinger, E. A., J. Van Loo, and G. C. Fahey, Jr. 2003. Nutritional responses to the presence of inulin and oligofructose in the diets of domesticated animals: a review. Crit. Rev. Food Sci. Nutr. 43:19–60.

Frei, B. 1994. Reactive oxygen species and antioxidant vitamins: mechanisms of action. Am. J. Med. 97(3, Suppl 1):5S–13S.

Friberg, C. A., and D. Logas. 1999. Treatment of Culicoides hypersensitive horses with high-dose n-3 fatty acids: a double-blinded crossover study. Vet. Dermatol. 10:117–122.

Glade, M. J. 1991a. Dietary yeast culture supplementation of mare during late gestation and early lactation: effects on dietary nutrient digestibilities and fecal nitrogen partitioning. J. Equine Vet. Sci. 11:10–16.

Glade, M. J. 1991b. Dietary yeast culture supplementation of mares during late gestation and early lactation: effects on milk production, milk composition, weight gain and linear growth of nursing foals. J. Equine Vet. Sci. 11:89–95.

Glade, M. J. 1991c. Effects of dietary yeast culture supplementation of lactating mares on the digestibility and retention of the nutrients delivered to nursing foals via milk. J. Equine Vet. Sci. 11:323–329.

Glade, M. J., and L. M. Biesik. 1986. Enhanced nitrogen retention in yearling horses supplemented with yeast culture. J. Anim. Sci. 62:1635–1640.

Glade, M. J., and M. D. Sist. 1988. Dietary yeast culture supplementation enhances urea recycling in the equine large intestine. Nutr. Rep. Int. 37:11–17.

Glade, M. J., and M. D. Sist. 1990. Supplemental yeast culture alters the plasma amino acid profiles of nursing and weanling horses. J. Equine Vet. Sci. 10:369–379.

Godbee, R. 1983. Effect of yeast culture on apparent digestibility and nitrogen balance in horses. Res. Bull., Clemson Univ., Clemson, SC.

Goodwin, D., H. P. B. Davidson, and P. Harris. 2005a. Sensory varieties in concentrate diets for stabled horses: effects on behavior and selection. Appl. Anim. Behav. Sci. 90:337–349.

Goodwin, D., H. P. B. Davidson, and P. Harris. 2005b. Selection and acceptance of flavours in concentrate diets for stabled horses. Applied Anim. Behav. Sci. 95:223–232.

Gross, K. L., R. Bollinger, P. Thawnghmung, and G. F. Collings. 1994. Effect of three different preservative systems on the stability of extruded dog food subjected to ambient and high temperature storage. J. Nutr. 124(Suppl.):S2638–S2642.

Gunter, S. A., P. A. Beck, and J. M. Phillips. 2003. Effects of supplementary selenium source on the performance and blood measurements in beef cows and their calves. J. Anim. Sci. 81:856–864.

Hainze, M. T. M., R. B. Muntifering, and C. A. McCall. 2003. Fiber digestion in horses fed typical diets with and without exogenous fibrolytic enzymes. J. Equine Vet. Sci. 23:111–115.

Hainze, M. T. M., R. B. Muntifering, C. W. Wood, C. A. McCall, and B. H. Wood. 2004. Faecal phosphorus excretion from horses fed typical diets with and without added phytase. Anim. Feed Sci. Technol. 117(3-4): 265–279.

Hall, J. A., R. J. Van Saun, and R. C. Wander. 2004a. Dietary (n-3) fatty acids from Menhaden fish oil alter plasma fatty acids and leukotriene B synthesis in healthy horses. J. Vet. Intern. Med. 18:871–879.

Hall, J. A., R. J. Van Saun, S. J. Tornquist, J. L. Gradin, E. R. Pearson, and R. C. Wander. 2004b. Effect of type of dietary polyunsaturated fatty acid supplement (corn oil or fish oil) on immune responses in healthy horses. J. Vet. Intern. Med. 18:880–886.

Hall, J. O. 2001. Toxic feed constituents in the horse. Vet. Clin. North Am. Equine Pract. 17:479–489.

Hall, M. M., and P. A. Miller-Auwerda. 2005. Effect of *Saccharomyces cerevisiae* pelleted product on cecal pH in the equine hindgut. Pp. 45–46 in Proc. 19th Equine Sci. Soc., Tucson, AZ.

Hall, R. P., S. G. Jackson, J. P. Baker, and S. R. Lowry. 1990. Influences of yeast culture supplementation on ration digestion by horses. J. Equine Vet. Sci. 10:130–134.

Hansen, R. A., C. J. Savage, K. Reidlinger, J. L. Traub-Dargatz, G. K. Ogilvie, D. Mitchell, and M. J. Fettman. 2002. Effects of dietary flaxseed oil supplementation on equine plasma fatty acid concentrations and whole blood platelet aggregation. J. Vet. Intern. Med. 16:457–463.

Hanson, L. J., H. G. Eisenbeis, and S. V. Givens. 1981. Toxic effects of lasalocid in horses. Am. J. Vet. Res. 42:456–461.

Hanson, R. R., L. R. Smalley, G. K. Huff, S. White, and T. A. Hammad. 1997. Oral treatment with a glucosamine-chondroitin sulfate compound for degenerative joint disease in horses: 25 cases. Equine Pract. 19:16–22.

Hanson, R. R., W. R. Brawner, M. A. Blaik, T. A. Hammad, S. A. Kincaid, and D. G. Pugh. 2001. Oral treatment with a nutraceutical (Cosequin®) for ameliorating signs of navicular syndrome in horses. Vet. Therap. 2:148–159.

Hargreaves, B. J., D. S. Kronfeld, J. N. Waldron, M. A. Lopes, L. S. Gay, K. E. Saker, W. L. Cooper, D. J. Skan, and P. A. Harris. 2002. Antioxidant status and muscle cell leakage during endurance exercise. Equine Vet. J. Suppl. 34:116–121.

Hempe, J. M., and R. J. Cousins. 1989. Effect of EDTA and zinc-methionine complex on zinc absorption by rat intestine. J. Nutr. 119:1179–1187.

Henry, M. M., J. N. Moore, and J. K. Fischer. 1991. Influence of an ω-3 fatty acid-enriched ration on in vivo responses of horses to endotoxin. Am. J. Vet. Res. 52:523–527.

Hill, D. A., E. R. Peo, and A. J. Lewis. 1987. Influence of picolinic acid on the uptake of ^{65}Zn-amino acid complexes by the everted rat gut. J. Anim. Sci. 65:173–178.

Hintz, H. F., H. F. Schryver, J. Mallette, and K. Houpt. 1989. Factors affecting rate of grain intake by horses. Equine Pract. 11:35–42.

Hoestenbach, R. D. 2004. Nutraceuticals—a regulatory paradox? Pp. 147–151 in Proc. Conf. on Equine Nutrition Research, May 22–23, Texas A&M University, College Station.

Hoffman, R. M., K. L. Morgan, A. Phillips, J. E. Dinger, S. A. Zinn, and C. Faustman. 2001. Dietary vitamin E and ascorbic acid influence nutritional status of exercising polo ponies. Pp. 129–130 in Proc. 17th Equine Nutr. Physiol. Soc. Symp., Lexington, KY.

Houpt, K.A. 1990. Ingestive behavior. Vet. Clin. North Am. Equine Pract. 6:319–337.

Huang, S. W., E. N. Frankel, and J. B. German. 1994. Antioxidant activity of α- and γ-tocopherols in bulk oils and in oil-in-water emulsions. J. Agric. Food Chem. 42:2108–2114.

Huang, S. W., E. N. Frankel, and J. B. German. 1995. Effects of individual tocopherols and tocopherol mixtures on the oxidative stability of corn oil triglycerides. J. Agric. Food Chem. 43:2345–2350.

Hynes, M. J., and M. P. Kelly. 1995. Metal ions, chelates and proteinates. Pp. 233–248 in 1995 Alltech Symposium., St. Paul, MN.

Janicki, K. M. 2001. The effect of dietary selenium source and level on broodmares and their foals. M.S. Thesis. University of Kentucky, Lexington.

Johnson, K. G., J. Tyrrell, J. B. Rowe, and D. W. Pethick. 1998. Behavioural changes in stabled horses given nontherapeutic levels of virginiamycin. Equine Vet. J. 30:139–143.

Jondreville, C., and P. S. Revy. 2002. An update on use of organic minerals in swine nutrition. Pp. 1–16 in Proc. Eastern Nutr. Conf., Montreal, Quebec.

Kantor, M. 1996. Food additives. Maryland Cooperative Extension Circular, FS-632, University of Maryland, College Park, MD.

Keir, A. A., H. R. Stampfli, and J. Crawford. 1999. Outbreak of acute colitis on a horse farm associated with tetracycline-contaminated sweet feed. Can. Vet. J. 40:718–720.

Kiessling, K. H, and H. Pettersson. 1991. Chemical preservatives. Pp. 765–775 in Mycotoxins and Animal Feeds, J. E. Smith and R. S. Henderson, eds. Boca Raton, FL: CRC Press.

Kirker-Head, C. A., and R. P. Kirker-Head. 2001. Safety of an oral chondroprotective agent in horses. Vet. Therap. 2:345–353.

Kirschvink, N., T. Art, B. de Moffarts, N. Smith, D. Marlin, C. Roberts, and P. Lekeux. 2002a. Relationship between markers of blood oxidant status and physiological variables in healthy and heaves-affected horses after exercise. Equine Vet. J. Suppl. 34:159–164.

Kirschvink, N., N. Smith, L. Fievez, V. Bougnet, T. Art, G. Degand, D. Marlin, C. Roberts, B. Genicot, P. Lindsey, and P. Lekeux. 2002b. Effect of chronic airway inflammation and exercise on pulmonary and systemic antioxidant status of healthy and heaves-affected horses. Equine Vet. J. 34:563–571.

Kirschvink, N., L. Fievez, V. Bougnet, T. Art, G. Degand, N. Smith, D. Marlin, C. Roberts, P. Harris, and P. Lekeux. 2002c. Effect of nutritional antioxidant supplementation on systemic and pulmonary antioxidant status, airway inflammation and lung function in heaves-affected horses. Equine Vet. J. 34:705–712.

Krusic, L., J. D. Pagan, J. Lorenz, and A. Pen. 2001. Influence of high carbohydrate and high fiber diet on cecum content of organic matter and volatile fatty acids. Pp. 425–434 in Proc. 17th Equine Nutr. Physiol. Soc. Symp., Lexington, KY.

Larsen, J. 1997. Acute colitis in adult horses: a review with emphasis on aetiology and pathogenesis. Vet. Quart. 19:72–80.

Lattimer, J. M., S. R. Cooper, D. W. Freeman, and D. A. Lalman. 2005. Effects of *Saccharomyces cerevisiae* on *in vitro* fermentation of a high concentrate or high fiber diet in horses. Pp. 168–173 in Proc. 19th Equine Sci. Soc., Tucson, AZ.

Laverty, S., J. D. Sandy, C. Celeste, P. Vachon, J. F. Marier, and A. H. K. Plaas. 2005. Synovial fluid levels and serum pharmacokinetics in a large animal model following treatment with oral glucosamine at clinically relevant doses. Arthrit. Rheumatol. 52:181–191.

Löscher, W., G. Jaeschke, and H. Keller. 1984. Pharmacokinetics of ascorbic acid in horses. Equine Vet. J. 16:59–65.

Marlin, D. J., K. Fenn, N. Smith, C. D. Deaton, C. A. Roberts, P. A. Harris, C. Dunster, and F. J. Kelly. 2002. Changes in circulatory antioxidant status in horses during prolonged exercise. J. Nutr. 132:1622S–1627S.

Mason, T. R. 1983. Effect of tall oil and yeast culture on growth rate of wild horses. Res. Bull., McNeese State University, Lake Charles, LA.

Matsuoka, T. 1976. Evaluation of monensin toxicity in the horse. J. Am. Vet. Med. Assoc. 169:1098–1100.

McCann, M. E., and J. B. Carrick. 1998. Potential uses of ω-3 fatty acids in equine diseases. Comp. Cont. Ed. Pract. Vet. 20:637–641.

McDaniel, A. L., S. A. Martin, J. S. McCann, and A. H. Parks. 1993. Effects of *Aspergillus oryzae* fermentation extract on *in vitro* equine cecal fermentation. J. Anim. Sci. 71:2164–2172.

McIlwraith, C. W. 2004. Licensed medications, "generic" medications, compounding, and nutraceuticals—What has been scientifically validated, where do we encounter scientific mistruth, and where are we legally? Pp. 459–475 in Proc. 50th Am. Assoc. Equine Pract., Denver, CO.

McLean, B. M. L., R. S. Lowman, M. K. Theodorou, and D. Cuddeford. 1997. The effects of YEA-SACC 1026 on the degradation of two fiber sources by caecal incola in vitro, measured using the pressure transducer technique. Pp. 45–46 in Proc. 15th Equine Nutr. Physiol. Soc. Symp., Ft. Worth, TX.

Medina, B., I. D. Girard, E. Jacotot, and V. Julliand. 2002. Effect of a preparation of *Saccharomyces cerevisiae* on microbial profiles and fermentation patterns in the large intestine of horses fed a high fiber or a high starch diet. J. Anim. Sci. 80:2600–2609.

Miles, E. A., and P. C. Calder. 1998. Modulation of immune function by dietary fatty acids. Proc. Nutr. Soc. 57:277–292.

Miller, E. D., L. A. Baker, J. L. Pipkin, R. C. Bachman, J. T. Haliburton, and G. O. Veneklasen. 2003. The effect of supplemental inorganic and organic forms of copper and zinc on digestibility in yearling geldings in training. Pp. 107–112 in Proc. 18th Equine Nutr. Physiol. Soc. Symp., East Lansing, MI.

Moore, B. E., and K. E. Newman. 1993. Influence of feeding yeast culture (Yea-Sacc) on cecum and colon pH of the equine. J. Anim. Sci. 71(Suppl. 1):261 (Abstr.).

Moore, B. E., K. E. Newman, P. Spring, and V. E. Chandler. 1994. The effect of yeast culture (YeaSacc1026) in microbial populations and digestion in the cecum and colon of the equine. J. Anim. Sci. 72(Suppl. 1):252 (Abstr.).

Morris, D. D., M. M. Henry, J. N. Moore, and J. K. Fischer. 1991. Effect of dietary α-linolenic acid on endotoxin-induced production of tumor necrosis factor by peritoneal macrophages in horses. Am. J. Vet. Res. 52:528–532.

Morris-Stoker, L. B., L. A. Baker, J. L. Pipkin, R. C. Bachman, and J. C. Haliburton. 2001. The effect of supplemental phytase on nutrient digestibility in mature horses. Pp. 48–52 in Proc. 17th Equine Nutr. Physiol. Soc. Symp., Lexington, KY.

Naile, T. L., S. R. Cooper, D. W. Freeman, and C. R. Krehbiel. 2005. Effects of trace mineral source on growth and mineral balance in yearling horses. Prof. Anim. Scientist 21:121–127.

Neil, K. M., J. P. Caron, and M. W. Orth. 2005. The role of glucosamine and chondroitin sulfate in treatment for and prevention of osteoarthritis in animals. J. Am. Vet. Med. Assoc. 226:1079–1088.

Nel, P. W., T. S. Kellerman, R. A. Schultz, N. van Aarde, J. A. W. Coetzer, A. T. Basson, N. Fourie, and J. J. van der Walt. 1988. Salinomycin poisoning in horses. J. S. Afr. Vet. Assoc. 59:103.

Nicpon, J., P. Czerw, O. Harps, and E. Deegen. 1997. Salinomycin poisoning in a Polish stud horse. Tierarztl. Prax. Ausg. G. Grosstiere Nutztiere 25:438–441.

NRC (National Research Council). 1987. Vitamin Tolerance of Animals. Washington, DC: National Academy Press.

NRC. 1989. Nutrient Requirements of Horses, 5th rev. ed. Washington, DC: National Academy Press.

NRC. 1998. Nutrient Requirements of Swine, 10th rev. ed. Washington, DC: National Academy Press.

NRC. 1999. The Use of Drugs in Food Animals: Benefits and Risks. Washington, DC: National Academy Press.

O'Connor, C. I., B. D. Nielsen, and R. Carpenter. 2005. Cellulase supplementation does not improve the digestibility of a high forage diet in horses. Pp. 192–198 in Proc. 19th Equine Sci. Soc., Tucson, AZ.

Ofek, I., and E. H. Beachey. 1978. Mannose binding and epithelial cell adherence of Escherichia coli. Infect. Immun. 22:247–254.

Officer, D. I. 2000. Feed enzymes. Pp. 405–426 in Farm Animal Metabolism and Nutrition, J. P. F. D'Mello, ed. Wallingford, UK: CABI Publishing.

Ohshima, T., V. V. Yankah, H. Ushio, and C. Kiozumi. 1998. Antioxidizing potentials of BHA, BHT, TBHQ, tocopherol, and oxygen absorber incorporated in a Ghanaian fermented fish product. Adv. Exp. Med. Biol. 434:181–188.

O'Neill, W., S. McKee, and A. F. Clarke. 2002. Flaxseed (*Linum usitatissimum*) supplementation associated with reduced skin test lesional area in horses with Culicoides hypersensitivity. Can. J. Vet. Res. 66:272–277.

Orth, M. W., T. L. Peters, and J. N. Hawkins. 2002. Inhibition of articular cartilage degradation by glucosamine-HCl and chondroitin sulphate. Equine Vet. J. Suppl. 34:224–229.

Ott, E. A. 2002. Use of mannan oligosaccharides in diets of mares and their suckling foals. Pp. 367–371 in Nutritional Biotechnology in the Feed and Food Industries, Proc. Alltech's 18th Annu. Symp., T. P. Lyons and K. A. Jacques, eds. Nottingham, UK: Nottingham University Press.

Ott, E. A., and R. L. Asquith. 1994. Trace mineral supplementation of broodmares. J. Equine Vet. Sci. 14:93–101.

Ott, E. A., and E. L. Johnson. 2001. Effect of trace mineral proteinates on growth and skeletal and hoof development in yearling horses. J. Equine Vet. Sci. 21:287–292.

Oyofo, B. A., R. E. Droleskey, J. O. Norman, H. H. Mollenhauer, R. L. Ziprin, D. E. Corrier, and J. R. DeLoach. 1989a. Inhibition by mannose of in vitro colonization of chicken small intestine by Salmonella typhimurium. Poult. Sci. 68:1351–1356.

Oyofo, B. A., J. R. DeLoach, D. E. Corrier, J. O. Norman, R. L. Ziprin, and H. H. Mollenhauer. 1989b. Prevention of Salmonella typhimurium colonization of broilers with d-mannose. Poult. Sci. 68:1357–1360.

Packer, L., E. H. Witt, and H. J. Tritschler. 1995. Alpha-lipoic acid as a biological antioxidant. Free Radic. Biol. Med. 19:227–250.

Pagan, J. D. 1990. Effect of yeast culture supplementation on nutrient digestibility in mature horses. J. Anim. Sci. 68(Suppl. 1):371 (Abstr.).

Pagan, J. D., P. Karnezos, M. A. P. Kennedy, T. Currier, and K. E. Hoekstra. 1999. Effect of selenium source on selenium digestibility and retention in exercised Thoroughbreds. Pp. 135–140 in Proc. 16th Equine Nutr. Physiol. Soc. Symp., Raleigh, NC.

Parraga, M. E., S. J. Spier, M. Thurmond, and D. Hirsh. 1997. A clinical trial of probiotic administration for prevention of *Salmonella* shedding in the postoperative period in horses with colic. J. Vet. Intern. Med. 11:36–41.

Patterson, D. P., S. R. Cooper, D. W. Freeman, and R. G. Teeter. 2002. Effects of varying levels of phytase supplementation on dry matter and phosphorus digestibility in horses fed a common textured ration. J. Equine Vet. Sci. 22:456–459.

Patterson, R., and L. G. Young. 1993. Efficacy of hydrated sodium calcium aluminosilicate, screening and dilution in reducing the effects of mold contaminated corn in pigs. Can. J. Anim. Sci. 73:616–624.

Pearson, W., H. J. Boermans, W. J. Gettger, B. W. McBride, and M. I. Lindinger. 2005. Association of maximum voluntary intake of freeze-dried garlic with Heinz body anemia in horses. Am. J. Vet. Res. 66:457–465.

Peek, S. F., F. D. Marques, J. Morgan, H. Steinberg, D. W. Zoromski, and S. McGuirk. 2004. Atypical acute monensin toxicosis and delayed cardiomyopathy in Belgian draft horses. J. Vet. Intern. Med. 18:761–764.

Pehrson, B., K. Ortman, N. Madjid, and U. Trafikowska. 1999. The influence of dietary selenium as selenium yeast or sodium selenite on the concentration of selenium in the milk of suckler cows and on the selenium status of their calves. J. Anim. Sci. 77:3371–3376.

Philips, T. D., L. F. Kubena, R. B. Harvey, D. R. Taylor, and N. D. Heidelbaugh. 1987. Mycotoxin hazards in agriculture: new approach to control. J. Am. Vet. Med. Assoc. 190:1617 (Abstr.).

Philips, T. D., L. F. Kubena, R. B. Harvey, D. R. Taylor, and N. D. Heidelbaugh. 1988. Hydrated sodium calcium aluminosilicate: a high affinity sorbent for aflatoxin. Poult. Sci. 67:243–247.

Pollack, G., and J. H. Burton. 1991. Feed flavors, diet palatability and parotid saliva secretion. Pp. 245–246 in Proc. 12th Equine Nutr. Physiol. Soc. Symp., Calgary, Alberta.

Poppenga, R. H. 2001. Risks associated with the use of herbs and other dietary supplements. Vet. Clin. North Am. Equine Pract. 17:455–477.

Raisbeck, M. F., and G. D. Osweiler. 1981. Lincomycin associated colitis in horses. J. Am. Vet. Med. Assoc. 179:362–363.

Ramey, D. W., N. Eddington, and E. Thonar. 2002. An analysis of glucosamine and chondroitin sulfate content in oral joint supplement products. J. Equine Vet. Sci. 22:125–127.

Randall, R. P., W. A. Schurg, and D. C. Church. 1978. Response of horses to sweet, salty, sour and bitter solutions. J. Anim. Sci. 47:51–55.

Raymond, S. L., T. K. Smith, and H. V. Swamy. 2003. Effects of feeding a blend of grains naturally contaminated with Fusarium mycotoxins on feed intake, serum chemistry, and hematology of horses, and the efficacy of a polymeric glucomannan mycotoxin adsorbent. J. Anim. Sci. 81:2123–2130.

Raymond, S. L., T. K. Smith, and H. V. Swamy. 2005. Effects of feeding a blend of grains naturally contaminated with Fusarium mycotoxins on feed intake, metabolism, and indices of athletic performance of exercised horses. J. Anim. Sci. 83:1267–1273.

Roberfroid, M. B. 1997. Health benefits of non-digestible oligosaccharides. Adv. Exp. Med. Biol. 427:211–219.

Robinson, P. H. 2002. Yeast products for growing and lactating dairy cattle: impacts on rumen fermentation and performance. Pp. 74–106 in Proc. XII International Program on Production of Meat and Milk in Hot Climates, L. Avendano, ed. Mexicali, Mexico: University of Baja California.

Rollinson, J. F., G. R. Taylor, and J. Chesney. 1987. Salinomycin poisoning in horses. Vet. Rec. 121:126–128.

Rowe, J. B., M. J. Lees, and D. W. Pethick. 1994. Prevention of acidosis and laminitis associated with grain feeding in horses. J. Nutr. 124(12 Suppl):2742S–2744S.

Russell, A. S., A. Aghazadeh-Habashi, and F. Jamali. 2002. Active ingredient consistency of commercially available glucosamine sulfate products. J. Rheumatol. 29:2407–2409.

Russell, J. B., and H. J. Strobel. 1989. Effect of ionophores on ruminal fermentation. Appl. Environ. Microbiol. 55:1–6.

Short, C. R., R. A. Sams, L. R. Soma, T. Tobin. 1998. The regulation of drugs and medicines in horse racing in the United States. The Association of Racing Commissions international uniform classification of foreign substances guidelines. J. Vet. Pharmacol. Ther. 21:144–153.

Siciliano, P. D., A. L. Parker, and L. M. Lawrence. 1997. Effect of dietary vitamin E supplementation on the integrity of skeletal muscle in exercised horses. J. Anim. Sci. 75:1553–1560.

Siciliano, P. D., K. D. Culley, and T. E. Engle. 2001a. Effect of trace mineral source (inorganic vs. organic) on hoof wall-growth rate, hardness, and tensile strength. Pp. 143–144 in Proc. 17th Equine Nutr. Physiol. Soc. Symp., Lexington, KY.

Siciliano, P. D., K. D. Culley, and T. E. Engle. 2001b. Effect of trace mineral source (inorganic vs. organic) on trace mineral status in horses. Pp. 419–420 in Proc. 17th Equine Nutr. Physiol. Soc. Symp., Lexington, KY.

Siciliano, P. D., T. E. Engle, and C. K. Swenson. 2003a. Effect of trace mineral source on hoof wall characteristics. Pp. 96–97 in Proc. 18th Equine Nutr. Physiol. Soc. Symp., East Lansing, MI.

Siciliano, P. D., T. E. Engle, and C. K. Swenson. 2003b. Effect of trace mineral source on humoral immune response. Pp. 269–270 in Proc. 18th Equine Nutr. Physiol. Soc. Symp., East Lansing, MI.

Snow, D. H., and M. Frigg. 1989. Oral administration of different formulations of ascorbic acid to the horse. J. Equine Vet. Sci. 9:30–33.

Snow, D. H., and M. Frigg. 1990. Bioavailability of ascorbic acid in horses. J. Vet. Pharmacol. Ther. 13:393–403.

Snow, D. H., S. P. Gash, and J. Cornelius. 1987. Oral administration of ascorbic acid to horses. Equine Vet. J. 19:520–523.

Spears, J. W. 1996. Organic trace minerals in ruminant nutrition. Anim. Feed Sci. Technol. 58:151–163.

Sumner, S. S., and J. D. Eifert. 2002. Risks and benefits of food additives. Pp. 27–42 in Food Additives, 2nd ed., A. L. Branen, R. M. Davidson, S. Salminen, and J. H. Thorngate, eds. New York: Marcel Dekker, Inc.

Swanson, C. A., R. M. Hoffman, D. S. Kronfeld, and P. A. Harris. 2003. Effects of diet and probiotic supplementation on stress during weaning in Thoroughbred foals. P. 243 in Proc. 18th Equine Nutr. Physiol. Soc. Symp., East Lansing, MI.

Switzer, S. T., L. A. Baker, J. L. Pipkin, R. C. Bachman, and J. C. Haliburton. 2003. The effect of yeast culture supplementation on nutrient digestibility in aged horses. Pp. 12–17 in Proc. 18th Equine Nutr. Physiol. Soc. Symp., East Lansing, MI.

Tsao, C. S., and M. Young. 1989. Effect of exogenous ascorbic acid intake on biosynthesis of ascorbic acid in mice. Life Sci. 45:1553–1557.

Ullrey, D. E., P. S. Brady, P. A. Whetter, P. K. Ku, and W. T. Magee. 1977. Selenium supplementation of diets for sheep and beef cattle. J. Anim. Sci. 45:559–565.

Van Doorn, D. A., H. Everts, H. Wouterse, and A. C. Beynen. 2004. The apparent digestibility of phytate phosphorus and the influence of supplemental phytase in horses. J. Anim. Sci. 82:1756–1763.

Van Soest, P. J. 1994. Nutritional Ecology of the Ruminant. Ithaca, NY: Cornell University Press.

Videla, D. I., and R. C. Guerrero. 1998. Effects of oral and intramuscular use of chondroitin sulfate in induced equine aseptic arthritis. J. Equine Vet. Sci. 18:548–555.

Wagner, E. L., G. D. Potter, E. M. Eller, P. G. Gibbs, and D. M. Hood. 2005. Absorption and retention of trace minerals in adult horses. Prof. Anim. Scientist 21:207–211.

Ward, M. P., C. A. Alinori, L. L. Couetil, L. T. Glickman, and C. C. Wu. 2004. A randomized clinical trial using probiotics to prevent *Salmonella* fecal shedding in hospitalized horses. J. Equine Vet. Sci. 24:242–247.

Webb, S. P., G. D. Potter, and K. J. Massey. 1985. Digestion of energy and protein by mature horses fed yeast culture. Pp. 64–67 in Proc. 5th Equine Nutr. Physiol. Soc. Symp., St. Louis, MO.

Weese, J. S. 2002a. Probiotics, prebiotics, and synbiotics. J. Equine Vet. Sci. 22:357–380.

Weese, J. S. 2002b. Microbial evaluation of commercial probiotics. J. Am. Vet. Med. Assoc. 220:794–797.

Weese, J. S., and J. Rousseau. 2005. Evaluation of *Lactobacillus pentosus* WE7 for prevention of diarrhea in neonatal foals. J. Am. Vet. Med. Assoc. 226:2031–2034.

Weese, J. S., M. E. Anderson, A. Lowe, and G. J. Monteith. 2003. Preliminary investigation of the probiotic potential of *Lactobacillus rhamnosus* strain GG in horses: fecal recovery following oral administration and safety. Can. Vet. J. 44:299–302.

Weese, J. S., M. E. Anderson, R. Penno, T. M. da Costa, L. Button, and K. C. Goth. 2004. Screening of the equine intestinal microflora for potential probiotic organisms. Equine Vet. J. 36:351–355.

Weiss, W. P. 2003. Selenium nutrition of dairy cows: comparing responses to organic and inorganic selenium forms. Pp. 333–343 in Nutritional Biotechnology in the Feed and Food Industries Proc. Alltech's 19th Ann. Symp., T. P. Lyons, and K. A. Jacques, eds. Nottingham, UK: Nottingham Univ. Press.

Werner, H. K., L. M. Lawrence, and T. Barnes. 2001. Effect of administration of an oral arabinogalactan supplement on mares and foals. Pp. 93–98 in Proc. 17th Equine Nutr. Physiol. Soc. Symp., Lexington, KY.

White, A., M. Estrada, K. Walker, P. Wisnia, G. Filgueira, F. Valdes, O. Araneda, C. Behn, and R. Martinez. 2001. Role of exercise and ascorbate on plasma antioxidant capacity in Thoroughbred race horses. Comp. Biochem. Physiol. A Mol. Integr. Physiol. 128:99–104.

White, G. W., E. W. Jones, J. Hamm, and T. Sanders. 1994. The efficacy of orally administered sulfated glycosaminoglycan in chemically induced equine synovitis and degenerative joint disease. J. Equine Vet. Sci. 14:350–353.

Williams, C. A. 2004. Studies show supplementation with antioxidants may reduce oxidative stress in the exercising horse. Feedstuffs 76(13):11–14.

Williams, C. A., R. M. Hoffman, D. S. Kronfeld, T. M. Hess, K. E. Saker, and P. A. Harris. 2002. Lipoic acid as an antioxidant in mature Thoroughbred geldings: a preliminary study. J. Nutr. 132:1628S–1631S.

Williams, C. A., D. S. Kronfeld, T. M. Hess, J. N. Waldron, K. E. Saker, R. M. Hoffman, and P. A. Harris. 2003. Oxidative stress in horses in three 80 km races. Pp. 47–52 in Proc. 18th Equine Nutr. Physiol. Soc. Symp., East Lansing, MI.

Williams, C. A., D. S. Kronfeld, T. M. Hess, K. E. Saker, and P. A. Harris. 2004a. Lipoic acid and vitamin E supplementation to horses diminishes endurance exercise induced oxidative stress, muscle enzyme leakage, and apoptosis. Pp. 105–119 in The Elite Race and Endurance Horse, A. Lindner, ed. Oslo, Norway: CESMAS.

Williams, C. A., D. S. Kronfeld, T. M. Hess, K. E. Saker, J. N. Waldron, K. M. Crandell, R. M. Hoffman, and P. A. Harris. 2004b. Antioxidant supplementation and subsequent oxidative stress of horses during an 80-km endurance race. J. Anim. Sci. 82:588–594.

10

Feed Analysis

GENERAL CONSIDERATIONS

Feed analysis is necessary to determine the nutrient content of the feeds used in horse diets. There are many kinds of laboratory analysis for feeds: chemical evaluation, in vitro digestion systems, and near infrared reflectance (NIR) methods. Analyses using wet chemistry are the most used, but they do not give a direct estimate of nutritive value. Feed analysis could be costly depending on the type of analysis requested. Ideally all feeds should be analyzed, particularly those nontraditional feeds or commercial mixed feeds for which table values are not available. Also, forage chemical composition varies with state of maturity, climate, season, soil type, and fertilization (Ralston, 1991). Feed analysis should be performed if there is a suspicion of nutritional problems based on clinical signs and poor animal performance. Accurate results depend on good sampling techniques, proper handling of the samples after collection, and good analytical procedures. The feed composition tables found in this publication represent average values, and variations in the composition of some of these feeds are expected as indicated above. When balancing feeds for horses, the most common nutrient concerns are water, energy, fiber, protein, calcium, and phosphorus. However, most laboratories will also provide analysis of other nutrients including vitamins, essential amino acids, fatty acids, microminerals, and sugars (total or single sugars) if needed. Other important dietary components for the horse, such as fructans, are not routinely analyzed by many laboratories because of the costs of the equipment required for the analysis and/or difficulties of the method. Chemical analytical techniques are always evolving, but most feed testing laboratories will use approved procedures recognized by organizations such as the National Forage Testing Association (NFTA), Association of Official Analytical Chemists (AOAC), American Association of Cereal Chemists (AACC), and American Oil Chemists Society (AOCS), among others. The selection of the laboratory is very important if good results are expected. Some laboratories are certified and/or participate in check-sample programs that ensure accuracy among participating laboratories. Accuracy of the analytical method and the chosen laboratory technique should be the focus when selecting laboratories.

ANALYSIS OF CARBOHYDRATES: FIBER

Analytical procedures for fiber are still under development despite a long history (DeVries et al., 1999). Fiber is a unique and complex nutritional entity often defined as the indigestible or slowly fermenting components of feeds. Chemically, fiber has been defined as a variable mixture of cellulose, hemicelluloses, some pectins, and lignin, plus indigestible protein and lipids (Mertens, 1992). In human nutrition, dietary fiber has been defined as the nondigestible carbohydrates and lignin that are intrinsic and intact in plants (NRC, 2000). Several authors have reviewed the methodologies to measure fiber in feeds including Van Soest et al. (1991) and Van Soest (1994), who described the advantages and limitations of the different analytical procedures for fiber. Most of the methods to measure fiber have been developed for the ruminant animal and for humans, but not for hindgut fermenters like horses. However, neither the ruminant nor the human system fits well with the digestive physiology and intermediary metabolism of the horse (Hoffman, 2004). Different protocols might be used to measure fiber content depending on the type of feed. Thus, the actual definition of fiber becomes method-dependent. Fiber can be determined as crude fiber (CF), total dietary fiber (TDF), neutral detergent fiber (NDF), and acid detergent fiber (ADF). Associated analyses include: neutral detergent insoluble nitrogen (NDIN), acid detergent insoluble nitrogen (ADIN), acid detergent lignin (ADL), or ADF Klason lignin. For further reading on forage fiber analysis, refer to Van Soest (1994), NRC (1996, 2000, 2001, 2003), and Mertens (1997, 2002).

Total Dietary Fiber

Total dietary fiber consists of the remnants of edible plant cells, polysaccharides, lignin, and associated substances resistant to digestion by the alimentary mammalian digestive system (Trowell, 1985). Included in TDF by definition are cellulose, hemicellulose, oligosaccharides (non-α-glucose polymers), lignin, pectins, mucilages, gums, waxes, cutin, and suberin, among others. Thus, TDF is relevant to most monogastric animals with hindgut fermentation (Van Soest et al., 1991). The TDF concept arose as a result of interest in fiber and human nutrition and is an analytical method recognized as an official method of the AOAC (method 991.43, 2002) and used extensively in human nutrition (Prosky et al., 1988). TDF has also been recognized as an official method by the AACC (1995a,b). The quantification of insoluble fibers by the Van Soest methods (NDF, ADF, ADL) is comparable to the insoluble fiber determined by the TDF method (Lee et al., 1992; Popovich et al., 1997). Soluble dietary fiber might be estimated by subtracting NDF from TDF (Baer et al., 1997) or by the AOAC method (991.43; AOAC, 2002). The analytical method for determining TDF recovers more fiber components than the NDF method but it does recover carbohydrates soluble in 78 to 80 percent ethanol, such as the fructooligosaccharides (NRC, 2000).

Neutral Detergent Fiber

The Van Soest detergent system (Van Soest et al., 1991) is the most popular method for measuring cell wall constituents in forages. The detergent system is not a method for isolating cell walls per se, but rather a method of partitioning forage dry matter (DM) into fractions based upon its bioavailability to ruminants (Van Soest, 1994). The original NDF method represents the percentage of cell wall material or plant structure in a feed, including cellulose, hemicellulose, and lignin as its major components (Van Soest and Wine, 1967; Goering and Van Soest, 1970). Sodium sulfite is used to remove contaminating nitrogen from NDF and was optional in the method described by Van Soest et al. (1991). However, Hintz et al. (1996) suggested that the use of sodium sulfite was crucial for the removal of contaminated nitrogen from heat-damaged feeds. Amylase-treated NDF (aNDF) is a modification of the original method and is used to minimize the contamination by starch in all feeds (Van Soest et al., 1991; Mertens, 2002). The aNDF method described by Mertens (2002) includes the use of amylase and sulfite and is applied for the determination of aNDF in forages, grains, grain byproduct feeds, oil seeds, oilseed meals, and mixed feeds. The NDF concentrations for dairy feeds in the NRC (2001) nutrient composition table were determined using amylase and sulfite. The aNDF method is the recommended method by the National Forage Testing Association (Undersander et al., 1993). The NDF method does not recover fructans, pectins, gums, mucilages, and β-glucans (Van Soest et al., 1991), which are resistant to mammalian digestive enzymes but rapidly fermented. In addition, the NDF fraction will not recover any hemicellulose that is soluble in neutral detergent.

Some feed laboratories use a filter-bag method commonly named the ANKOM system for analyzing forages including NDF, ADF, lignin, and in vitro dry matter digestibility (IVDMD) (Komarek, 1993; Komarek et al., 1994). The filter-bag system can produce results similar to the conventional methods with the advantage that the method is easier to use and safer than conventional methods (Vogel et al., 1999).

Acid Detergent Fiber

Acid detergent fiber (ADF) analyzed according to Van Soest and Wine (1967) is intended as a sample preparation for the determination of the sum of cellulose, lignin, ADIN, acid insoluble ash (AIA), and silica (Van Soest, 1994). ADF may not be a valid fiber fraction for nutritional use or for predicting digestibility (Van Soest, 1991). Hemicelluloses can be estimated by subtracting ADF from NDF (Robertson and Van Soest, 1981), but the accuracy of the estimations will depend on the sample (e.g., beet pulp, citrus pulp, etc.) and the botanical origin of the sample. To avoid errors, a sequential analysis for NDF and then ADF on the same sample is recommended (Bailey and Ulyatt, 1970).

Cell Wall Phenolics (Lignin)

The presence of phenolic compounds within the cell wall matrix limits the digestion of polysaccharides (Akin and Chesson, 1989). The cell wall phenolics consist primarily of lignin and phenolic acids chemically bound to lignin or to cell wall polysaccharides. True lignin appears to be a polymerized product of phenylpropanoid alcohols and ferulic and para-coumaric acids (Van Soest, 1994). The composition of lignin preparations varies according to the method of isolation. It is generally defined as the residue obtained by the Klason two-stage sulfuric acid hydrolysis method (Van Soest, 1994) or one of its many modifications. However, the potential presence of nonlignin components in the Klason residue has been a subject of criticism of the method (Van Soest, 1994). The ADL method includes both hydrolytic (sulfuric acid) and oxidative (potassium permanganate) procedures (Van Soest, 1965). Jung et al. (1997) reported that the Klason lignin method showed higher values than the ADL method for grasses (2 to 4 times higher) and up to 30 percent higher in legumes. However, both methods were equally correlated with digestibility of forages. ADL has been criticized for underestimating the lignin content of forages due to the ADF step of ADL, losing acid soluble lignin (Lowry et al., 1994).

Crude Fiber

Crude fiber is one of the components analyzed when performing the proximate analysis, the others being moisture, ash, crude protein, ether extract, and nitrogen-free extract (NFE). Henneberg and Stohmann of the Weende Experimental Station in Germany developed the "Proximate Analysis" or "Weende system" of feed analysis more than a century ago. For analyzing CF, samples are treated with dilute acid and then with alkali to mimic digestion of gastric secretions (Method 962.09; AOAC, 2002). The Weende CF procedure is still being used by regulatory agencies despite the errors in the determination of the structural and nonstructural carbohydrates. The most significant error of the Weende system is due to the solubilization and loss of part of the lignin, cellulose, and hemicellulose in the preparation of CF and its inclusion in the NFE (Van Soest, 1994). The Weende system is still being used in Europe for the evaluation of feeds for horses (Martin-Rosset et al., 1994; Gudmundsson, 1998).

ANALYSIS OF CAROBOHYDRATES: NONFIBER FRACTIONS

Nonfiber Carbohydrates (NFC)

The more readily digestible carbohydrates in animal feeds lack a satisfactory system of classification, particularly for the horse, but they constitute a major energy-yielding component of feeds. They comprise those carbohydrates not included in the cell wall matrix and not recovered in NDF as described for the ruminant system of analysis (Van Soest et al., 1991; Mertens, 1997; Hall and Van Horn, 2001; Hall, 2003). The NFC are calculated by difference: 100 − (protein + (NDF − NDICP) + fat + ash), where NDICP = neutral detergent insoluble crude protein, and include sugars, starches, fructans, galactans, pectins, β-glucans, and organic acids (Van Soest et al., 1991). Nonstarch polysaccharides (NSP, non-α-glucan polysaccharides) are broadly defined in human nutrition as the fiber in plant material that includes cellulose, hemicellulose, and pectic substances, without inclusion of nonfibrous entities (Englyst and Cummings, 1990). From an analytical perspective, the NSP component does not include lignin, which might present a limitation for horse diets although a filtration step of the residue after cell wall hydrolysis gives a value for Klason lignin, which with the total NSP gives a total fiber value. The NSP does not include fructan but does include galactan (Theander and Aman, 1982). Starch is measured by an enzymatic method (Salomonsson et al., 1984) modified by Herrera-Saldana et al. (1990). Mertens (1997) and Hall and Van Horn (2001) divided the nonfibrous or non-NDF carbohydrates into four general categories: organic acids, sugars (mono and oligosaccharides), starch, and neutral detergent soluble fiber. The NFC values for feeds are calculated by subtracting from 100 the addition of CP, NDF, ether extract (EE), and ash. The nonstructural carbohydrate (NSC) fraction is measured by hydrolytic methods using a modified procedure by Smith (1981). The terms NSC and NFC are not synonymous and should not be used interchangeably. Some fiber components such as pectins and gums are included in NFC but not in NSC (Mertens, 1997). Recently, there has been an interest in determining specific NSC components such as fructans (oligo- and polyfructosyl sucrose) in fresh forages fed to horses because of their potential effects on laminitis (Longland et al., 1999). Methods to determine oligofructans and fructan polysaccharides in foodstuffs have been reported by Cairns and Pollock (1988), McCleary et al. (2000), and McCleary and Rossiter (2004).

Water-Soluble Carbohydrates (WSC)

Water-soluble carbohydrates (WSC) include compounds soluble in cold water or in gastrointestinal contents such as monosaccharides (e.g., glucose, fructose, galactose), disaccharides (e.g., sucrose, melibiose), oligosaccharides (e.g., raffinose, stachyose), and some polysaccharides (Van Soest, 1994). Fructans are included within the WSC fraction (Figure 10-1).Glucose and fructose generally constitute virtually all of the free-reducing sugars and, with sucrose and maltose, all of the free total sugars found in grass and legume species (Smith, 1981). Extraction with 80-percent ethanol is the most common method used to remove sugars such as glucose, fructose, and sucrose, and the extracts can then be analyzed using nonspecific colorimetric or titrimetric assays (Smith, 1981; Sturgeon, 1990). Further fractionation of these carbohydrates can be accomplished by chromatographic techniques (Fales et al., 1982) or by enzyme-coupled assays (Avigad, 1990). A WSC analysis can be also determined by NIR spectoscopy (NIRS) as reported by Jafari et al., (2003). From an analytical perspective, the NSC is approximated to the sum of WSC and starch, depending on the methodology used (Figure 10-1).

Starch

Starch in forages can be measured by either acid or enzyme hydrolysis on residues that have been previously extracted with ethanol to remove soluble sugars (Smith, 1981). Enzymatic hydrolysis is preferred because of its specificity. The enzyme α-amylase hydrolyzes the starches to glucose without hydrolyzing the fructosans. Glucose concentrations are then converted into equivalent starch concentrations (Smith, 1981; Moore and Hartfield, 1994). Determination of starch in animal feeds is described by the AOAC method 920.40 (AOAC, 2002) and in plants by the method 948.02 (AOAC, 2002). Starch analysis in a variety of plant material is described also by Hall et al. (1999).

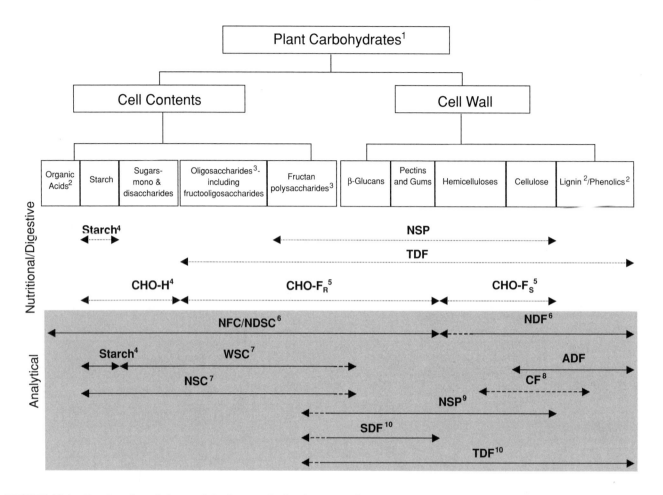

FIGURE 10-1 Fractionation of plant carbohydrates and related compounds

Current and proposed systems for partitioning dietary carbohydrates based on current analytical methods (lower/shaded bracket; solid/dashed lines) and nutritional or physiologic definitions (upper bracket; dotted lines) relative to equine digestive function. Adapted from Hall, 2003 and Hoffman, 2004. In the analytical bracket, dashed lines indicate that recovery of included compounds may be incomplete.

Abbreviations: ADF = acid detergent fiber; CF = crude fiber; CHO-H = hydrolyzable carbohydrates; $CHO-F_S$ = slowly fermentable carbohydrates; $CHO-F_R$ = rapidly fermentable carbohydrates; NDF = neutral detergent fiber; NDSC = neutral detergent soluble carbohydrates; NFC = nonfiber carbohydrates; NSC = nonstructural carbohydrates; NSP = nonstarch polysaccharides; SDF = soluble dietary fiber; TDF = total dietary fiber; WSC = water-soluble carbohydrates

[1] Major categories of carbohydrates and associated substances are shown. These categories may not include all carbohydrates produced by plants.
[2] Some noncarbohydrate components are included here as they are components of the specific analytical fractions.
[3] Specific fructans can be categorized as either fructooligosaccharides or fructan polysaccharides depending on degree of polymerization.
[4] A variable fraction of total starch can be resistant to enzymatic hydrolysis and thus some starch may appear in other nutritional fractions.
[5] Fermentability of gums may be variable.
[6] Some hemicellulose may be soluble in neutral detergent and thus recovered in the NFC/NDSC fraction, rather than the NDF fraction.
[7] Recovery of compounds in the analytical WSC fraction (and thus the NSC fraction when NSC is approximated as starch + WSC) may depend on methodology used.
[8] Amount of cell wall constituents included in CF analysis varies by feed.
[9] From a nutritional perspective, NSP includes all polysaccharides except starch. However, the analytical method for NSP may recover a variable amount of fructan polysaccharide.
[10] From a nutritional perspective, TDF includes all carbohydrates resistant to mammalian digestion. However, the analytical method for TDF (and SDF) does not recover oligosaccharides and may recover a variable amount of fructan polysaccharides.

CRUDE PROTEIN AND AMINO ACID ANALYSES

Crude Protein

The percent of crude protein (CP) reflects the total nitrogen (N) content of feeds (N × 6.25). Official methods for nitrogen determinations in feeds include several modifications of the Kjeldahl method for plants and animal feeds (methods 976.05, 976.06; 977.02; AOAC, 2002). Total nitrogen provides a good estimate of digestible protein in forages that are not heat damaged. For heat-damaged feeds, adjustments of the total protein content are necessary to account for the bound protein unavailable to the animal.

Acid Detergent Insoluble Nitrogen

The acid detergent insoluble nitrogen, also called ADFN in forages, represents heat-damaged browning (Maillard) products or bound protein that are indigestible or poorly digested by animals (Van Soest, 1965; Goering and Van Soest, 1970; Goering et al., 1972; Weiss et al., 1986; Van Soest and Mason, 1991). Acid detergent insoluble nitrogen can also be measured in forages that have not been exposed to heat and is related to lignin and to a fraction of protein in forages (Mertens, 1979). This author found that between 5 and 12 percent of the nitrogen in nonheat-damaged forages is isolated as ADIN, representing the truly indigestible protein in feeds. The ADIN fraction is determined as the nitrogen in the ADF residue using sodium sulfate. Acid detergent insoluble crude protein (ADICP) is ADIN expressed as crude protein on a dry matter basis. The quantitative subtraction of ADIN from crude protein to estimate available nitrogen seems justified (Waters et al., 1992).

Neutral Detergent Insoluble Nitrogen

The neutral detergent insoluble nitrogen, or NDICP, measured without the use of sodium sulfite represents ADIN plus insoluble fibrous proteins and cell wall protein. The difference between NDIN and ADIN represents an estimate of the slowly degraded protein in the rumen or bypass protein that can be digested in the lower digestive tract (Van Soest, 1994; Licitra et al., 1996). The NDIN or NDICP as a percentage of NDF for certain feeds can be as high as 40 percent (Weiss et al., 1989) and between 8 and 12 percent of the NDF for unheated forages (NRC, 2001).

Amino Acid Analysis

Most amino acids in feeds and feed ingredients are measured by AOAC methods (e.g., 994.12; AOAC, 2002). Samples are derivatized and amino acids measured using high performance liquid chromatography (HPLC). This method can be applied to measure alanine, arginine, aspartic acid, cystine, glutamic acid, glycine, histidine, isoleucine, leucine, lysine, methionine, phenylalanine, proline, serine, threonine, and valine. The AOAC method 999.13 (AOAC, 2002) is applicable to the determination of the free nonprotein-bound amino acids lysine, methionine, and threonine in feeds and premixes. Tryptophan in feeds can be determined by the AOAC method 988.15 (AOAC, 2002).

ANALYSES OF FAT AND FATTY ACIDS

Ether Extract (Crude Fat)

The ether extract (EE) or crude fat is one of the components of the Proximate Analysis of feeds and commonly is used to represent the total fat in a diet or ingredient. However, using the term EE might be an oversimplification, as EE also contains organic acids, oils, pigments, alcohols, and the fat-soluble vitamins. Crude fat is determined by a solvent extraction method using a Soxhlet apparatus (method 920.29; AOAC, 1990) or modifications of the latter such as the Soxtec method (Randall, 1974). Another method to determine crude fat used mainly with extruded feeds is the gravimetric method 954.02 (AOAC, 2002).

Fatty Acid Analysis

Free fatty acid (FFA) content is measured after extraction of fat by petroleum ether. The method includes fatty acid methyl ester derivatization followed by gas chromatography (GC) analysis (AOAC method 996.06, 2002). The profiles will include saturated FFA such as C_{12} (lauric), C_{14} (myristic), C_{16} (palmitic), and C_{18} (stearic), and unsaturated FFA such as $C_{18:1,\omega-9}$ (oleic), $C_{18:2,\omega-6,9}$ (linoleic), and $C_{18:3,\omega-3,6,9}$ (α-linolenic), among others.

CARBOHYDRATE ANALYSIS IN HORSE NUTRITION

Neither the ruminant (Van Soest et al., 1991) nor human (Englyst and Cummings, 1990) systems of carbohydrate classification and analysis fit well with the digestive physiology and metabolism of horses (Hoffman, 2004). The ruminant system of carbohydrate analysis will divide carbohydrates as cell wall (measured as NDF) and cell contents (measured as NSC). On the other hand, the human system uses fractions that can be applied to the horse such as TDF and NSP. However, NSP ignores the lignin and lignocellulose fractions present in horse diets that might have an effect on retarding the rate of fermentation. Hoffman et al. (2001) suggested that it would be helpful to develop a scheme of proximate analysis components for the horse that better relates to the digested fractions. The authors proposed to use the following terminology: (1) hydrolysable carbohydrates (CHO-H) measured by direct analysis (e.g., Davis, 1976; Smith, 1981); and (2) fermentable carbohydrates (CHO-F) that can be divided into rapidly fermentable carbohydrates (CHO-F_R) and slowly fermentable carbohydrates (CHO-F_S).

Values for CHO-F_R are calculated as the difference between NFC and CHO-H, representing gums, mucilages, β-glucans, pectins, and/or storage polysaccharides such as fructans. In the Hoffman et al. (2001) system, CHO-F_S is equated with the NDF values of the Van Soest et al. (1991) ruminant system. The breakdown of dietary carbohydrates is given in Figure 10-1 (adapted from Hall, 2003 and Hoffman, 2004).

FEED ANALYSIS USING NEAR INFRARED REFLECTANCE

Near infrared reflectance spectroscopy (NIRS) relates a sample's reflectance of near infrared light to its chemical composition. It relies on prediction equations of nutrient levels rather than direct measurements. The technique was first applied to measure moisture content and was developed at the U.S. Department of Agriculture, Beltsville, Maryland (Norris, 1964). In the last 20 years, NIRS has gained acceptance as an analytical tool for feeds and forages because of its quickness, low operating costs, safety, and accuracy to measure chemical composition. The near infrared region of the spectrum (700 nm to 2,500 nm) includes molecular absorptions of overtone and combination bands (Birth and Hecht, 1987). Since 1973, with the application of NIRS to the analysis of cereals and oilseeds (Williams, 1975), NIRS technology has become widely accepted in food analysis. Its potential for rapidly evaluating forage quality was first demonstrated by Norris et al. (1976). A complete review of the NIRS application to forage analysis has been given by Shenk and Westerhaus (1994). Most feed testing laboratories will offer analysis of feeds and forages by NIRS and at a lower cost. The AOAC official method of analysis 989.03 (AOAC, 1990) describes the application of NIRS to measure protein and ADF in feed and forages. NIRS is also applied to measure NDF or aNDF of feed and forages (Martin et al., 1989). Because all energy-yielding components of feeds absorb in the near infrared region of the spectrum, NIRS has the potential to be a fast alternative method to predict metabolizable energy in feeds. Thus, Valdes and Leeson (1992, 1994) successfully applied NIRS to measure apparent metabolizable energy in poultry feeds and feed ingredients, reducing the need and the cost for bioassays. NIRS has been used to estimate animal response and, according to Abrams et al. (1987), NIRS could be more accurate in predicting animal response than any single reference method or combination of these methods. The application of NIRS to predict organic matter digestibility of forages fed to horses has been reported by Andrieu and Martin-Rosset (1995) and Andrieu et al. (1996). NIR predictions of hydrolysable carbohydrates in forages have been reported by Hoffman et al. (2001) and by Jafari et al. (2003). Ideally, minerals should not be analyzed using NIRS as they do not absorb light energy in the near infrared region. However, some minerals can be measured indirectly by NIRS due to association with organic molecules (Shenk and Westerhaus, 1994). Biological components such as ADIN might be more difficult to measure using NIRS because of its complex composition.

REFERENCES

AACC. 1995a. Method 32-05: Total Dietary Fiber. Approved Methods of the American Association of Cereal Chemists, 9th ed. St. Paul, MN: American Association of Cereal Chemists.

AACC. 1995b. Method 32-07: Determination of Soluble, Insoluble and Total Dietary Fiber in Foods and Food Products. Approved Methods of the American Association of Cereal Chemists, 9th ed. St. Paul, MN: American Association of Cereal Chemists.

Abrams, S. M., J. S. Shenk, M. O. Westerhaus, and F. E. Barton II. 1987. Determination of forage quality by near infrared reflectance spectroscopy (NIRS): efficacy of broad based calibration equations. J. Dairy Sci. 70:806–813.

Akin, D. E., and A. Chesson.1989. Lignification as the major factor limiting forage feeding value especially in warm conditions. Pp. 1753–1760 in Proc. 16th Intl. Grassl. Congr., October 4–11, Nice, France, French Grassl. Soc.

Andrieu, J., and W. Martin-Rosset. 1995. Chemical, biological and physical (NIRS) methods for predicting organic matter digestibility of forages in horse. Pp. 76–77 in Proc. 14th Equine Nutr. Physiol. Soc. Symp., Ontario, CA.

Andrieu, J., M. Jestin, and W. Martin-Rosset. 1996. Prediction of the organic matter digestibility (OMD) of forages in horse by near infrared spectrophotometry (NIRS). P. 299 in Proc. of the 47th European Assoc. of Animal Production, Lillehammer, Norway

AOAC Method 920.29. 1990. Fat (Crude) or Ether Extract in Animal Feed. Official Methods of Analysis, 15th ed. Gaithersburg, MD: Assoc. Official Anal. Chem.

AOAC Method 989.03. 1990. Fiber (Acid Detergent) and Protein (Crude) in Animal Feed and Forages: Near-infrared Reflectance Spectroscopy Method. Official Methods of Analysis, 15th ed. Gaithersburg, MD: Assoc. Official Anal. Chem.

AOAC Method 920.40. 2002. Starch in Animal Feed. Official Methods of Analysis, 17th ed. Gaithersburg, MD: Assoc. Official Anal. Chem.

AOAC Method 948.02. 2002. Starch in Plants. Official Methods of Analysis, 17th ed. Gaithersburg, MD: Assoc. Official Anal. Chem.

AOAC Method 954.02. 2002. Fat (Crude) or Ether Extract in Pet Foods. Official Methods of Analysis, 17th ed. Gaithersburg, MD: Assoc. Official Anal. Chem.

AOAC Method 962.09. 2002. Fiber (Crude) in Animal Feed and Pet Food. Official Methods of Analysis, 17th ed. Gaithersburg, MD: Assoc. Official Anal. Chem.

AOAC Method 976.05. 2002. Protein (Crude) in Animal Feeds and Pet Foods. Official Methods of Analysis, 17th ed. Gaithersburg, MD: Assoc. Official Anal. Chem.

AOAC Method 976.06. 2002. Protein (Crude) in Animal Feeds and Pet Foods. Official Methods of Analysis, 17th ed. Gaithersburg, MD: Assoc. Official Anal. Chem.

AOAC Method 977.02. 2002. Nitrogen (Total) (Crude Protein) in Plants. Official Methods of Analysis, 17th ed. Gaithersburg, MD: Assoc. Official Anal. Chem.

AOAC Method 988.15. 2002. Tryptophan in Foods and Food and Feed Ingredients—Ion Exchange Chromatographic Method. Gaithersburg, MD: Assoc. Official Anal. Chem.

AOAC Method 991.43. 2002. Total Soluble and Insoluble Dietary Fiber in Foods. Official Methods of Analysis, 17th ed. Gaithersburg, MD: Assoc. Official Anal. Chem.

AOAC Method 994.12. 2002. Amino Acids in Feeds. Official Methods of Analysis, 17th ed. Gaithersburg, MD: Assoc. Official Anal. Chem.

AOAC Method 996.06. 2002. Fat (total, saturated and unsaturated in foods). Official Methods of Analysis, 17th ed. Gaithersburg, MD: Assoc. Official Anal. Chem.

AOAC Method 999.13. 2002. Lysine, Methionine and Threonine in Feed Grade Amino Acids and Premixes. Official Methods of Analysis, 17th ed. Gaithersburg, MD: Assoc. Official Anal. Chem.

Avigad G. 1990. Disaccharides. Pp.112–188 in Methods in Plant Biochemistry, vol. 2, P. M. Dey, ed. New York: Academic Press.

Baer, D. J., W. V. Rumpler, C. W. Miles, and G. C. Fahey, Jr. 1997. Dietary fiber decreases the metabolizable energy content and nutrient digestibility of mixed diets fed to humans. J. Nutr. 127:579–586.

Bailey, R. W., and M. J. Ulyatt. 1970. Pasture quality and ruminant nutrition. II. Carbohydrate and lignin composition of detergent-extracted residues from pasture grasses and legumes. N. Z. J. Agric. Res. 13:591–594.

Birth, G. S., and H. G. Hecht. 1987. The physics of near-infrared reflectance. Pp. 1–15 in Near Infrared Technology in the Agricultural and Food Industries, P. Williams and K. Norris, eds. St. Paul, MN: American Association of Cereal Chemists.

Cairns, A. J., and C. J. Pollock. 1988. Fructan biosynthesis in excised leaves of *Lolium temulentum* L. I. Chromotographic characterization of oligofructans and their labeling patterns following $^{14}CO_2$ feeding. New Phytol. 109:399–405.

Davis, R. E. 1976. A combined automated procedure for the determination of reducing sugars and nicotine alkaloids in tobacco products using a new reducing sugar method. Tob. Sci. 20:139–144.

DeVries, J. W., L. Prosky, B. Li, and S. Cho. 1999. A historical perspective on defining dietary fiber. Cereal Food World 44:367–369.

Englyst, H., and J. Cummings. 1990. Dietary fibre and starch: definition, classification and measurement. Pp. 3–26 in Dietary Fibre Perspectives– Reviews and Bibliography, A. R. Leeds, ed. London: John Libbey and Co.

Fales, S. L., D. A. Holt, V. L. Lechtenberg, K. Johnson, M. R. Ladisch, and A. Anderson. 1982. Fractionation of forage grass carbohydrates using liquid (water) chromatography. Agronom. J. 74:1074–1077.

Goering, H. K., and P. J. Van Soest. 1970. Forage fiber analysis (apparatus, reagents, procedures and some applications). Agric. Handbook No 379. Washington, DC: ARS-USDA.

Goering, H. K., C. H. Gordon, R. W. Hemken, D. R. Waldo, P. J. Van Soest, and L. W. Smith. 1972. Analytical estimates of nitrogen digestibility in heat damaged forages. J. Dairy Sci. 55:1275–1280.

Gudmundsson, O. 1998. Evaluation of feeds for horses. Pp. 1–30 in Nova Course on the Icelandic Horse and Horse Breeding and Management, August 9–20, Hvanneyri Agricultural College, Iceland.

Hall, M. B. 2003. Challenges with nonfiber carbohydrate methods. J. Anim. Sci. 81:3226–3232.

Hall, M. B., and H. H. Van Horn. 2001. How should we formulate for non-NDF carbohydrates? Pp. 44–49 in 12th Annual Florida Ruminant Nutrition Symposium Proceedings.

Hall, M. B., W. H. Hoover, J. P. Jennings, and T. K. Miller Webster. 1999. A method for partitioning neutral detergent-soluble carbohydrates. J. Sci. Food Agric. 79:2079–2086.

Herrera-Saldana, R. E., J. T. Huber, and M. H. Poore. 1990. Dry matter, crude protein and starch degradability of five cereal grains. J. Dairy Sci. 73:2386–2393.

Hintz, B. W., D. R. Mertens, and K. A. Albrecht. 1996. Effect of sodium sulfite on recovery and composition of detergent fiber and lignin. J. AOAC Int. 79:16–22.

Hoffman, R. M. 2004. Carbohydrate in horse nutrition. Pp. 21–37 in Proceedings, Conference on Equine Nutrition Research, May 22–23, Texas A&M University, Equine Science Section, Department of Animal Science.

Hoffman, R. M., J. A. Wilson, D. S. Kronfeld, W. L. Cooper, L. A. Lawrence, D. Sklan, and P. A. Harris. 2001. Hydrolyzable carbohydrates in pasture, hay and horse feeds: direct assay and seasonal variation. J. Anim. Sci. 79:500–506.

Jafari, A., V. Connolly, A. Frolich, and E. J. Walsh. 2003. A note on estimation of quality parameters in perennial ryegrass by near infrared reflectance. Irish J. Agric. Food Res. 42:293–300.

Jung, H. G., D. R. Mertens, and A. J. Payne. 1997. Correlation of acid detergent and Klasson lignin with digestibility of forage dry matter and neutral detergent fiber. J. Dairy Sci. 80:1622–1628.

Komarek, A. R. 1993. A filter bag procedure for improved efficiency of fiber analysis. J. Dairy Sci. 76 (Suppl. 1):250.

Komarek, A. R., J. B. Robertson, and P. J. Van Soest. 1994. A comparison of methods for determining ADF using the filter bag technique versus conventional filtration. J. Dairy Sci. 77 (Suppl. 1):114.

Lee, S., L. Prosky, and J. DeVries. 1992. Determination of total, soluble and insoluble dietary fiber in foods. Enzymatic gravimetric-method, MEW-TRIS buffer: collaborative study. J. AOAC Int. 75:395–416.

Licitra, G., T. M. Hernandez, and P. J. Van Soest. 1996. Standardization of procedures for nitrogen fractionation of ruminant feeds. Anim. Feed Sci. Technol. 57:347–358.

Longland, A. C., A. J. Cairns, P. I. Thomas, and M. O. Humphreys. 1999. Seasonal and diurnal changes in fructan concentration in *Lolium Perenne*: implications for the grazing management of equines predisposed to laminitis. Pp. 258–259 in Proc. 16th Equine Nutr. Physiol. Soc. Symp., Raleigh, NC.

Lowry, J. B., L. L. Conlan, A. C. Schlink, and C. S. McSweeney. 1994. Acid detergent dispersible lignin in tropical grasses. J. Sci. Food Agric. 65:41–49.

Martin, G. C., J. S. Shenk, and F. E. Barton II. 1989. Near infrared reflectance spectroscopy (NIRS) analysis of forage quality. Agricultural Handbook No 643, U.S. Department of Agriculture, Agricultural Research Service.

Martin-Rosset, W., M. Vermorel, M. Doreau, J. L. Tisserand, and J. Andrieu. 1994. The French horse feed evaluation system and recommended allowances for energy and protein. Livest. Prod. Sci. 40:37–56.

McCleary, B. V., and P. Rossiter. 2004. Measurement of novel dietary fibres. J. AOAC Int. 87:707–711.

McCleary, B. V., A. Murphy, and D. C. Mugford. 2000. Determination of oligofructans and fructan polysaccharides in foodstuffs by an enzymatic/spectrophotometric method: collaborative study. J. AOAC Int. 83:356–364.

Mertens, D. R. 1979. Adjusting heat-damaged protein to a CP basis. J. Anim. Sci. 42:259.

Mertens, D. R. 1992. Critical conditions in determining detergent fiber. Pp. C1–C8 in Proc. NFTA Forage Analysis Wkshp., Denver, CO.

Mertens, D. R. 1997. Creating a system for meeting the fiber requirements of dairy cows. J. Dairy Sci. 80:1463–1481.

Mertens, D. R. 2002. Gravimetric determination of amylase-treated neutral detergent fiber in feeds with refluxing in beakers or crucibles: collaborative study. J. AOAC Int. 85:1217–1240.

Moore, K. J., and R. D. Hatfield. 1994. Carbohydrates and forage quality. Pp. 229–280 in Forage Quality, Evaluation and Utilization, G. C. Fahey Jr., ed. Univ. Nebraska, Lincoln: Am. Soc. of Agronomy.

Norris, K. H. 1964. Simple spectroradiometer for 0.4 to 1.2 micron region. Trans. Am. Soc. Agri. Eng. 7:240–242.

Norris, K. H., R. F. Barnes, D. E. Moore, and J. S. Shenk. 1976. Predicting forage quality by infrared reflectance spectroscopy. J. Anim. Sci. 43:889–897.

NRC (National Research Council). 1996. Nutrient Requirements of Beef Cattle, 7th rev. ed. Washington, DC: National Academy Press.

NRC. 2000. Dietary Reference Intakes: Proposed Definition of Dietary Fiber. Washington, DC: National Academy Press.

NRC. 2001. Nutrient Requirements of Dairy Cattle, 7th rev. ed. Washington, DC: National Academy Press.

NRC. 2003. Nutrient Requirements of Nonhuman Primates, 2nd rev. ed. Washington DC: The National Academies Press.

Popovich, D. G., D. J. A. Jenkins, C. W. C. Kendall, E. S. Dierenfeld, R. W. Carroll, N. Tariq, and E. Vidgen. 1997. The western lowland gorilla diet has implications for the health of humans and other hominoids. J. Nutr. 127:2000–2005.

Prosky, L., N. G. Asp, T. F. Schweizer, L. Furda, J. W. DeVries, and I. Furda. 1988. Determination of insoluble, soluble, and total dietary fiber in foods and food products: inter-laboratory study. J. AOAC Int. 71:1017–1023.

Ralston, S. I. 1991. Principles of ration analysis. Pp. 131–137 in Large Animal Clinical Nutrition, J. M. Naylor and S. L. Ralston, eds. St. Louis, MO: Mosby-Yearbook.

Randall, E. L. 1974. Improved method for fat and oil analysis by a new process of extraction. J. AOAC Int. 57:1165–1168.

Robertson, J. B., and P. J. Van Soest. 1981. The detergent system of analysis and its application to human foods. Pp. 123–158 in The Analysis of Dietary Fiber in Food, W. P. T. James and O. Theander, eds. New York: Marcel Dekker.

Salomonsson, A. C., O. Theander, and E. Westerlund. 1984. Chemical characterization of some Swedish cereal, whole meal and bran fractions. Swed. J. Agric. Res. 14:111–118.

Shenk, J. S., and M. O. Westerhaus. 1994. The application of near infrared reflectance spectroscopy (NIRS) to forage analysis. In Forage Quality, Evaluation and Utilization, J. C. Fahey, ed. Univ. Nebraska, Lincoln: Am. Soc. of Agronomy.

Smith, D. 1981. Removing and analyzing total non-structural carbohydrates from plant tissues. Wisconsin Ag. Exp. Stn. Rep. No. R2107, Madison.

Sturgeon, R. J. 1990. Monosaccharides. Pp. 1–37 in Methods in Plant Biochemistry, vol 2, P. M. Dey, ed. New York: Academic Press.

Theander, O., and P. Aman. 1982. Studies in dietary fibre. A method for the analysis and chemical characterization of total dietary fibre. J. Sci. Fd. Agric. 33:340–344.

Trowell, H. 1985. Dietary fibre: a paradigm. Pp. 1–20 in Dietary Fibre, Fibre Depleted Foods and Disease, H. W. Trowell, D. Burkitt, and K. W. Heaton, eds. London: Academic Press.

Undersander, D., D. R. Mertens, and N. Thiex. 1993. Forage Analyses Procedures. Pp. 95–103 in National Forage Testing Association Proceedings, Omaha, NE.

Valdes, E. V., and S. Leeson. 1992. Near infrared reflectance analysis as a method to measure metabolizable energy in complete poultry feeds. Poult. Sci. 71:1179–1187.

Valdes, E. V., and S. Leeson. 1994. Measurement of metabolizable energy, gross energy, and moisture in feed grade fats by near infrared reflectance spectroscopy. Poult. Sci. 73:163–171.

Van Soest, P. J. 1965. Use of detergents in analysis of fibrous feeds. III. Study of effects of heating and drying on yield of fiber and lignin in forages. J. AOAC Int. 48:785–790.

Van Soest, P. J. 1994. Nutritional Ecology of the Ruminant. Ithaca, NY: Cornell University Press.

Van Soest, P. J., and V. C. Mason. 1991. The influence of the Maillard reaction upon the nutritive value of fibrous feeds. Anim. Feed Sci. Technol. 32:45–53.

Van Soest, P. J., and R. H. Wine. 1967. Use of detergents in the analysis of fibrous feeds. IV. J. AOAC Int. 50:50–55.

Van Soest, P. J., J. B. Robertson, and B. A. Lewis. 1991. Methods for dietary fiber, neutral detergent fiber, and nonstarch polysaccharides in relation to animal nutrition. J. Dairy Sci. 74:3583–3597.

Vogel, K. P., J. F. Pedersen, S. D. Masterson, and J. J. Toy. 1999. Evaluation of a filter bag system for NDF, ADF and IVDMD forage analysis. Crop Sci. 39:276–279.

Waters, C. J., M. A. Kitcherside, and A. J. F. Webster. 1992. Problems associated with estimating the digestibility of undergraded dietary nitrogen from acid-detergent insoluble nitrogen. Anim. Feed Sci. Technol. 39:279–291.

Weiss, W. P., H. R. Conrad, and W. L. Shockey. 1986. Digestibility of nitrogen in heat-damaged alfalfa. J. Dairy Sci. 69:2658–2670.

Weiss, W. P., D. O. Erickson, G. M. Erickson, and G. R. Fisher. 1989. Barley distillers grains as a protein supplement for dairy cows. J. Dairy Sci. 72:980–987.

Williams, P. C. 1975. Application of near infrared reflectance spectroscopy to analysis of cereal grains and oilseeds. Cereal Chem. 5:561–576.

11

Feeding Behavior and General Considerations for Feeding Management

FEEDING BEHAVIOR

Equine feeding behavior affects feed intake and feeding management of horses. Horses are herbivores; therefore, they may require a forage supply to lessen the risks of clinical disorders such as colic (Archer and Proudman, 2005), laminitis (Rowe et al., 1994), and oral and locomotory behavioral problems (Mills et al., 2005). By acknowledging the normal feeding behaviors of the equine, appropriate feed management decisions can be made to minimize these important clinical problems and contribute to the well-being of the horse. The following discussion is not intended to be a comprehensive treatise on equine behavior, which can be found in books by Waring (2002), McGreevy (2004), and Mills and McDonnell (2005).

Energy Balance

A commonly held nutritional maxim is that horses eat to meet their energy requirements. In actuality, patterns of seasonal feed intake plotted against weight gain or body weight (BW) have not totally upheld this concept. The body weight–time plots of pastured Przewalski's horses and mature and young Quarter horse mares (Berger et al., 1999; Fitzgerald and McManus, 2000) showed increasing weight gains through spring, reaching a maximum weight in summer, followed by progressive weight loss through the autumn and winter. Weight gains through spring and summer averaged about 0.5 kg/d, followed by similar weight loss through autumn and winter. A high feeding rate coincided with low body weight in spring, followed by low feeding activity during peak body weights in summer with a return to high feeding activity in autumn and winter (Berger et al., 1999). The study did not determine if weight loss in autumn and winter was due to poor quality feed, a reduction in voluntary feed intake, or cold weather extremes. Similar body weight–time patterns are typical of wild ruminants, which deposit fat and soft tissue in summer and use stored energy (fat) during colder weather conditions rather than increasing voluntary feed intake in times of poor feed supply (Loudon et al., 1989; Rhind et al., 1998).

Some semblance of the eat-for-energy maxim was evident in ponies fed pelleted diets whose energy content was diluted by adding sawdust (Laut et al., 1985). Ponies responded to the dietary caloric dilution by increasing their total daily feed intake and thereby maintained energy intake until gut capacity became limiting (Laut et al., 1985). However, voluntary energy intake can be greatly distorted by the palatability and composition of the diet. When offered, Thoroughbred and Standardbred racehorses consumed about 1.58 to 1.76 kg concentrate/100 kg BW, representing about 65–71 percent of total feed intake (Southwood et al., 1993). Young pony mares (average weight 238 kg) fed a 60 percent grass hay–40 percent concentrate mix as a chaff or pellet ate excessive amounts of diet and, hence, energy for 6–7 weeks (peak intake of 4.5 kg DM/100 kg BW), with the result that all mares gained considerable weight (45 kg over 4 weeks) (Argo et al., 2002). Following this period of greed, the mares self-limited their feed consumption to maintenance energy amounts resulting in no further weight gain. This overindulgence of palatable feeds occurs despite the risk of clinical disorders (colic, laminitis) (Rowe et al., 1994; Tinker et al., 1997; Cohen et al., 1999; Hudson et al., 2001).

Dulphy et al. (1997a,b) summarized forage intakes by horses and found a considerable range of voluntary intakes of hays by horses. Based on 17 INRA studies and 42 published papers, Dulphy et al. (1997b) provided summary data that showed that lucerne (alfalfa) hay was consumed at average rates of 2.24–2.44 kg/100 kg BW (range 2–2.7), amounts that were higher than average voluntary feed intake (VFI) of some grass hays (2.01–2.12 kg/100 BW; range 1.3–2.7) and/or straws (1.28 kg/100 kg BW; range 0.9–1.8) (Dulphy et al., 1997b). In a separate study, barley straw and maize silage had a low acceptability by horses and were eaten in small amounts (< 1 kg/100 kg BW) despite providing subnormal energy intakes (Dulphy et al., 1997a). Evidently, simply providing feed to a horse is not sufficient to make the horse eat it, but providing palatable feed ad libitum may contribute to undesired consequences.

Typical Feeding Behavior

Foals

Dam's milk is the main source of nutrients for the newborn foal. Normal foals began suckling within 1 to 2 hours after birth (Kubiak et al., 1988; Houpt, 2002) and nursed 10 times an hour to 1 day old, gradually decreasing this rate to 1.5 bouts/h by 17 weeks of age (Smith-Funk and Crowell-Davis, 1992). Successful suckling bouts by mule foals lasted 47–54 seconds regardless of age (Smith-Funk and Crowell-Davis, 1992), compared to 57–79 seconds for Thoroughbred foals (Cameron et al., 1999). The average daily time spent nursing by Thoroughbred foals was 46 minutes (range 27–78 minutes) and milk consumption, estimated by using isotope dilution methods, was determined to be 14.7 kg milk/d (Cameron et al., 1999).

Feral neonates suckled for 6–8 percent of the day, then rapidly decreased time spent suckling to 2.3 percent of the day over the next 8 weeks, plateaued at 2 percent of the day until week 29, and self-weaned at week 35 (Duncan et al., 1984). Some foals started eating solid feeds as early as 1 day of age, although 1-week-old foals spent only about 8 percent of the day eating solid feed (Crowell-Davis et al., 1985; Boyd, 1988). By 21 weeks, foals spent 47 percent of daylight hours eating solid feeds. Similarly, feral foals were reported to spend only 18–25 percent of the day grazing at 2–4 weeks old, then 42–45 percent by 20–28 weeks of age, and up to 73 percent at 5 months of age (Duncan et al, 1984; Boyd, 1988). Dams allowed their foals to eat grain with them (Boyd, 1991), which is a behavior that can be exploited to introduce foals to grain and/or other solid feeds. Foals confined with their dams in box stalls will learn relatively quickly to consume grain mixes and hays. Realistically, foals kept continuously on pasture with their dams are unlikely to consume much grain or hay. Coleman et al. (1999) reported that 2-month-old foals, whose dams were grazing good-quality pastures, ate only 48–75 percent of the 0.9–1.35 kg creep feed offered to them daily.

Mature Horses on Pasture

Forages are the main component of feral horse diets. Typically, the forage diets consumed by feral horses have considerable variety: 65 percent grasses and sedges, 25 percent shrubs, and minor amounts of forbs (Salter and Hudson, 1979; Krysyl et al., 1984). This feral horse preference for variety has been shown to be mimicked by domesticated horses (see below; Goodwin et al., 2005a). Horses are highly selective grazers and have grazed pastures to ground level (Goold, 1991), which can cause considerable pressure on palatable species and which, if sustained, can lead to the disappearance of the preferred species from the sward (Archer, 1973; Wallace, 1977; Archer, 1978a,b; Elphinstone, 1981). Studies on pasture species preference by equines have yielded inconsistent results, and this may at least in part reflect differences in the maturity of the herbage at the time of study. As plants mature, they become less palatable. Fleurance et al. (2001) suggested that horses selected herbage on the basis of stage of growth rather than botanical species. As a consequence, differential maturation rates between species may result in those which mature rapidly being selected less frequently as the season advances in favor of those which mature more slowly (McMeniman, 2003). In addition to changes in acceptance with seasonal changes in plant development, palatability is affected by plant nutrient status, which is under environmental influence. Nevertheless, despite the difficulties of interpreting data of studies on species preference by horses due to the dynamic nature of herbage palatability, it has generally been found that pastures of mixed species were preferred to monocultures (Archer, 1973) and grasses were preferred to legumes and herbs (Archer, 1973; Odberg and Francis-Smith, 1976; Archer, 1978a,b; Rogalski, 1982, 1984a; Krysyl et al., 1984; Chenost and Martin-Rosset, 1985). Reported palatable cool-season pasture species for horses include perennial ryegrass (*Lolium perenne*), meadow fescue (*Festuca pratensis*), timothy (*Phleum pratense*), orchardgrass (*Dactylis glomerata*), creeping red fescue (*F. rubra*), white bent (*Agrostis gigantea*), smooth stalked meadow grass, Italian ryegrass (*Lolium multiflorum*), hybrid ryegrass (*L. perenne × multiflorum*), tall fescue (*F. arundinacea*), Kentucky bluegrass (*Poa pratensis*), and smooth brome grass (*Bromus inermis*). Other pasture species acceptable to horses include several cereals grown as forage crops such as barley (*Hordeum vulgare*) and oats (*Avena sativa*). Legumes in horse pastures may include red and white clover (*Trifolium pratense, T. repens*), strawberry clover (*T. fragiferum*), sainfoin (*Onobrychis vicifolia*), alfalfa (*Medicago sativa*), and vetch (*Vicia atropurpurea*). Herbs such as dandelion (*Taraxacum officinale*), ribgrass (*Plantago lanceolata*), and chicory (*Cichorium intybus*) may also be eaten. Warm-season species include Bermudagrass (*Cynadon dactylon*), crabgrass (*Digitaria* spp.), Eastern gamagrass (*Tripsacum dactyloides*), blue couch (*Digitaria didactylis*), bahiagrass (*Paspalum notatum*), Rhodes grass (*Chloris gayana*), setaria (*Setaria anceps*), elephantgrass (*Pennisetum purpureum*), pearl millet (*Pennisetum glaucum*), Kikuyu grass (*Pennisetum clandestinum*), paspalum (*Paspalum dilantatum*), prairiegrass (*Bromus* spp.), India grass (*Sorgastrum nutans* L.), switchgrass (*Panicum virgatum* L.), big bluestem (*Andropogon geradi*), matua bromegrass (*Bromus willldenowii*), altai wildrye (*Leysum angustus* Trin), crested wheatgrass (*Agrypynon cristatum*), and reed canarygrass (*Phalaris arundinaceae*) (Archer, 1973;

Rogalski, 1977, 1984b; Templeton, 1979; Elphinstone, 1981; Falkowski et al., 1983; Williams, 1987; Gallagher and McMeniman, 1988; Hunt, 1991; McCann and Hoveland, 1991; Lieb et al., 1993; Almeida et al., 1999; Friend and Nash, 2000; Guay et al., 2002). Further information on the relative intakes and nutritive value of some of these species is given in Chapter 8, Tables 8.1–8.4.

There have been a number of reports on sward height preferences by grazing horses, which have yielded conflicting results. Although horses showed a distinct preference for timothygrass swards of 5 cm to those 20 cm tall (Hayakawa, 1991) and preferred seminatural herbage in lawns less than 4 cm high (Fleurance et al., 2001), Naujeck et al., (2005) reported that horses preferred perennial ryegrass swards 15 cm high to those less than 4.5 cm. Grass, 6.6–9.4 cm in height, was equally well eaten (1.5–1.7 kg DM/100 kg body weight [BW]) by yearling and 2-year-old horses, although 2-year-old horses ate more forage per bite (9.9 vs. 7.6 g organic matter [OM]) and spent less time foraging (59 percent vs. 66 percent of the day) than yearlings (Mesochina et al., 1998). Nonpregnant draft mares pastured on wet grasslands consumed 166.2 g OM/kg $W^{0.75}$, an intake of about 3.3 kg/100 kg BW (Fleurance et al., 2001). In addition, forage selection and intake may be dictated by seasonal sward growth. In spring, horses moved to areas where the first pasture grew irrespective of its height or thickness (Salter and Hudson, 1979).

Such equivocal results suggest that fresh herbage intake is governed by the interaction of a number of factors, including plant maturity/herbage quality and sward characteristics, which dictate herbage bite mass, rather than sward height per se. Indeed, Hughes and Gallagher (1993) found that herbage dry matter (DM) intakes by horses did not change with increasing sward height, for although herbage bite mass increased, bite rate decreased, maintaining constant intakes. Quality and quantity of vegetation in a grazing area affect grazing rate and time spent grazing. Time budget experiments have shown that horses at pasture generally graze for 10–17 hours daily (Martin-Rosset et al., 1978; Crowell-Davis et al., 1985; Gallagher and McMenniman, 1989; Duncan, 1992; Fleurance et al., 2001). Hughes and Gallagher (1993) and Gallagher and McMeniman (1989), studying horses pastured on warm-season species and perennial ryegrass, respectively, concluded that horses needed to graze for approximately 17 hours daily to meet their nutritional needs. Gender, age, and breed all influenced time spent grazing. Thus, stallions grazed for lesser periods than mares, weanlings less than mature horses (Crowell-Davis et al., 1985), and 2-year-olds less than yearlings (Mesochina et al., 2000). Furthermore, single animals grazed for shorter periods than when in a herd (Kusonose et al., 1986) and Arabians grazed for longer periods than Thoroughbreds (Rogalski, 1977). Nocturnal intakes may account for between 20–50 percent of the total time spent grazing (Doreau et al., 1980; Fleurance et al., 2001), but this is also seasonally dependent. Horses spent more time in nocturnal feeding in summer than winter (Kaseda, 1983).

Feral horses in Alberta spent nearly 75 percent of the day in foraging activities (Salter and Hudson, 1979), while Camargue mares spent 71 percent of daylight hours and 49–56 percent of nighttime hours (sunset to sunrise) grazing during winter and spring (Duncan, 1985). Ponies in Iceland and Thoroughbred geldings in Scotland spent 62 percent time grazing, 12–29 percent resting, and 9 percent walking on late-summer pastures (Marsden, 1993; Magnusson and Thorhallsdottir, 1994). Lactation, which increases energy demands of mares, might be expected to increase foraging durations, yet studies showed that lactating mares were similar to other pastured horses, spending about 61–70 percent of their time feeding (Crowell-Davis et al., 1985; Duncan, 1985). As pasture availability increased, there was a linear decrease in time spent grazing (Arnold, 1984). With grass senescence, horses decreased both pasture intakes (1.8–2 kg DM/100 kg BW) and grazing time (52–58 percent of the day) (Shingu et al., 2000). Voluntary intakes of fresh forages by various classes of equids are summarized in Chapter 8 (Table 8.1). Daily pasture intakes ranged from 15–32 g DM/kg BW (average 20 g DM/kg BW).

Horses are constant feeders. When grazing, horses take a bite of grass, then move forward one or two steps, followed by another bite (Feist and McCullough, 1976). Exmoor ponies walked 3–5 km daily in winter and 3.8–4.9 km in summer (Booth, 1998). Similarly, Shingu et al. (2000) reported that pastured horses moved a distance of 2.6–3 km daily, of which 50–60 percent occurred during grazing. Consequently, horses eat and/or trample more pasture than cattle. Dry matter intake (144 g DM/kg $W^{0.75}$) by horses on pasture was 63 percent higher than by cattle (88 g DM/kg $W^{0.75}$) (Menard et al., 2002). The time spent grazing by nonpregnant horses (47 percent of the day or 11 hours) was longer than by cattle (32 percent) or sheep (37.5 percent) sharing the same pastures (Arnold, 1984). Menard et al. (2002) observed that breeding mares spent 54 percent of the day grazing in summer compared to cattle, which grazed for 36 percent of the day. Autumnal grazing time increased to 68 percent for mares and 45 percent for cattle, suggesting a sparser pasture supply. Although horses graze or eat for longer periods than ruminants, if time spent ruminating is added to active foraging by cattle, the time budgets of both species is very similar.

The range of DM intakes of selected feeds by horses, ponies, and donkeys is given in Table 11-1. Mature and young horses appear to have a maximal daily DM feed intake of about 3–3.2 percent of their body weight, although average intakes appear to be lower. Ponies may have higher voluntary dry matter intake (VDMI) than horses. Ponies ate 3.9 kg/100 kg BW alfalfa hay (Pearson et al., 2001) and up to 5.1 kg fresh weight/100 kg BW of 60 percent hay–40 percent concentrate pellets (Argo et al., 2002). In the latter study, the feed intakes seem atypically high, but these ob-

TABLE 11-1 Summary of Ranges of Reported Average Voluntary Dry Matter Intakes (AVDMI) of Selected Feedstuffs

Classification	Ranges of AVDMI (kg/100 kg BW/d)	References
Mature horses Fresh forage, all hay, mixed concentrate and hay and complete, processed mix diets	1.8–3.2	Aiken et al. (1989); Crozier et al. (1997); Dulphy et al. (1997a); Dulphy et al. (1997b); Heusner (1993); Marlow et al. (1983)
Mature ponies Hay and complete, processed mix diets	1.5–5.2	Argo et al. (2002); Bergero et al. (2002); Hale and Moore-Colyer (2001); Moore-Colyer and Longland (2000); Pearson and Merritt (1991); Pearson et al. (2001)
Mature ponies Straw diets	1.5–2.4	Pearson and Merritt (1991); Pearson et al. (2001)
Growing horses Fresh forage, all hay and mixed concentrate–hay diets	2.0–3.0	Aiken et al. (1989); Cymbaluk et al. (1989); Guay et al. (2002); LaCasha et al. (1999); McMeniman (2000)
Donkeys Alfalfa hay	2.3–2.6	Pearson et al. (2001)
Donkeys Oat-straw diet	0.8–1.6	Pearson and Merritt (1991); Pearson et al. (2001)

servations might not be unexpected after a period of feed restriction or when the feed is exceptionally palatable. Typical voluntary intakes of various hays by mature horses were reported at about 2 kg DM/100 kg BW (Dulphy et al., 1997a) and were remarkably similar despite differences in hay nutrient composition (Martin-Rosset and Dulphy, 1987; Dulphy et al., 1997b). Ad libitum-fed legume and grass hays containing 52 percent and 66 percent neutral detergent fiber (NDF), respectively, were consumed at the rate of 2–2.4 kg DM/100 kg BW by both young and mature horses (Martin-Rosset and Dulphy, 1987; Dulphy et al., 1997b). The exceptions were barley straw, whose VDMI by horses was 0.9 kg DM/100 kg BW (Dulphy et al., 1997a); oat straw, whose VDMI by ponies was 2.4 kg DM/100 kg BW (Pearson et al., 2001); and corn silage, which was eaten at the rate of 0.97 kg/100 kg BW (Martin-Rosset and Dulphy, 1987). The low intake of straw by ponies compared to that of alfalfa hay was attributed to an increased mean gastrointestinal particle retention time (Pearson et al., 2001).

Meal length on pasture by feral horses ranged from a few minutes to 13.5 hours (Mayes and Duncan, 1986). The average duration of all hay or straw meals by light horse geldings ranged from 151–188 min/meal (Dulphy et al., 1997a) and was considerably longer than the 21–30.6 minutes that pony mares needed to consume a meal of 60 percent hay–40 percent concentrate chaff or pellets (Argo et al., 2002). The time taken to consume 0.5 g hay/kg BW was 617 seconds; doubling the feeding rate to 1 g/kg BW increased feeding time to 1,065 seconds (Lorenzo-Figueras et al., 2002), whereas the time taken to eat 0.5 g or 1 g grain/kg BW was considerably shorter at 176 and 281 seconds, respectively. The average time taken by mature horses to eat 1 kg of dry hay, moist hay, whole oats, barley, and corn was 36.5, 29.7, 9.3, 9.1, and 13.8 minutes, respectively (Bergero and Nardi, 1996). Crushed or pelleted grains took less time to consume than whole, dry grains.

Meal size and frequency for horses are affected by diet type. Ponies ate a 60 percent grass hay–40 percent concentrate pellet more often (30 meals/d) than the same diet fed as chaff (23.8 meals/d) (Argo et al., 2002). Geldings ate 8.4–13 meals daily consuming 52–1,179 g/meal when fed alfalfa hay, grass hays, or barley straw (Dulphy et al., 1997a). Horses spent an average daily time grazing either a woodland or summer pasture of 938 and 980 minutes, respectively, compared to only 856 minutes eating hay when kept in a drylot (Kondo et al., 1993).

The form and composition of the diet and age of the horse affect bite size, bites/minute, and chews/bite. The relationship between diet type and various eating criteria are given in Table 11-2. Ponies fed a pellet comprised of 60 percent chopped forage (voluntary feed intake [VFI] of 5.1 kg fresh weight/100 kg BW) ate the pellet 54 percent more rapidly than the same diet offered as chaff (Argo et al., 2002). A similar amount of diet was consumed per bite (about 5 g DM/bite), but the number of bites was significantly greater for pellets (5.2 bites/min) than chaff (3.8 bites/min). However, eating chaff required more chews per bite (22.8/min) than pellets (16.1/min), with the result that

TABLE 11-2 Foraging Criteria by Horses Provided Various Feeds

Feed Type	DM Intake (kg/100 kg BW)	Bite or Chew Frequency (bites/min)	DM Intake (g/min)	Reference
60% forage pellet	Variable, maximum 4.5	5.2	26.2	Argo et al. (2002)
60% chaff pellet	Variable, up to 2.2	3.8	17	Argo et al. (2002)
Legume hay	2–2.35		12.6–14.2	Dulphy et al. (1997a)
Grass hay	2–2.43		12.3–14.4	Dulphy et al. (1997a)
Grass hay		4.7–5.5	4.6–5.2	Shingu et al. (2001)
Barley straw	0.91–1.0		7.6–7.9	Dulphy et al. (1997a)
Orchardgrass pasture		11–12	10–12.4	Duren et al. (1989)
Mixed grass pasture	1.54–1.71		7.6–9.9	Mesochina et al. (2000)
Endophyte pasture		16–18		Pfister et al. (2003)
Alfalfa pasture		8		Pfister et al. (2003)
Fresh alfalfa		15	40.4	Gross et al. (1993)
Kentucky bluegrass		30.3–54.1		Kawai et al. (2004b)
Native grass hay and concentrate Pregnant Lactating	1.88 3.13		10.2 15.2	Boulot et al. (1987)
Pellet (50%)–alfalfa chaff (15%)–beet pulp (35%)		77 ± 12.8	147 ± 36.8	Ellis et al. (2005)
Pellet only as above		65 ± 11.6	140 ± 19.4	Ellis et al. (2005)
Trial pellet (TP; 80%)–molasses (10%)– short chopped alfalfa (10%)		69 ± 9.3	161 ± 32.1	Ellis et al. (2005)
TP + 10% chopped straw 2.5 or 4 cm		68 ± 9.2 to 71 ± 8.6	94 ± 15.7 99 ± 19.4	Ellis et al. (2005)
TP + 20% chopped straw 2.5 or 4 cm		66–68 ± 10	75 ± 13.1 77 ± 15.6	Ellis et al. (2005)
TP + 30% chopped straw 2.5 or 4 cm		68 ± 9.1 69 ± 9.7	64 ± 15.2 66 ± 15.4	Ellis et al. (2005)

less chaff DM was eaten per minute (17 g DM) than pellets (26.2 g DM). The applicability of using short chaff (< 2 cm) to slow sweet-feed intake was examined by Harris et al. (2005) who found that the addition of 35 percent chaff to a sweet-feed meal effectively doubled the time to consume the meal, but it also increased the minute intake rate, which may be undesirable.

Bite size and maximal intake rates (g DM/min) increase in proportion to body mass, but grazing rate (min/bite) has similarity irrespective of animal species (Gross et al., 1993). Diet affects bite size and minute intake rates in horses (Duren et al., 1989; Gross et al., 1993; Dulphy et al., 1997a; Shingu et al., 2001; Pfister et al., 2002; Kawai et al., 2004b). Geldings ate about 12.2–14.3 g DM grass or alfalfa hay/min but only 7.6 g DM barley straw/min (Dulphy et al., 1997a). Horses fed straw spent less time eating daily (559–605 min/d) than horses fed hay (748–852 min/d). Consequently, total intake of barley straw was significantly lower than for hay. Lactating mares consumed 15.2 g/min of a hay-concentrate diet compared to 10.2 g/min by pregnant mares (Boulot et al., 1987), likely reflective of the higher energy demands imposed by lactation. These authors observed that lactating mares spent 1,087 ± 105 min/d eating compared to pregnant mares, which spent 944 ± 195 min/d eating. Horses overwintered in paddocks consumed hay at the rate of 4.6–5.2 g DM/bite (Shingu et al., 2001). Bites occurred at the rate of 4.7–5.5 /min with a chewing rate of 64–68. The addition of chopped straw either of 2.5 or 4 cm in length at rates of 10, 20, and 30 percent to a pelleted diet mixed with chopped alfalfa produced no effect on chews/min, increased ($P < 0.001$) time taken to consume 1 kg wet matter and decreased intake rates, but not significantly (Ellis et al., 2005).

Widely divergent minute intake rates are evident for green forage (Table 11-2), which may reflect differences in methodology. Forage biting rates by exercised and nonexercised yearling horses grazing orchardgrass were 11–12/min with a DM intake rate of 0.86 g/bite and a minute intake rate of about 10 g/min (Duren et al., 1989). Forage biting rates decreased over the allotted 3-hour grazing period. Conversely, Kawai et al. (2004b) observed a much higher bite frequency and lower chew rates. Biting rate increased from 30.3 to 54.1 bites/min as sward height of a Kentucky bluegrass pasture decreased with a concomitant reduction in chewing rate from 84.5 to 66.5 times/min. The chewing rate of fresh alfalfa was similar (91 chews/min) (Gross et al., 1993). Horses grazing endophyte-infected forage had more bites/min (16–18) than horses grazing alfalfa (8 bites/ min) (Pfister et al., 2002), which suggests horses do not have the innate ability to discriminate forages that might be potentially harmful.

Animal Factors Affecting Feed Intake

Young horses appear to eat more per unit BW than mature horses (Table 11-1), but feed intake comparisons between young and mature horses may be misleading unless both groups are fed similar diets. Boyd (1988) confirmed that foals from the age of 5 months to the age of 14 months spent more time in feeding activity than mature horses. However, the age-feed intake response of Danish Warmblood weanlings fed a total mixed ration (TMR) varied with energy content of the diet (Sondergaard, 2003). Feed intake of a TMR containing about 1.24 Mcal net energy (NE)/kg DM decreased from about 2 kg/100 kg BW by 5-month-old foals to 1.7 kg/100 kg DM when the foals were 1 year of age. By comparison, 5-month-old foals fed a TMR containing 1.04 Mcal NE/kg DM ate about 1.5 kg DM/100 kg BW, which increased to about 2 kg DM/100 kg BW by 1 year of age. From 16.5 months through 24 months, feed intake decreased from about 2 to 1.8 kg/100 kg BW irrespective of diet caloric content.

Forage eating rates may be breed-related. Hokkaido native horses consumed a similar amount of feed (1.5 kg DM/100 kg BW) over a shorter period of time (6.7 hours) than cross-bred light horses (9.3 hours) (Shingu et al., 2001). Light pregnant mares maintained in straight stalls spent significantly more time eating (57.9 percent of the day) than similarly housed draft mares (50.2 percent) (Flannigan and Stookey, 2001). Yet, the voluntary DM intake of 90 percent hay–10 percent concentrate by pregnant light and heavy mares was similar at 1.73 and 1.82 kg/100 kg BW, respectively (Doreau et al., 1991).

Feeding activity was marginally increased immediately after strenuous exercise, whereas time spent drinking water increased markedly (Caanitz et al., 1991). However, exercise had no long-term impact on time spent eating.

Regulating feed intake in grouped, meal-fed horses presents unique challenges. Herd social orders, as well as variation in appetites and intake rate of individual horses, can cause differences between amounts allotted and amounts actually consumed. Age along with residency time in the herd have been identified as the main factors in the social rank of wild equids and Icelandic horses and was established by biting and/or kicking aggression (Keiper and Receveur, 1992; Sigurjonsdottir et al., 2003; Pluhacek et al., 2006). Horses grazed, ate hay, and rested with preferred individuals when competition for feed was unlimited, but aggressive interaction by horses became evident when feed was limited (Arnold and Grassia, 1982; Wood-Gush and Galbraith, 1987). Pregnant and barren mares typically had at least one partner whose close proximity was tolerated over other horses, whereas mares with foals diverted their social attachment to their offspring (Estep et al., 1993; van Dierendonck et al., 2004). Kinship and familiarity have a significant impact on partner preference and dominance within a herd (Keiper and Sambraus, 1986). Consequently, related horses or horses that have resided together will likely tolerate closer proximity to each other within the feeding area. Hierarchy among horses has been documented (Ellard and Crowell-Davis, 1989; Boyd, 1991), so vigilant oversight of group dynamics is necessary to avoid malnutrition or obesity as a result of submissiveness and dominance in the group structure. Holmes et al. (1987) observed that subordinate horses had an extended latency period (> 200 sec) when eating in close proximity to dominant pen-mates. This behavioral situation was solved by providing a wire partition on the feeders, which allowed subordinate horses to eat while continuously observing their dominant pen-mates. However, isolation of subordinate horses in competitive feeding situations may be contraindicated because horses appear to be stimulated to eat by visual contact of companion horses. Visibility of other horses, particularly in the afternoon, reportedly increased the time spent feeding by pony mares (Sweeting et al., 1985). Houpt and Houpt (1988) confirmed that horses isolated from direct visual contact of others were three times more active and spent 51.5 percent less time eating compared to being housed together or separately but in visual contact of other horses.

Growing horses, exercising horses, pregnant mares, lactating mares, and stallions during the breeding season require more nutrients than horses at maintenance. Heavy or draft horses require more total feed than light horses by virtue of body weight. Lactation increased the voluntary forage intake by 65 percent compared to the same mares during pregnancy (Boulot et al., 1987). Feeding strategies should consider these differences, and farm facilities should separate group-housed horses into different production classes. Use of individual feeding containers may help some horses to consume allotted amounts in group-fed situations. Distance between feeding containers should be determined by observing each group's eating behaviors. Likewise, size of the group-fed herd may need to be reduced to decrease horse density in the eating area and to reduce the time required to deliver the portions to every feeding container. Horses requiring significantly less or more time than the herd's average to consume feeds may need to be fed separately.

Confinement can aggravate dominance behavior in horses. Przewalski's horses kept in a small pen showed a

46–76 percent increase in aggressive behavior (threats, bites, and kicks) compared to horses housed in large paddocks (Hogan et al., 1988). Young or timid horses may be driven away from feed if inadequate feeding space is given. However, spacing feeders at distances ranging from 2.4–9.7 meters had less effect than the arrangement of the feeders (Janicki et al., 1999). Placing feeders in a triangle appeared to improve the feeding opportunities of submissive horses. Dominance behavior should be considered whenever designing feeding arrangements for two or more horses that will be kept in a confined area. To avoid competitive problems among group-fed horses, it may be necessary to increase the availability of feed and/or to increase the feeding area. Timid animals may need to be fed separately but in visual contact of other horses to ensure that sufficient feed is ingested to maintain a satisfactory body weight.

Fever, anorexia, and depression are common signs of illness in all animals (Hart, 1988). The most common recognizable clinical symptom of illness in horses is inappetence. Sick horses eat little or do not eat at all. Usually, horses that reduce their feed intake will also reduce their water intake (see Chapter 7). Dental and head pain have specific behavioral indicators, including altered eating patterns, anorexia, feed refusal, quidding, and food pocketing that may contribute to weight loss (Ashley et al., 2005).

Environmental Effects on Feed Intake

Grazing time can be affected by environmental conditions. High rainfall and high winds resulted in decreased time spent grazing (Rogalski, 1975) as did high temperatures, but increased relative humidity increased grazing time (Rogalski, 1974). Horses spent more time feeding during cold weather and less during hot weather (Booth, 1998). Horses grazing on pastures during a Scottish winter had a higher bite rate (61.4 vs. 52.4/min), step rate (6.7 vs. 4.2 steps/min), and step distance (0.058 vs. 0.021 m/step), but fewer bites/step (10 vs. 12) than in summer (Booth, 1998). Snowfall at sub-zero temperatures typically did not disrupt feeding if supplementary feed was available, but shelter-seeking behavior occurred when cold weather was coupled with wind (Booth, 1998). Where winter grazing is practiced, the impact of snow on feed intake is related to the depth of the snow cover. Horses grazing on pastures with 20 cm of snow reduced daily grazing time to 416 min/d and reduced DM intake to 2.1 kg/100 kg BW compared to the 544 min/d spent grazing on nonsnowy pastures and intakes of 2.7 kg/100 kg BW on nonsnowy pasture (Kawai et al., 2004a). The decreased DE intake created by snow on pastures resulted in weight loss of the horses. Horses generally seek out areas with less snow cover because deep snow (40–50 cm) required 10 times the activity in pawing ("cratering") compared to that needed to uncover grass with a light snow cover (10 cm) (Salter and Hudson, 1979). Pawing through snow cover for feed has a high energy cost. The combination of this added work to get feed and the poor nutritional quality of the feed under snow underscores the need to monitor horses daily on winter pastures and to provide supplementary hay (and perhaps grain) when needed (see Chapter 12, Feeding Management of Horses in Cold or Hot Weather).

Horses graze in a diurnal pattern with an early morning and dusk component (Salter and Hudson, 1979; Duncan et al., 1984; Crowell-Davis et al., 1985; Berger et al., 1999). Peak feeding by pastured Welsh ponies occurred between 5:00 to 9:00 am then again at dusk from 5:00 to 9:00 pm (Crowell-Davis et al., 1985). Natural patterns of feeding are modified in modern husbandry systems of confinement and restricted feed access. Horses kept in a drylot and fed orchardgrass hay spent 90 percent more time lying down (63 min/d vs. 33 min/d) and spent 8–12 percent less time feeding than horses grazing similar pastures (Kondo et al., 1993).

Seasonal changes in ambient temperature and day length altered the absolute ultradian and daily patterns (Berger et al., 1999). In French wetland pastures, grazing by barren mares occurred principally (74 percent) at night (Fleurance et al., 2001) and grazing time was generally greatest in spring and autumn (Rogalski, 1975). Fleurance et al. (2001) reported horses spent 12 and 16 hours grazing in summer and autumn respectively, while Kaseda (1983) found that horses grazed less in winter than summer. During warm weather in summer, horses increased the time spent standing (Berger, 1977; Booth, 1998). Lactating pony mares reduced feeding activity in summer, typically spending more time resting in the shade during late mornings and afternoons (Crowell-Davis et al., 1985). Camargue and Przewalski's horses rested during peak heat periods of the day, and any grazing during the heat of the day was considered atypical and was concluded to be an indicator of undernourishment (Mayes and Duncan, 1986; Klimov, 1988). Rainfall did not significantly affect foraging by Camargue horses, but horses spent more time in standing rest and less time lying down (Duncan, 1985).

Infestations of mosquitoes, ticks, horseflies, and other external parasites disrupt feeding activities of horses. Horses reduced the length of feeding bouts when biting flies were active (Mayes and Duncan, 1986) and shifted feeding activities to periods of the day when lower ambient temperature reduced irritating insects (Duncan, 1985). Insect activity was positively related to ambient temperature but decreased with wind speed (Keiper and Berger, 1982). During periods of high fly activity (typically from 10:00 am to 4:00 pm), Assateague ponies spent time on beaches or dunes and reduced feeding activity by 11–16 percent compared to other periods of the day (Keiper and Berger, 1982). By comparison, feral horses in mountainous areas moved to higher elevations and stood in snow patches to avoid flies. Booth (1998) reported that Exmoor ponies preferred to stand on bare ground when Tabanids (horse flies) were active, which reduced their time spent grazing. The nuisance effect of flies, ticks, and lice on feeding behavior of horses, and associated weight loss, can result in large economic costs associated with unthriftiness, reproductive failure, and disease (Steelman, 1976). Insect annoyance should always be considered as a potential cause of weight loss when pasture quality is not a contributing cause.

Feed Effects on Feeding Behavior

Orosensory sensations are equated to palatability, which has been defined as the smell, texture, and taste characteristics of a feed that determines its rate of intake (Dulphy et al., 1997a). Coarseness and brittleness are examples of textures that can negatively affect hay intake by horses. Textures can be altered by feed processing, which can lead to very different feed intakes (Haelein et al., 1966; Hintz et al., 1985). Flavorings and sweeteners have been used to increase feed intake by horses (Goodwin et al., 2005b). The impact of physical forms of feed, criteria of feed quality, and chemical/physical properties of grasses, hays, and pastures on feed intake are discussed elsewhere in this publication (Chapters 8 and 14).

As indicated above, horses prefer certain pastures, hays, and grains, but they also appear to like variety in their diet as evidenced by the wide range of forages consumed by feral horses (Salter and Hudson, 1979). Feeding preferences exist for forages and roughages (Archer, 1978a; Carson and Wood-Gush, 1983). Although constant feeding of the same diet may help reduce digestive problems (Lewis, 1995), it may also lead to long-term monotony, which may lower feed intake and contribute to abnormal stall behaviors (McGreevy et al., 1995a). Long-term monotony may have caused stall-housed horses to reject hay they had previously preferred in favor of other roughage choices (Goodwin et al., 2002; Thorne et al., 2005). In these studies, horses provided with an array of forage choices reduced their bedding intake, and increased the time and frequency of foraging activity.

Horses become accustomed to the tastes and textures of feeds to which they are exposed during growth, i.e., a learned behavior. Horses born and raised in upstate New York preferred oats over corn and corn over barley (Hawkes et al., 1985), but in western Canada, where horses are rarely exposed to whole or cracked corn, oats were the most preferred grain but barley was preferred over corn (Cymbaluk, 1983). For this reason, horses that have been recently moved to a new region may reject local feeds. Knowing the types and preferences of feeds the horse received at its previous stable and supplying similar feeds can help ease the transition of the horse to its new environment. Horses may need a period of adaptation before they accept novel feeds.

Sucrose and other sweeteners and flavorings are added to improve intake of feed by horses by taste alone or to mask distasteful feeds. Adding even small amounts (2 percent) of sucrose to oats increased the quantity of oats eaten by ponies compared to plain oats, as did the addition of 2.5 percent molasses for four of five ponies (Hintz, 1980; Hawkes et al., 1985). The authors reported that 67 percent of the test ponies preferred oats with 10 percent sucrose compared to plain oats or oats with 2 percent sucrose. Horses also preferred the taste of sugar solutions to plain water (Randall et al., 1978). Sidedness or handedness, i.e., preference for eating grain from the left or right hand side of the manger, was observed in one of six ponies (Hintz, 1980) and has been confirmed by others (Bottom et al., 2004), who found that older horses had a stronger side preference than younger horses.

Hawkes et al. (1985) also tested the preferences of other feed ingredients and their threshold acceptability. A basal mixed feed was preferred to the same feed to which 20 percent blood meal, meat and bone meal, or beet pulp were added, whereas 20 percent alfalfa meal and 5 or 10 percent meat and bone meal additions were equally palatable to the ponies as the basal mix.

Ponies preferred a basal mixed feed with 20 percent added dry distillers' grains over the basal diet (Hawkes et al., 1985), yet the substitution of dry wheat distillers' grain for a cereal-based concentrate in increments of 25 percent reduced intake and the rate of ingestion by horses in a near linear fashion (Hill, 2002). Intakes were based on access of horses to 1-kg concentrate mixture over 10 minutes and, thus, this study did not evaluate whether the horses would consume the mix over an extended period. Nevertheless, acceptance of the distillers' grain did not appear to occur over time. Soaking the concentrate with water lowered palatability of the basal concentrate, which was further reduced when distillers' grains were added, thus resulting in a lowered feed intake (Hill, 2002).

Fats have been added to horse diets to increase energy supply and added in smaller amounts to reduce feed dustiness. At the concentrations needed to influence energy intake, flavor of oil/fat may influence feed intake. Horses fed diets to which various oils and fats had been added preferred diets containing only added corn oil (Holland et al., 1998). Diets to which peanut, safflower, cottonseed, or mixtures of either corn oil, soy, or corn lecithin were added to either corn or soy oil, various animal-vegetable oil blends, fancy bleached tallow, hydrolyzed tallow flakes, or inedible tallow were eaten less well. Horses rejected inedible tallow and fancy bleached tallow diets. Horses fed diets containing 10 percent corn oil, corn oil–soy lecithin, or soy lecithin–soy oil consumed all of the diets well and showed reduced reactivity to a startle test compared to horses fed a control diet of chopped hay–concentrate (Holland et al., 1996).

Flavorings and additives are occasionally used to mask unpalatable ingredients or to enhance intake of livestock feeds (Kunkle et al., 1997). Garlic, an additive in pet diets, increased the concentrate intake by horses when added at the rate of 1.5–3 g/kg (Horton et al., 1990). Garlic apparently has moderate palatability to horses but has been consumed in amounts causing toxicosis (Pearson et al., 2005). These authors reported that horses that voluntarily ate more than 0.25 g/kg BW freeze-dried garlic twice daily developed Heinz body anemia. The amounts of garlic typically added to concentrate mixtures are considerably below this amount.

Preference and foraging studies in which horses were offered four low-energy concentrate mixes showed that horses would eat some feed from each container, but tended to eat more of a high-fiber concentrate than mixes with a lower fiber content (Goodwin et al., 2005a). Adding flavors and sweeteners to the diet altered concentrate preferences. Horses provided with an array of concentrates ate more often, had shorter eating bouts, and collectively ate longer each day than those offered only one concentrate. The correct combination of garlic, flavorings, and sweeteners appeared key to whether horses rejected or preferred a diet (Goodwin et al., 2005a). In some combinations, horses ate more of the seasoned feed; other combinations were less popular. Mint-flavored diets were preferred over garlic-flavored diets when added to pelleted grain with the same energy content (Cairns et al., 2002). However, when the energy content of the pellet was varied, the high-energy diets, which contained 20 percent more dietary energy than the low-energy pellets, were preferred irrespective of flavor added. Under the conditions of the study, the associated hay was high quality. Whether the preferences would hold true if low-quality hay had been provided was not examined.

In a subsequent study, Goodwin et al. (2005b) examined the effect of 15 flavorings on consumption of 100 g of cereal byproduct. These authors found that the flavored byproduct was eaten well in most cases and that preferences of the top eight flavorings were fenugreek > banana > cherry > rosemary > cumin > carrot > peppermint > oregano. When the consumption rate of unflavored mineral pellets was compared to banana- and fenugreek-flavored pellets, the flavored pellets were eaten at rates 3 to 3.75 times more rapidly. This supports the observation that horses accept variety in their diet. Although these data suggest that flavorings stimulate intake of certain feeds by horses, flavorings should be added judiciously. Horses naïve to certain feed flavors and textures may require gradual exposure to a flavored diet.

Feed Contaminants and Taste Aversions

Taste aversion of feeds is a learned behavior, occurring when horses become sick immediately after feed is consumed but not if illness is delayed (Houpt et al., 1990). Horses exposed to feed contaminated with monensin, an ionophore toxic to horses, became anorexic or ate the diet reluctantly after an initial exposure (Matsuoka et al., 1996). Similarly, horses reduced their intakes of mycotoxin-contaminated feed. Horses ate about one-third of a grain mix (1 kg/d) contaminated with 14 µg/kg deoxynivalenol, 0.7 µg/kg 15-acetyldeoxynivalenol, 6.4 µg/kg fusaric acid, and 2 µg/kg zearalenone compared to horses fed uncontaminated grain (2.8 kg/d) (Raymond et al., 2003). Intake of the contaminated feed did not increase over a period of 3 weeks so adaptation did not occur. Continued reluctance to eat any feed should always be investigated.

Aversion learning, however, is limited in horses. With a few exceptions, horses given lithium-chloride by stomach-tube, which causes nausea, could be taught to avoid eating locoweed under hay-fed and grazing conditions (Pfister et al., 2002). However, horses grazing early pastures contaminated with spotted locoweed were unable to discriminate between nontoxic plants and locoweed (Pfister et al., 2003). In fact, horses ate more bites of locoweed (toxic component, swainsone) than cattle, resulting in high serum swainsone concentrations and, ultimately, depression and anorexia, signs indicative of clinical swainsone toxicity (Pfister et al., 2003). Although horses are selective grazers, they differ in their ability to discriminate between normal and toxic weeds (Marinier and Alexander, 1992). Pony mares fed pelleted rations comprised of 45 to 60 percent perennial ryegrass contaminated with *Penicillium cyclopium* continued to eat the diet despite development of neurological signs of ryegrass staggers (Blythe and Holtan, 1983). Therefore, innate intelligence should not be relied on to prevent ingestion of toxic plants or contaminated diets.

Adult horses appear to have an aversion to eating grass that has been contaminated by equine feces (Odberg and Francis-Smith, 1977). Horses restricted to pastures may perform "latrine" behavior whereby they graze and defecate in separate areas. This behavior produces a pasture containing "roughs and lawns," in which the "lawn" areas are preferentially grazed and the toilet areas are comparatively lightly grazed, leading to rank overgrowth of pasture (Odberg and Francis-Smith, 1976). However, horses accepted grass cut from roughs as long as no feces were present, indicating an aversion to feces rather than the herbage in roughs per se (Odberg and Francis-Smith, 1977). Horses have been reported to reject pastures where feces have contacted the grass for longer than 24 hours (Archer, 1978b), despite the greater canopy growth in latrine areas compared to those in noncontaminated areas (Loucougaray et al., 2004).

It has been suggested that such a grazing pattern reduces the parasite load to the grazed areas by spatial separation of feeding and defecating areas (Taylor, 1954). However, Fleurance et al. (2001) proposed that this behavior resulted in a constantly producing vegetative regrowth with greater nutritional value in the grazed area than that of more mature ungrazed forage in the rough latrine areas. However, with time, some nutrients, particularly potassium and phosphorous, may become deficient in lawns through their gradual transfer to the roughs in the feces (Archer, 1973; Odberg and Francis-Smith, 1977). Truly free-ranging horses, however, may not have latrine behavior and tend to defecate where they graze (Lamoot et al., 2004). Defecations and urinations by mares in a grazing area were positively correlated to grazing time. That is, if horses grazed in an area for a long time, they also soiled the area more often. In grazed pastures, latrine areas can occupy from 30 percent of wetland pastures to 89 percent of flatland pastures (Loucougaray et al., 2004). Thus, horses have no conception that they are contaminating the pasture they will have to eat. Therefore, efficient management of small pastures may require removal or harrowing of feces on a regular basis to prevent rejection of the pasture.

UNUSUAL ORAL BEHAVIOR

Coprophagy, Geophagia, and Wood-Chewing

Unusual oral behaviors include coprophagy, geophagia, and wood-chewing that are not defined as stereotypic behaviors because they appear to represent a normal physiological or foraging response (Francis-Smith and Wood-Gush, 1977; Salter and Hudson, 1979; Crowell-Davis and Houpt, 1985; Mills et al., 2005). Coprophagy, or feces eating, is an apparently normal activity of foals as young as 5 days of age extending to about 2 months of age (Francis-Smith and Wood-Gush, 1977; Crowell-Davis and Houpt, 1985). Typically, the foal consumes its dam's feces, but occasionally the foal may eat its own feces or that of an unrelated adult. Under controlled, stall-housing conditions, coprophagy occurred infrequently, once every 20.6 hours, (Crowell-Davis and Caudle, 1989), but under grazing situations, eating of feces occurred on average every 4.3 hours for the first 2 months of age (Crowell-Davis and Houpt, 1985). Thereafter, as the foal matured, the occurrence of feces-eating declined and was rarely seen by 6 months of age (Crowell-Davis and Houpt, 1985). The purpose of coprophagy has been speculated to be a mechanism of populating the neonatal gut with bacteria and protozoa (Crowell Davis and Houpt, 1985), but an alternative hypothesis has been proposed that foals eat feces to learn feed preferences (Marinier and Alexander, 1995). No nutrient motivation has been identified for feces consumption by foals, but mature horses that eat feces were suggested to lack sufficient feed, fiber, or other nutrients (Feist and McCullough, 1976). The latter claims have been poorly researched, but several studies have reported consumption of feces when alternative feeds (whole corn plant, ryegrass straw) were fed either as pellets, as cubes, or in long form at intakes below 1.3 kg/100 kg BW/d (Schurg et al., 1977; Schurg et al., 1978). Subnormal protein intakes existed in the latter study, which confounded the interpretation of which stimulus initiated the coprophagy.

Geophagia or dirt-eating is not uncommon in feral and domesticated horses (Salter and Hudson, 1979; McGreevy et al., 2001; Weise and Lieb, 2001; Husted et al., 2005). In feral horses, soil-licking was felt to be a method of acquiring salt (Salter and Hudson, 1979), although this has not been further studied. In domesticated horses, geophagia occurred in clinically normal horses that had access to mineral mixes (54 percent) and/or access to supplementary feed (71 percent) (McGreevy et al., 2001). Soil iron and copper in licked soils were higher, but the mineral concentration among and between licked and unlicked soils was so widely variable that it suggests that geophagia may not be a simple pursuit for trace minerals.

Although dirt-eating is generally innocuous, consumption of sandy soil can cause colic or diarrhea (Bertone et al., 1988; Husted et al., 2005). Sand-eating has been estimated to cause up to 30 percent of colic cases, particularly in regions with sandy soils such as the southern United States (Lieb and Weise, 1999). These authors found that feeding concentrate on sand resulted in inadvertent sand consumption by horses, whereas feeding hay on sand resulted in little to no sand intake. Subsequently, Weise and Lieb (2001) evaluated the effect of feeding a low-protein diet (70 percent of basal requirements), a low-energy diet (75 percent of basal requirements), and a combination low energy–low protein diet on sand intake. No differences were found in sand intake when energy or protein intakes were below requirements. However, horse effects were highly significant ($P < 0.001$). That is, some horses were prone to eating sand, whereas others were not. Although mineral intake also varied among horses, the amount of mineral consumed was unrelated to sand intake. In a Danish study that evaluated sand intake by Icelandic horses, Husted et al. (2005) identified both soil type and pasture quality as important variables in sand-eating. Feeding horses off the ground when pastures were sparse or had no grass increased the probability of detecting sand in the feces. The authors also noted a trend for thinner and younger horses to have detectable amounts of sand in their feces. This study supported the recommendation that horses kept in outdoor paddocks with sparse or little grass growth should only be fed from cribs or hay racks.

Wood-chewing occurs in stabled and free-living horses in which the horse gnaws on fencing, trees, or any similar wooden object and either discards or swallows bits of wood. Bark-eating has been reported to be not uncommon in feral horses (Ashton, 2005), and about one-third of young Thoroughbreds chewed wood (Waters et al., 2002), which has led to the assessment that this oral behavior may be a normal, functional foraging behavior (Mills et al., 2005). Most often, wood-chewing has an economic rather than a clinical impact, but Nicol (1998) reported that wood-chewing appeared to precede cribbing in some horses and infrequently causes small intestinal obstruction due to wood splinters (Green and Tong, 1988).

Although the incidence of wood-chewing in foals was as high as 30 percent (Waters et al., 2002), pastured or stabled horses wood-chewed only 5.1 and 8.1 percent, respectively (Pell and McGreevy, 1999). The inciting causes of wood-chewing in horses are many and varied. Wood-chewing increased during inclement weather (Jackson et al., 1985), when diets were limit-fed, processed, or low in fiber content (Haelein et al., 1966; Krzak et al., 1991; Johnson et al., 1998), during confinement (Krzak et al., 1991; Boyd, 1991), and after weaning (Waters et al., 2002). High-concentrate diets or pelleted feeds increased wood-chewing activity compared to horses fed long hay (Haelein et al., 1966; Willard et al., 1977; Marsden, 1993; McGreevy et al., 1995a). High-starch (concentrate) intakes have also been implicated in aggressive behavior when feeding horses, which was eliminated by feeding at least 1 kg hay/100 kg BW (Zeyner et al., 2004). Jackson et al. (1985) fed mature Quarter horse mares either long alfalfa hay twice daily or cubed alfalfa hay two and three times per day at the rate of 2.5 kg/100 kg BW/d and found no difference in the amount of wood chewed but noted a correlation of wood-chewing with inclement weather. During periods of cold, wet weather (−2.6°C and 39.8 cm rain), wood-chewing increased in the mares compared to periods of warm, dry weather (9.8°C and 0.4 cm rain).

Horses fed long hay either ad libitum or in amounts to provide 100 percent of maintenance energy requirements spent 58–64 percent of their normal daily budget eating and showed few abnormal behaviors (0–2 percent) (Marsden, 1993). Feeding pelleted or processed feeds reduced the time spent eating to 10–12 percent of the day with a concurrent increase to 58–66 percent of time spent in abnormal behaviors. Similarly, Houpt et al. (2004) reported that horses fed hay spent 50 percent of their daily time budget eating compared to only 10 percent when pellets were fed. Horses fed hay chewed 40,000 times per day compared to 10,000 times per day for pellet-fed horses. In this study, motivation for forage or pellets was tested when pellets were fed or when hay was fed. The number of presses for pellets when hay was fed had a median number of 25 compared to 12 presses for hay when horses were fed the pelleted diet. These data suggest that horses are motivated for variety but also for forage when pellets are fed, and for pellets when forage is fed.

Feeding high amounts of concentrates or processed diets stimulates wood-chewing activity. Willard et al. (1977) observed a 5-fold increase in wood-chewing by concentrate-fed horses compared to hay-fed horses, which was accompanied by a reduction in post-feeding cecal pH from 6.97 in hay-fed horses to 6.64 in concentrate-fed horses. The wood-chewing activity may have been related to the decrease in cecal pH but may have also been a response to a low-fiber intake. Similarly, a dramatic increase was observed in wood-chewing and eating of bedding after the diet was gradually increased in grain over a 4-week period to account for 75 percent of the total diet (Johnson et al., 1998). Wood-chewing occurred in 30 percent of weaned foals by 30 weeks of age, and a higher incidence was observed in foals born to dominant mares and confined to barns or stables at weaning (Waters et al., 2002). Lack of exercise increased wood-chewing several-fold in yearling horses fed principally pelleted feeds (Krzak et al., 1991). Weanlings confined to stables showed increased behavioral abnormalities such as cribbing, box-walking, and wood-chewing compared to weanlings kept in paddocks (Waters et al., 2002). Use of a high-fat and high-fiber supplement at weaning appeared to relax the foals compared to those fed a high-sugar and high-starch concentrate (Redgate et al., 2004). However, the durability of the behavioral effect of a high-fat and high-fiber diet to prevent wood-chewing has not yet been reported. The best predictor of wood-chewing has been reported to be roughage intake (Mills et al., 2005), which implies that to minimize wood-chewing, an adequate supply of roughage should be available to the horse.

Cribbing

Stable vices or stereotypies are defined as apparently functionless, repetitive behaviors and include cribbing (crib-biting), weaving, and stall-walking (Nicol, 1998; Mills et al., 2005). Detailed descriptions of these conditions can be found in McGreevy (2004) and Mills et al. (2005). The incidence of stereotypic behavior and factors associated in their occurrence were established in part by using research surveys (Vecchiotti and Galanti, 1986; McGreevy et al., 1995a,b; Luescher et al., 1998; Pell and McGreevy, 1999; McBride and Long, 2001), which have led to some conflicting conclusions due to unavoidable confounding of data collected on horses located in different geographies, in various athletic or nonathletic disciplines, fed varying diets, and kept under a wide range of environmental conditions. Controlled studies have also produced conflicting outcomes, but the important contribution made by behavioral research has been the increased awareness of the complexity of stereotypical and/or normal feeding behavior of horses. As a result, many of the interventions once used to arrest stereotypic behavior, such as punishment or physical prevention, have been recognized to be mostly ineffective and potentially detrimental to the horse's welfare, especially if no attempt has been made to resolve the instigating cause (Cooper and Mason, 1998; McGreevy and Nicol, 1998a,b; Nicol, 1998; McBride and Cuddeford, 2001; Mills et al., 2005).

Cribbing or crib-biting, stall-walking, and weaving are stereotypies that may have a breed, function, environmental, feed management, age, or disease condition (Vecchiotti and Galanti, 1986; Luescher et al., 1998; Bachman et al., 2003; Archer et al., 2004; Nicol et al., 2005; Mills et al., 2005). Based on a survey of trainers, Vecchiotti and Galanti (1986) reported a 7.4 percent cribbing incidence in Thoroughbred horses with a higher than usual prevalence in some families that suggested a hereditary predisposition to cribbing. Luescher et al. (1998), using survey data obtained from pleasure horse and racehorse stables, found a cribbing incidence of 5.1–5.5 percent in pleasure and Thoroughbred horses but no reports of cribbing in Standardbred horses. A similar incidence of cribbing (5.5 percent) was reported in young racehorses (McGreevy et al., 1995a) and in young Thoroughbreds (10.5 percent) (Waters et al., 2002). The athletic pursuits of dressage, eventing, and endurance created risks of having abnormal oral or locomotory behaviors at a prevalence rate of 32.5, 30.8, and 19.5 percent, respectively (McGreevy et al., 1995b). The time spent in the stable, not the activity, contributed to the abnormal behavior. However, the frequency of turnout or type of exercise did not affect cribbing occurrence in pleasure or racehorses (Luescher et al., 1998). Moreover, Marsden (1993) concluded that housing method, whether pasture, box stalls, or tie stalls, had little effect on eliciting abnormal behaviors, but that the form of the diet clearly affected behavior.

Mares were less likely than stallions or geldings to crib, and risk of cribbing increased with age (Luescher et al., 1998). However, wood-chewing and cribbing behaviors have been observed early in life, and 9.7 percent of preweaned foals and 22.5 percent of post-weaned foals were reported to have these behaviors (Nicol and Badnell-Waters, 2005). Post-weaned foals fed concentrate had a 4-fold increased risk of becoming cribbers (Waters et al., 2002), and cribbing foals had a higher incidence of gastric ulceration than non-cribbing foals (Nicol et al., 2002). Nicol and Badnell-Waters (2005) observed that foals that developed abnormal oral behavior preweaning had more fragmented suckling intervals and spent more time bunting, whereas those that developed cribbing behavior postweaning spent 44.8 percent more time suckling and nuzzling than foals with no abnormal behavior. The authors suggested that the extended suckling activity may have occurred in response to a developing gastric problem or due to insufficient milk supply from the dam. As a consequence, it was predicted that hungry foals offered creep feed might consume more concentrate feed resulting in the gastric pathology that may stimulate cribbing. Murray (1997) reported that 50 percent of foals have gastric ulcers during the 1st month of life, a time period when gastric epithelium is in rapid development. The use of antacids in some foals not only improved gastric ulceration, but also reduced or removed the abnormal oral behavior (Nicol et al., 2002). Thus, feed management such as use of a concentrate-based creep feed might aggravate an existing ulcerative condition or predispose the foal to gastric ulceration, thereby leading to abnormal oral behavior.

Wood-chewing and cribbing have been associated with a lack of fiber or roughage. In addition to low-fiber intake, physiological changes in the gut, including a more acidic stomach pH (Lillie et al., 2003), cecal acidity (Willard et al., 1977), and fecal acidity (Nicol et al., 2002) in cribbing horses, have been implicated in these oral behaviors. Cribbing horses had a gastric pH of 3.3 compared to normal horses whose stomach acidity was 5.5 (Lillie et al., 2003). Prevention of cribbing using a cribbing collar eliminated the drop in stomach pH (pH 5.5) seen in horses that continued to crib (pH 3.3) (Lillie et al., 2003). Cribbing horses have a low basal saliva production, and it has been postulated that the cribbing stimulated the production of saliva (Nicol, 1998). McCall et al. (2001) confirmed the lower saliva production by cribbing horses compared to normal horses but suggested that cribbing did not produce sufficient excess saliva to effectively buffer the stomach or gastrointestinal tract acidity. Antacid therapy has been used to ameliorate gastric acidity and cribbing in some horses (Nicol et al., 2002; Mills and Macleod, 2002), but this outcome may be inconstant. Garcia et al. (2005) found that antacid therapy reduced gastric acidity in cribbing horses, but had no effect on cribbing duration or frequency (Garcia et al., 2005). Overall, these studies suggest that high-concentrate diets may contribute to cribbing in predisposed horses by creating an acidic gastrointestinal tract.

Feeding less than 6.8 kg forage/d and feeding hay rather than providing pasture increased the risk of wood-chewing and cribbing (McGreevy et al., 1995a). Feeding only one type of forage induced stereotypic behavior in horses that showed no such behavior when fed a choice of hays (Thorne et al., 2005). Feeding forage three times daily increased cribbing relative to feeding hay twice daily or feeding more often than three times per day (McGreevy et al., 1995a). Bachman et al. (2003) identified a risk for cribbing associated with feeding more than four times per day. Evidently, there are confounding factors that influence how feed management contributes to stereotypic behavior.

Cooper et al. (2005) observed that all horses, whether prone to stereotypic behavior or not, showed more stereotypic behavior as feeding frequencies of grain increased from two, to four, to six times per day. Although high-concentrate diets were implicated as a potential cause of cribbing (Cooper et al., 2005), cribbers spent the same amount of time eating as normal horses but displaced resting time with cribbing activity (McGreevy and Nicol, 1998b). Cribbers fed hay had similar concentrations of β-endorphin to noncribbing horses, whereas concentrate-fed cribbers had β-endorphin concentrations less than half of those found in normal horses (Gillham et al., 1994). This suggests that cribbing may have a neurochemical origin in addition to the predisposition that may arise through nutritional management. Mills et al. (2005) recommended the following nutritional methods for prevention of cribbing: avoid creep feeding preweaning, minimize concentrates, supplement with antacid, or manage horses on pasture. Slightly different management techniques have been posited by McBride and Long (2001), including increasing the hay ration, feeding the affected horse before other horses, reducing the time the horse spends in the stable, increasing its exercise, increasing social contact, and using stable chain instead of a solid door so that the horse has a varied view from its stall. The practicality of these management tools may be difficult to implement in many parts of the world where feeding practices based on high-concentrate diets have been engrained or are necessary. Data are not necessarily available to support these recommendations and the percentage of horses that might respond to these interventions is unknown.

GENERAL FEEDING CONSIDERATIONS

The goal of feeding management is to efficiently supply dietary ingredients in amounts that will meet the horse's nutrient needs, while still retaining the horse's normal feeding behavior as discussed above. Meeting a horse's dietary nutrient needs requires awareness of practices that manage feed intake and dietary ingredients that are safe, efficiently utilized sources of nutrients.

Horses are fed a variety of diets, ranging from continuous access to forage (e.g., pasture) to high amounts of concentrates. The type of diets fed, housing of horses, and how the feeding plan integrates with other routine management practices influences feeding management routines. Meal feeding of high-energy concentrate feeds requires intense management and a large amount of control, which routinely necessitates individually housing horses during feeding periods. Horses fed solely forage-based diets are felt to have a safer, more predictable feed intake because gutfill limitations will precede the physiological controls of energy intake that control satiety in horses fed high amounts of concentrate.

Regardless of feeding system used, there are several management principles that support efficient, healthy utilization of diets. The first important factor in managing nutrient intake is to provide ingredients that supply a nutritionally balanced diet and to provide nutrients in amounts that meet or marginally exceed nutrient requirements for the class of horse in question. Pasture should be managed to supply utilizable nutrients in amounts aligned with the horse needs. Prepared mixes should be nutritionally balanced to meet needs of specific classes of horses, when fed as the complete nutrient source or as a supplement to an expected daily intake of long-stem forage. As noted in Chapter 14, ration balancing requires knowledge of requirements, nutrient content of feedstuffs, feeding strategies, and physiology of horses. Common errors of on-site formulation or supplementation include making adjustments without knowledge of the horse's nutrient requirements or expected intakes, supplementing without knowing the amounts of nutrients already supplied by the diet, adding ingredients with little or no nutritional value, and creating dietary imbalances by adjusting for a single nutrient with a feedstuff or supplement that contains other nutrients.

Feeding by weight of feedstuffs rather than volume is recommended because of variation in the density of feeds (see Chapter 8). As most feeding routines use volume to apportion diets, it is recommended to schedule periodic checks by weighing allotted amounts. This is especially important when there are changes with feed sources or with the personnel assigned to feeding.

Changes in the amount given or in the physical form of dietary ingredients should be implemented gradually. This practice allows the digestive tract time to adapt to different levels and forms of diet, and it is especially important when feeding energy-dense diets. Large increases in daily concentrate intakes should occur in increments over a period of several days to weeks. Although there was no experimental evidence cited, Lewis (1995) suggested that mature horses should only be fed in increments of 0.2–0.3 kg concentrate per day to allow the horse sufficient time to adapt to concentrate. For similar reasons, horses should be introduced to lush, nutrient-dense pastures by limit-grazing for several days.

Reducing the rate of feed intake may be desirable if horses tend to bolt feed and to reduce competition in group-fed horses. Methods that have been recommended to slow feed intake in fast-eating horses include spreading grain out in shallow troughs, placing several large stones in the feed trough requiring the horse to eat around them, or using spaced bars or feeding rings to partially limit access to the feed trough. Processing method also affects rate of intake (see Chapter 8), so moving from pelleted to textured or extruded forms of concentrates (Hintz et al., 1985) or adding long-stem forage or short, chopped chaff (2–5 cm) can be beneficial (Harris et al., 2005; Ellis et al., 2005).

Meal Feeding Concentrates

Voluntary intake in horses appears to be influenced by a number of factors, including weather, palatability of feed, interaction with other horses, and energy intake (see above). Regardless, if allowed free access to unlimited amounts, horses may consume enough starchy, nonfibrous carbohydrates to cause digestive upset, colic, and/or laminitis (see specific disease entity in Chapter 12).

Horses efficiently digest starch. Research trials cited in Chapters 1, 2, and 8 have shown nearly 100 percent total tract digestion of starch. Prececal digestion of starch is at best a constant percent of ration as intake of starch is increased (Hinkle et al., 1983). The more starch fed, the more will be presented to the microbes of the cecum and colon, and the more digested by these microbes. Significant levels of starch in the hindgut may cause short- and long-term changes in the microbial populations, decrease intestinal pH, disrupt normal gut motility, cause shifts in water absorption, result in a build-up of toxins, and consequentially increase the incidence of laminitis and colic (Garner et al., 1978; Goodson et al., 1988; de Fombelle et al., 2004).

With the noted ill consequences of overfeeding starch, it is advantageous to determine what levels can be fed safely in a meal-feeding system. Trials done with different sizes of horses and ponies ingesting different levels of starch suggest that single meal starch intakes over 0.2 to 0.4 percent of body weight greatly increase the amount of starch presented to the cecum and large intestine (Potter et al., 1992; Meyer et al., 1993; Kienzle, 1994).

The level of starch in different feeds can vary greatly; however, typical grain-based mixes may contain as much as 30–50 percent starch (see Chapter 2). If meals are distributed to maximize the time between feedings, confining single meal intakes of a concentrate containing these amounts of starch to below 0.5–0.6 percent of body weight per day should safely limit the meal-fed intake of starch. Those horses prone to digestive or metabolic dysfunction associated with starch intakes should be restricted below the upper limit of a single meal of starch at 0.2–0.4 percent of body weight (see Chapter 8). High-quality forage diets and diets containing significant amounts of digestible fiber and added fat reduce the need for starch as an energy source. Individual horse responses to meal-fed concentrates will vary, and additional influences such as rate of flow of ingesta, processing of feedstuffs, and addition of feedstuffs such as long-stem and chopped forage will alter the suggested recommendation for limiting starch levels of meals, as well as the amounts fed per meal and the meal frequency.

Increased intake resulting from the feeding of low-energy-dense, high-fiber feedstuffs decreases the total tract mean retention time (Cuddeford et al., 1995; Drogoul et al., 2001). Slowing the rate of flow of nutrients through the small intestine by feeding less hay or indigestible dry matter with high-starch feedstuffs may increase prececal starch digestion (Meyer et al., 1993; Yoder et al., 1997). The transit rate of high-fiber feedstuffs through the small intestine has been shown to be faster than when feeding similarly processed levels of high-starch feedstuffs (Varloud et al., 2004). Even so, starch disappearance in the small intestine may not be affected with differences in transit rate (Varloud et al., 2004).

Altering the relative proportions of hay and grain and the feeding frequency may affect prececal starch digestion. Using the mobile-bag technique, de Fombelle et al. (2004) fed high-fiber or high-starch pellets with hay in two different feeding patterns. Similar rations were offered five times daily, alternating proportionate amounts of pellets and hay over a 12-h period, or three times daily by feeding two-thirds of the pellets in the morning, all the hay 4 hours following, and the remaining pellets at the end of the 12-hour period. Transit time through the small intestine was faster when the diets were fed five times per day; however, small intestine dry matter disappearance was higher when the rations were split into five meals. Starch disappearance in the small intestine was not affected by the two different feeding patterns. Prececal starch disappearance was most affected by the botanical source of starch.

Starch digestion in the small intestine is dependent on the action of the pancreatic enzyme, α-amylase. Addition of supplemental amylase enzyme from bacterial sources has been shown to increase small intestinal digestion of ground corn (Meyer et al., 1993). Addition of amylase enzymes has elevated the glycemic response in horses fed triticale diets (Richards et al., 2004), leading to conclusions that some horses may have increased ability to digest starch when supplemental amylase is incorporated in the ration. However, reports are limited, and prececal starch digestion has been shown to be influenced by many factors, so more research is necessary to clarify if α-amylase supplementation is warranted.

Based on the above studies and recommendations, it is recommended to limit single-meal intakes of starch to levels below 0.2–0.4 percent of body weight. Adjustments made to increase the nonfibrous energy concentration in the ration should be made gradually over several days in a step-wise fashion until targeted intakes are met. Starch intake per meal can be reduced by replacement of starch with feeds containing larger proportions of digestible fiber with added fat.

Feeding Forages

Commonly fed high-fiber feedstuffs include grain byproducts, pasture, and harvested forage. As noted in Chapters 8 and 10, the term "fiber" encompasses a diverse group of feedstuffs that differ in nutrient content, particle size, and degree of utilization.

There are advantages for feeding diets high in fiber. The feeding of palatable harvested feeds high in fiber allows for more continual access to feed by horses, which may reduce boredom and stress. Vices such as wood-chewing may increase when long-stem fiber is restricted. Fiber, especially long-stem roughage, adds bulk to rations, which slows intake time (Argo et al., 2001). Increased dry matter intake also encourages water intake.

As levels of fibrous compounds increase as a portion of the diet, the relative amount of nonfibrous carbohydrate decreases. Reducing the level of starch by utilizing more fiber as an energy source may reduce the incidence of colic and founder. Also, treatment of horses with certain clinical conditions such as polysaccharide storage myopathy routinely includes recommendations to reduce starch intake by feeding high fiber and by adding fat to rations (McKenzie et al., 2003; Ribeiro et al., 2004; Valentine, 2005).

Fibrous carbohydrates are digested more slowly than nonfibrous carbohydrates (Argo et al., 2001). Although research in horses is lacking, there may be a need for larger particle, slower digested fiber to maintain hindgut homeostasis. Nutritional recommendations for cattle are incorporating minimally acceptable levels of effective neutral detergent fiber (NRC, 2001). Physically effective neutral detergent fiber is a measurement used to guard against too high a level of small particle-sized fiber in rations.

The need to partition the energy source away from rapidly digestible, highly soluble carbohydrate is even apparent in some high-quality, spring-growth pastures. These pastures can contain high levels of hydrolysable and rapidly fermentable fibrous carbohydrates. These levels, even when fed without supplemental grain, may cause digestive upset because of too rapid a rate of hindgut fermentation (Hoffman et al., 2001; Longland and Murray, 2003; Watts and Chatterton, 2004). These concerns, coupled with the use of numerous byproduct feeds containing high levels of different types of fiber, emphasize the need to better define fiber by partitioning into hydrolysable, rapidly fermentable, slowly fermentable, and resistant fractions.

Many nutritionists support the use of fiber-based rations using long-stem harvested or growing roughage. Among the reported benefits, horses can receive a continuous supply of nutrients and the potential for soluble carbohydrate overload is lessened. The question of how much fiber is minimally essential is not easily answered. Horses grazing pasture to meet their energy needs can consume diets three times higher in crude fiber than horses receiving high concentrate-to-forage ratio diets. Horses have been safely fed rations in research trials with as little as 11–12 percent acid detergent fiber under research situations with no gastric disturbances (Yoder et al., 1997; Williams et al., 2001) and, in some feeding situations, especially with young, rapidly growing horses, much less.

There are concerns with feeding too high a level of fibrous carbohydrates. Some horses may require more energy-dense sources of feedstuffs to ingest sufficient energy within limits of dry matter intake. Starch digestion in the small intestine may be more energetically efficient as more adenosine triphosphate (ATP) is produced per glucose molecule than when fibrous carbohydrate is catabolized to volatile fatty acids in the hindgut (Maynard et al., 1979; McDonald et al., 1995). Also, there may be limits to restricting the level of particular energy-containing substrates. Although research is limited and results suggest varying responses, reducing starch in the diet may decrease the levels of stored glucose in the body to levels that negatively affect exercise activities that preferentially use glucose as substrate (Lawrence et al., 1991; McKenzie et al., 2003).

There is also concern about depressing digestibility when feeding diets containing both concentrate and long-stem roughage. Reports detecting negative associative effects with mixed diets indicate fiber digestion may be most affected (Thompson et al., 1984; Karlsson et al., 2000). Negative associative effects of feeding grain with long-stem roughage are not as apparent in horses as in ruminants (Hintz et al., 1971; Martin-Rosset and Dulphy, 1987). Young horses can be fed a range of hay:grain ratios and have similar growth characteristics as long as the capacity for dry matter intake does not limit the supply of energy. Weanlings fed similar levels of nutrients with diets containing 50:50 or 35:65 hay:grain ratios have been shown to have similar weight and height gain and bone strength (Ott and Kivipelto, 2003). A wide variety of feedstuffs have been successfully used for growing horses (Coleman et al., 1997; Hoffman et al., 1999; LaCasha et al., 1999; Heusner et al., 2001).

The previous NRC committee provided a general guideline for minimal intake of long-stem roughage or pasture at 1 percent of body weight per day (NRC, 1989). Even though there are several benefits for diets based on the use of long-stem forage, the absolute minimal needs for intake of long-stem forage is unclear. A variety of feeding strategies are used for feeding horses, ranging from all-forage diets to complete rations containing high levels of fiber as part of a ground, reformed, processed mix. Additional studies are needed to further quantify minimal needs of long-stem roughage. Nonetheless, because of the noted advantages of using fibrous sources of energy, the general guidelines of minimally supplying long-stem roughage or pasture at 1 percent of body weight per day and recommending roughage and pasture-based diets have nutritional merit. Forage-based diets guard against excessive starch ingestion by reducing or eliminating the need for concentrates. In many instances, forages can be offered free-choice, without increasing the risk of colic or laminitis.

Managing Body Condition

If energy supplies are in surplus, the horse's body will store portions of the unneeded energy as fat. If energy supplies are deficient, the horse will mobilize energy-containing compounds in the body and burn stored energy for fuel. Observable body fat, such as rump fat, has been used to indicate total body fat (Westerfelt et al., 1976). Body condition scoring methods use fat cover to quantify the amount of body fat. The most recognized body scoring system uniformly rates body condition in a scale from 1 to 9 (Henneke et al., 1983), as described in Chapter 1.

The optimal condition score for an individual horse depends on the health, production, and use status of the horse. Broodmares maintained in moderate to fleshly condition have increased reproductive performance as compared to mares maintained in a moderately thin body condition (Henneke et al., 1984; Morris et al., 1987; Gentry et al., 2002). Varying body condition scores may also affect athletic performance. Energy-containing compounds in muscle may be decreased in exercising horses in thin body condition (Scott et al., 1992) and correlations between body condition scores and endurance race performance have been noted (Garlinghouse and Burrill, 1999).

As noted in Chapter 1, energy balance may be manipulated to produce weight loss or weight gain. The most common means of increasing energy expenditure is to increase activity. The most common way to facilitate weight gain is to increase energy intake.

Managing Weight

Whether a horse is considered too fat or too thin varies between different classes of horses. For example, broodmares will typically be best managed in slightly higher body condition score than many growing or exercising horses. To date, there is not a universally agreed-upon definition for overweight or obesity related to body condition score in horses.

Best management guidelines for weight reduction in horses will be specific to the individual horse's health status and history. Horses consuming high-calorie diets while receiving little to no forced or voluntary exercise are more apt to become overweight. As such, weight loss management with horses should include lowering the amount of ration, consuming diets lower in energy concentration, and increasing caloric expenditure through exercise.

Some of the frequently recommended methods for weight reduction include reducing the levels of nonfibrous carbohydrate and fat in rations by feeding higher proportions of fibrous feedstuffs. One method would be to feed bulkier feedstuffs, such as grass hay, instead of more energy-dense concentrate mixtures. Reducing the total caloric intake is also achieved by reducing the total amount fed of meal-fed concentrates and forage. Supplementation of other nutrients will be affected with changes or decreases in intake of the major ingredients of the diet, i.e., forage and/or concentrate. Consequently, when diets are adjusted to reduce energy intake, it is necessary to ensure adequate intake of other associated nutrients. Overweight horses on lush pasture may require restricted grazing to adequately reduce caloric intake. It is desirable to combine dietary alterations with structured exercise programs that increase caloric expenditure. There are no proven regimens to ensure weight loss in horses.

Horses will lose weight and body condition when energy-yielding nutrients are restricted. When nutritional restrictions are prolonged, horses may become emaciated and, if continued, subsequently die from starvation. Extreme weight loss, low body condition scores, and emaciated appearance are usually associated with insufficient energy or protein. However, malabsorption, parasitic infestations, old age, senility, and various diseases also lead to emaciation (Kronfeld, 1993). As such, nutritional programs must be coordinated with the correct diagnosis of the cause and with the total rehabilitation procedures. Nutritional programs to rehabilitate emaciated horses should consider the administration route, physical form, and nutrient content of the nutritional support. If the horse is unable or unwilling to eat, intragastric administration or enteral support may be the only alternatives.

If the horse is willing and able to eat, nutritional programs must consider the physical form and nutrient profile of the diet, and patterns and level of intake. As such, recommendations tend to vary between reports, including the need to adjust procedures based on animal response, and are somewhat qualitative in nature. Regardless, nutritional programs for starved or emaciated horses should be aligned with the total rehabilitation program, thus emphasizing the need for frequent, close veterinary care and intervention.

Witham and Stull (1998) have reported on the metabolic responses of chronically starved horses re-fed with either alfalfa hay, oat hay, or a combination of oat hay and an extruded, complete commercially prepared ration. The diets were initially offered at 50 percent of the calculated dietary energy need per day, and gradually increased over 10 days to 100 percent. Energy density of the oat hay was lowest, and the combined grain and hay ration highest. Horses consumed more of the grain and hay ration as compared to oat hay as a percent of the amounts offered.

Weight gains over the 10-day period were not different between treatments. Little to no difference was observed in most of the measured metabolic responses: red blood cell count, total bilirubin, glucose, free fatty acid, and venous concentration of various minerals. Horses fed the grain and hay ration had higher insulin concentrations. The general conclusions were supportive of gradually refeeding emaciated horses with roughage-based diets. Alfalfa hay was considered to have the best results because it had a high concentration of nutrients and less bulk than oat hay, and it produced a lower insulin response than the combination diet (Stull, 2003). In a subsequent study, Stull (2003) compared an alfalfa hay diet with a combination of alfalfa hay and corn oil diet when refeeding starved horses for 10 days. The addition of corn oil lowered the dietary intake of phosphorus, and those horses were reported to have lower blood phosphorus levels. As such, the suggestion of initially refeeding with alfalfa hay was reinforced.

Nutritional programs to refeed emaciated horses should be coordinated with total health rehabilitation using veterinary assistance. Methods used to provide nutrients will depend on appetite, severity of emaciation, prevalence of disease, and advice from the attending veterinarian. Ration amounts should be gradually introduced by closely regulating intake amounts and feeding schedules. Ration amounts should be offered initially in small amounts and frequent feedings. Generally, use of high-fiber feedstuffs is preferred for the initial refeeding period. Uniformly accepted practices are largely unavailable, partially because of limited amounts of controlled research and clinical reports, the specific nature of individual cases, and the variety of associated medical conditions that are possible.

ENVIRONMENTAL CONSIDERATIONS

Most dietary nutrients that are not retained in the body are excreted in the urine and feces. Therefore, the nutrient composition of the diets consumed by horses will affect the amount and composition of waste excreted by horses into the environment (Topliff and Potter, 2002). The desire to feed diets that maximize production and performance is understandable. No one wants to feed a diet that prevents a horse from achieving its genetic potential. However, diets are regularly formulated to cover any potential shortfall of most nutrients on a "worst case scenario" basis, often with little regard as to the environmental impact. The goal of this section is to review the current environmental regulations that pertain to horses, horse owners, and horse facilities and to further heighten awareness of the specific areas where horses may contribute significantly to the nutrient and pathogen load in the environment.

Current Regulations

The U.S. Environmental Protection Agency (EPA) promulgated new regulations under the Clean Water Act (CWA) in 2003 (40 CFR–Chapter 1–Part 122). These new regulations update the definition of Animal Feeding Operations (AFO) and regulation of certain AFOs as Concentrated Animal Feeding Operations (CAFO). The regulations contain provisions that have potentially serious implications for the horse industry. The EPA has adopted a three-tiered plan for regulation of CAFOs that classify them as Large, Medium, or Small and places the number of confined horses necessary to qualify for a particular status at 500 and 150 for the Large and Medium categories and authority of regional directors to specify operations for the Small category. Any AFO that discharges pollutants directly into the waters of the United States or has animals in direct contact with waters of the United States may be designated as a CAFO regardless of the number of animals confined. Data were provided to EPA from the American Horse Council (Topliff and Potter, 2002) in response to a Notification of Data Availability (NODA), requesting that horses be counted in the same manner as feedlot cattle; however, the EPA chose to continue counting each horse as two animal units. Thus, any operation that has 150 or more horses in confinement (including stalls or drylots) for a total of 45 days or more in any 12-month period or is otherwise designated as a CAFO has a duty to seek coverage under a National Pollution Discharge Elimination System (NPDES) permit. Many stables, breeding farms, and exhibition facilities that have not previously been affected may now have to meet the requirements of the new regulations, including a provision to be able to contain all of the runoff from a 25-year, 24-hour storm event.

Effects of Diet Composition on Nutrient Excretion

The main environmental challenges created by animals and their waste products are nitrogen, minerals, fecal bacteria, and land erosion from overgrazing. Nitrogen is eliminated from the horse as urea in the urine and protein in the feces. Urea is easily converted to ammonia, a volatile and toxic gas, by urease, an enzyme that is abundant in the environment. Ammonia is a health concern to horses as well as to humans. High ammonia concentrations in stalls have been associated with upper respiratory disease and poor performance in horses (Pratt et al., 1999). Additionally, ammonia is a significant contributor to the particulate matter (PM) 2.5 load in the atmosphere. The designation 2.5 refers to fine particles less than 2.5 micrometers in diameter. This aspect of air quality is one that is relatively new, but one that has serious consequences for the animal industry. The nitrogen found in feces is mostly in the form of microbial protein and nitrate. This nitrogen usually stays with the manure until spread on pastures or composted. When manure is spread in a fresh state, the nitrates can leach into ground water or run off into surface water. Nitrates have been associated with "blue baby" syndrome in humans (US EPA, 1999). The EPA has set the allowable limits of nitrates in ground water at 10 mg/L. Many rural water supplies now exceed this limit and those communities have been forced to search for new supplies. The exact source of these nitrates has not been identified. Although it is likely that nitrogen fertilizers are a significant contributor, livestock waste may contribute as well. Composting of manure is often touted as a solution; however, much of the nitrogen fraction in composted manure is volatilized and released depending on the degree of composting. The result is a nitrogen:phosphorus ratio that is very low, necessitating the use of an additional nitrogen source to support ideal plant growth (Havlin et al., 1999). Some of the nitrogen is captured in the organic matter and is often termed organic nitrogen. It tends to be released very slowly and is less available to support plant growth.

Of the minerals found in fecal material, phosphorus is generally of greatest concern. It is usually found in the highest concentration and is the most stable and mobile of the minerals. Phosphorus in the form of phosphate is soluble in water and moves freely among soil particles. Surface application of manure in high-rainfall areas results in surface water contamination that is usually manifested as algae blooms in streams and rivers. As the algae growth proceeds unchecked, the dissolved oxygen levels in the water decline and massive kills of marine and aquatic life can occur. Phosphorus concentrations are not significantly affected by composting, which, as previously stated, necessitates the addition of nitrogen to produce a balanced fertilizer product. In some areas of the United States, the phosphorus content of the soil is sufficient to support plant growth for the next 100 years. In many areas, the problem is so severe that it is currently illegal to apply manure or commercial fertilizers containing phosphorus to that land.

Other minerals are also of concern. Copper and zinc are toxic to certain aquatic microorganisms and will likely become a target for nutrient management plans. Sodium is contained mostly in the urine and can reach significant concentrations in composted manure. In some areas of the United States, the sodium content of surface water is becoming problematic. In those areas, water is being blended from several sources to achieve a sodium level acceptable for drinking (US EPA, 1996).

Bacteria of fecal origin are currently a major health concern. Recent disease outbreaks from *Escherichia coli*, *Listeria*, and *Salmonella* that have resulted in the deaths of children and the elderly have heightened the awareness of animal waste. Horses are not likely a source of the most deadly *E. coli* strain (0157:H7) or of *Listeria*, which is found mainly in sausage-type products. Horses do, however, harbor *Salmonella*. One study estimated that 80 percent of all horses harbor *Salmonella* and that up to 20 percent are active shedders (NAHMS, 2001). Certainly the opportunity for transmission to the human population exists. *Clostridium* spp. may also pose zoonotic risks but are uncommon inhabitants of the feces of normal horses, although moderately prevalent in diarrheic horses (Garrett et al., 2002). There are proposals circulating within regulatory agencies that would require fencing of all riparian waterways from all livestock and establishment of filter strips along those waterways that would take up nutrients from potential runoff.

The final environmental challenge is soil erosion as a result of overstocking, overgrazing, and undermanagement. While the small horse owner with limited land area is the most often seen example, large reputable breeding farms are often guilty as well. If the Total Maximum Daily Load (TMDL) standards are adopted as currently proposed by EPA, nonpoint source pollution will be regulated. Horse owners along with other entities in a particular watershed may be assessed fees based on the proportion they contribute to the TMDL, even if they do not have CAFO status (US EPA, 2005).

Waste Management Considerations

There are several options to manage waste from horse operations. Proper composting methods are well described in a number of publications. Composting has the advantage of reducing the volume of material to be disposed of by reducing the moisture content, reducing the particle size of any bedding that may be present, and, if done properly, reducing the potential pathogen load through heating during the process. The end product of a good composting system is a uniform, semi-dry product that is high in organic matter, phosphorus, and trace elements, depending on the diet. The main disadvantage of composted waste is that much of the nitrogen is lost through volatilization into ammonia, resulting in an unfavorable nitrogen:phosporus ratio for plant growth. Composted waste may be land applied or could potentially be sold to local homeowners. If land application is chosen, soil phosphorus concentrations should be monitored yearly to avoid excess buildup and potential runoff.

Land application of animal waste is the traditional method of waste management. Recycling of nutrients by this method has been used for centuries as a way to improve crop production, maintain soil quality, and manage animal waste. The main consideration in modern animal production is the amount of land available on which to spread animal waste in a manner that does not result in leaching or runoff of excess nutrients into U.S. waters. A nutrient management plan that considers the lay of the land, soil type, crop nutrient uptake, cultural practices, and rainfall is vital to successfully managing animal waste. In certain cases, a NPDES permit may be required and a certified planner must do the nutrient management plan. It is the responsibility of the owner of the property to know whether or not a permit is necessary.

If land application is not possible, such as in urban or suburban settings, waste may need to be taken to a landfill. Owners should check local laws and regulations concerning this practice and may need to hire a commercial firm to dispose of the waste.

In spite of the method of waste disposal chosen, horse owners have the opportunity to be more environmentally friendly by feeding horses as closely to their nutrient requirements as possible. Feeding diets that are excessively high in protein and minerals, particularly phosphorus, copper, and zinc, puts the industry at significant risk for regulation by federal agencies in the future.

REFERENCES

Aiken, G. E., G. D. Potter, B. E. Conrad, and J. W. Evans. 1989. Voluntary intake and digestion of coastal Bermuda grass hay by yearling and mature horses. J. Equine Vet. Sci. 9:262–264.

Almeida, M. I. V., W. M. Ferreira, F. Q. Almeida, C. A. S. Just, L. C. Goncalves, and A. S. C. Rezende. 1999. Nutritive value of elephant grass (*Pennisetum purpureum* Schum) alfalfa hay (*Medicago sativa*) and coast-grass cross hay (*Cynodon dactylon L.*) for horses. Zootech. Doutorando Zootecnica, Brazil.

Archer, D. C., D. E. Freeman, A. J. Doyle, C. J. Proudman, and G. B. Edwards. 2004. Association between cribbing and entrapment of small intestine in the epiploic foramen in 2 hospital populations: 68 cases. J. Am. Vet. Med. Assoc. 224:563–564.

Archer, D. C., and C. J. Proudman. 2005. Epidemiological clues to preventing colic. Vet. J. 172:29–39.

Archer, M. 1973. The species preference of grazing horses. J. Br. Grassland Soc. 28:123–128.

Archer, M. 1978a. Further studies on palatability of grasses to horses. J. Br. Grassland Soc. 33:239–243.

Archer, M. 1978b. Studies on producing and maintaining balanced pastures for studs. Equine Vet. J. 10:54–59.

Argo, C. McG., Z. Fuller, and J. E. Cox. 2001. Digestible energy intakes, growth and feeding behavior of pony mares offered ad libitum access to a complete diet in a pelleted or chaff-based form. Pp. 170–172 in Proc. 17th Equine Nutr. Physiol. Soc. Symp., Lexington, KY.

Argo, C. McG., J. E. Cox, C. Lockyear, and Z. Fuller. 2002. Adaptive changes in the appetite, growth and feeding behaviour of pony mares offered ad libitum access to a complete diet in either a pelleted or chaff-based form. Anim. Sci. 74:517–528.

Arnold, G. W. 1984. Comparison of the time budgets and circadian patterns of maintenance activities in sheep, cattle and horses grouped together. Appl. Animal Behav. Sci. 13:19–30.

Arnold, G. W., and A. Grassia. 1982. Ethogram of agonistic behavior for Thoroughbred horses. Appl. Anim. Ethol. 8:5–25.

Ashley, F. H., A. E. Waterman-Pearson, and H. R. Whay. 2005. Behavioral assessments of pain in horses and donkeys: application to clinical practice and future studies. Equine Vet. J. 37:565–575.

Ashton, A. 2005. Bark-chewing by the wild horses of Guy Fawkes River National Park: impacts and causes. Pp. 1–124 in B.Sc. Thesis. University of New England, New South Wales, Australia.

Bachman, I., P. Bernasconi, R. Herrmann, M. A. Weishaupt, and M. Stauffacher. 2003. Behavioral and physiological responses to an acute stressor in crib-biting and control horses. Appl. Anim. Behav. Sci. 822:297–311.

Berger, A., K. M. Scheibe, K. Eichhorn, A. Scheibe, and J. Streich. 1999. Diurnal and ultradian rhythms of behavior in a mare group of Przewalski horse (*Equus ferus przewalskii*), measured through one year under semi-reserve conditions. Appl. Anim. Behav. Sci. 64:1–17.

Berger, J. 1977. Organizational systems and dominance in feral horses in the Grand Canyon. Behav. Ecol. Sociobiol. 2:131–146.

Bergero, D., and S. Nardi. 1996. Eating time of some feeds for saddle horses reared in Italy. Obiettivi e Documenti Vet. 17:63–67.

Bergero, D., P. G. Peiretti, and E. Cola. 2002. Intake and apparent digestibility of perennial ryegrass haylages fed to ponies either at maintenance or at work. Livestock Prod. Sci. 77:325–329.

Bertone, J. J., J. L. Traub-Dargtz, R. W. Wrigley, D. G. Bennett, and R. J. Williams. 1988. Diarrhea associated with sand in the gastrointestinal tract of the horse. J. Am. Vet. Med. Assoc. 193:1409–1412.

Blythe, L., and D. W. Holtan. 1983. Ryegrass staggers in ponies fed processed ryegrass straw. J. Am. Vet. Med. Assoc. 182:285–286.

Booth, M. E. 1998. Factors influencing the energy requirements of native ponies living outdoors in the United Kingdom. PhD Thesis. University of Edinburgh. 223 pp.

Bottom, S. H., H. Owen, R. E. Lawson, P. A. Harris, and S. Hall. 2004. Equine feeding side preference–incidence and age effect. P. 45 in Emerging Equine Science, J. Alliston, M. Moore-Colyer, A. Hemmings, and J. Hysplop, eds. BSAS Publication No. 32. UK: Nottingham University Press.

Boulot, S., J. P. Brun, M. Doreau, and W. Martin-Rosset. 1987. Activites alimentaires et niveau d'ingestion chez la jument gestante et allaitainte. Reprod. Nutr. Develop. 27:205–206.

Boyd, L. E. 1988. Ontogeny of behavior in Prezwalski horses. Appl. Anim. Behav. Sci. 21:41–69.

Boyd, L. E. 1991. The behavior of Przewalski's horses and its importance to their management. Appl. Anim. Behav. Sci. 29:301–318.

Caanitz, H., L. O'Leary, K. Houpt, K. Peterson, and H. Hintz. 1991. Effect of exercise on equine behavior. Appl. Anim. Behav. Sci. 31:1–12.

Cairns, M. C., J. J. Cooper, H. P. Davidson, and D. S. Mills. 2002. Association in horses of orosensory characteristics of foods with their post-ingestive consequences. Anim. Sci. 75:257–265.

Cameron, E. Z., K. J. Stafford, W. Linklater, and C. J. Veltman. 1999. Suckling behavior does not measure milk intake in horses, Equus caballus. Anim. Behav. 57:673–678.

Carson, K., and D. G. M. Wood-Gush. 1983. Behavior of Thoroughbred foals during nursing. Equine Vet. J. 15:257–262.

Chenost, M., and W. Martin-Rosset. 1985. Comparison between species (sheep, horses, cattle) on intake and digestibility of fresh herbage. Ann. Zootech. 34:291–312.

Cohen, N. D., P. G. Gibbs, and A. M. Woods. 1999. Dietary and other management factors associated with colic in horses. J. Am. Vet. Med. Assoc. 215:53–60.

Coleman, R. J., G. W. Mathison, L. Burwash, and J. D. Milligan. 1997. The effect of protein supplementation of alfalfa cube diets on the growth of weanling horses. Pp. 59–64 in Proc. 15th Equine Physiol. Nutr. Soc. Symp., Fort. Worth, TX.

Coleman, R. J., G. W. Mathison, and L. Burwash. 1999. Growth and condition at weaning of extensively managed creep-fed foals. J. Equine Vet. Sci. 19:45–49.

Cooper, J. J., and G. J. Mason. 1998. The identification of abnormal behaviour and behavioural problems in stable horses and their relationship to horse welfare: a comparative review. Equine Vet. J. Suppl. 27:5–9.

Cooper, J. J., N. McCall, S. Johnson, and H. P. B. Davidson. 2005. The short-term effects of increasing meal frequency on stereotypic behavior of stable horses. Appl. Anim. Behav. Sci. 90:351–364.

Crowell-Davis, S. L., and A. B. Caudle. 1989. Coprophagy by foals. Recognition of maternal feces. Appl. Anim. Behav. Sci. 24:267–272.

Crowell-Davis, S. L., and K. A. Houpt. 1985. Coprophagy by foals: effect of age, and possible functions. Equine Vet. J. 17:17–19.

Crowell-Davis, S. L., K. A. Houpt, and J. Carnevale. 1985. Feeding and drinking behavior of mares and foals with free access to pasture and water. J. Anim. Sci. 60:883–889.

Crozier, J. A., V. G. Allen, N. E. Jack, J. P. Fontenot, and M. A. Cochran. 1997. Digestibility, apparent mineral absorption and voluntary intake by horses fed alfalfa, tall fescue and Caucasian bluestem. J. Anim. Sci. 75:1651–1658.

Cuddeford, D., R. A. Pearson, R. F. Archibald, and R. H. Muirhead. 1995. Digestibility and gastro-intestinal transit time of diets containing different proportions of alfalfa and oat straw given to Thoroughbreds, Shetland ponies, highland ponies and donkeys. Anim. Sci. 61:407–477.

Cymbaluk, N. F. 1983. Grain preferences of ponies. Pp. 58–62 in Dept. Anim. Poult Sci. Res. Rept. Publication No. 460. University of Saskatchewan, Saskatoon.

Cymbaluk, N. F., G. I. Christison, and D. H. Leach. 1989. Energy uptake and utilization by limit and ad libitum-fed growing horses. J. Anim. Sci. 67:403–413.

de Fombelle, A., L. Veiga, C. Drogoul, and V. Julliand. 2004. Effect of diet composition and feeding pattern on the prececal digestibility of starches from diverse botanical origins measured with the mobile nylon bag technique in horses. J. Anim. Sci. 82:3625–3634.

Doreau, M., W. Martin-Rosset, and D. Petit. 1980. Nocturnal feeding activities of horses at pasture. Ann. Zootech. 29:299–304.

Doreau, M., S. Boulot, and W. Martin-Rosset. 1991. Effect of parity and physiological state on intake, milk production and blood parameters in lactating mares differing in body size. Anim. Prod. 53:111–118.

Drogoul, C., A. de Fombelle, and V. Julliand. 2001. Feeding and microbial disorders in horses: 2: Effect of three hay:grain ratios on digesta passage rate and digestibility in ponies. J. Equine Vet. Sci. 21:487–490.

Dulphy, J. P., W. Martin-Rosset, H. Dubroeucq, J. M. Ballet, A. Detour, and M. Jailler. 1997a. Compared feeding patterns in ad libitum intake of dry forages by horses and sheep. Livest. Prod. Sci. 52:49–56.

Dulphy, J. P., W. Martin-Rosset, H. Dubroeucq, and M. Jailler. 1997b. Evaluation of voluntary intake of forage trough-fed to light horses. Comparison with sheep. Livest. Prod. Sci. 52:97–104.

Duncan, P. 1985. Time-budgets of Camargue horses. III. Environmental influences. Behaviour 92:188–208.

Duncan, P. 1992. Horses and Grasses: The Nutritional Ecology of Equids and Their Impact on the Carmargue. Ecological Studies 87. New York: Springer.

Duncan, P., P. H. Harvey, and S. M. Wells. 1984. On lactation and associated behavior in a natural herd of horses. Anim. Behav. 32:255–263.

Duren, S. E., C. T. Dougherty, S. G. Jackson, and J. P. Baker. 1989. Modification of ingestive behavior due to exercise in yearling horses grazing orchardgrass. Appl. Anim. Behav. Sci. 22:335–345.

Ellard, M. E., and S. L. Crowell-Davis. 1989. Evaluating equine dominance in draft mares. Appl. Anim. Behav. Sci. 24:55–75.

Ellis, A. D., S. Thomas, K. Arkell and P. Harris. 2005. Adding chopped straw to concentrate feed: the effect of inclusion rate and particle length on intake behavior of horses. Pferdeheilkunde 21:35–37.

Elphinstone, G. D. 1981. Pastures and fodder crops for horses in southern coastal Queensland. Queensland Agric. J. 107:122–126.

Estep, D. Q., S. L. Crowell-Davis, S. A. Earl-Costello, and S. A. Beatey. 1993. Changes in the social behaviour of drafthorse (Equus caballus) mares coincident with foaling. Appl. Anim. Behav. Sci. 35:199–213.

Falkowski, M., M. Rogalski, J. Kryszak, S. Kozlowski, and I. Kukulka. 1983. Intensive grassland management and the problem of animal behavior and grazing. Roczniki Akademii Rolniczej Poznaniu, Ogrodnictwo. 26:85–92.

Feist, J. D., and D. R. McCullough. 1976. Behavior patterns and communication in feral horses. Z. Tierpsychol. 41:337–371.

Fitzgerald, B. P., and C. J. McManus. 2000. Photoperiodic versus metabolic signals as determinants of seasonal anestrus in the mare. Biol. Reprod. 63:335–340.

Flannigan, G., and J. M. Stookey. 2001. Day-time time budgets of pregnant mares housed in tie stalls: a comparison of draft versus light mares. Appl. Anim. Behav. Sci. 78:125–143.

Fleurance, G., P. Duncan, and B. Mallevaud. 2001. Daily intake and the selection of feeding sites by horses in heterogeneous wet grasslands. Anim. Res. 50:149–156.

Francis-Smith, K., and D. G. Wood-Gush. 1977. Coprophagia as seen in Thoroughbred foals. Equine Vet. J. 9:15–18.

Friend, M., and D. Nash. 2000. Pasture intake by grazing horses. Final report for the Rural Industries Research and Development Corporation, Project UCS-22A.

Gallagher, R., and N. P. McMeniman. 1988. The nutritional status of pregnant and non-pregnant mares grazing South East Queensland pastures. Equine Vet. J. 20:414–416.

Gallagher, R., and N. P. McMeniman. 1989. Grazing behavior of horses on SE Queensland pastures. In Recent Advances in Animal Nutrition in Australia, 11A, D. Farrell, ed. New South Wales: University of New England.

Garcia, L. N., C. A. McCall, W. H. McElhenney, J. S. Taintor, and J. Schumacher. 2005. The effect of oral antacid on gastric pH and cribbing frequency in the horse. P. 214 in Proc. 19th Equine Sci. Soc., Tucson, AZ.

Garlinghouse, S. E., and M. J. Burrill. 1999. Relationship of body condition score to completion rate during 160 km endurance races. Equine Vet. J. Suppl. 30:591–595.

Garner, H. E., J. N. Moore, J. H. Johnson, L. Clark, J. F. Amend, L. G. Tritschler, J. R. Coffmann, R. F. Sprouse, D. P. Hutcheson, and C. A. Salem. 1978. Changes in the caecal flora associated with the onset of laminitis. Equine Vet. J. 10:249–252.

Garrett, L. A., R. Brown, and I. R. Poxton. 2002. A comparative study of the intestinal microbiota of healthy horses and those suffering from equine grass sickness. Vet. Microbiol. 87:81–88.

Gentry, L. R., D. L. Thompson, Jr., G. T. Gentry, Jr., K. A. Davis, R. A. Godke, and J. A. Cartmill. 2002. The relationship between body condition, leptin, and reproductive and hormonal characteristics of mares during the seasonal anovulatory period. J. Anim. Sci. 80:2695–2703.

Gillham, S. R., N. H. Dodman, L. Shuster, R. Kream, and W. Rand. 1994. The effect of diet on cribbing behavior and plasma β-endorphin in horses. Appl. Anim. Behav. Sci. 41:147–153.

Goodson, J., W. J. Tyznik, J. H. Cline, and B. A. Dehority. 1988. Effects of an abrupt diet change from hay to concentrate on microbial numbers and physical environment in the cecum of the pony. Appl. Environ. Microbiol. 54:1946–1950.

Goodwin, D., H. P. Davidson, and P. Harris. 2002. Foraging enrichment for stabled horses: effects on behavior and selection. Equine Vet. J. 34:686–691.

Goodwin, D., H. P. B. Davidson, and P. Harris. 2005a. Sensory varieties in concentrated diets for stabled horses: effects on behavior and selection. Appl. Anim. Behav. Sci. 90:337–349.

Goodwin, D., H. P. B. Davidson, and P. Harris. 2005b. Selection and acceptance of flavors in concentrated diets for stabled horses. Appl. Anim. Behav. Sci. 95:223–232.

Goold, G. J. 1991. Problems of pasture management. Pp. 115–116 in Proc. Equine Nutr. Seminar, Nut. Soc. Aust. Canberra.

Green, P., and J. M. J. Tong. 1988. Small intestinal obstruction associated with wood chewing in two horses. Vet. Rec. 123:196–198.

Gross, J. E., L. A. Shipley, N. T. Hobbs, D. E. Spalinger, and B. A. Wunder. 1993. Functional response of herbivores in food-concentrated patches: tests of a mechanistic model. Ecology 74:778–791.

Guay, K. A., H. A. Brady, V. G. Allen, K. R. Pond, D. B. Wester, L. A. Janecka, and N. L. Heninger. 2002. Matua bromegrass hay for mares in gestation and lactation. J. Anim. Sci. 80:2960–2966.

Haelein, G. F., R. D. Holdren, and Y. M. Yoon. 1966. Comparative response of horses and sheep to different physical forms of alfalfa hay. J. Anim. Sci. 25:740–743.

Hale, C., and M. J. S. Moore-Colyer. 2001. Voluntary feed intakes and apparent digestibilities of hay, big bale grass silage and red clover silage by ponies. Pp. 470–471 in Proc. 17th Equine Nutr. Physiol. Soc. Symp., Lexington, KY.

Harris, P. A., M. Sillence, R. Inglis, C. Siever-Kelly, M. Friend, K. Munn, and H. Davidson. 2005. Effect of short (<2 cm) lucerne chaff addition on the intake rate and glycaemic response of sweet feed. Pferdeheilkunde 21:87–88.

Hart, B. L. 1988. Biological basis of the behavior of sick animals. Neurosci. Biobehav. Rev. 12:123–137.

Havlin, J. L., J. D. Beaton, S. L. Tisdale, and W. L. Nelson. 1999. Soil fertility and fertilizers. Pp. 136–138 in An Introduction to Nutrient Management. Upper Saddle River, NJ: Prentice-Hall, Inc.

Hawkes, J., M. Hedges, P. Daniluk, H. F. Hintz, and H. F. Schryver. 1985. Feed preferences of ponies. Equine Vet. J. 17:20–22.

Hayakawa, Y. 1991. Grazing management of yearling racehorses. 2. Sward canopy height in set grazing. J. Japan. Soc. Grassland Sci. 31:337–342.

Henneke, D. R., G. D. Potter, J. L. Kreider, and B. F. Yeates. 1983. Relationship between condition score, physical measurements and body fat percentage in mares. Equine Vet. J. 15:371–372.

Henneke, D. R., G. D. Potter, and J. L. Kreider. 1984. Body condition during pregnancy and lactation and reproductive efficiency rates of mares. Theriogenology. 21:897–909.

Heusner, G. L. 1993. Ad libitum feeding of mature horses to achieve rapid weight gain. Pp. 86–87 in Proc. 13th Equine Nutr. Physiol. Symp., Gainesville, FL.

Heusner, G. L., M. A. Froetschel, and C. A. McPeake. 2001. The utilization of cottonseed hulls as the single fiber source in rations for the growing horse. P. 330 in Proc.17th Equine Nutr. Physiol Soc. Symp., Lexington, KY.

Hill, J. 2002. Effect of the inclusion and method of presentation of a single distillery by-product on the processes of ingestion of concentrate feeds by horses. Livest. Prod. Sci. 75:209–218.

Hinkle, D. K., G. D. Potter, and J. L. Kreider. 1983. Starch digestion in different segments of the digestive tract of ponies fed varying levels of corn. Pp. 227–230 in Proc. 8th Equine Nutr. Physiol. Soc., Univ. of Kentucky, Lexington, KY.

Hintz, H. F. 1980. Feed preferences of horses. Pp. 113–116 in Proc. Cornell Nutr. Conf., Syracuse, NY.

Hintz, H. F., R. A. Argenzio, and H. F. Schryver. 1971. Digestion coefficients, blood glucose levels and molar percentage of volatile acids in intestinal fluid of ponies fed varying forage-grain ratios. J. Anim. Sci. 33:992–995.

Hintz, H. F., J. Scott, L. V. Soderholm, and J. Williams. 1985. Extruded feeds for horses. Pp. 174–176 in Proc. 9th Equine Nutr. Physiol. Soc. Symp., East Lansing, MI.

Hoffman, R. M., L. A. Lawrence, D. S. Kronfeld, W. L. Cooper, D. J. Sklan, J. J. Dascanio, and P. A. Harris. 1999. Dietary carbohydrates and fat influence radiographic bone mineral content of growing foals. J. Anim. Sci. 77:3330–3338.

Hoffman, R. M., J. A. Wilson, D. S. Kronfeld, W. L. Cooper, L. A. Lawrence, D. Sklan, and P. A. Harris. 2001. Hydrolyzable carbohydrates in pasture, hay and horse feeds: direct assay and seasonal variation. J. Anim. Sci. 79:500–506.

Hogan, E. S., K. A. Houpt, and K. Sweeney. 1988. The effect of enclosure size on social interactions and daily activity patterns of captive Asiatic wild horse (Equus przewalskii). Appl. Anim. Behav. Sci. 21:147–168.

Holland, J. L., D. S. Kronfeld, and T. N. Meacham. 1996. Behavior of horses is affected by soy lecithin and corn oil in the diet. J. Anim. Sci. 74:1252–1255.

Holland, J. L., D. S. Kronfeld, G. A. Rich, K. A. Kline, J. P. Fontenot, T. N. Meacham, and P. A. Harris. 1998. Acceptance of fat and lecithin containing diets by horses. Appl. Anim. Behav. Sci. 56:91–96.

Holmes, L. N., G. K. Song, and E. O. Price. 1987. Head partitions facilitate feeding by subordinate horses in the presence of dominant pen-mates. Appl. Anim. Behav. Sci. 19:179–182.

Horton, G. M., D. B. Blethen, and B. M. Prasad. 1990. The effect of garlic (Allium sativum) on feed palatability of horses and feed consumption, selected performance and blood parameters in sheep and swine. Can. J. Anim. Sci. 71:607–610.

Houpt, K. A. 2002. Formation and dissolution of the mare-foal bond. Appl. Anim. Behav. Sci. 78:319–328.

Houpt, K. A., and T. R. Houpt. 1988. Social and illumination preference of mares. J. Anim. Sci. 66:2159–2164.

Houpt, K. A., D. M. Zahorik, and J. A. Swartzman-Andert. 1990. Taste aversion learning in horses. J. Anim. Sci. 68:2340–2344.

Houpt, K., J. Elia, and M. Stalker. 2004. Roughage craving in horses. P. 78 in Proc. 38th Intl. Cong., ISAE, Helsinki, Finland.

Hudson, J. M., N. D. Cohen, P. G. Gibbs, and J. A. Thompson. 2001. Feeding practices associated with colic in horses. J. Am. Vet. Med. Assoc. 219:1419–1425.

Hughes, T. P., and J. R. Gallagher. 1993. Influence of sward height on the mechanics of grazing and intake by racehorses. Pp. 1325–1326 in Proc. XVII International Grassland Cong, Palmerston North, NZ.

Hunt, W. F. 1991. Common grasses in New Zealand and their palatability and nutrient value for horses. The New Zealand Equine Research Foundation Biomac lecture series:1–9, Palmerston North, NZ.

Husted, L., M. S. Andersen, O. K. Borggaard, H. Houe, and S. N. Olsen. 2005. Risk factors for faecal sand excretion in Icelandic horses. Equine Vet. J. 37:351–355.

Jackson, S. A., V. A. Rich, S. L. Ralston, and E. W. Anderson. 1985. Feeding behavior and feed efficiency of horses as affected by feeding frequency and physical form of hay. Pp. 78–83 in Proc. 9th Equine Nutr. Physiol. Soc. Symp., East Lansing, MI.

Janicki, K. M., C. I. O'Connor, and L. M. Lawrence. 1999. The influence of feed tub placement and spacing on feeding behavior of mature horses. Pp. 360–361 in 16th Proc. Equine Nutr. Physiol. Soc. Symp., Raleigh, NC.

Johnson, K. G., J. Tyrrell, J. B. Rowe, and D. W. Pethick. 1998. Behavioral changes in stabled horses given nontherapeutic levels of virginiamycin. Equine Vet. J. 30:139–143.

Karlsson, C. P., J. E. Lindberg, and M. Rundgren. 2000. Associative effects on total tract digestibility in horses fed different ratios of grass hay and whole oats. Livestock Prod. Sci. 65:143–153.

Kaseda, Y. 1983. Seasonal changes in time spent grazing and resting of Misaki horses. Japan. J. Zoological Sci. 54:464–469.

Kawai, M., H. Hisano, Y. Yabu, N. Yabu, and S. Matsuoka. 2004a. Effects of fallen snow on the voluntary intake and grazing behavior of Hokkaido native horses in winter woodland with underlying Sasa Senanensis. Anim. Sci. 75:435–440.

Kawai, M., N. Yabu, T. Asa, K. Deguiche, and S. Matsuoka. 2004b. Biting and chewing behavior of grazing light breed horses on different pasture conditions. P. 167 in Proc. 28th Intl. Cong., ISAE, Helsinki, Finland.

Keiper, R. R., and J. Berger. 1982. Refuge-seeking and pest avoidance by feral horses in desert and island environments. Appl. Anim. Ethol. 9:111–120.

Keiper, R. R., and H. S. Sambraus. 1986. The stability of equine dominance hierarchies and the effects of kinship, proximity and foaling status on hierarchy rank. Appl. Anim. Behav. Sci. 16:121–130.

Keiper, R. R., and H. Receveur. 1992. Social interactions of free-ranging Przewalski horses in semi-reserves in the Netherlands. Appl. Anim. Behav. Sci. 33:303–318.

Kienzle, E. 1994. Small intestinal digestion of starch in the horse. Revue Med. Vet. 145:199–204.

Klimov, V. V. 1988. Spatial-ethological organization of the herd of Przewalski horses (Equus prezwalskii) in Askania-Nova. Appl. Anim. Behav. Sci. 21:99–115.

Kondo, S., T. Yasue, K. Ogawa, M. Okubo, and Y. Asahida. 1993. Behavior aspects of Hokkaido native horses kept outdoors all year round. Pp. 241–242 (Abst. 348) in World Conf. Anim. Prod., Edmonton, Alberta.

Kronfeld, D. S. 1993. Starvation and malnutrition of horses: recognition and treatment. J. Equine Vet. Sci. 13:298–303.

Krysyl, L. J., M. E. Hubbert, B. F. Sowell, G. E. Plumb, T. K. Jewett, M. A. Smith, and J. W. Waggoner. 1984. Horses and cattle grazing in the Wyoming Red Desert, I. Food habits and dietary overlap. J. Range Mgmt. 37:72–76.

Krzak, W. E., H. W. Gonyou, and L. M. Lawrence. 1991. Wood chewing by stabled horses: diurnal pattern and effects of exercise. J. Anim. Sci. 69:1053–1058.

Kubiak, J. R., W. Evans, G. D. Potter, P. G. Harms, and W. L. Jenkins. 1988. Parturition in the multiparous mare fed to obesity. J. Equine Vet. Sci. 8:135–140.

Kunkle, W. E., J. E. Moore, and O. Balbuena. 1997. Recent research on liquid supplements for beef cattle. Proc. Florida Ruminant Nutr. Symp. 15 pp.

Kusonose, R., H. Hatakeyama, F. Ichikawa, K. Kubo, A. Kiguchi, Y. Asai, and K. Ito. 1986. Behavioral studies on yearling horses in field environments. 2. Effects of group size on the behavior of horses. Bulletin of the Equine Research Institute No. 23:1–6.

LaCasha, P. A., H. A. Brady, V. G. Allen, and K. R. Pond. 1999. Voluntary intake, digestibility and subsequent selection of Matua bromegrass, coastal bermudagrass, and alfalfa hays by yearling horses. J. Anim. Sci. 77:2766–2773.

Lamoot, I., J. Callebaut, T. Degezelle, E. Demeulenaere, J. Laquiere, C. Vandenberghe, and M. Hoffmann. 2004. Eliminative behavior of free-ranging horses: do they show latrine behavior or do they defecate where they graze? Appl. Anim. Behav. Sci. 86:105–121.

Laut, J. E., K. A. Houpt, H. F. Hintz, and T. R. Houpt. 1985. The effects of caloric dilution on meal patterns and food intake of ponies. Physiol. Behav. 34:549–554.

Lawrence, L., S. Jackson, K. Kline, L. Moser, D. Powell, and M. Biel. 1991. Observations on body weight and condition of horses competing in a 150 mile endurance ride. Pp. 167–168 in Proc. 12th Equine Nutr. Phys. Soc. Symp., University of Calgary, Alberta.

Lewis, L. D. 1995. Equine Clinical Nutrition. Feeding and Care of the Horse, 1st ed. Media, PA: Williams and Wilkins.

Lieb, S., and J. Weise. 1999. A group of experiments on the management of sand intake and removal in the equine. P. 257 in Proc. 16th Equine Nutr. Physiol. Soc. Symp., Raleigh, NC.

Lieb, S., E. A. Ott, and E. C. French. 1993. Digestible nutrients and voluntary intakes of rhizomal peanut, alfalfa, Bermudagrass and bahiagrass hays in equine. Pp. 98–99 in Proc. 13th Equine Nutr. Physiol. Soc. Symp., Gainesville, FL.

Lillie, H. C., C. A. McCall, W. H. McElhenney, J. S. Taintor, and S. J. Silverman. 2003. Comparison of gastric pH in crib-biting and normal horses. P. 247 in Proc. 18th Equine Nutr. Physiol. Soc. Symp., East Lansing, MI.

Longland, A. C., and J. M. D. Murray. 2003. Effect of two varieties of perennial ryegrass (Lolium perenne) differing in fructan content on fermentation parameters in vitro when incubated in vitro with a pony faecal inoculum. Pp. 144–145 in Proc. 18th Equine Nutr. Phys. Soc. Symp., East Lansing, MI.

Lorenzo-Figueras, M., G. Jones, and A. M. Merritt. 2002. Effects of various diets on gastric tone in the proximal portion of the stomach of horses. Am. J. Vet. Res. 63:1275–1278.

Loucougaray, G., A. Bonis, and J. B. Bouzille. 2004. Effects of grazing by horses and/or cattle on the diversity of coastal grasslands in western France. Biol. Conservation 116:59–71.

Loudon, A. S., I. Milne, J. D. Curlewis, and A. S. McNeilly. 1989. A comparison of seasonal changes and patterns of growth, voluntary feed intake and reproduction in juvenile and adult red deer (Cervus elaphus) and Pere David's deer (Elaphurus davidiamus) hinds. J. Endocrinol. 122:733–745.

Luescher, U. A., D. B. McKeown, and H. Dean. 1998. A cross-sectional study on compulsive behavior (stable vices) in horses. Equine Vet. J. Suppl. 27:14–18.

Magnusson, J., and A. G. Thorhallsdottir. 1994. Horse grazing in northern Iceland–behavior and habitat selection. Livest. Prod. Sci. 40:83 (Abstr.).

Marinier, S. L., and A. J. Alexander. 1992. Use of field observations to measure individual grazing ability in horses. Appl. Anim. Behav. Sci. 33:1–10.

Marinier, S. L., and A. J. Alexander. 1995. Coprophagy as an avenue for foals of the domestic horse to learn food preferences from their dams. J. Theor. Biol. 173:121–124.

Marlow, C. H. B., E. M. van Tonder, F. C. Hayward, S. S. van der Merwe, and L. E. G. Price. 1983. A report on the consumption, composition and nutritional adequacy of a mixture of lush green perennial ryegrass (*Lolium perenne*) and cocksfoot (*Dactylis glomerata*) fed ad libitum to thoroughbred mares. J. S. Afr. Vet. Assoc. 54:155–157.

Marsden, M. D. 1993. Feeding practices have greater effect than housing practices on the behavior and welfare of the horse. Pp. 314–318 in Am. Soc. Agric. Eng., Livest. Env. IV. 4th Internat. Symp., E. Collins and C. Boon, eds., University of Warwick, Coventry, England.

Martin-Rosset, W., and J. P. Dulphy. 1987. Digestibility interactions between forages and concentrates in horses: influence of feeding level-comparison with sheep. Lives. Prod. Sci. 17:263–276.

Martin-Rosset, W., M. Doreau, and J. Cloix. 1978. Activities of a herd of draught brood mares and their foals on pasture. Annl. Zootech. 27:33–45.

Matsuoka, T., M. N. Novilla, T. D. Thomson, and A. L. Donoho. 1996. Review of monensin toxicosis in horses. J. Equine. Vet. Sci. 16:8–15.

Mayes, E., and P. Duncan. 1986. Temporal patterns of feeding behavior in free-ranging horses. Behav. 96:105–129.

Maynard, L. A., J. K. Loosli, H. F. Hintz, and R. G. Warner. 1979. Animal Nutrition, 7th ed. New York: McGraw-Hill Book Co.

McBride, S. D., and D. Cuddeford. 2001. The putative welfare reducing effects of preventing equine stereotypic behaviour. Animal Welfare 10:173–189.

McBride, S. D., and L. Long. 2001. Management of horses showing stereotypic behaviour, owner perception and the implications for welfare. Vet. Rec. 148:799–802.

McCall, C. A., B. A. Moeller, S. J. Silverman, and W. H. McElhenney. 2001. Saliva production in crib-biting and normal horses. P. 358 in Proc. 17th Equine Nutr. Physiol. Soc. Symp., Lexington, KY.

McCann, J. S., and C. S. Hoveland. 1991. Equine grazing preferences among winter annual grasses and clovers adapted to south-eastern United States. J. Equine Vet. Sci. 11:275–277.

McDonald, P., R. A. Edwards, J. F. Greenhalgh, and C. A. Morgan. 1995. Animal Nutrition, 5th ed. New York: John Wiley & Sons.

McGreevy, P. D. 2004. Equine Behavior. A Guide for Veterinarians and Equine Scientists. Edinburgh: Saunders, 412 pp.

McGreevy, P., and C. Nicol. 1998a. Prevention of crib-biting: a review. Equine Vet. J. 27:35–38.

McGreevy, P. D., and C. J. Nicol 1998b. The effect of short-term prevention on the subsequent rate of crib-biting in Thoroughbred horses. Equine Vet. J. Suppl. 27:30–34.

McGreevy, P. D., P. J. Cripps, N. D. French, L. E. Green, and C. J. Nicol. 1995a. Management factors associated with stereotypic and redirected behavior in the thoroughbred horse. Equine Vet. J. 27:86–91.

McGreevy, P. D., N. D. French, and C. J. Nicol. 1995b. The prevalence of abnormal behaviours in dressage, eventing and endurance horses in relation to stabling. Vet. Rec. 137:36–37.

McGreevy, P. D., L. A. Hawson, T. C. Habermann, and S. R. Cattle. 2001. Geophagia in horses: a short note on 13 cases. Appl. Anim. Behav. Sci. 71:119–125.

McKenzie, E. C., S. J. Valberg, S. M. Godden, J. D. Pagan, J. M. MacLeay, R. J. Geor, and G. P. Carlson. 2003. Effect of dietary starch, fat, and bicarbonate content on exercise responses and serum creatine kinase activity in equine recurrent exertional rhabdomyolysys. J. Vet. Intern. Med. 17:693–701.

McMeniman, N. P. 2000. Nutrition of grazing broodmares, their foals, and young horses. A report for the Rural Industries Research and Development Corporation, RIDRC publication No. 00/28, Melbourne, Australia.

McMeniman, N. P. 2003. Pasture intake by young horses. A report for the Rural Industries Research and Development Corporation, RIDRC publication No. 00W03/005, Melbourne, Australia.

Menard, C., P. Duncan, G. Fleurance, J. Y. Georges, and M. Lila. 2002. Comparative foraging and nutrition of horses and cattle in European wetlands. J. Appl. Ecol. 39:120–133.

Mesochina, P. M., W. Martin-Rosset, J. L. Peyraud, P. Duncan, D. Micol, and S. Boulot. 1998. Prediction of digestibility of the diet of horses: evaluation of faecal indices. Grass Forage Sci. 53:159–196.

Mesochina, P. M., J. L. Peyraud, P. Duncan, D. Micol, and C. Tillaud-Geyl. 2000. Grass intake by growing horses at pasture: a test on the effect of the horse's age and sward biomass. Ann. Zootech. 49:505–515.

Meyer, H., S. Radicke, E. Kienzle, S. Wilke, and D. Kleffken. 1993. Investigations on preileal digestion of oats, corn and barley starch in relation to grain processing. Pp. 92–97 in Proc. 13th Equine Nutr. Phys. Soc. Symp, Gainesville, FL.

Mills, D. S., and C. A. Macleod. 2002. The response of crib-biting and windsucking horses to treatment with antacid mixture. Ippologia 13:33–41.

Mills, D. S., and S. M. McDonnell. 2005. The Domestic Horse. The Origins, Development and Management of Its Behavior. Cambridge: Cambridge University Press. 264 pp.

Mills, D. S., K. D. Taylor, and J. J. Cooper. 2005. Weaving, headshaking, cribbing and other stereotypies. Am. Assoc. Equine Pract. 51:22–229.

Moore-Colyer, M. J. S., and A. C. Longland. 2000. Intake and in vivo apparent digestibilities of four types of conserved grass forage by ponies. Anim. Sci. 71:527–534.

Morris, R. P., G. A. Rich, S. L. Ralston, E. L. Squires, and B. W. Pickett. 1987. Follicular activity in transitional mares as affected by body condition and dietary energy. Pp. 93–97 in Proc. 10th Equine Nutr. Phys. Soc. Symp., Fort Collins, CO.

Murray, M. J. 1997. Overview of equine gastroduodenal ulceration. Proc. Am. Assoc. Equine Pract. 43:382–387.

NAHMS (National Animal Health Monitoring System). 2001. *Salmonella* and the U.S. Horse Population. Washington, DC: U.S. Department of Agriculture, Animal and Plant Health Inspection Service.

Naujeck, A., J. Hill, and M. J. Gibb. 2005. Influence of sward height on diet selection by horses. Appl. Anim. Behav. Sci. 90:49–63.

Nicol, C. 1998. Understanding equine stereotypies. Equine Vet. J. Suppl. 28:20–25.

Nicol, C. J., and A. J. Badnell-Waters. 2005. Suckling behaviour in domestic foals and the development of abnormal oral behaviour. Anim. Behav. 70:21–29.

Nicol, C. J., H. P. B. Davidson, P. A. Harris, A. J. Waters, and A. D. Wilson. 2002. Study of crib-biting and gastric inflammation and ulceration in young horses. Vet. Rec. 151:658–662.

Nicol, C. J., A. J. Badnell-Waters, R. Bice, A. Kelland, A. D. Wilson, and P. A. Harris. 2005. The effects of diet and weaning method on the behaviour of young horses. Appl. Anim. Behav. Sci. 95:205–221.

NRC (National Research Council). 1989. Nutrient Requirements of Horses, 5th rev. ed. Washington, DC: National Academy Press.

NRC. 2001. Nutrient Requirements of Dairy Cattle, 7th rev. ed. Washington, DC: National Academy Press.

Odberg, F. O., and K. Francis-Smith. 1976. A study on eliminative and grazing behavior—the use of the field by captive horses. Equine Vet. J. 8:147–149.

Odberg, F. O., and K. Francis-Smith. 1977. Studies on the formation of ungrazed eliminative areas in field used by horses. Appl. Anim. Ethol. 3:27–34.

Ott, E. A., and J. Kivipelto. 2003. Influence of concentrate:hay ratio on growth and development of weanling horses. In Proc. 18th Equine Nutr. Physiol. Soc. Symp., East Lansing, MI.

Pearson, R. A., and J. B. Merritt. 1991. Intake, digestion and gastrointestinal transit time in resting donkeys and ponies and exercised donkeys given ad libitum hay and straw diets. Equine Vet. J. 23:339–343.

Pearson, R. A., R. F. Archibald, and R. H. Muirhead. 2001. The effect of forage quality and level of feeding on digestibility and gastrointestinal transit time of oat straw and alfalfa given to ponies and donkeys. Br. J. Nutr. 85:599–606.

Pearson, W., H. J. Boermans, W. J. Bettger, B. W. McBride, and M. I. Lindinger. 2005. Association of maximum voluntary dietary intake of

freeze-dried garlic with Heinz body anemia in horses. Am. J. Vet. Res. 66:457–465.
Pell, S. M., and P. D. McGreevy. 1999. Prevalence of stereotypic and other problem behaviours in Thoroughbred horses. Austral. Vet. J. 77:678–679.
Pfister, J. A., B. L. Stegelmeir, C. D. Cheney, M. H. Ralphs, and D. R. Gardner. 2002. Conditioning taste aversions to locoweed (Oxytropis sericea) in horses. J. Anim. Sci. 80:79–83.
Pfister, J. A., B. L. Stegelmeir, D. R. Gardner, and L. F. James. 2003. Grazing of spotted locoweed (Astralagus lentiginous) by cattle and horses in Arizona. J. Anim. Sci. 81:2285–2293.
Pluhacek, J., L. Bartos, and L. Culik. 2006. High-ranking mares of captive plains zebra Equus burchelli have greater reproductive success than low-ranking mares. Appl. Anim. Behav. Sci. 99:315–329.
Potter, G. D., F. F. Arnold, D. D. Householder, D. H. Hansen, and K. M. Brown. 1992. Digestion of starch in the small or large intestine of the equine. Pp. 107–111 in European Conf. on Nutrition for the Horse, Hannover, Germany.
Pratt, S. E., L. M. Lawrence, T. Barnes, D. Powell, and L. K. Warren. 1999. Measurement of ammonia concentrations in horse stalls. P. 334 in Proc. 16th Equine Nutr. Physiol. Soc. Symp., Raleigh, NC.
Randall, R. P., W. A. Schurg, and D. C. Church. 1978. Response of horses to sweet, salty, sour and bitter solutions. J. Anim. Sci. 47:51–55.
Raymond, S. L., T. K. Smith, and H. V. Swamy. 2003. Effects of feeding a blend of grains naturally contaminated with Fusarium mycotoxins on feed intake, serum chemistry, and hematology of horses, and the efficacy of a polymeric glucomannan mycotoxin adsorbent. J. Anim. Sci. 81:2123–2130.
Redgate, S. E., A. L. Ordakowski-Burk, H. P. B. Davidson, P. A. Harris, and D. S. Kronfeld. 2004. A preliminary study to investigate the effect of diet on the behaviour of weanling horses. P. 154 in Proc. 38th Intl. Cong., ISAE, Helsinki, Finland.
Rhind, S. M., S. R. McMillen, E. Duff, D. Hirst, and S. Wright. 1998. Seasonality of meal patterns and hormonal correlates in red deer. Physiol. Behav. 65:295–302.
Ribeiro, W. P., S. J. Valberg, J. D. Pagan, and B. E. Gustavsson. 2004. The effect of varying dietary starch and fat content on serum creatine kinase activity and substrate availability in equine polysaccharide storage myopathy. J. Vet. Intern. Med. 18:887–894.
Richards, N., M. Choct, G. N. Hinch, and J. B. Rowe. 2004. Examination of the use of exogenous α-amylase and amyloglucosidase to enhance starch digestion in the small intestine of the horse. Anim. Feed Sci. Tech. 114:295–305.
Rogalski, M. 1974. The comparison of some characteristic interdependent factors between the sward and the grazing animal. Proc. 12th Int. Grassland Congress. Grassland Utilization. Moscow, USSR.
Rogalski, M. 1975. Effect of weather conditions and grazing management on the behavior of horses on pasture. Rocz-Nauk-Roln. Ser-B. Zootech 97:7–16.
Rogalski, M. 1977. Behaviour of animals on pasture. Roczniki Akademii Rolniczej Poznaniu, Rozprawny Naukowe. 78:41.
Rogalski, M. 1982. Testing the palatability of pasture sward for horses based on the comparative grazing intensity unit. Herbage Abstracts 1984, 054–00602.
Rogalski, M. 1984a. Preferences for some types of grasses and intake of pasture by English thoroughbred mares. Herbage Abstracts 1986, 056–07146.
Rogalski, M. 1984b. Effect of carbohydrates or lignin on preferences for and intakes of pasture plants by mares. Roczniki Akademii Rolniczej Poznaniu 27:183–193.
Rowe, J. B., M. J. Lees, and D. W. Pethick. 1994. Prevention of acidosis and laminitis associated with grain feeding in horses. J. Nutr. 124:2742S–2744S.
Salter, R. E., and R. J. Hudson. 1979. Feeding ecology of feral horses in western Alberta. J. Range Manage. 32:221–225.

Schurg, W. A., D. L. Frei, P. R. Cheeke, and D. W. Holtan. 1977. Utilization of whole corn plant pellets by horses and rabbits. J. Anim. Sci. 45:1317–1321.
Schurg, W. A., R. E. Pulse, D. W. Holtan, and J. E. Oldfield. 1978. Use of various quantities and forms of ryegrass straw in horse diets. J. Anim. Sci. 47:1287–1291.
Scott, B. D., G. D. Potter, L. W. Greene, P. S. Hargis, and J. G. Anderson. 1992. Efficacy of a fat-supplemented diet on muscle glycogen concentrations in exercising thoroughbred horses maintained in varying body conditions. Equine Vet. Sci. 12:109–113.
Shingu, Y., M. Kawai, H. Inaba, S. Kondo, H. Hata, and M. Okubo. 2000. Voluntary intake and behavior of Hokkaido native horses and light halfbred horses in woodland pasture. J. Equine Sci. 11:69–73.
Shingu, Y., S. Kondo, H. Hata, and M. Okubo. 2001. Digestibility and number of bites and chews on hay at fixed level in Hokkaido native horses and light half-bred horses. J. Equine Sci. 12:145–147.
Sigurjonsdottir, H., M. C. van Dierendonck, S. Snorrason, and A. G. Thorhallsdottir. 2003. Social relationships in a group of horses without a mature stallion. Behaviour 140:783–804.
Smith-Funk, E. D., and S. L. Crowell-Davis 1992. Maternal behavior of draft mares (Equus caballus) with mule foals (Equus asinus × Equus caballus). Appl. Anim. Behav. Sci. 33:93–119.
Sondergaard, E. 2003. Activity, feed intake and physical development of young Danish Warmblood horses in relation to the social environment. Pp. 55–75, PhD Thesis, Danish Institute of Agricultural Sciences, Tjele, Denmark.
Southwood, L. L., D. L. Evans, W. L. Bryden, and R. J. Rose. 1993. Nutrient intake of horses in Thoroughbred and Standardbred stables. Aust. Vet. J. 70:164–168.
Steelman, C. D. 1976. Effects of external and internal arthropod parasites on domestic animal production. Ann. Rev. Entomol. 21:155–178.
Stull, C. 2003. Nutrition for rehabilitating the starved horse. J. Equine Vet. Sci. 23:456.
Sweeting, M. P., C. E. Houpt, and K. A. Houpt. 1985. Social facilitation of feeding and time budgets in stabled horses. J. Anim. Sci. 60:369–374.
Taylor, E. J. 1954. Grazing behavior and helminthic disease. Br. J. Anim. Behav. 2:61–62.
Templeton, W. C. 1979. Forages for horses. Proc. Annu. Ky. Horsemen's Shortcourse 3:81.
Thompson, K. N., S. G. Jackson, and J. P. Baker. 1984. Apparent digestion coefficients and associative effects of varying hay:grain rations fed to horses. Nutr. Rep. Int. 30(1):189–197.
Thorne, J. B., D. Goodwin, M. J. Kennedy, H. P. B. Davidson, and P. Harris. 2005. Foraging enrichment for individually housed horses: practicality and effects on behavior. Appl. Anim. Behav. Sci. 94:14–164.
Tinker, M. K., N. A. White, P. Lessard, C. D. Thatcher, K. D. Pelzer, B. Davis, and D. K. Carmel. 1997. Prospective study of equine colic risk factors. Equine Vet. J. 29:454–458.
Topliff, D. R., and G. D. Potter. 2002. Comparison of Dry Matter, Nitrogen, and Phosphorus Excretion From Feedlot Steers and Horses in Race/Performance Training. Written testimony submitted to the United States Environmental Protection Agency.
U.S. Environmental Protection Agency (US EPA). 1996. Managing nonpoint source pollution from agriculture. Pointer No. 6. EPA841-F-96-0004F. Washington, DC: U.S. EPA, Office of Wetland, Oceans, and Watersheds, Office of Water.
U.S. EPA. 1999. Children and drinking water standards. Publication 815-K-99-001. Washington, DC: U.S. EPA Office of Water.
U.S. EPA. 2005. Guidance for 2006 assessment, listing and reporting requirements pursuant to sections 303(d), 305(b) and 314 of the Clean Water Act. Washington, DC: U.S. EPA, Watershed Branch, Assessment and Watershed Protection Division, Office of Wetland, Oceans, and Watersheds, Office of Water.
Valentine, B. A. 2005. Diagnosis and treatment of equine polysaccharide storage myopathy. Equine Vet. Sci. 25:52–61.

Van Dierendonck, M. C., H. Sigurjonsdottir, B. Colenbrander, and A. G. Thorhallsdottir. 2004. Differences in social behavior between late pregnant, post-partum and barren mares in a herd of Icelandic horses. Appl. Anim. Behav. Sci. 89:283–297.

Varloud, M., A. de Fombelle, A. G. Goachet, C. Drogoul, and V. Julliand. 2004. Partial and total apparent digestibility of dietary carbohydrates in horses as affected by diet. Anim. Sci. 79:61–72.

Vecchiotti, G. G., and R. Galanti. 1986. Evidence of heredity of cribbing, weaving and stall-walking in Thoroughbred horses. Livest. Prod. Sci. 14:91–95.

Wallace, T. 1977. Pasture management on Waikato equine studs. N. Z. Vet. J. 25:346–350.

Waring, G. H. 2002. Horse Behavior, 2nd ed. Norwich, NY: William Andrew Publishing.

Waters, A. J., C. J. Nicol, and N. P. French. 2002. Factors influencing the development of stereotypic and redirected behaviors in young horses: findings of a four year prospective epidemiological study. Equine Vet. J. 34:572–579.

Watts, K. A., and N. J. Chatterton. 2004. A review of factors affecting carbohydrate levels in forage. J. Equine Vet. Sci. 24:84–86.

Weise, J., and S. Lieb. 2001. The effects of protein and energy deficiencies on voluntary sand intake and behavior in the horse. Pp. 103–105 in Proc. 17th Equine Nutr. Physiol. Soc. Symp., Lexington, KY.

Westerfelt, R. G., J. R. Stouffer, H. F. Hintz, and H. F. Schryver. 1976. Estimating fatness in horses and ponies. J. Anim. Sci. 43:781–784.

Willard, J. G., J. C. Willard, S. A. Wolfram, and J. P. Baker. 1977. Effect of diet on cecal pH and feeding behavior of horses. J. Anim. Sci. 45:87–93.

Williams. M. C. 1987. Nitrate and soluble oxalate accumulation in Kikuyugrass (*Pennisetum clandestinum*). Proc. Western Soc. Weed Sci. 40:78–79.

Williams, C. A., D. S. Kronfeld, W. B. Staniar, and P. A. Harris. 2001. Plasma glucose and insulin responses of Thoroughbred mares fed a meal high in starch and sugar or fat and fiber. J. Anim. Sci. 79:2196–2201.

Witham, C. L., and C. L. Stull. 1998. Metabolic responses of chronically starved horses to refeeding with three isoenergetic diets. J. Am. Vet. Med. Assoc. 212:691–696.

Wood-Gush, D. G. M., and F. Galbraith. 1987. Social relationship in a herd of 11 geldings and two female ponies. Equine Vet. J. 19:129–132.

Yoder, M. J., E. Miller, J. Rook, J. E. Shelle, and D. E. Ullrey. 1997. Fiber level and form: effects on digestibility, digesta flow and incidence of gastrointestinal disorders. Pp. 24–30 in Proc. 15th Equine Nutr. Physiol. Soc. Symp., Ft. Worth, TX.

Zeyner, A., C. Geißler and A. Dittrich. 2004. Effect of hay intake and feeding sequence on variables in feces and faecal water (dry matter, pH value, organic acids, ammonia, buffering capacity) of horses. J. Anim. Physiol. Anim. Nutr. 88:7–19.

12

Unique Aspects of Equine Nutrition

NURSING AND ORPHAN FOALS

During the first week of life, healthy foals will nurse up to seven times per hour, with each nursing bout lasting 1 to 2 minutes (Carson and Wood-Gush, 1983). Subsequently, there is a decrease in the frequency and duration of nursing bouts; at 4 weeks of age, foals nurse about three times per hour (Carson and Wood-Gush, 1983). During the first 24 hours of life, foals consume approximately 15 percent of body weight (BW) as milk, increasing to 22–23 percent on day 2, and approximately 25 percent of BW (15 liters for a 50 kg-foal) by 7 days postpartum (Ousey et al., 1996). One study of Thoroughbred foals indicated that the digestibility of mare's milk is 98 percent (Ousey et al., 1997). Although the dam's milk will normally supply all the nutritional needs of foals for the first 6–8 weeks of life, foals will begin to consume small portions of solid feed within days of birth. Foals will increasingly seek solid feed sources to supply their nutrient needs by consumption of the dam's feed, or if available, feed supplied by creep feeding. Creep feeding has advantages of supplying a nutrient-dense source of feed to foals that is protected from ingestion by mares.

Average daily gain of foals fed creep feed before weaning can be higher when compared to foals not receiving creep rations (Coleman et al., 1999). Additionally, foals that become accustomed to consuming dry feed prior to weaning have reduced weaning stress (McCall et al., 1985; Hoffman et al., 1995). Creep rations are typically formulated to contain 16–20 percent high-quality crude protein (CP), 0.8–1 percent calcium, and 0.6–0.8 percent phosphorus, although there has been limited research to assess the optimal nutrient composition of creep feeds for foals.

The decision to provide creep feed will depend on desired growth rates and post-weaning nutritional programs. Voluntary intake of creep feed is expected to vary between foals and to be influenced by factors such as herd behavior, placement of creep feeders, and presence of other foals consuming feeds. One trial reported that orphan foals receiving liquid milk replacer consumed less than 1 kg grain mix per 100 kg BW daily up to 1 month of age, then increased intake to 1.5–2 kg grain mix per 100 kg BW daily at 7 weeks of age (Cymbaluk et al., 1993). Foal body weight averaged about 60 kg at birth, and average daily gains ranged from a low of 0.18 kg/d during the first 2 weeks of age to 1.43 kg/d between 16 and 24 weeks of age. In another trial, creep feed intakes of extensively managed nursing foals averaged 0.56–0.84 kg/d (Coleman et al., 1999). Initially, foals were approximately 2 months of age with a mean BW of 140 kg. At 4 months of age (the end of the study), mean BW was approximately 200 kg.

Management of the orphan foal is dependent upon the age at which the foal loses its dam. Young foals should be fed a milk-based diet to ensure satisfactory growth and development, whereas older foals may develop adequately with a diet of high-quality forage and creep feed. For foals orphaned on the 1st day of life, an important consideration is provision of high-quality colostrum that contains immunoglobulins vital to competency of the foal's naïve immune system. Following ingestion by the foal, immunoglobulins in colostrum are absorbed by specialized cells throughout the epithelium of the small intestine. The absorption process is most efficient following the first few feedings postpartum, with a rapid decline in uptake efficiency over the first 12 hours of life. By 24 hours, the small intestine is no longer permeable to colostral immunoglobulins (Jeffcott, 1972). Colostrum should be fed before any milk replacers to ensure maximal absorption of immunoglobulins (Stoneham, 2005). The immunoglobulin content of colostrum declines rapidly after the onset of nursing in postpartum mares. Milk samples collected 4–8 hours after birth have 15 percent of the immunoglobulin concentration of samples collected in the first 3 hours postpartum (Naylor, 1979). Therefore, the colostrum fed to orphan foals should have been harvested from mares soon after parturition.

Fostering to a nurse mare is the preferred option for management of orphan foals less than 6 to 8 weeks of age. Foals that cannot be fostered should be fed a mare's milk substitute. Fortified cow's milk, goat milk, and commercially available milk replacer products specifically designed for foals have been used (Naylor and Bell, 1985; Pugh and Williams, 1992). Milk substitutes should be designed to mimic the nutrient concentrations in mare's milk (Naylor and Bell, 1985). Research findings on composition of mare's milk are provided in Table 16-8. On a dry matter (DM) basis, foal milk replacers should contain approximately 15 percent fat and 22 percent CP, with a fiber content of less than 0.5 percent (Naylor and Bell, 1985). Milk replacers should be fed as a 10–15 percent solution. Milk from farm animal species (i.e., goat, pig, sheep, and cow) is dissimilar to mare's milk. Therefore, commercially available milk replacers are the preferred milk substitute for foals. However, cow's milk is suitable if some of the fat is removed and sugar added. One recommendation is to feed 2-percent-fat skimmed milk to which dextrose has been added at the rate of 20 g/L (40 ml of 50 percent dextrose per liter of milk) (Naylor and Bell, 1985).

It is advisable to gradually increase the volume of milk fed over a 7- to 10-d period. One recommendation is to start at 5–10 percent BW at day 1, increasing to 20–25 percent BW by day 10 (Naylor and Bell, 1985). Initially, many small meals should be provided to somewhat mimic natural feeding patterns (e.g., every hour). As the foal begins to eat solid feed, the frequency of feedings can be gradually reduced. Alternatively, the foal can be given free choice access to milk in a pail or by use of an automated feeding device designed for calves. Fresh water should be available at all times (Cymbaluk et al., 1993). Orphan foals can be weaned from milk at 10–12 weeks of age (Naylor and Bell, 1985).

OLD AGE

Several challenges exist in defining nutrient requirements of old horses. The first challenge is to establish criteria that define the threshold for old age in horses. Secondly, nutrient requirements are a function of metabolic requirements and the efficiency of nutrient digestion, absorption, and metabolism. Therefore, knowledge of age-related changes in digestion, absorption, and metabolism is necessary to define the nutrient requirements of old horses. Finally, the effect of aging-associated disease on nutrient requirements must be determined and should be viewed separately from the effects of aging itself. Old age is not synonymous with the term "geriatric," which refers to diseases of the aged.

Defining Old Age

Paradis (2002) described three types of age that may be useful in establishing old age threshold for horses: chronologic, physiologic, and demographic. Chronologic age is the actual number of years of life from birth. Physiologic age relates to physiological function and uses the decline in physiological function as a threshold for old age. Demographic age reflects survivorship of an age-group subpopulation relative to the whole. No exact chronological threshold for old age in horses has been identified. Several investigators have used 20 years of age to define the threshold of old age (Ralston et al., 1988, 1989; Malinowski et al., 1997; Brosnahan and Paradis, 2003). The 1998 National Animal Health Monitoring Systems study (USDA, 1998) estimated that 7.5 percent of the horse population (total horse population estimated at approximately 7 million) was 20 years of age or older.

Although 20 years of age may serve as an estimate of the threshold for old age, the degree of variation of this estimate is not known. Therefore, the combination of chronological age and physical signs of aging may be the most effective means of establishing the "old-age" threshold for individual horses. Physical signs of aging may include chronically low body condition score, loss of muscle mass over the top line yielding a sway-backed appearance, hollowing out of the grooves above the eyes, graying of the coat, and dental disease (Ralston et al., 1988, 1989; Ralston and Breuer, 1996; Paradis, 2002).

Energy Requirements of Aged Horses

Energy requirements are a function of energy expenditure and the efficiency with which gross energy (GE) present in feeds is converted to net energy (NE). Both of these factors have the potential to be affected by age.

Maintenance energy requirements typically constitute the largest proportion of total energy expenditure. Maintenance energy requirements in aged humans and dogs have been reported to be 15–20 percent lower when compared to younger populations (Harper, 1998a; Bosy-Westphal et al., 2003). The decline in maintenance energy expenditure is thought to be a function of declining fat-free mass associated with aging (Bosy-Westphal et al., 2003). Decreased physical activity is thought to be a primary factor in the age-related decline in fat-free mass (Harper, 1998a; Roubenoff, 1999). Whether an age-related decline in maintenance energy requirement occurs in horses is unknown. Although apparent loss of muscle mass has been observed in old horses (Ralston et al., 1989), age-related change in fat-free mass and subsequent changes in maintenance energy requirement have not been quantified in horses. Nor is the effect of age on physical activity in horses well characterized. Therefore, the extent to which aging alters the maintenance energy requirements of horses is not known. Some disease conditions may increase energy requirements. Mean resting energy expenditure was increased by approximately 41 percent in horses with recurrent airway obstruction as compared to controls (Mazan et al., 2004).

Fecal energy typically accounts for the largest proportion of gross energy lost from feedstuffs. Therefore, factors that influence DM digestibility have a large impact on digestible energy yield. Mean crude fiber apparent digestibility tended (P = 0.10) to be lower (~ 5 percent) in a group (n = 7) of old horses (26 ± 5 years of age) when compared to a small group (n = 5) of younger horses (2.3 ± 0.5 years of age) (Ralston et al., 1989). Because the magnitude of this change in crude fiber apparent digestibility was similar to that of the young horses used in the study following resection of left and right colons, the authors suggested that aged horses have a reduced absorptive and/or digestive function in the large intestine (Ralston et al., 1989). This is in contrast to findings in humans and dogs that suggest gastrointestinal function, at least with regard to macronutrients, is well preserved with aging (Harper, 1998b; Russell, 2000). It is also likely in some instances that age-related changes to teeth may impair a horse's ability to masticate feed, subsequently decreasing digestibility in the remainder of the digestive tract.

Another area of potential interest in old horses is the effect of caloric restriction on aging and age-related disease. Caloric restriction has been demonstrated to extend the lifespan in a variety of species (Heilbronn and Ravussin, 2003). Larson et al. (2003) reported that lifetime dietary restriction improved glucose tolerance and had a favorable effect on disease and survival in dogs.

Equine Cushing's disease is a chronic progressive disease of the intermediate pituitary gland of older horses. This disease is discussed in detail elsewhere (McCue, 2002). Hyperglycemia and hyperinsulinemia are common findings in horses with equine Cushing's disease (Garcia and Beech, 1986). Therefore, providing calories from sources that do not contribute substantial quantities of glucose to the blood stream (e.g., fiber) appears prudent.

Protein and Amino Acid Requirements

The effect of aging and age-related disease on protein requirements of horses is unknown. Ralston et al. (1989) reported lower crude protein apparent digestibility (67 ± 3 vs. 73 ± 3 percent) in aged horses (26 ± 5 years of age) when compared to younger horses (2.3 ± 0.5 years of age). Whether this finding reflects the old horse population in general and significantly impacts protein requirements of old horses remains to be determined. Supplemental lysine and threonine (0.25 percent on a DM basis or approximately 20.0 g/d and 0.2 percent of DM or 15 g/d, respectively) have been suggested to maintain muscle mass in old (22.4 ± 0.87 years) as well as younger horses (9.1 ± 0.29 years) undergoing light exercise (Graham-Thiers and Kronfeld, 2005). Healthy humans appear to have a decreased protein requirement with aging. Millward et al. (1997) reported a 33 percent reduction in protein metabolic demand and no significant impairment in efficiency of protein utilization in healthy, mobile, elderly persons, suggesting a decline in protein requirements with aging.

Micronutrient Requirements

Requirements for micronutrients in old horses remain relatively uninvestigated. Only two reports related to the effect of aging on micronutrient nutrition were identified as of this writing. Ralston et al. (1989) found decreased phosphorus apparent digestibility (–4 ± 19 vs. 11 ± 6 percent) in old (26 ± 5 years of age) vs. younger (2.3 ± 0.5 years of age) horses. Additionally, initial reports suggested vitamin C status may be different between young and old horses (Ralston et al., 1988), but more recent evidence does not support this idea (Deaton et al., 2004).

Feed Form

Dental abnormalities, which are common in older horses (Paradis, 2002; Graham, 2002), can limit the ability to prehend and chew feed, decrease the digestibility of nutrients, and lead to substantial loss of body weight. Alterations in the physical form of the ration can be beneficial for old horses with dental disease. A common approach is to feed older horses processed, complete feeds. In one study, the feeding of a complete feed containing extruded ingredients was more effective at maintaining the body weight of old horses with low body condition (condition score less than 3) when compared to a more traditional ration consisting of a grain mix and timothy-alfalfa hay (Ralston and Breuer, 1996). Other options include the feeding of ensiled forage (haylage) or chopped hay (e.g., early cut alfalfa) or forage cubes that have been soaked in water. Oil can be added to increase the energy density of the ration.

Conclusion

The true effect of aging and age-related disease on nutrient requirements remains to be determined in horses. There appears to be a large degree of variation in the way old horses respond to similar diets (Ralston and Breuer, 1996), suggesting chronological age alone is not sufficient to categorize horses relative to age-related changes in nutrient requirements.

FEEDING MANAGEMENT OF HORSES IN COLD OR HOT WEATHER

Chapter 1 includes a discussion of the effects of climate on heat production in horses and also describes factors that affect upper critical temperature (UCT) and lower critical temperature (LCT) for horses. The UCT is the upper range of the thermoneutral zone and is the temperature above which evaporative heat loss must be increased to control body temperature. The LCT is the lowest temperature in the thermoneutral zone and is the temperature below which metabolic heat production must be increased to maintain body temperature. For horses kept in environments outside of the thermoneutral zone, adjustments in nutrient require-

Feeding in Cold Weather

Two studies with growing horses reared in cold, outdoor weather gave differing results concerning voluntary feed intake (Cymbaluk and Christison, 1989a; Cymbaluk, 1990). As temperatures fell below LCT, yearling horses in the first study were found to eat less, not more, feed and, therefore, consumed less digestive energy (DE). Although decreases in DE intakes were only 5.7 percent and 8.8 percent less at temperatures below −10° and below −20°C compared to above −10°, weight gains were lower than expected (Cymbaluk and Christison, 1989a). In the second study, growing horses ate 0.2 percent more feed per Celsius degree decrease in ambient temperature below LCT (Cymbaluk, 1990). Based on this study, DE intakes for growing horses must be increased by 1.3 percent per Celsius degree below LCT. By comparison, maintenance DE for adult horses must be increased 2.5 percent per Celsius degree below their LCT of −15°C (McBride et al., 1985). The disparity between feeding recommendations for adults and growing horses is that the LCT for adults was based on maintenance only, and those for young horses was based on energy intakes for maintenance and gain. Young, thin, or aged mature horses are less cold-tolerant than mature horses. When cold weather occurs, diet changes for susceptible horses must be made much sooner than for mature horses in good body condition.

The overall conclusion from the preceding data is that cold weather creates an increased demand mainly for energy. Modified guidelines to those previously published for feeding horses in cold weather are given in Table 12-1 (Cymbaluk and Christison, 1990). Feeding good-quality hay free-choice may be the simplest way to supply additional DE for most idle, adult horses during cold weather. The influence of diet composition and nutrient content on energy metabolism during cold weather is described in Chapter 1. In addition to diet, the effects of cold weather on nonacclimated horses can be ameliorated through physical modifications including housing or application of a rug or blanket. Shelters, rugs or blankets, and shelters plus rugs or blankets reduced heat loss during cold exposure by 9, 18, and 26 percent, respectively (MacCormack and Bruce, 1991).

Feeding in Hot Weather

Water intake is markedly increased (30–75 percent) by both acute and chronic heat loads (Geor et al., 1996; Marlin et al., 2001). The high intake of water compensates for water lost through rapid respiration and increased sweating rate when conditions are hot and dry but not hot and humid (McCutcheon et al., 1995). The increased sweating rate in hot conditions, especially when superimposed with exercise, results in substantial electrolyte losses (McCutcheon et al., 1995, 1999; McCutcheon and Geor, 1996). The primary electrolytes lost in sweat are sodium, potassium, and chloride. The amount and type of electrolyte supplementation depends on the extent of heat stress and the amount and duration of physical stress that is imposed. At a minimum, free-choice access to salt should be available to horses during hot weather (McCutcheon and Geor, 1996). General guidelines for feeding horses during hot weather are given in Table 12-2.

In hot weather conditions, the feeding program for idle horses should be designed to minimize heat load. Although high-fat diets may prove potentially useful in reducing heat load in hot weather (Kronfeld, 1996; Kronfeld et al., 1998), few studies have critically examined the metabolic effects of high-fat diets on thermoregulation of idle horses in hot weather conditions. Under normal thermal conditions, horses fed high-fat diets reportedly had lower respiratory exchange ratios than those fed high-carbohydrate diets (Pagan et al., 2002). Lower blood pH, higher blood glucose, a calculated reduction in urine volume, reduced feed and water intake, and weight gain have also been reported (Zeyner et al., 2002). Mathiason-Kochan et al. (2001) observed that horses fed a fat-supplemented diet (a concentrate with 10 percent fat of DM, fed in a 65:35 ratio with hay) had higher sweat losses after a high-intensity standard exercise test (SET) but lower packed cell volumes than horses fed a high-hay diet (60 percent hay) or the basal diet with no added fat. The authors suggested this might reflect an increase in extracellular fluid, but in the absence of plasma

---

TABLE 12-1 Guidelines for Feeding Horses during Cold Weather[a]

1. The lower critical temperature (LCT) for young horses can range from −11 to 0°C and for adult horses can be as low as −15°C in northern continental climates. In more temperate climates, LCT was reported to be 5°C. Specific horses may have higher or lower LCT. If cold weather persists at temperatures below LCT, then an increased provision of dietary energy may become necessary.
2. Growing horses may require an additional 1.3 percent digestible energy (DE) for each degree below LCT plus the DE required for weight gain (Cymbaluk, 1990). Adult horses should be given an additional 2.5 percent DE for maintenance per degree below LCT (McBride et al., 1985).
3. Hays should be provided free-choice to allow horses to eat to their energy demands. Use of digestible hays facilitates higher total intake (Dulphy et al., 1997). Concentrate may need to be added to ensure adequate energy intake especially for growing, thin, worked, or aged horses. If a concentrate is to be fed, the horse must be fully adapted to this feed.
4. Additional mineral and vitamin supplementation does not appear to be necessary during cold weather beyond the requirements needed for the specific production level of the horse.
5. Water should be provided ad libitum and can be heated up to 20°C to maximize intake (Kristula and McDonnell, 1994).
6. Well-bedded and wind-protected shelter should be provided to minimize energy loss.

[a]SOURCE: Modified from Cymbaluk and Christison (1990).

TABLE 12-2 Guidelines for Feeding Horses during Hot Weather

1. The upper critical temperature (UCT) for horses is about 38°C for foals and 25°C for adults, depending on duration of exposure to hot ambient temperatures. Climatic conditions of an area will determine the absolute value of the UCT of the horses living in those regions.
2. At ambient temperatures that exceed UCT, water should be supplied in a manner that allows voluntary intake by the horse. There appears to be no preference for iced water by horses exposed to warm ambient temperatures (McDonnell and Kristula, 1996).
3. Although the benefit of feeding grain-based and fat-supplemented diets to horses in hot weather is unclear, these types of diets may be theoretically useful for horses.
4. Salt should be available to horses during hot weather (McCutcheon and Geor, 1996).
5. A shade, preferably that allows unimpeded air movement, may reduce heating effects of direct sunlight. Coat clipping may help dissipate heat in horses with a long hair coat (Morgan et al., 2002).

protein data, the effect on body fluid distribution is difficult to interpret.

Conflicting data have been reported on the impact that fat may have on utilization of other nutrients (see Chapter 3; Beynen and Hallebeek, 2002). Although soybean oil added to provide dietary fat at 5–10.8 percent resulted in reduced dry matter, fiber, and protein digestibility by horses (Worth et al., 1987; Jansen et al., 2001), no effect of fat was found on nutrient digestion coefficients derived by various methods (Meyers et al., 1987; Bush et al., 2001). Others have found an increase in fiber utilization (Hughes et al., 1995; Julen et al., 1995). Fat supplementation of diet did improve utilization of either natural or β-carotene or α-tocopherol by horses (Keinzle et al., 2003). More importantly, the stability and effects of long-term storage of high-fat horse diets under high heat conditions have not been fully explored.

NUTRITIONAL MANAGEMENT OF SPECIFIC DISEASE CONDITIONS

Hyperkalemic Periodic Paralysis

Hyperkalemic periodic paralysis (HYPP) is a co-dominant single autosomal gene disorder that appears to have originated as a point mutation in the Quarter horse stallion Impressive (Spier et al., 1994). The genetic nature of this condition has been well documented and a highly reliable test based on polymerase chain reaction (PCR) technology has been developed to identify horses with this condition (Meyer et al., 1999). The test was developed originally for a condition in humans that is essentially the same genetic abnormality (Lehmann-Horn et al., 2002). To be affected, the horse must have inherited the defective gene from an affected parent descended from Impressive. Affected horses are either heterozygous (H/N) or homozygous (H/H) for HYPP. Horses that are homozygous are more severely affected than those that are heterozygous (Carr et al., 1996). The gene in question codes for the sodium channel, a membrane protein involved in the regulation of cellular sodium and potassium content. This ion channel facilitates movement of potassium into the cell and outward movement of sodium.

Etiology and Genetic Basis

In normal muscle cells, an electrical gradient is established across the cell membrane as sodium is pumped outside of the cell and potassium into the cell. That electrical gradient is typically on the order of 85 millivolts (mV) and is maintained in part by the ability of the sodium channel to restrict entry of sodium into the cell. As long as that gradient is maintained, the cell is at rest and no muscle contraction occurs. During excitation, a nerve impulse is received by the muscle cell that results in a conformational change of the sodium ion channel and the generation of an "action potential." During this event, sodium rushes into the cell, potassium rushes out, and the electrical gradient approaches 0 mV. This action potential, in a coupled reaction, causes the release of calcium from storage sites within the sarcoplasmic reticulum of the muscle cell, with movement of calcium ions to the area of the muscle fibrils actin and myosin. Calcium binds to sites on myosin, and the muscle contracts and remains contracted until the calcium is resequestered in the storage sites by the action of a calcium pump.

In the muscle cells of horses with the HYPP trait, regulation of the movement of sodium and potassium ions via the sodium channel is disturbed such that there is a constant "back leakage" of sodium ions into the cell. As a consequence, there is repetitive depolarization of some muscle cells. Under certain conditions, these repetitive contractions become more severe and are clinically recognized as muscle fasiculations. During clinical episodes of HYPP, fasiculations are often first evident over the rib cage and flank areas, but may spread to other muscle groups. There can be prolapse (eversion) of the third eyelid and the horse may show signs similar to colic. In severe episodes, the contractions become tetanic; the horse may sit like a dog and later become recumbent. Death due to respiratory failure is possible. In horses that experience severe episodes, serum potassium concentrations may increase from 3 to 4 mEq/L to as much as 12 mEq/L or higher (Meyer et al., 1999). Recognition of such a marked increase in serum potassium concentration is useful in differentiating HYPP from other muscle diseases.

Nutritional Management

Treatment and management of HYPP aims to limit increases in serum potassium concentration by one or a combination of three methods: (1) limiting the dietary intake of potassium, (2) promoting entry of potassium into cells, or (3) eliminating excess extracellular potassium from the body via the urine.

The most important management practice for HYPP-positive horses is a restriction in potassium intake. Recent work has demonstrated that the risk of clinical episodes is heightened when dietary potassium exceeds 1 percent of the total diet (Reynolds, 1997; Reynolds et al., 1998a,b). When dietary potassium content is maintained below this 1 percent threshold, HYPP episodes can often be controlled without other preventative measures.

The largest single source of potassium in a horse's diet is forage (hay). Grains contain potassium, but are generally less than 0.5 percent potassium. Forages may, on the other hand, contain in excess of 3 percent potassium. Forages vary widely in their potassium content by type, region of the country, and even different areas within a single field. Fertility level of the field, rainfall or irrigation, and stage of maturity all have an effect on the potassium content of forages. Higher fertility levels, increased moisture, and cutting hay at an early stage of maturity all tend to increase the potassium concentration of the forage (Minson, 1990). Given this wide variation in potassium content, even within forage types, laboratory analysis is required for accurate estimation of potassium content. However, in general, grass forages tend to have less potassium than legume forages.

In view of the potassium concentrations in feeds, the use of grass hays or pastures such as Bermudagrass, prairie hay, or timothy instead of legume hays or pastures such as alfalfa seems prudent. If alfalfa must be included in the diet, then other preventative measures may be necessary. Also, the use of cereal grains as a major portion of the diet will reduce the overall potassium content of the ration. In addition, grain intake will stimulate insulin release that may facilitate the uptake of potassium by muscle cells. However, the inclusion of commercially prepared concentrates that contain large amounts of molasses, soybean meal, or dehydrated alfalfa should be monitored, as these feed ingredients may be relatively high in potassium (> 2 percent).

In cases where control of potassium intake is insufficient to manage episodic events, additional interventions may be required. The uptake of potassium by the cells is enhanced by a number of factors, including mild exercise, insulin release, and administration of other cations into the extracellular fluid. Insulin concentrations can be increased by oral or intravenous (IV) glucose administration, or the feeding of cereal grains high in starch. Cations such as sodium and calcium-administered IV promote the intracellular movement of potassium in order to maintain electrical neutrality of the extracellular fluid (ECF). As a further preventive measure, a diuretic such as acetazolimide may be administered under the supervision of a veterinarian. This drug increases the excretion of potassium in urine.

Exertional Rhabdomyolysis Syndromes

Exertional rhabdomyolysis (ER) in horses is a syndrome of muscle pain and cramping associated with exercise. It can be categorized into sporadic exertional rhabdomyolysis, in which horses have sporadic or infrequent episodes of muscle necrosis and pain associated with exercise, or chronic exertional rhabdomyolysis, in which affected horses have repeated episodes (Valberg et al., 1999a). Two forms of chronic exertional rhabdomyolysis have been described: (1) recurrent exertional rhabdomyolysis (RER), which commonly afflicts Thoroughbreds but also may affect other breeds such as Standardbreds and Arabians; and (2) polysaccharide storage myopathy (PSSM), which predominantly affects Quarter horses but also has been described in other breeds including Paints, European Warmbloods, Appaloosas, Morgan horses, and draft breeds (Valberg et al. 1999a). In Thoroughbreds, RER has been identified as a heritable defect in intracellular calcium regulation that leads to muscle necrosis during exercise (MacLeay et al., 1999). Polysaccharide storage myopathy involves increased storage of glycogen and abnormal polysaccharide in skeletal muscle. In both RER and PSSM, there is some evidence that a reduction in dietary starch and sugar and/or an increase in dietary fat are beneficial in the management of affected horses (see McKenzie et al., 2003).

Polysaccharide Storage Myopathy

Polysaccharide storage myopathy is characterized by high concentrations of glycogen and glucose-6-phosphate in muscle and the accumulation of amylase-resistant, periodic acid Schiff (PAS)-positive inclusions in up to 30 percent of type II muscle fibers (Valberg et al., 1992). Clinical signs include ER, exercise intolerance, muscle stiffness, back pain, shifting lameness, gait changes, muscle atrophy, a camped-out stance, and colic-like signs. Detection of amylase-resistant polysaccharide in muscle of horses with a history of recurrent ER is considered diagnostic for PSSM. However, the accumulation of polysaccharide may be a gradual process. In a small group of Quarter horse foals with clinical and laboratory evidence of chronic, intermittent ER, polysaccharide accumulation in skeletal muscle was not apparent until 2 years of age (De La Corte et al., 2002).

A glycogen storage disorder also has been described in Warmblood horses (Hunt et al., 2005), draft horses and related breeds, and Welsh ponies (Valentine et al., 1997, 2000, 2001a,b). In draft horses, this disorder has been termed equine polysaccharide storage myopathy (EPSM) (Valentine et al., 2001a).

Clinical signs of polysaccharide myopathy in draft horses and related breeds include muscle soreness of the hindquarters and back, stiffness, muscle atrophy, and occasionally overt ER. In Belgian draft horses, PSSM may occur concurrently with "shivers," a disorder characterized by muscle tremors and hindlimb hyperflexion that may progress to muscle atrophy, weakness, and recumbency (Firshman et al., 2005). The results of one epidemiologic study indicated that PSSM and shivers are common but unrelated disorders of Belgian draft horses (Firshman et al., 2005).

Nutritional Factors

There is evidence that diet modifies the clinical expression of PSSM (and EPSM). In clinical reports, the frequency and severity of ER episodes were higher when PSSM-affected horses received little exercise and were fed energy concentrates containing moderate amounts of starch and sugar such as straight grains or sweet feed mixes (Valentine et al., 2001b; McKenzie et al., 2003). Conversely, controlled laboratory experiments in Quarter horses with PSSM (Ribeiro et al., 2004) and uncontrolled clinical trials in Quarter horses (Firshman et al., 2003), Warmblood horses (Hunt et al., 2005), and draft horses (Valentine et al., 2001a) with evidence of muscle polysaccharide accumulation have shown that the feeding of a ration with restricted starch and sugar content (on a total ration basis, < 8 percent DE from starch and sugar) and added fat (> 10 percent of total DE from fat) resulted in clinical improvement of affected horses.

In one study, Quarter horse mares (n = 4) were fed isocaloric diets ranging in DE from 21.2 percent (diet A), 14.8 percent (B), 8.4 percent (C), to 3.9 percent (D) for starch, and 7.2 percent DE (diet A), 9.9 percent (B), to 12.7 percent DE (diet C and D) for fat (Ribeiro et al., 2004). The diets were fed for 6-week periods in a 4 × 4 Latin square design. During the last 4 weeks of each period, the horses underwent 15–30 minutes of treadmill exercise (trotting). Blood samples for measurement of serum creatine kinase (CK) activity were taken 4 hours after each exercise session. The log of serum CK activity was significantly ($P < 0.05$) higher when horses were fed diets A, B, and C when compared to diet D. Postprandial glucose and insulin responses were lower in diet D when compared with diet A, while serum free fatty acid (FFA) concentrations (measured 4 hours after exercise) were consistently higher in diet A when compared to the other diets. However, muscle glycogen and glucose-6-phosphate concentrations and the percentage of muscle fibers with abnormal polysaccharide accumulation did not differ among the diets (Ribeiro et al., 2004).

Whereas there are reports that draft horses with PSSM can show clinical improvement with diet change alone (Valentine et al., 2001b), studies in Quarter horses (Firshman et al., 2003) and Warmbloods (Hunt et al., 2005) have demonstrated that both a change in diet and institution of daily exercise (including turnout) are necessary for a favorable response. In a study of 65 Warmblood or Warmblood-cross horses with PSSM, only horses that received regular exercise and/or turnout, in addition to diet change, showed significant clinical improvement (Hunt et al., 2005). Quarter horses with PSSM also were more likely to show improvement in the severity and frequency of ER when changes in both diet and physical activity were instituted vs. a change in diet only (Firshman et al., 2003).

Pathogenesis

The mechanisms underlying enhanced glycogen storage in Quarter horses with PSSM have been partially elucidated. Unlike skeletal muscle glycogenoses in humans and other species (DiMauro and Lamperti, 2001), excessive glycogen storage is not due to reduced capacity for glycogen utilization. During controlled exercise protocols, net glycogen breakdown and accumulation of lactate in skeletal muscle (middle gluteal m.) were similar in affected Quarter horses and controls (Valberg et al., 1999a,b). Similarly, the activities of key glycolytic enzymes, measured in homogenates of muscle biopsies, did not differ between affected and control horses (Valberg et al., 1998). Instead, excessive muscle glycogen storage may be related to enhanced insulin sensitivity and uptake of glucose into skeletal muscle. Glucose clearance following bolus intravenous administration of glucose (0.5 g/kg BW) was 1.5 times faster in affected Quarter horses when compared to healthy control horses, while glucose concentrations after oral glucose administration were significantly lower (De La Corte et al., 1999a). Affected horses had lower resting insulin concentrations and lower insulin concentrations than controls after intravenous or oral administration of glucose. Furthermore, intravenous insulin resulted in a more profound hypoglycemia when compared to controls (De La Corte et al., 1999a). Blood glucose and insulin concentrations were also lower in affected horses than in healthy controls after consumption of a meal of sweet feed (De La Corte et al., 1999b), findings consistent with enhanced glucose clearance and insulin sensitivity. The strongest evidence of enhanced insulin sensitivity in PSSM was provided by a more recent study that demonstrated a 2-fold higher rate of glucose clearance in affected vs. control horses during a euglycemic-hyperinsulinemic clamp (Annandale et al., 2004).

Nutritional Management

Dietary recommendations (Firshman et al., 2003; McKenzie et al., 2003) for management of horses with PSSM include: (1) feeding a minimum of 1.5 percent of BW as forage per day, ideally a grass or oat hay as these forages have lower nonfiber carbohydrate content when compared to legumes; (2) removal of all concentrates containing grain and molasses from the ration; and (3) use of alternative energy sources such as vegetable oil, rice bran, and/or non-molassed beet pulp when DE requirements are higher than that provided by forage alone. Clinical improvement of horses with PSSM may be dependent upon the addition of fat to the ration. It has been reported that signs of muscle dysfunction can persist when affected horses are fed an all-forage ration with low starch and sugar content (< 10 percent DE) content, whereas clinical signs of muscle dysfunction abate when even a small amount of vegetable-source fat is added to the ration (McKenzie et al., 2003). There are conflicting views on the amount of dietary fat required for clinical improvement of horses with PSSM. Valentine et al. (2001b) reported that horses with ESSM showed greatest improvement when fed a ration that provided, on a total diet basis, at least 20–25 percent of DE from fat. Other researchers have reported clinical improvement when affected horses were fed rations with only 10–15 percent of DE provided by fat (Firshman et al., 2003; Ribeiro et al., 2004). As some horses with PSSM are overweight, the feeding of a high-oil diet is problematic without instigation of an exercise program. On balance, it appears that a reduction in dietary starch and simple sugar is the most important dietary recommendation for horses with PSSM. When forage alone does not meet daily DE needs, a source of fat such as vegetable oil (as much as 600 ml/d for a 500-kg horse), rice bran (0.5–2 kg/d), or other sources of fat should be added to the diet. For horses in heavy training, other feedstuffs such as nonmolassed beet pulp may be needed to meet DE requirements and ensure palatability of the diet.

As mentioned, the implementation of a daily exercise regimen is also important for successful management of Quarter horses and Warmbloods with PSSM. A combination of a low-starch, high-fat diet and regular exercise may result in clinical improvement via a decrease in muscle glycogen storage (Firshman et al., 2003) and/or an increase in lipid metabolism in muscle (Ribeiro et al., 2004).

Developmental Orthopedic Disease

Developmental orthopedic disease (DOD) is a complex of musculoskeletal abnormalities that can afflict growing horses. These conditions include angular limb deformities (ALD, or "crooked-legged foals"), physitis, subchondral bone cysts, osteochondrosis (OC), flexural limb deformities ("contracted tendons"), and cervical vertebral malformation ("wobbler syndrome") (Pool, 1993; McIlwraith, 2004). Congenital contracted tendons are not considered part of the DOD complex (Kidd and Barr, 2002) and will not be discussed here, nor will cervical vertebral malformation.

The incidence of DOD disorders (physitis and OC) submitted to a North American veterinary hospital and in young Irish Thoroughbreds was 68–81 percent (Gabel, 1986; O'Donohue et al., 1992). Of these foals, 11.3 percent required treatment (O'Donohue et al., 1992). Conformational leg abnormalities in the neonate are high (Aldred, 1998; Leibsle et al., 2005). Aldred (1998) reported that 80 percent of Thoroughbred foals born in Australia annually have some degree of ALD. It was predicted that 40 percent of these foals would need corrective hoof trimming, 8 percent would need surgical correction, 3–5 percent would develop contracted tendons, 6 percent would become wobblers, 5 percent would develop OC, and 10 percent would be unsold as yearlings because of the bone abnormalities. Leibsle et al. (2005) found that only 3 percent of newborn (average age 2 days) Thoroughbred foals had "straight" carpal conformations compared to 55 percent with correct fetlocks. At 1 to 1.5 years of age, only 7 percent of the same foals were considered straight at the carpus (knee), while 79 percent were straight at the fetlock. Since a considerable number of young horses are born with less than perfectly aligned joints, subsequent mismanagement of the dietary program and husbandry of the foal could potentially exacerbate any developing osteochondral problems.

Bone growth disorders in young horses have multifactorial causes. Pool (1993) divided the causes of OC into those that are idiopathic or acquired. Idiopathic causes are constitutional and hereditary; acquired causes are associated with biomechanically induced trauma or nutritional, toxic, iatrogenic, and other determinable causes. Thus, the collective risks for bone growth disorders in a foal originate with breed risk, the conformation of the foal inherited from its dam and sire, its prenatal and postnatal diet, and the husbandry methods and housing practices used during the critical growth period from birth to at least 2 years of age. Future studies to elucidate the etiology and pathogenesis of DOD will continue to provide conflicting and nonedifying conclusions until all of these factors are controlled and all criteria used to confirm the clinical and pathological diagnoses of DOD are standardized. The extent to which these criteria were controlled and standardized should be considered in the interpretations of conclusions in the studies described below.

Pathogenesis

Developmental orthopedic diseases originate from abnormalities of endochondral ossification in one or both of the growing areas of bone, articular-epiphyseal cartilage complex and the growth plates (physis) (Pool 1993; McIlwraith, 2004). Osteochondrosis is the pathologic description of bone diseases of young horses in which there is failure of or abnormal cartilage maturation. The abnormalities of joint cartilage and subchondral bone in osteochondrosis dissecans (OCD) have progressed to cracks and fissures in the cartilage. If osteochondrotic cartilage loosens, bone chips or joint mice may occur within the joint or synovial space (McIlwraith, 2004). Although OC and OCD are often used interchangeably, the pathology associated with OCD is more advanced than that seen in OC. Clinical symptoms and pathologies are different depending on the affected site and affected bone. A detailed review of the cellular pathogenesis of equine osteochondrosis can be found in Jeffcott and Henson (1998) and some of the site specific modulators of the physeal growth zones including dietary nutrients were reviewed by Orth (1999).

Osteochondrosis has been described as a dynamic bone disorder that can develop or regress in specific joints depending on the joint's "window of susceptibility" (Pool, 1987; Dik et al., 1999; Barneveld and van Weeren, 1999). In 1987, Pool suggested that the pathologic insult to a susceptible bone likely was of short duration and occurred randomly during the period of joint vulnerability. This hypothesis appears to be supported by subsequent studies. Mild to moderate radiographic abnormalities were observed in the intermediate ridge of the distal tibia in 67.4 percent of 1-month-old Dutch Warmblood foals (Dik, 1999; Dik et al., 1999; van Weeren et al., 2003), but tended to regress over time so that at 11 months of age, only 18.4 percent of hocks were still abnormal. Stifle abnormalities occurred between 3–4 months of age but reverted to normal by 8 months of age. Similarly, Sondergaard (2003) observed an age-related decrease in radiographic OCD from weaning through 2 years. Although most lesions were temporary, the "age of no return" when regression was less likely to occur in the hock was after 5 months of age and for the stifle was after 8–12 months of age (Dik, 1999; Dik et al., 1999). The important nutritional conclusion from these observations is that dietary mismanagement preceding and during these critical ages may tip the balance from regression to progression of subclinically abnormal cartilage and bone to clinical lesions. Hence, a balanced and appropriately managed diet is necessary prior to and at the time of weaning.

Genetics and Growth Rate

The genetic growth potential of the foal, including its conformational traits and growth, are governed by the genotype of the dam and sire (Saastamoinen, 1990; Preisinger et al., 1991; Árnason and Bjarnason, 1994; Koenen et al., 1995; Molina et al., 1999; Zechner et al., 2001; Leibsle et al., 2005). Skeletal dimensions and conformation were moderately to highly heritable traits in Andalusian and Lipizzaner horses (Molina et al., 1999; Zechner et al., 2001) and Trakehner foals (Preisinger et al., 1991). Associations between parent and progeny were found for carpal but not fetlock conformation (Leibsle et al., 2005). These authors also reported a significant relationship between heavier birth weights and an offset carpal conformation (P < 0.01) and fetlock inward deviation at 46 days (P < 0.005), effects that persisted beyond 1 year of age (Leibsle et al., 2005). Foals with hock OC and palmar/plantar osteochondral fragments tended to have outwardly rotated limb axes and periodically had a more upright pastern (Sandberg, 1993). The high incidence of conformational imperfections in foals (Leibsle et al., 2005), coupled with the relative immaturity of the radiocarpal physis at birth (Mase, 1987), and/or a high body mass could exacerbate abnormal biomechanical pressure, asymmetrical growth, or direct trauma occurring at the physis (Mase, 1987; Firth and Hodge, 1997; Whitton, 1998) leading to carpal physitis or other forms of DOD.

The impact of genotype on osteochondrosis has been reported in several studies. Based on a survey of 753 Swedish Standardbred trotters aged 6–21 months, 14.3 percent had tibiotarsal OC while 11.8 percent had fetlock joint involvement (Grondahl and Dolvik, 1993). The incidence of fetlock, hock, and stifle OC ranged from 17, 6, and 3 percent and 24, 6, and 11 percent, respectively, in nonlame and clinically lame Swedish Warmblood horses (Beneus, 2005). Radiographic evidence of OC was found in 16.6 percent of 350 Maremmano Warmblood horses with a heritability index of 0.14, which increased with inbreeding (Pieramati et al., 2003). These authors predicted that through genetic selection, OC in their studied population could be reduced from 16 percent to 2 percent within five generations.

In North America, the breeds with the highest incidence of DOD were Quarter horses, Thoroughbreds, Arabians, and Paints (Wagner, 1986), while Standardbred followed by Thoroughbred horses were at highest risk of OC (Mohammed, 1990). Ponies and draft horses have been suggested to have a low incidence of osteochondrotic bone disorders (Stromberg, 1979). In a veterinary hospital, only 5 percent of the admitted draft horse population had OCD and/or subchondral bone cysts (Riley et al., 1998). The heavy breeds most often presented in the latter study were Clydesdale and Percheron horses.

Foals at risk for osteochondrosis were described as those that are the most rapidly growing foals in the group (Turner and Fretz, 1977; Stromberg, 1979; Thompson et al., 1988a,b), which is consistent to observations in other species (Olsson, 1978; Stromberg and Rejno, 1978; Stromberg, 1979). Some ambiguity between the association of weight gain with DOD has been raised (McIlwraith, 2004), and this uncertainty is supported by the conflicting data presented in studies examining these relationships. Foals affected with hock OC tended to have heavier birth weights, had higher average daily gain (ADG), and were heavier at 1.5 years of age, but those with palmar/plantar osteochondral fragments tended to weigh less than nonaffected foals (Sandgren, 1993). Foals with stifle OC were significantly taller at the withers and had 7–20 percent higher weight gains only at 3 and 5 months of age; there was no relationship between rates of weight gain and OC in the hock joint (van Weeren et al., 1999). The average incidence of DOD in Thoroughbred foals evaluated between 4 through 18 months of age was 16.1 percent (range 12.9–28.8 percent) and the highest incidence was recorded at 4 months of age (Jelan et al., 1996). Body weights were not statistically different between affected and nonaffected foals, although the authors noted that affected foals were generally heavier. Based on farm data, OCD-affected and normal Thoroughbred or Hanoverian foals did not differ in body weight (Pagan, 2003; Vervuert et al., 2003). The total incidence of hock and fetlock osteochondrotic lesions in the latter study was 31.5 percent. Foals in controlled studies fed excess energy or starch did not differ in final body weights or average daily gain, although dyschondroplasia was prevalent in one study (Savage et al., 1993a) but not the other (Ott et al., 2005).

That genotype affects the rate of weight gain is evident from the wide range of weight gains of various breeds of horses (see Chapter 1), but certain lines of horses within breeds are also recognized to have different body dimensions (Zechner et al., 2001). A highly positive correlation (0.97) was found between body weight and growth rate at 12 months in Finnhorses indicating that selection for rapid growth rates is possible in horses (Saastamoinen, 1990). The heritability for body weight from birth to 2 years of age was 0.22–0.88 (SE = 0.46 to 0.87); the overall heritability from birth to 48 months was 0.86 ± 0.32 (Saastamoinen, 1990). The variance in growth rates exceeded variance in absolute body measurements. Variation in absolute body weight ranged from 7.3–14.9 percent and from 2.4–4.6 percent for withers height. Variance in ADG in the age categories from birth–6 months, 6–12, 12–24, 24–36, 36–48, and 0–48 months was 10.9, 26.8, 24.1, 64, 45.3, and 7.9 percent, respectively. The calculated variances in biweekly ADG for weanlings fed a high-forage diet (70 percent alfalfa) in limited amounts or free-choice, or a high-concentrate diet (34.7 percent alfalfa) fed free-choice were 7.8, 14.2, and 17 percent, respectively, indicating a more fluctuating weight gain with ad libitum feeding (Cymbaluk, 1989). Thus, rate and amplitude of weight gain are not only affected by diet but by method of feeding, which is further confounded by heritability of gain.

Fluctuating growth rate may be a precursor to DOD (Barneveld and van Weeren, 1999), yet fluctuating biweekly weight gains are evident even in normal Thoroughbred foals between birth and 1 year of age (Thompson, 1995). Although erratic weight gains were more prevalent in free-choice than in limit-fed foals (Cymbaluk, 1989), it was unclear whether this alone would contribute a sufficient biomechanical insult during the critical window of susceptibility to alter endochondral ossification. Other management conditions that have been reported to result in nonuniform growth rates are dietary stress (Hintz et al., 1976), environmental stress (Rooney, 1984; Cymbaluk and Christison, 1989a; Cymbaluk, 1990), season (Jelan et al., 1996; Hoffman et al., 1999), hormonal maturation (Noguiera et al., 1997), and unidentified factors (Jelan et al., 1996). Contracted tendons and/or physitis in young horses followed a suspected compensatory gain following a switch from nutritionally marginal to abundant diets (Hintz et al., 1976), following environmental stress either as extreme cold (Cymbaluk and Christison, 1989a) or prolonged inclement weather (Rooney, 1984).

Seasonal growth spurts were associated with an increased occurrence of bone abnormalities in young horses (O'Donohue et al., 1992; Hoffman et al., 1999). The peak incidence (4.1 percent) of clinical musculoskeletal conditions in young Thoroughbreds monitored from birth through 2 years occurred post-weaning in early winter and gradually resolved over the next year (O'Donohue et al., 1992). Seasonal fluctuations in DOD were also evident in yearlings fed high starch (SS) or high fat-fiber (FF) diets (Hoffman et al., 1999). The most severe clinical physitis in suckling foals occurred over 2 months in late summer and autumn, and were not influenced by the foal's growth rate or sex (Finkler-Schade et al., 1999; Gee et al., 2005b). However, in other studies the seasonal clinical observations were coincident with changes in serum bone markers, including osteocalcin, carboxypropeptide of type 1 collagen and type III collagen propeptide, and with average daily gain (Price et al., 1997, 2001). The production of sex hormones may also stimulate growth spurts. Weight gains increased abruptly in 14-month-old Thoroughbred fillies concurrent with a pubertal spike in progesterone secretion (Nogueira et al., 1997).

Thus, sustained modest growth rates may be preferred for young horses to minimize some DOD-like conditions, especially prior to the earliest window of susceptibility for specific joints. Supplying creep feed to suckling foals at 2–3 months of age has been suggested as a method to maintain growth during the suckling period and to minimize the immediate post-weaning weight loss seen in foals (Coleman et al., 1999; Peterson et al., 2003). Although creep feeding did not entirely prevent weight loss post-weaning, creep-fed foals were perceived to be less stressed than noncreep-fed foals just after weaning (Coleman et al., 1999).

Dietary Nutrients and Bone Growth Disorders

The potential effect of dietary nutrient intake on bone growth in foals has been reviewed by Jeffcott and Savage (1996) and Harris et al. (2005). Documented evidence has confirmed that horses kept under pratical management situations are often fed diets that may not be adequately designed to meet the predicted nutrient requirements (Knight et al., 1985; Hacklander et al., 1996; Finkler-Schade et al., 1999; Gibbs and Cohen, 2001; Paragon et al., 2003). The most common nutrient imbalances identified included excess energy intake, and excesses or deficiencies in protein, macromineral, and trace mineral content, as well as calcium/phosphorus imbalances. Feeding programs on Thoroughbred and Quarter horse breeding farms were well managed on about half of the farms, but the remaining farms were felt likely to be using unbalanced diets (Gibbs and Cohen, 2001). Although the role of diet in foal growth cannot be disputed, the complexity of the relationships among nutrients and their interactions in abnormal bone growth are not yet fully elucidated. It is, however, important to recognize that when formulating practical diets, nutrient concentrations can deviate from NRC recommendations without causing abnormal growth in young horses (Ott and Kivipelto, 2002). However, all variances in dietary nutrient concentrations in horse diets should be evaluated to ensure that the nutrient concentration falls into an accepted normal range for the class of horse for which the diet is intended.

Energy, Protein, and Fat Intake

Excessive energy intake has received considerable interest in the etiology of equine DOD in part based on the hypothesis that excessive amounts of nonfiber carbohydrates may contribute to hormonal abnormalities in foals, specifically through modified insulin responses (Kronfeld et al., 1990). High-energy diets were felt to cause OCD irrespective of feed composition (Stromberg, 1979). The data of Savage et al. (1993a), who fed weanling foals diet containing 29 percent more energy than recommended by NRC (1989), supported this hypothesis. Histological dyschondroplastic changes in the stifle, hock, and fetlock joints were observed in all foals fed high-energy diets (29 percent above control) created by adding 0.25 kg of corn oil to a basal diet of 13 percent oaten chaff and 77 percent rice-based pellets (Savage et al., 1993a). The source of the additional dietary energy in the high-energy diet in this study was derived from corn oil, but all diets were based on rice concentrate, a feed that is high in starch, and the foals were partially confined. The foals in this study had similar net gains in skeletal and weight growth to control foals (Savage et al., 1993c); consequently, the dyschondroplastic bone lesions may have been induced through a hormonal alteration, although this was not verified.

Dietary composition, in addition to absolute nutrient content, of foal diets has also been scrutinized as a possible influence on the incidence of DOD. The assumption that rapid growth obtained through use of grain-based, high nonfiber carbohydrates has contributed to a higher incidence of DOD has led to examination of dietary effects on the insulin-glucose axis and the role of insulin sensitivity in foals. The plasma insulin-glucose response to feeding a diet of 50:50 textured grain:alfalfa-grass hay was compared in OCD-affected to normal young horses (Ralston, 1996). Although glucose:insulin ratios did not differ, plasma insulin concentration was 29–79 percent higher in OCD-affected horses than controls. Pagan (2003) correlated the post-meal feeding (2 h) plasma insulin concentrations of 218 10-month-old foals to surgical OCD lesions present at the time of blood sampling or which developed over the next 6–10 months and observed that the 27 OCD-affected foals had higher plasma glucose and insulin concentrations but no difference in the glucose:insulin ratio compared to normal cohorts. Yearling Thoroughbreds fed a 72 percent hydrolysable carbohydrate diet had a significantly higher glycemic ($P < 0.043$) and insulinemic ($P < 0.031$) response than foals fed a high fat-fiber concentrate (Staniar, 2002). That high nonfiber carbohydrate concentrates modify the insulin responsiveness was shown by Treiber et al. (2005), who observed a 37 percent reduction in insulin sensitivity in weanlings fed a 49 percent nonfiber carbohydrate (SS) concentrate compared to foals fed a fat-fiber (FF) concentrate. However, Ropp et al. (2003) compared the insulin-glucose responses of weanling Quarter horses fed a more typical concentrate containing 33.9 percent nonfiber carbohydrates vs. a concentrate containing 10 percent fat and 24 percent nonfiber carbohydrate for 75 days and found no treatment by time interactions on day 0 or 60 for glucose and no interaction effect for insulin on day 0 or 30. There was no change in growth hormone secretion or plasma insulin-like growth factor I (IGF-I) concentrations, and only a minor glucose sparing effect. Ott et al. (2005) fed weanling horses either a medium- (2.9 starch/kg BW) or high- (6.5 starch/kg BW) starch diet without inducing changes in bone mineral content or creating new osteochondrotic bone lesions. During the study, the incidence of preexisting radiographic OCD bone lesions decreased about 29 percent irrespective of whether the foals were fed hay plus a concentrate containing either 17 or 37.5 percent starch. These data confirm that foals fed some types of grain-based concentrates can have altered insulin responses. Unlike growing horses, ponies were significantly more hyperglycemic and hyperinsulinemic when fed a high-fat (11.1 percent) diet than when fed a high-sugar diet (Schmidt et al., 2001). The role of insulin resistance in developmental bone disorders is unclear and conflicts with the observation that ponies are more insulin resistant than horses (Rijnen and van der Kolk, 2003), yet have an apparently low incidence of DOD or osteochondrosis (Stromberg, 1979).

The suspicion that insulin resistance may contribute to developmental bone disorders (Kronfeld et al., 1990) has stimulated interest in finding alternative energy sources to nonstructural carbohydrates. Fat, in limited amounts (< 11 percent), was added to highly fibrous constituents (oat straw, soybean hulls–FF) (Hoffman et al., 1999; Staniar, 2002) or to concentrate-based supplements (Ropp et al., 2003) to lower the nonfiber carbohydrate while maintaining energy content of the diet. Carpal physitis scores and joint effusion did not differ between FF and SS foals, but hind fetlock physitis was higher ($P < 0.5$) for the SS group at 8 and 12 months (Hoffman et al., 1999). Foals in the FF group had higher ($P < 0.05$) scores for angular limb deformities at 1 month, 8 months, and 10 months of age.

The conflicting data obtained on the effects of energy intake on the incidence of DOD have in part arisen through different methods of feeding. Regulated feeding of concentrate mixes has not resulted in increased bone abnormalities (Ott and Asquith, 1989; Reynolds et al., 1992; Ott et al., 2005). Quarter horse weanlings fed a diet of 25 percent Bermudagrass hay plus 75 percent concentrate (given twice daily) from 6 to 12 months of age gained weight at 0.65 kg/d, and all subchondral and cystic lesions, except for the cystic carpal lesions, identified radiographically at 6 months had regressed by 1 year of age (Reynolds et al., 1992). Unregulated feeding of any diet, whether high in fiber or not, has led to transient physitis and flexural limb deformities (Cymbaluk and Christison, 1989b). In addition to the effect on the somatotrophic axis, the use of FF concentrates (Hoffman et al., 1999) requires further study to verify its usefulness in preventing developmental bone disease.

High-protein diets do not appear to influence the occurrence of DOD. Although feeding excessive protein, specifically soybean meal, has previously been proposed as a cause of flexural limb deformities in growing horses (Fackelman, 1980), others have suggested minimal to no effect of high dietary protein intake on DOD occurrence (Stromberg, 1979; Boren et al., 1987; Savage et al., 1993a). Addition of 0.2 percent lysine or 0.2 percent lysine and 0.1 percent threonine to diets of yearling horses had no effect on bone mineral content or skeletal growth rates (Graham et al., 1994).

Mineral Intake

The effect of excesses and deficiencies of minerals on foal growth has been reviewed in Chapter 5. Macrominerals, especially calcium (CA), phosphorus (P), and magnesium, form the mineral complex in bone. Bone mineral density, ash, and calcium content in subchondral and trabecular bone increased in horses up to 4 years old (van der Harst et al., 2005), suggesting that an inadequate or an imbalanced macromineral intake could affect bone development and strength up to this age. Dietary mineral content may affect the severity of OCD as shown by Firth et al. (1999), who observed comparatively lower bone mineral density in the third carpal bone and the distal radial bone of young horses with severe signs of OCD. Imbalances in dietary calcium and phosphorus also increased the risk of DOD. Weanling Warmblood foals fed diets with either a normal Ca:P ratio (2.5:1) or a low Ca:P ratio (1:2.5) had normal weight gains, but all foals developed physitis, synovial distension, and, except for one foal, all others developed OCD in two or more joints (Staun et al., 1989). Savage et al. (1993b) observed that weaned foals fed a high-calcium diet (1.95 percent) had a similar number (33 percent) of histological dyschondroplastic lesions as foals (17 percent) fed a control diet with a Ca:P ratio of 1.3:1. A companion study in which weaned foals were fed a diet containing adequate calcium and excess phosphorus (1.7 percent) whose calcium:phosphorus ratio was imbalanced resulted in an 83 percent incidence of histological dyschondroplasia of the shoulder, hock, and/or intervertebral joints (Savage et al., 1993c). Joint lesions were attributed to a nutritional secondary hyperparathyroidism induced by a Ca:P imbalance. These data support the need for an adequate macromineral intake and an acceptable Ca:P ratio during postnatal growth, but they also indicate that even when macrominerals are supplied in adequate amounts, some foals may develop bone abnormalities.

Dietary micromineral content, particularly copper through lysyl oxidase, has been shown necessary for formation and repair of collagen, the main component of bone matrix. Copper (Cu) was first linked to OC and physitis in an epidemiological study, which found a higher incidence of clinically diagnosed disorders in foals fed low-copper diets (Knight et al., 1985). Although copper was implicated in the clinical conditions, foals on farms with a higher incidence of OC and physitis also fed diets low in calcium and high in phosphorus. Subsequently, controlled studies on DOD (Knight et al., 1990; Hurtig et al., 1993; Pearce et al., 1998a,b,c; Grace et al., 2002; van Weeren et al., 2003; Gee et al., 2005a,b, 2006) have examined the role of copper in foal bone development with contradictory outcomes. Knight et al. (1990) evaluated bone development in 21 foals whose dams were either fed 13 (control) or 32 mg Cu/kg BW (supplemented) during the last 3–6 months of gestation and during lactation. Foals received a creep ration containing 15 mg Cu/kg concentrate (control) or 55 mg Cu/kg concentrate (supplemented). Postmortem findings of 90-day-old foals revealed predominantly physeal abnormalities that were not different between groups. Equal numbers of physeal lesions occurred in the forelimbs of 180-day-old foals although control foals had more physeal and articular-epiphyseal lesions in the hindlimbs. Notably, at both 90 and 180 days of age, one individual in the control group accounted for 59 percent or 35 percent of the bone lesions, respectively. Hurtig et al. (1993) fed 18 foals, including 2 with preexisting DOD, diets containing either 8 or 25 mg Cu/kg feed. A higher incidence of cartilaginous flaps and/or thinning was observed for foals fed the diet containing 8 mg Cu/kg feed. No significant difference was observed between treatment groups in the tibial or radial growth plates, calcified cartilage area, metaphyseal bone formation, or epiphyseal bone formation rates or in the biochemical properties of the bone or growth plate cartilage.

Pearce et al. (1998a,b,c) compared feeding supplemental copper to pregnant mares (0.5 mg/kg BW or 28 mg Cu/kg diet) to a control group grazing pasture containing 4.4–8.6 mg Cu/kg. Foals born to these mares were randomly allocated to either a copper-supplemented or a copper-control group. Copper-supplemented foals received 0.2 mg Cu/kg BW from 21 to 49 days of age and 0.5 mg Cu/kg BW to 150 days of age. Only those foals whose dams were given supplemental copper in the latter part of pregnancy had a lower incidence of OC (Pearce et al., 1998c). The incidence of bone and cartilage lesions was low in all foals irrespective of copper intake by dam or foal. Providing the foals with supplemental copper (0.5 mg/kg BW) from 1.5–5 months of age did not further eliminate bone or cartilage lesions (Pearce et al., 1998c). Subsequently, Grace et al. (2002) supplemented yearling horses on pasture (7.9 mg Cu/kg DM) with 130 mg copper daily so that copper-supplemented yearlings consumed a total of 186 mg Cu/d compared to 56 mg/d for controls. Neither weight gain nor incidence of physitis differed between copper-supplemented and control yearlings. Gee et al. (2006) administered injectable copper (calcium copper edentate) to pregnant mares starting at about 7 months through parturition and observed no difference in osteochondral abnormalities between foals born to the treated and untreated mares. All osteochondral lesions were considered minor and there were no differences in foal or dam hepatic copper concentrations. The authors concluded that injectable copper was an unsuitable method of copper supplementation and did not confer the protective effect against the development of osteochondrotic bone lesions observed in foals born to dams given oral copper three times weekly (Pearce et al., 1998c).

Hepatic copper decay in neonatal foals followed a pattern of rapid decline in concentration from birth to weaning (Gee et al., 2000; van Weeren et al., 2003). Two distinctive patterns of hepatic copper decay were observed; a normal and an accumulator pattern (Gee et al., 2000). Neonatal hepatic copper concentration (374 mg/kg DM liver) in normal foals declined to adult values (21 mg/kg DM liver) by 160 days of age. Accumulator foals had a much slower rate of hepatic copper decay. At weaning, liver copper concentrations were still high (162 mg/kg DM liver). Although hepatic liver copper concentrations and OCD status in foals were not correlated (van Weeren et al., 2003), a higher hepatic copper status at birth appeared to promote the regression of OCD lesions present in the stifle at 11 months of age but not at 5 months of age. Van Weeren et al. (2003) proposed that copper deficiency may not initiate OC lesions but rather may stimulate the repair mechanism in abnormal cartilage. The collective conclusions of copper studies in foals support the following: (1) copper supplementation of the pregnant dam, not the weanling foal, may have reduced incidence of DOD in foals; (2) experimental copper deficiency in foals produced inconsistent cartilage pathology, which may differ to that of clinical OC; and (3) copper deficiency may not initiate OC, but supplemental copper may be beneficial for OC-affected foals by promoting repair of developing osteochondral lesions.

Dietary trace mineral supplementation of diets for foals did not dramatically change the incidence of bone abnormalities in foals fed diets marginally adequate in trace minerals. The addition of a trace mineral and/or calcium mixture to a concentrate mix fed with a Bermudagrass hay containing 7 mg Cu/kg and 57 mg Zinc (Zn)/kg to yearling horses had no effect on feed intake ($P < 0.1$) but increased bone mineral content of the third metacarpal bone only when the basal diet was supplemented to provide 11 mg Cu/kg and 69 mg Zn/kg (Ott and Asquith, 1989). A subsequent study in which a basal diet, marginal in calcium (0.36 percent) and phosphorus (0.29 percent), but which contained 11 mg Cu/kg and 40 mg Zn/kg, was compared to the same diet supplemented to supply the following mineral concentrations: calcium (0.53 percent), phosphorus (0.38 percent), copper (14 mg/kg), and zinc (45 mg/kg). None of the yearlings showed any clinical abnormalities in either study, and there was no effect on bone mineral content of yearlings fed the diets for 112 days.

Vitamins

The effect of deficient and excessive intake of vitamins has been described in Chapter 6. The fat-soluble vitamins A and D have been implicated in developmental abnormalities of the growth plate. Feeding vitamin A in amounts 1,000-fold greater than control (12 µg/kg BW) produced histological osteochondrotic lesions in growth plates of growing ponies (Donoghue, 1980). Deficiencies of vitamin D can lead to poorly mineralized bone but excesses also have been shown to result in weakened, porous bone. Unexpectedly, serum vitamin 1,25 $(OH)_2$ D and parathyroid hormone concentrations were higher in osteochondrotic foals than those without or with few lesions and, perhaps, indicate that higher hormone levels are needed to maintain plasma calcium concentration in this condition (Sloet van Oldruitenborgh-Oosterbaan et al., 1999).

Exercise and Training

Weight bearing and exercise have been shown to positively affect bone turnover and remodeling (Lanyon, 1992) and may also act as a stimulus for collagen development in subchondral bone of horses (Brama et al., 2002). In most of the Thoroughbred and Quarter horse breeding farms surveyed in Texas, young horses were kept in semiconfinement and received free exercise (Gibbs and Cohen, 2001). Voluntary exercise (foals kept on pasture) tended to protect the articular cartilage from development of OC lesions compared to complete confinement in 5-month-old Dutch Warmblood foals (Barneveld and van Weeren, 1999). Benefits in bone mineral content of the third metacarpal bone were also reported for weanling Arabians and Quarter horses given voluntary (pasture) or enforced exercise (82 m/d, 5 d/wk) (Bell et al., 2001; Hiney et al., 2004). Exercise produced site-specific increases in calcium and collagen cross-links in the subchondral bone of 5-month-old foals (Brama et al., 2001, 2002) and increased bone mineral density by 5–8 percent in 2-year-old Thoroughbred fillies compared to idle controls, suggesting a beneficial mechanical effect of exercise (Jackson et al., 2003). In contrast, bone mineral density did not differ whether foals were kept in box stalls, boxed and exercised, or on pasture for 5 months then turned out for voluntary exercise on pasture for an added 6 months (Firth et al., 1999). Sondergaard (2003) observed that group-housed growing horses were more active than foals housed alone, but the increased voluntary activity did not influence the incidence of radiographic OCD.

Intensive exercise may also cause negative effects. Enforced exercise of 2-month-old foals for 12 months reduced the number of thyroid C cells required for calcitonin secretion involved in calcium homeostasis and also produced a trend to lowered bone mineral density of the hind cannon bone (Ueki et al., 2003). Box-stalled foals required to do gallop sprints up to 5 months of age, then turned out to pasture until 11 months of age, had a reduced glycosaminoglycan content and hypermetabolic chondrocytes in articular cartilage compared to unexercised and pastured foals, suggesting that the enforced exercise regimen reduced the vitality of the chondrocyte (Barneveld et al., 1999; van den Hoogen et al., 1999). A positive effect, however, of enforced exercise was an enhancement in bone mineral density compared to foals given voluntary exercise (pasture) and sustained confinement.

Summary of Studies on Developmental Orthopedic Diseases in Foals

The following conclusions can be inferred about foal developmental bone disorders based on current information:

- The causes of DOD are numerous and likely interrelated.
- The incidence of DOD can be as low as 1 foal in 20 to as high as 1 foal in 3.
- Osteochondral abnormalities were observed early in life (1 month of age) but most lesions regress. Joints appear to have different windows of susceptibility after which regression of lesions may be less likely to occur. The "age of no return" was felt to occur about 5 months of age for the hock and 8–12 months for the stifle.
- Genotype affects growth rate and likely impact the incidence of DOD. Weight was highly heritable but rate of gain may or may not be directly related to the incidence of DOD.
- The normal variability seen in foal weight gain up to 1 year of age was increased when diets were fed ad libitum, irrespective of composition (either high concentrate or high forage). An irregular growth rate may be a factor in the occurrence of DOD and can be created through dietary and environmental stresses, seasonal and hormonal changes, and unidentified factors.
- Creep feeding may help smooth the growth pattern of foals in the transition from suckling through weaning.
- Practical diets fed to foals and broodmares may or may not be balanced in the critical nutrients—energy, protein, macrominerals, and trace minerals—required for bone growth.
- Diet composition can affect hormonal responses. Specifically, concentrates high in nonfiber carbohydrates have resulted in higher insulin-glucose responses to feeding and lower insulin sensitivity when compared to high-fat (> 10 percent) and fiber concentrates. However, the source of energy in the concentrate does not appear to affect the incidence of clinical osteochondral abnormalities.
- Feeding excess protein does not appear to affect DOD.
- Imbalances in calcium and phosphorus (Ca:P ratio < 1) can produce dyschondroplasia.
- Copper deficiency may not initiate osteochondral abnormalities. Supplementation of the pregnant dam, not the weanling foal, may reduce incidence of DOD in foals by promoting repair of developing osteochondral lesions.
- Voluntary exercise may be beneficial in reducing DOD compared to confinement. Enforced exercise may benefit bone mineral content but may negatively affect chondrocytic metabolism.

Practical nutritional management to prevent bone growth disorders was discussed by Lewis (1995). Although, the research data cited by this author are only current to 1995, many of the feeding management suggestions are still valid.

Laminitis

Laminitis is a systemic disease that manifests in the foot and results in significant pain and lameness. The junction between dermal and epidermal laminae serves to attach the distal phalanx to the hoof wall. Failure of the attachment between the dermo-epidermal junction is the signature lesion of laminitis (Pollitt et al., 2003). The progression of laminitis can be categorized into four phases: developmental, acute, subacute, and chronic. Hood (1999a) defines the four phases as follows. The developmental phase is the period between the initial causative insult and the first appearance of lameness and lasts an average of 40 hours (range 24–60). The acute phase follows the developmental phase and takes one of two courses: continuation for 72 hours without physical or radiographic collapse or termination abruptly upon occurrence of digital collapse (i.e., rotation or sinking of the distal phalanx). The subacute phase follows the acute phase in the absence of physical or radiographic collapse, lasts from 8–12 weeks, and is considered a period of recovery from the damage done during developmental and acute phases. The terms chronic laminitis and founder are frequently used synonymously and are reserved for the horse having mechanical collapse of the foot. Thus, any horse with radiographic or physical evidence of digital collapse is categorically considered to have chronic laminitis, regardless of the duration of the disease. Specific clinical features associated with acute and chronic laminitis have been discussed in detail (Herthel and Hood, 1999; Swanson, 1999).

Laminitis is considered a major disease of the horse due to the associated pain, lameness, and potential debilitation. There are limited data on the prevalence of laminitis in equids. Summary data from a survey involving 1,178 horse operations, totaling 28,026 horses, estimated that 13 percent of the operations had one or more horses with laminitis over a 12-month period, and the overall incidence of laminitis was 2.1 ± 0.3 percent (USDA, 2000). A slightly higher incidence (7.1 percent) was reported in a survey involving 113,000 horses in the United Kingdom (Hinckley and Henderson, 1996). The incidence of laminitis in geriatric horses (> 20 years of age) was 6.4 percent, according to a survey involving 467 geriatric horses (Brosnahan and Paradis, 2003).

Several factors have been implicated in the etiology of acute laminitis. These include excessive ingestion of rapidly fermentable carbohydrate (e.g., starch, sugars, and/or fructans) (Garner et al., 1978; Rowe et al., 1994; Pollitt et al., 2003), endotoxemia (Garner et al., 1978; Moore et al., 1989; Rowe et al., 1994; Pollitt et al., 2003), black walnut shavings (Minnick et al., 1987), excessive concussion (Hood, 1999a), obesity and insulin resistance (Jeffcott et al., 1986; Treiber et al., 2005, 2006), glucocorticoid administration (Johnson et al., 2004a), and endocrine disturbances (Johnson et al., 2004b). Although several factors have been associated with the onset of laminitis, the exact mechanism(s) by which these factors trigger laminitis is unknown.

Pathogenesis

The pathogenesis of acute laminitis is uncertain (Bailey et al., 2004; Moore et al., 2004). Three primary theories exist: (1) vascular hemodynamic theory; (2) toxic, metabolic, or enzymatic theory; and (3) traumatic or mechanical overload theory. These theories have been discussed in detail (Hood, 1999b; Moore et al., 2004; Bailey et al., 2004). Briefly, the vascular theory states that a yet to be identified factor(s) initiates a change in digital vascular function, resulting in impaired blood supply to the laminae and subsequent damage resulting in the failure of the dermal-epidermal junction (Moore et al., 2004). One research group (Bailey et al., 2004) proposed that vasoactive monoamines formed and released from the hindgut might be the link between ingestion of feedstuffs rich in rapidly fermentable carbohydrates and the digital ischemic events thought to precede the onset of laminitis. The toxic, metabolic, or enzymatic theory states that an unknown trigger factor delivered in the bloodstream activates metallic matrix metalloproteinases (MMPs), which leads to the breakdown of the basement membrane and separation of the dermo-epidermal junction (Moore et al., 2004; French and Pollitt, 2004). The traumatic or mechanical overload theory states that trauma or mechanical overload and/or associated inflammation and altered blood flow through the foot leads to separation of the dermo-epidermal junction (Hood, 1999b).

Nutritional Management and the Prevention of Acute Laminitis

Strict nutritional guidelines for the prevention of acute laminitis have not been determined. It is well documented that disturbance of normal fermentation pattern in the hindgut resulting from the fermentation of rapidly fermentable carbohydrates (e.g., starch, fructans) can precipitate laminitis (Garner et al., 1977, 1978; Pollitt et al., 2003). However naso-gastric bolus was the means of delivering the rapidly fermentable carbohydrate used in these experiments, which makes extrapolation to oral ingestion of a meal or meals difficult. Potter et al. (1992) suggested that the starch intake per meal (assuming 2 to 3 meals/d) should not exceed 2 to 4 g starch/kg BW in order to minimize postileal starch digestion and the subsequent potential for disturbance of normal fermentation patterns. Garner et al. (1977) induced clinical signs of laminitis in 23 of 31 horses following administration of a cornstarch-wood flour gruel (mean 40 hours; range 24–48 hours), via stomach tube, that delivered approximately 15 g starch/kg BW. Rowe et al. (1994) reported lameness, characteristic of laminitis, in 4 of 4 horses after 4 days of consuming 2 meals/d, 12 hours apart, each containing approximately 3.75 to 6.8 g starch/kg BW (calculation assumes corn contains 75 percent starch). Therefore, the recommendation by Potter et al. (1992) of no more than 2 to 4 g starch/kg BW/meal (assuming 2 to 3 meals/d) may be prudent in the prevention of acute laminitis. However, it should be noted that not all starch is created equal in terms of prececal digestion as stated in Chapter 8.

The ingestion of pasture grasses rich in water-soluble carbohydrates (glucose, fructose, sucrose, and fructan) may precipitate laminitis (Bailey et al., 2004). It has been proposed that ingestion of fructans can result in disturbances to hindgut function in a similar way to undigested starch (Longland and Cairns, 2000), with triggering of laminitis. However, a direct relationship between the onset of laminitis and ingestion of specific pasture carbohydrates has not been demonstrated. Furthermore, there is limited information on the quantities of pasture fructan or other storage carbohydrate required to cause significant changes in hindgut function that may increase risk of laminitis. Longland et al. (1999) reported fructan concentrations in specific varieties of perennial ryegrass (*Lolium perenne*) ranging from 100–420 g fructan/kg DM, depending on environmental conditions. In general, pasture content of storage carbohydrates (including fructans) is highest in spring, lowest in midsummer, and intermediate in autumn. However, there also can be marked daily fluctuations that coincide with patterns of energy storage (photosynthetic activity) and utilization. Thus, pasture water-soluble carbohydrate tends to rise during the morning, reaching maxima in the afternoon, and declining overnight. Horses grazing in the afternoon, when compared to nighttime or morning, may ingest between 2 and 4 times as much water-soluble carbohydrate. Assuming a dry matter intake of 2.5 percent of body weight for a 500-kg horse, the fructan intake from the perennial ryegrass pasture studied by Longland et al. (1999) could range from 2.5–10.5 g fructan/kg BW. The upper end of this range falls within a range of oral fructan dosage (7.5–12.5 g/kg BW) reported to induce laminitis in horses (French and Pollitt, 2004). Smaller dosages of fructan also may alter the hindgut environment and increase risk of laminitis. In ponies, the consumption of inulin (a fructan extracted with chicory root) at 1 g or 3 g/kg BW resulted in a significant decrease in fecal pH (Crawford et al., 2005). Vervuert et al. (2005) reported fructan concentrations in cool-season grass-legume pasture ranging from 18 ± 8 to 57 ± 17 g/kg DM. Using similar assumptions on DM intake as above, the fructan intake from the cool-season grass-legume mix pasture studied by Vervuert et al. (2005) is considerably lower (0.45–1.4 g fructan/kg BW) than the range reported capable of inducing laminitis by French and Pollitt (2004). Hoffman et al. (2001)

reported that the rapidly fermentable carbohydrate content of grass-legume pasture (a large proportion of which was assumed to be fructan) ranged from 22.9–145 g/kg DM which could result in an intake of approximately 0.57–3.6 g rapidly fermentable carbohydrate/kg BW. Although the role of pasture carbohydrates in the pathogenesis of laminitis has not been unequivocally demonstrated, the disease occurs most commonly in equids kept at pasture (USDA, 2000). Therefore, for horses and ponies with a history of pasture-associated laminitis, there is rationale for restricted access to pasture, particularly during the growing seasons.

Nutritional Management and Chronic Laminitis

Specific, objective information regarding nutritional management of horses with chronic laminitis is not available. However, a logical approach to feeding horses with chronic laminitis is to prevent excess body weight in order to minimize mechanical stress on the foot and supply nutrients necessary for hoof growth and repair (Hood, 1999c). Rations having low-caloric density (e.g., low-quality forage only) are often recommended in an effort to prevent excess body weight. If unsupplemented, low-calorie rations may have the potential to be deficient in protein, amino acids, and various micronutrients (Hood, 1999c). Hoof wall growth has been demonstrated to be influenced by overall plane of nutrition (Butler and Hintz, 1977), as well as biotin supplementation (Buffa et al., 1992; Reilly et al., 1998). Therefore, based on limited information, providing a ration that does not exceed digestible energy requirements but contains at least adequate protein and micronutrients should be a feasible approach to promote hoof wall growth and repair.

Nutritional Secondary Hyperparathyroidism

Nutritional secondary hyperparathyroidism (NSH) is a metabolic bone disease associated with the feeding of rations with an excess of phosphorus or a deficiency of available calcium (Joyce et al., 1971; Capen, 1983; Bertone, 1992). Although associated skeletal lesions are generalized, bony changes do not occur uniformly or consistently within skeletal regions. Horses from weaning up to 7 years of age are most often affected. Early signs of the disease include a shifting lameness of one or more legs, tenderness of joints, reluctance to move, and a stiff, stilted gait. These signs are associated with bone demineralization and resultant development of subepiphyseal microfractures, loss of trabecular bone integrity with disruption of articular cartilage, and tearing or detachment of tendons and ligaments. In advanced cases, spontaneous fractures may occur, most often of the sesamoids, phalanges, or both.

Bones of the head are most often visibly affected. Mineral content of facial bones and mandible is replaced with increased amounts of osteoid and fibrous tissue, a process termed osteodystrophia fibrosa. Subsequent bone thickening results in physical distortion of the head, accounting for the disease's descriptive name "big head." Changes to maxillary and mandibular bones are bilateral, but not necessarily symmetrical. Affected horses may first present with clinical signs associated with upper airway breathing difficulty or noise (Clarke et al., 1996). As the disease progresses, horses may have difficulty chewing as a result of decreased bone integrity of dental alveoli and associated dental pain. Reduced feed intake results in weight loss and poor body condition.

Nutritional secondary hyperparathyroidism was prevalent among working horses in the early 1900s. Working horses fed large amounts of bran byproduct, especially those used to mill wheat, were most often afflicted, hence the names "bran disease" and "miller's disease" were used to describe the condition. Presently, NSH is not considered a common condition, but inappropriate dietary management relative to calcium and phosphorus intake can lead to lesion development in individual or groups of horses.

Nutritional Factors

Nutritional situations in which available dietary calcium is insufficient to meet daily requirements can result in development of NSH. Inadequate dietary calcium can result from a primary or secondary deficiency. Diets consisting of mature grass forage with large amounts of cereal grain-based supplements are often low to deficient in dietary calcium with adequate to slightly excessive phosphorus. Grass forages vary in calcium content, but generally have a Ca:P ratio less than 2:1 compared to legume forages that have Ca:P ratios greater than 4:1. Cereal grains of all varieties contain very low calcium (< 0.1 percent DM) and high phosphorus (0.3–0.4 percent DM), resulting in a Ca:P ratio of 1:6 or more. Mature warm-season grasses may have a Ca:P ratio of 1:1 or slightly less, and their feeding with large amounts of cereal grain supplements has been implicated in reported cases of NSH (Joyce et al., 1971; Ronen et al., 1992; David et al., 1997; Wisniewski et al., 1999).

Excessive dietary phosphorus can induce a secondary calcium deficiency. Diets supplemented with large amounts of wheat or rice bran have been reported to induce NSH (Joyce et al., 1971; Clarke et al., 1996). Fiber bran byproducts of wheat and rice contain between 1.3 and 2.3 percent DM phosphorus and low calcium (< 0.2 percent DM). Diets containing large amounts of wheat or rice bran contain either adequate or slightly deficient calcium with excessive phosphorus, resulting in a dietary Ca:P ratio less than 1:1. Supplementing a diet with a high phosphorus mineral without calcium could also result in a dietary calcium and phosphorus imbalance (Lewis, 1995). Feed byproducts of cereal grain processing also contain high concentrations of phosphorus and have low calcium to phosphorus ratios. For example, corn distillers' byproducts and corn gluten feed contain high concentrations of phosphorus (> 1 percent DM) with low calcium (< 0.15 percent DM). Dietary supplements containing large amounts of these byproducts can result in excessive phosphorus intake and a low dietary Ca:P ratio.

Availability of dietary calcium is reduced in the presence of dietary oxalates resulting in a secondary calcium deficiency (Swartzman et al., 1978; Blaney et al., 1981; McKenzie et al., 1981a), and NSH has been reported in horses that consumed oxalate-containing plants as their primary forage source over a prolonged period of months (Walthall and McKenzie, 1976; Blaney et al., 1981; McKenzie, 1988). A number of tropical warm-season grasses (Table 12-3) can contain potentially harmful amounts of oxalate (Walthall and McKenzie, 1976; McKenzie, 1988; Lewis, 1995; David et al., 1997). Alfalfa hay (n = 11; mean ± standard deviation [SD], 0.56 ± 0.15 percent DM) and pelleted alfalfa meal (n = 22; mean ± SD, 0.36 ± 0.1 percent DM) were found to contain variable oxalate concentration, but comparable in magnitude to grasses shown to induce NSH (Hintz et al., 1984). Cymbaluk et al. (1986) reported total oxalate concentration in legume hays (n = 68; mean ± SD, 0.83 ± 0.27 percent DM) and showed legume hay oxalate concentration to be greater compared to mixed legume-grass, various grass, or cereal grain hays. Diets containing more than 0.5 percent DM total oxalate and with a Ca:oxalate ratio of 0.5:1 or less pose greater risk for induction of calcium deficiency and NSH (Blaney et al., 1981; McKenzie et al., 1981a). As a result of higher calcium content associated with legume forages, Ca:oxalate ratios range from 1.7 to over 7:1 (Hintz et al., 1984; Cymbaluk et al., 1986), which are well above ratios associated with greater risk. Conversely, native and other grass species were found to have lower available calcium, due to their lower calcium content, and posed a greater risk for dietary calcium deficiency (Cymbaluk et al., 1986). Calcium digestibility was not found to be adversely affected by oxalate content of alfalfa (Hintz et al., 1984; Cymbaluk et al., 1986). Oxalate-induced calcium deficiency can occur in any horse, but lactating mares and weanlings are most susceptible as a result of their higher calcium requirements and greater feed intake (Lewis, 1995).

Pathogenesis

Clinical signs of NSH are the result of sustained secretion of parathyroid hormone (PTH) and mobilization of bone calcium in an effort to maintain normal blood ionized calcium concentration in the face of dietary imbalances that induce a state of hypocalcemia (Joyce et al., 1971; Capen, 1983; Bertone, 1992; Hunt and Blackwelder, 2002). Ionized calcium plays critical roles in muscle contraction, neuromuscular activity, blood coagulation, and membrane permeability, as well as many other intracellular regulatory processes (Capen, 1983). Consequently, plasma-ionized calcium con-

TABLE 12-3 Grasses That May Contain Excessive Amounts of Oxalates

Common Name	Scientific Name
Buffel grass	*Cenchrus cilaris*
Blue or green panic grasses	*Panicum* spp.
Dallis grass	*Paspalum* spp.
Foxtail millet	*Setaria italica*
Kikuyu grass	*Pennisetum clandistinum*
Napier, mission grass	*Pennisetum* spp.
Purple pigeon grass	*Setaria incrassate*
Pangola grass	*Digitaria recumbens*
Setaria grass	*Setaria sphacelata*

centration is tightly controlled by the counterregulatory hormones PTH and calcitonin (CT). A primary or secondary calcium deficiency results in decreased plasma-ionized calcium and increased PTH secretion. PTH in conjunction with biologically active vitamin D promotes increased calcium uptake from the gut, bone, and kidneys. In dietary situations of limited calcium availability, bone resorption becomes the primary source of calcium. PTH promotes increased resorption of bone by activation of osteoclasts. The result is loss of skeletal calcium and phosphorus (bone demineralization). In the kidney, PTH promotes phosphorus excretion and calcium reabsorption.

Blood phosphorus concentration is directly related to dietary phosphorus intake (Capen, 1983). Therefore, consumption of a diet with excessive phosphorus will result in a state of hyperphosphatemia. Hyperphosphatemia will reduce blood calcium concentration, by law of mass action, and suppress PTH's ability to stimulate renal activation of vitamin D, further decreasing digestive absorption efficiency (Capen, 1983; Bertone, 1992). Insoluble dietary oxalates bind dietary calcium forming indigestible calcium oxalates, which are excreted in the feces (Swartzman et al., 1978; Blaney et al., 1981). Lowered availability of dietary calcium induces hypocalcemia and subsequent stimulation of PTH secretion. Prolonged exposure to the imbalanced diet results in hypertrophy and hyperplasia of parathyroid glands in support of increased secretory activity (Fujimoto et al., 1967; Capen, 1983).

Although NSH is induced by a dietary imbalance of calcium and phosphorus, blood concentrations of these minerals are not useful for diagnosis. Increased PTH concentration with normal to slightly low blood calcium and normal to slightly high blood phosphate concentrations are typical in horses with NSH (Roussel et al., 1987; Benders et al., 2001; Estepa et al., 2003). This is in contrast to primary hyperparathyroidism where elevated PTH concentrations are associated with hypercalcemia (Frank et al., 1998; Peauroi et al., 1998). Increased urinary fractional clearance of phosphate (4 percent or greater, normal 0–0.5 percent) results from PTH effects on increased renal clearance of phosphorus and is suggestive of NSH (Ronen et al., 1992; David et al., 1997; Ramirez and Seahorn, 1997). Serum alkaline phosphatase activity will be elevated as a result of increased bone osteoclastic activity, but this is not specific for NSH. Ration evaluation in conjunction with presenting clinical signs is the best method for diagnosis of NSH.

Nutritional Management and Prevention

Horses affected by NSH can be effectively treated by dietary alterations to increase available dietary calcium intake to meet daily requirements, along with a reduction in dietary phosphorus to an appropriate ratio with calcium. High Ca:P ratios in the range 3:1 to 6:1 have been advocated in the early treatment of the disease (David et al., 1997; Ramirez and Seahorn, 1997). Reversal of clinical signs associated with bony changes occurs over a period of months. Prognosis for recovery is good in older horses, although some facial distortion may be permanent, and guarded in young growing horses depending upon severity of bony lesions and remodeling of long bones (Hunt and Blackwelder, 2002).

Prevention of this disease can be accomplished by feeding a diet appropriately balanced to provide sufficient amounts of available calcium and phosphorus and maintain a dietary Ca:P ratio of between 1 to 2.5:1 (David et al., 1997; Ramirez and Seahorn, 1997). Diets containing large amounts of cereal grains or bran products must have the total dietary calcium content evaluated to ensure adequate intake and balance relative to total dietary phosphorus. Dietary calcium supplementation may be achieved by increasing or substituting legume for grass forages. Alfalfa hay can provide an excellent source of calcium (Lewis, 1995). Dietary calcium can also be increased with addition of calcium carbonate in a mineral or grain supplement. Dietary Ca:P ratio greater than 2.5:1 is not warranted unless dietary factors impeding calcium availability (i.e., oxalates) are documented. Removal of feed containing high amounts of oxalates would be desired; however, feeding supplemental dietary calcium and phosphorus has been shown to control the disease in grazing horses where alternative feed resources were not available (McKenzie et al., 1981b).

Gastric Ulcer Syndrome

Equine gastric ulcer syndrome (EGUS) refers to a group of distinct disorders that includes neonatal gastric ulceration, gastroduodenal ulcer disease of suckling foals, gastric glandular ulceration, and squamous mucosal ulceration (Andrews and Nadeau, 1999; Lester, 2004). The neonatal condition generally occurs in foals with concurrent severe illness such as generalized sepsis or peripartum asphyxia syndrome, and it may be clinically inapparent or result in perforation and fatal peritonitis. Gastroduodenal ulcer disease in suckling foals is characterized by ulceration of the proximal duodenum, pylorus, stomach, and/or distal esophagus. It has been suggested that inflammation of the duodenum results in functional impairment of gastric emptying, with irritation and ulceration of the gastric and esophageal mucosa probably due to prolonged exposure to acidic luminal contents. This condition may occur in mini-outbreak form on an individual farm and may be preceded by episodes of diarrhea, leading to speculation that a viral or bacterial infection precipitates disease. Gastric mucosal inflammation and ulceration in foals post-weaning has been associated with cribbing (Nicol et al., 2002). Cribbing behavior in these foals was decreased after administration of antacids and ulcer healing, suggesting a cause-and-effect relationship between gastric ulceration and cribbing (see Chapter 11).

Erosion or ulceration of the squamous mucosa is the predominant form of EGUS in mature horses (Andrews and Nadeau, 1999; Lester, 2004). The squamous mucosa adjacent to the margo plicatus is most frequently affected, particularly on the lesser curvature. The pathogenesis of these lesions is likely multifactorial (see below), but it has been suggested that diet and feeding practice may alter risk for development of squamous ulcer disease. Ulceration of the gastric glandular mucosa, alone or in combination with nonglandular squamous lesions, also occurs in mature horses but is much less common than the squamous form of EGUS. Clinical signs of EGUS, such as poor appetite and abdominal pain after feed ingestion, have been described to be more severe with glandular as compared to squamous lesions. Concurrent disease and other stress factors, such as prolonged transportation, may predispose to development of glandular ulceration. Experimentally high doses of nonsteroidal anti-inflammatory drugs induce ulceration of the glandular mucosa.

The remainder of this discussion deals with gastric ulceration in mature horses.

Epidemiology and Risk Factors

Squamous mucosal ulceration is common in performance horses, with prevalence ranging from approximately 40–90 percent in various studies (Murray et al., 1996; McClure et al., 1999; Vatistas et al., 1999b; Rabuffo et al., 2002; Dionne et al., 2003; Andrews et al., 2005). The prevalence and severity of gastric ulceration appears to be dependent on several factors, including feeding and housing management, and the form and level of physical activity. However, intense exercise appears to play a major role in the development of squamous gastric ulcers. In an epidemiological study of Thoroughbreds, the prevalence of gastric ulcers was 100 percent in actively racing horses and 91 percent for horses in race training (Murray et al., 1996). A high prevalence (67 percent) was also reported in one study of endurance horses after 50- and 80-km races (Nieto et al., 2004). In an experimental study, gastric ulceration developed soon after the start of simulated race training and was maintained during the period of active training (Vatistas et al., 1999a). In contrast, there is low prevalence of gastric lesions in horses given limited controlled exercise and kept at pasture (Andrews et al., 2005). In a study of 275 Standardbreds, horses in race training were nine times more likely to have gastric ulcers than horses not in training (Dionne et al., 2003).

Exposure of the squamous mucosa to gastric acid is thought to be the primary cause of ulceration, although other acids (short-chain or volatile fatty acids produced by fermentation in the stomach or reflux of bile acids from the duodenum) and pepsin also may play a role (Andrews et al., 2005). In vitro experiments using strips of nonglandular squamous mucosa have shown that hydrochloric acid, alone and in combination with volatile fatty acids, cause dose-dependent inhibition of cellular sodium transport, cell swelling, and ulceration (Nadeau et al., 2003a,b). Therefore, factors that alter gastric acid secretion, production of volatile fatty acids in the stomach, and exposure of the squamous mucosa to these organic acids may alter risk for development of mucosal injury and ulceration.

Repeated oral administration of hypertonic electrolyte solutions, a common practice in horses during endurance competitions, may be another risk factor for ulceration of the squamous mucosa in horses. In a study of 14 horses, oral administration of 56.7 g of commercial electrolyte supplement mixed with 60 ml of water once an hour for 8 hours (approximately 11 g sodium, 24 g chloride, 7.5 g potassium, 1.5 g calcium, and 300 mg magnesium per dose) resulted in a significant increase in mean ulcer number ($P = 0.017$) and severity ($P = 0.0006$) scores in the nonglandular stomach (Holbrook et al., 2005).

Nonnutritional Factors

Exercise

Exercise may favor prolonged exposure of the squamous mucosa to gastric glandular secretions (hydrochloric acid, pepsin) and bile acids due to alterations in gastric volume. In a study of horses exercising on a treadmill, there was a sudden and marked decrease in gastric volume after the onset of trotting in concert with an increase in intra-abdominal pressure (Lorenzo-Figueras and Merritt, 2002). The authors surmised that the exercise-induced increase in intra-abdominal pressure was responsible for the decrease in gastric volume. Furthermore, the decrease in volume resulted in exposure of the squamous mucosa to the acidic contents (pH 1–2) of the dependent area of the gastric lumen. It also has been suggested that an exercise-associated decrease in gastric emptying rate increases exposure of the squamous mucosa to acidic gastric fluid (Lester, 2004). Other researchers have reported that exercise training results in an increase in the serum gastrin response to meal feeding (Furr et al., 1994). Such an increase in serum gastrin concentration might result in enhanced acid secretion and lower stomach pH.

Stall Confinement

Confinement housing has been implicated in the development of gastric ulcer disease. In one study, squamous mucosal lesions were apparent 7 days after relocating horses from pasture to a stall environment (Murray and Eichorn, 1996). It has been proposed that lack of socialization with other horses, changes in dietary composition, and intermittent rather than continuous feeding could contribute to the increased risk of gastric ulceration after confinement (Lester, 2004).

Temperament

Some studies have reported a higher prevalence of ulceration in horses with nervous temperaments. One unproven hypothesis is that horses with nervous dispositions maintain reduced gastric volume in response to persistent tension of the abdominal muscles, forcing acidic gastric fluid to the dorsal (squamous) region of the stomach (Lester, 2004).

Putative Nutritional Factors

There is no definitive evidence implicating diet in the development of squamous ulcer disease. Possible dietary influences include the effects of diet composition, meal size, and feeding frequency on saliva production; the rate and extent of intragastric fermentation; and gastric emptying rate (Andrews et al., 2005). Saliva production during the consumption of a hay meal is approximately double that produced during intake of the equivalent DM as grain, in part due to the longer period of mastication required for ingestion of forage (Meyer et al., 1985). As the flow of salivary fluid and masticated feed into the stomach may buffer the acidity of gastric contents, the lower volume of salivary fluid with ingestion of grain may favor mucosal injury due to exposure to hydrochloric acid. Another consideration is the potentially ulcerogenic effects of volatile fatty acids (VFA) produced by the fermentation of starch and other readily fermentable substrate in the nonglandular region of the stomach (Nadeau et al., 2003a,b; Andrews et al., 2005). In studies of harvested equine gastric squamous mucosa, the addition of 60 nmol/L VFA (butyric, propionic, acetic, and valeric acids) resulted in decreased chloride-dependent sodium transport, cell swelling, and tissue damage (Nadeau et al., 2003a). In the acidic conditions of the equine stomach (pH ≤ 4), these organic acids will be predominantly in nonionized forms and therefore able to penetrate and damage squamous epithelial cells. In a previous study (Nadeau et al., 2000), this research group compared the effects of a grass hay (bromegrass) diet vs. a combination of legume hay (alfalfa) and grain on gastric squamous epithelial ulceration and the pH and VFA contents of gastric juice in horses with surgically implanted gastric cannulae. Surprisingly, the number and severity of squamous ulcers were greater in horses that received the grass hay-only diet. In this group, postprandial pH was lower and butyric acid concentration higher when compared to the alfalfa/grain diet, whereas acetic, propionic, valeric, and isovaleric acid concentrations were higher in the alfalfa/grain diet group, consistent with a higher rate of intragastric fermentation in grain-fed horses. In a subsequent analysis of these data, the presence of VFA (butyric, propionic, and valeric acids) and low stomach pH (gastric acidity) were found to be significant predictors of ulcer severity (Andrews et al., 2005).

The size of grain meals may affect the extent of intragastric fermentation and thus VFA production (Metayer et al., 2004; Lorenzo-Figueras et al., 2005). Metayer et al. (2004) compared gastric emptying rate in horses fed a small (300 g/100 BW) vs. large (700 g/100 kg BW) high-starch concentrate. Although the calculated rate of gastric emptying (g/min) was higher with the large meal, gastric emptying in terms of percent of the total meal was much slower. Thus, with large starch-rich meals, intragastric fermentation and volatile fatty production may be favored due to the large load of fermentable substrate and longer residence time in the stomach.

Feeding frequency also may affect the risk of gastric squamous ulceration (Murray and Schusser, 1993; Lester, 2004). In grazing horses, the continuous flow of saliva and ingesta may provide a buffering effect such that gastric pH remains above 4 for most of the day. On the other hand, given that horses are continuous secretors of gastric acid, stomach pH falls when feed is withheld and the nonglandular mucosa is exposed to an acid environment. In healthy horses, squamous ulceration was induced by alternating 24-hour periods of feed deprivation and ad libitum access to hay over an 8-day period (Murray and Schusser, 1993). Ulceration developed after 24 hours of cumulative feed deprivation. The median intragastric pH during a 24-hour period with ad libitum access to grass hay was 3.1, whereas median pH was 1.6 during feed deprivation. These findings confirm that gastric acidity is the primary mechanism of squamous mucosal ulceration and suggest that the typical practice of twice daily meal feeding may be a contributing factor.

Further studies are needed to better elucidate the role of diet composition in ulcer development and to identify feeds and feeding methods that reduce risk of squamous ulcer disease. For example, it has been suggested that the feeding of lower starch and higher oil and fiber concentrates is beneficial, but this hypothesis remains unproven. Interestingly, corn oil supplementation (45 ml/d) in ponies was associated with a significant decrease in gastric acid production and increased prostaglandin E_2 concentration in gastric juice (Cargile et al., 2004).

Colic

Colic is defined as abdominal pain and is used to describe symptoms resulting from intestinal ileus or inflammation (White, 1999). Worldwide, colic is one of the most frequent causes of emergency treatment of horses (White, 1990; Proudman, 1991; Traub-Dargatz et al., 2001) and is reported as a leading cause of equine mortality in the United States (Tinker et al., 1997a; USDA, 2001). Estimates of the annual incidence of colic range from 3.5 to 10.6 colic cases per 100 horses (Kaneene et al., 1997; Tinker et al., 1997a; USDA, 2001). Mortality rate among horses with colic has been estimated in two large-scale studies at 6.6 percent (Tinker et al., 1997a) and 11 percent (Traub-Dargatz et al., 2001).

Colic can be classified according to the disease causing it. These classifications include ileus (e.g., spasm, intraluminal obstruction, paralytic ileus, displacement/strangulation); inflammation (e.g., enteritis); ulcer (e.g., gastric ulcers, intestinal ulcers, dorsal colitis); and false colic (e.g., pregnancy, rhabdomyolitis, liver disease, renal/bladder disease) (White, 1999). However, in many cases, the cause of colic is unknown (Kaneene et al., 1997; Tinker et al., 1997a; White, 1999).

Several factors have been reported to influence the risk of colic. These risk factors include diet and feeding characteristics, internal parasitism, intrinsic factors (e.g., sex, age, and breed), medical history (e.g., previously affected by colic), management (e.g., housing, activity level), and weather-related factors (Goncalves et al., 2002). It should be noted that risk factors do not imply a direct cause-and-effect relationship and that the relationship between risk factors and colic is not always clear (Cohen, 1997; Goncalves et al., 2002). Among the various risk factors identified, diet and feeding characteristics are often associated with the greatest risk for colic (Tinker et al., 1997b; Cohen et al., 1999; Hudson et al., 2001). The diet and feeding characteristics associated with the risk of colic include changes in feeding program, amount of concentrate fed, access to pasture, type of forage, and characteristics of water delivery.

Diet change and change of hay were reported to increase the risk of colic by 5 and 9.8 times, respectively, according to the results of a prospective matched case-control study involving 2,060 horses (Cohen et al., 1999); however, no specifics describing the change were provided (e.g., increase, decrease, change in type, or change in source). In a follow-up study, the same group reported that a recent change in batch of hay (i.e., different source), but not type of hay (e.g., legume vs. grass), increased the risk of colic by 4.9 times (Hudson et al., 2001). Additionally, a recent change in type (e.g., pelleted vs. textured) of grain or concentrate fed increased the risk of colic 2.6 times. The authors of these studies noted that both experiments were conducted during drought conditions, which may have influenced the outcome. However, others have also reported increased risk of colic associated with a change in concentrate or hay feeding (Tinker et al., 1997b).

Concentrate intakes between 2.5 and 5 kg/d and those greater than 5 kg/d increased the risk of colic 4.8 and 6.3 times compared to horses on pasture receiving no concentrate (Tinker et al., 1997b). Concentrate intake of less than 2.5 kg/d was not significantly associated with the incidence of colic compared to horses on pasture receiving no concentrate. However, the association between amounts of grain fed per day and colic is not always clear. Hudson et al. (2001) reported that feeding greater than 2.7 kg/d of oats increased the risk of colic 5.9 times, but noted that this factor may not be causative, but only a marker for some other factor (e.g,. level of exercise). Reeves et al. (1996) reported an increased risk of colic associated with feeding increased amounts of whole corn grain, but a decreased risk associated with increased amounts of nonroughage concentrate feed. Interestingly, the amount of whole corn grain fed was relatively low (i.e., colic affected and nonaffected horses consumed 1.3 ± 0.18 and 0.7 ± 0.13 kg/d, respectively), as was the difference in amount of nonroughage concentrate. Colic affected and nonaffected horses consumed 3.4 ± 0.10 and 3.9 ± 0.11 kg/d, respectively (Reeves et al., 1996).

Hudson et al. (2001) reported that a recent decrease in pasture availability (i.e., either no pasture time or a decrease in pasture acreage or time at pasture) increased colic risk three times compared to horses in which no change in pasture was made. However, the association between colic risk and pasture access is not always clear (Reeves et al., 1996).

Based on an observation of a small group of horses, Pugh and Thompson (1992) suggested that feeding Coastal Bermudagrass hay was a factor in the development of impaction colic. However, this association has not been substantiated (Cohen et al., 1999). In addition, results of epidemiological studies implicated water source (e.g., bucket, pond, automatic waterer) as a colic risk factor, but the relationship is unclear (Reeves et al., 1996; Kaneene et al., 1997; Cohen et al., 1999).

Mechanisms by which various factors contribute to the development of colic are not clearly defined. Clarke et al. (1990) provided evidence supporting the hypothesis that meal feeding of concentrated diets leads to exaggerated fermentation characteristics in both the foregut and hindgut and altered fluid balance in the hindgut. Exaggerated fermentation, specifically that resulting in decreased pH, could result in damage to the intestinal mucosa and/or excess gas production leading to intestinal distention (Clarke et al., 1990). Rate of passage was increased with increased meal size when high-starch diets were fed to horses (Metayer et al., 2004). Feeding meals containing greater than 2 to 4 g starch/kg BW has been reported to increase postileal digestion of starch (Potter et al., 1992), which has been reported to decrease hindgut pH leading to mucosal damage (Garner et al., 1977). Meal feeding of concentrated meals may alter fluid balance in the hindgut, which could predispose horses to impaction colic (Clarke et al., 1990). Ingestion of sand can result in colic due to inflammation (Jones, 2004) and/or blockage (Blikslager and Jones, 2004) of the intestine.

Enterolithiasis

Enteroliths (intestinal calculi) are found in the large intestine, where they may cause obstruction and varying degrees of abdominal pain (colic). Enteroliths are composed of struvite, a mixture of magnesium ammonium phosphate (Hassel et al., 2001). The struvite crystals are laid down in concentric rings, typically surrounding a dense nidus or foreign body (e.g., cloth, metal, hair, or pebbles). Enteroliths may form singly or in large groups of small calculi. Large calculi tend to be located in the right dorsal colon, while smaller calculi may enter the transverse colon and descending colon. Clinical signs of abdominal pain can occur when calculi become lodged in a segment of large intestine, resulting in variable amounts of distention with gas and ingesta proximal to the obstruction. Alternatively, multiple small calculi may cause abdominal pain without obstruction, perhaps due to irritation of the bowel wall.

The occurrence of enterolithiasis has been reported over a wide geographic area. However, there is a high prevalence of enterolithiasis in certain geographic regions, such as California and in the southeastern United States (Florida, Louisiana) (Hassel et al., 1999). In one study, horses with enterolithiasis represented approximately 15 percent of horses admitted to the Large Animal Clinic at the University of California–Davis for evaluation of colic and 27.5 percent of patients undergoing celiotomy for treatment of colic (Hassel et al., 1999). In contrast, enterolithiasis was an uncommon (< 2 percent of cases) cause of colic at a referral clinic in Texas (Cohen et al., 2000). All breeds of horses can be affected. However, in one report, Arabian and Arabian crosses, Morgans, American Saddlebreds, and donkeys were significantly overrepresented in the study population (Hassel et al., 1999), while in another study, Arabian and miniature breeds were at increased risk for development of enteroliths (Cohen et al., 2000). A high prevalence in siblings also has been reported (Hassel et al., 1999), raising the possibility of a heritable component to the disease. In a study of 900 equids, the mean age of occurrence was 11.4 years (Hassel et al., 1999). However, colonic obstruction due to an enterolith has been recognized in horses less than 1 year of age (Lloyd et al., 1987), suggesting that intestinal calculi can grow to sufficient size to cause intestinal obstruction within a short time period.

Nutritional Factors

Several studies have identified increased alkalinity in the colonic contents of horses with enteroliths compared with a control population (Hintz et al., 1988, 1989; Hassel et al., 2004). Hassel et al. (2004) measured the pH and mineral contents of colonic ingesta in 43 horses with enterolithiasis and 19 horses with surgical colic due to nonstrangulating obstruction of the colon without enteroliths. Mean pH of colonic contents for horses with enteroliths (pH 7.32 ± 0.07) was significantly higher than for control horses (pH 6.93 ± 0.13), while percent colonic dry matter was lower in the horses with enteroliths (13.6 percent ± 0.7 percent vs. 20.9 percent ± 2.1 percent). Horses with enterolithiasis also had higher percent nitrogen and concentrations of magnesium, phosphorus, sulfur, sodium, calcium, and potassium in colonic ingesta (Hassel et al., 2004). The mechanisms of these differences in colonic pH and chemical composition are not known, but contributing factors might include diet composition, mineral content of water supply, and genetic differences in mechanisms for colonic luminal ion exchange. Alternatively, the observed differences in mineral content and dry matter of colonic ingesta may be attributable to the presence of enteroliths rather than the predisposing cause (Hassel et al., 2004). Nonetheless, the higher pH and mineral content of colonic ingesta might favor deposition of struvite. This hypothesis is consistent with findings in dogs and cats with struvite urolithiasis, wherein formation of calculi is promoted by alkaline conditions and high mineral concentrations in urine (Osborne et al., 1989).

An association between the feeding of alfalfa hay and development of enterolithiasis has been reported (Blue and Wittkopp, 1981; Lloyd et al., 1987; Murray et al., 1992; Cohen et al., 2000; Hassel et al., 2004). When compared to grass forages, alfalfa has both high protein and magnesium content, which could result in higher levels of ammonium nitrogen and magnesium in the large intestine. In addition, because alfalfa has high buffering capacity (Fadel, 1992), high-alfalfa diets could favor alkalinization of colonic contents and struvite deposition. In support of these considerations, Hassel et al. (2004) reported that horses with enterolithiasis were fed a higher proportion of alfalfa in their diet (91.9 percent ± 2.6 percent) compared with control horses (62.1 percent ± 7.7 percent). From univariate regression analysis, it was shown that horses on a diet of more than 70 percent alfalfa were at greater risk for enterolithiasis (odds ratio [OR] = 13; 95 percent confidence interval [CI], 3.5–48.7) than horses on a lower alfalfa (< 70 percent) diet (Hassel et al., 2004). In addition, the mean concentrations of magnesium, phosphorus, sulfur, sodium, calcium, and potassium in colonic contents of horses fed more than 70 percent alfalfa were 1.5–2 times higher than of horses on the lower alfalfa diet (Hassel et al., 2004). However, because most horses fed an alfalfa diet do not develop enteroliths, it is clear that alfalfa is not the only factor involved in enterolith formation. Indeed, in the report of Cohen et al. (2000), 14 of the 26 horses with enterolithiasis were not fed alfalfa.

In epidemiologic studies, stall confinement and/or lack of access to pasture have been identified as risk factors for enterolithiasis (Cohen et al., 2000; Hassel et al., 2004). In one study (Cohen et al., 2000), horses that spent less than 50 percent of the day outdoors were at increased risk (OR = 4.5; 95 percent CI, 1.4–13.9) for enterolithiasis, while Hassel et al. (2004) found that horses with enteroliths were one-tenth as likely (OR = 0.11; 95 percent CI, 0.03–0.45) to have daily access to pasture than horses without enterolithiasis. It was suggested that ingestion of grass might dilute the effects of alfalfa on the chemical composition of colonic contents, a speculation in part supported by observations of higher colonic mineral contents in horses without daily access to pasture grazing (Hassel et al., 2004). Alternatively, increased physical activity by horses at pasture might lower risk of enterolith formation via alterations in intestinal transit, colonic ion exchange, or diet digestibility (Orton et al., 1985; Pearson and Merritt, 1991; Hassel et al., 2004).

The feeding of wheat bran also has been proposed as a risk factor for the development of enteroliths because of its relatively high protein (CP 16–17 percent), phosphorus (1.2 percent–1.3 percent), and magnesium (0.6 percent–0.7 percent) content (Lloyd et al., 1987). However, in the study by Cohen et al. (2000), only 1 of 26 horses with enterolithiasis had been fed wheat bran. There are no published reports of the relationship between mineral content of the water supply and enterolithiasis.

Nutritional Management

Studies in dogs and cats have demonstrated that a diet with low magnesium, phosphorus, and protein that results in maintenance of low urine pH is effective for prevention or even dissolution of struvite calculi in the urinary tract. The results of epidemiologic and case-control studies (Hassel et al., 1999; Cohen et al., 2000; Hassel et al., 2004) that identified alkaline pH and higher mineral concentrations in samples of colonic fluid in horses with enterolithiasis also suggested that dietary modifications promoting acidification of colonic contents might be beneficial for prevention of enterolithiasis in horses. Specific dietary recommendations have included the exclusion of alfalfa and wheat bran from the diet, an increase in the grain:hay ratio, and supplementation with apple cider vinegar (Hintz et al., 1989; Murray et al., 1992; Lewis, 1995; Stratton-Phelps and Fascetti, 2003). However, there are limited data on the effectiveness of these approaches for modification of the colonic environment and no information regarding efficacy for prevention of enterolith formation. In laboratory experiments, a colonic pH of less than 6.6 reduced the weight of implanted enteroliths (Hintz et al., 1989). Daily supplementation of ponies with apple cider vinegar (one-half cup or 110 ml per day) also resulted in a modest decrease in the pH of colonic contents but did not appear to reduce the size of enteroliths (Hintz et al., 1989).

Based on current knowledge, grass rather than legume (alfalfa) forage, should be fed to horses with a history of enterolithiasis to reduce intake of nutrients that may promote struvite deposition. Wheat bran also should be avoided.

Feeding grain (e.g., 0.5 kg/100 kg BW) and about 1 cup (220 ml) of apple cider vinegar twice daily may be beneficial in promoting mild acidification of colonic contents. Finally, daily pasture turnout may reduce risk of enterolith formation.

Recurrent Airway Obstruction

Recurrent airway obstruction (RAO) is the accepted terminology for the disease entity in mature horses formerly known as chronic obstructive pulmonary disease (COPD) or heaves (Robinson, 2001). Approximately 9.2 percent of clinical cases referred to North American veterinary teaching hospitals have RAO (Ward and Couetil, 2005). Epidemiologic studies indicate that affected horses were typically 4 years or older and symptoms occurred more often in winter and spring and occurred more often in the southern than northern hemisphere (Couetil and Ward, 2003; Ward and Couetil, 2005). The monthly prevalence of RAO was significantly correlated to total pollen counts measured 3 months before clinical symptoms and to total mold counts occurring 1 month before or during the same month of clinic admission (Ward and Couetil, 2005). A genetic predisposition has been reported with exacerbation by environmental contaminants in stables and age of horse (Marti, 2001; Marti and Ohnesorge, 2002). The incidence of RAO in German Warmblood horses was 17, 48, and 69 percent when neither, one, or both parents, respectively, were affected by RAO symptoms. Using a relative risk analysis, Marti and Ohnesorge (2002) reported that the relative risk of RAO is low in offspring (13 percent) if neither dam nor sire is affected, but increased 3.2-fold ($P < 0.05$) if either parent was affected and 4.6-fold ($P < 0.05$) if both parents were affected.

Environmental pollutants, generically labeled as "stable dust," include airborne fungi, thermophilic actinomycetes, dust mites, endotoxins, and inorganic compounds (Clarke and Madelin, 1987; McGorum et al., 1998; Art et al., 2002) and typically enter the microenvironment (stall) and macroenvironment (stable) through feed and bedding. RAO symptoms are not exclusive to indoor-stabled horses. A condition known as "summer-pasture-associated obstructive pulmonary disease" (SPAOPD; also known as "summer-pasture associated allergy") has been recorded in horses on pasture (Seahorn and Beadle, 1993; Costa et al., 2000).

Nutritional Factors

Stable dusts have been classified as nonrespirable (> 10 mm) or respirable (large or small) particles (Clarke and Madelin, 1987). Large respirable particles are 5–10 mm and include particles such as plant structures, large pollen grains, and "fair weather" spores *(Alternaria, Cladosporium* spp). These particles typically are not inhaled because of rapid sedimentation to the stable floor. Small respirable particles are 0.1–5 mm and are typically comprised of actinomycetes spores, small fungal spores, and dust mites. The role of dust mites in exacerbating the allergenicity of molds is unclear. Storage mites infest many feedstuffs and were linked to the spread and growth of molds within those infected feeds. In addition to these usual allergens, endotoxins (lipopolysaccharides) can amplify the symptoms of RAO (Pirie et al., 2003). The small size of respirable particles allows escape from the turbinate trap in the upper respiratory tract (Art et al., 2002). If not captured by the bronchial mucociliary mechanism, these particles can traverse to the alveoli. The threshold limiting value (TLV) is the level of exposure of an agent above which disease or organic dysfunction can occur. The TLV of spores for horse stables has been calculated at 33 particles/cm^3 (Webster et al., 1987).

Thermotolerant and thermophilic fungal species (*Aspergillus*, *Rhizomucor*, *Penicillium*, and *Stachybotrys* spp.) produce the majority of small respirable, fungal spores in hays, straw, and shavings (Clarke and Madelin, 1987). The high temperature conditions (> 38°C) preferred by these fungi most often occur in poorly cured hay, which heats during storage. Fungal invasion was shown to occur in the stand-ing crop, during curing, and during storage, but growth during storage was enhanced in square alfalfa hay bales when moisture content of the hay was high (29 percent) at baling (Wittenberg et al., 1989). For horses with heaves, hay should contain few mold and fungi. Hay has been graded at levels I through III based on numbers of mold and fungi type. Grade I hay had less than 999 particles/mg source material, grade II ranged from 1,000–4,999 particles/mg source material, and grade III contained more than 5,000 particles/ mg source material (Clarke and Madelin, 1987). Hays and bedding with a grade III score are undesirable for horses because millions of spores can be inhaled from these materials by a horse.

Bedding has also been shown to contribute to horse stable dust. Harvesting conditions often determine the quality of the straw for bedding. Based on their mold content, straws used to bed horse stalls were generally classified as good or poor quality (Clarke and Madelin, 1987; Vandenput et al., 1997). Straws and shavings had a similar complement of molds as contaminated hays, whereas peat harbored few potential allergenic molds (Clarke and Madelin, 1987). By contrast, good-quality wheat and flax straw had fewer respirable particles and allergenic spores than wood shavings (Vandenput et al., 1997). All-natural bedding materials were inferior to cardboard bedding, which had low levels of respirable dust and spores (Kirschvink et al., 2002c). Pelleted newspaper may be an alternative to straw and shavings as bedding, although particle mass less than 10 µm was initially higher in the newspaper product than either natural bedding material when spread in the stall (Ward et al., 2001). This study also confirmed that microbial numbers in the breathing zone and on the legs of horses were greater in autumn than in summer. When bedding down the stall, horses should be removed from the barn. In one study, the high exposure to respirable dust particles during "bedding down" increased airborne particles in the breathing zone of the horse 3- to 6-fold (Webster et al., 1987). Good stable ventilation is indispensable in the control of respirable particles in the breathing zone of the horse, yet many stables were inadequately ventilated to accomplish this objective (Webster et al., 1987).

Pathogenesis and Clinical Symptoms

Exposure of a sensitized horse to excessive amounts of respirable dust particles or organic dust in hay and moldy bedding has been shown to initiate neutrophilic inflammation of the small airway (bronchioles) and/or the entire tracheobronchial tree (Robinson et al., 1996). Altered responses by the mucociliary system result in increased mucus and/or mucopus production in the bronchial and bronchiolar tree (Gerber et al., 2004), mucosal edema, and bronchospasm, eventually followed by varying degrees of fibrosis and fibroplasia of the submucosa. These pathologies reduce oxygen exchange and a progressively reduced exercise tolerance of the horse. Other symptoms, which can be mild to severe, include coughing, respiratory distress, mucus or mucopurulent nasal discharge, abnormal lung sounds, increased work in breathing, and an abdominal "heave" line after chronic and sustained respiratory impairment (Robinson et al., 2003). Importantly, the symptoms of RAO can be induced by a moldy hay/straw challenge in affected horses (McGorum et al., 1993).

The hypothesized causes for the airway hyperresponsiveness seen in RAO-affected, RAO-prone horses, and SPAOD-affected horses are numerous. Airway inflammation seen in RAO has been suggested to originate at a cellular level, in part from increased activity of transcription factors such as nuclear factor-κB and activator protein-1 (Bureau et al., 2000). The profound neutrophilia seen in RAO may promote the continued production of mucus by the mucociliary apparatus (Gerber et al., 2004), perhaps through upregulation of equine MUC5AC mucin mRNA (Gerber et al., 2003). Other pathologic indicators in RAO horses include an increased expression of IL-4 mRNA and IL-13 mRNA and a decreased expression of IFN-γ mRNA indicative of an IgE-mediated response (Robinson, 2001; Bowles et al., 2002), increased IL-1 β mRNA (Matera et al., 2005), higher systemic levels of endothelin-1 (Benamou et al., 1998), and reduced densities of the β-adrenergic receptors of the lung and bronchi particularly of the β-1 subtype, which may increase airway smooth muscle sensitivity (Abraham et al., 2006).

The upregulation of the inflammatory genes has been linked to the redox conditions initiated by the increase in reactive oxidant species (ROS) or free radicals during inflammation (Kirschvink and Lekeux, 2005). The overabundance of ROS in airway inflammation relative to the level of neutralizing oxidants has been speculated to exacerbate airway pathology. The concentrations of antioxidant indicators, oxidized and reduced glutathione, glutathione redox ratio, and ascorbic acid have been characterized in normal horses undergoing RAO episodes and those in remission (Art et al., 1999; Kirschvink et al., 2002a; Deaton et al., 2004). Horses with an induced RAO or clinical RAO crisis have increased production of elastase, decreased ascorbic acid concentration in bronchoalveolar lavage fluid, and epithelial lining fluid (Deaton et al., 2004, 2005a,b) and increased total glutathione and oxidized glutathione (Art et al., 1999). Although these data would indicate an increased production of free radicals or reactive oxygen species and that ascorbate might be protective, the acute neutrophilic episode did not result in a marked pulmonary oxidative stress (Deaton et al., 2005b; Deaton, 2006). When healthy horses were given antioxidant supplements including ascorbic acid, there was no effect on ascorbic acid concentrations in pulmonary epithelial lining fluid (Deaton et al., 2002), yet an antioxidant supplement containing vitamins C and E plus selenium given to heaves-affected horses in remission resulted in improved exercise tolerance and lower airway inflammation (Kirschvink et al., 2002b). Further data will be required to determine if dietary ascorbic acid supplementation ameliorates or protects the equine airway from pathology associated with the inflammatory responses seen in RAO.

Nutritional Management and Prevention

The best environment for RAO-prone horses has been to house them outdoors on pasture (Art et al., 2002). Horses with symptoms of heaves become asymptomatic within 4–6 days of being turned outdoors (Vandenput et al., 1998). Improvement in respiratory function was observed within 3 days after pasture turnout in horses who were induced into a RAO episode by environmental modification (Jackson et al., 2000). However, every precaution must be taken to minimize respiratory allergens even when the heaves-prone horses are kept outdoors. Supplementary hays and grains, if fed, should have minimal organic dust content. Despite the apparent benefit of housing RAO horses outside, the outdoor environment may not be acceptable for horses prone to SPAOPD.

Unfortunately, horse athletes, including RAO-affected horses, must often be stabled. If bedded and fed with feeds with low allergenicity, even RAO-affected horses appear to be able to stay asymptomatic indoors. Thompson and McPherson (1984) showed that horses with symptoms of RAO became asymptomatic within 4–24 days after measures were taken to control dust in the stable by bedding with shredded paper and feeding a complete pelleted diet. Similar observations were observed in heaves-affected horses bedded with cardboard or good-quality straw and fed a completed pelleted diet (Vandenput et al., 1998; Kirschvink et al., 2002c).

Good-quality hay for RAO-affected horses has low numbers of thermophilic and thermotolerant molds and fungi and dust mite allergens, but, contrary to popular belief, stable operators were less able to detect mold through smell or appearance than expected (Clarke and Madelin, 1987). Moreover, feed quality, based on allergenicity, cannot be guaranteed because weather conditions at the time of harvest, methods of harvest, and storage all profoundly influence mold growth in hays, straws, silage, and grains. Although pelleted or cubed alfalfa and grass silage can have low levels of aeroallergens and dust and have been effectively used in diets of stabled, heaves-affected horses (Raymond et al., 1994; Vandenput et al., 1997), these observations may not apply universally to similar feeds produced in other geographic areas. Poor-quality meals and uncoated pellets can expose animals to a large number of respirable particles (Li et al., 1993), so quality of these products should also be evaluated.

Management to prevent and control symptoms of RAO involves medical treatment, as well as eliminating or minimizing the respiratory tract allergens (stable dust, especially respirable particles) in the horse's macroenvironment (barn) and microenvironment (stall). There are several ways to reduce exposure of the horse to respirable dust: keep the horse outdoors, use only dust and mold-free feeds, moisten feeds, use nondusty bedding, wash stalls regularly to remove dust, and provide effective and sufficient ventilation to remove dust particles in barn and stall air (Thompson and McPherson, 1984; Webster et al., 1987; Raymond et al., 1994; Vandenput et al., 1998). Soaking or steaming can reduce respirable particles in hay. The major impact of soaking hay to reduce respirable particles was realized within 30 minutes; no further benefit was observed in soaking hay for 12 hours (Moore-Colyer, 1996). Although soaking hay up to 30 minutes or steaming for 80 minutes reduced 93 percent of respirable particles, steaming had no effect on nutrient loss whereas soaking reduced phosphorus, potassium, magnesium, sodium, and copper concentrations in hay (Blackman and Moore-Colyer, 1998). Horses affected with chronic and severe RAO are reported to be thinner than unaffected cohorts because of a 41 percent increase in resting energy expenditure (Mazan et al., 2004). Thus, in addition to controlling respirable dusts, horses with heaves may require a diet designed to provide a higher caloric intake.

REFERENCES

Abraham, G., C. Kottke, S. Dhein, and F. R. Ungemach. 2006. Agonist-independent alteration in β-adrenoceptor-G-protein-adenylate cyclase system in an equine model of recurrent airway obstruction. Pulm. Pharmacol. Therap. 19:218–229.

Aldred, J. 1998. Developmental orthopaedic disease in horses. Rural Ind. Res. Develop. Corp. Publ. 97/79:1–31.

Andrews, F. M., and J. A. Nadeau. 1999. Clinical syndromes of gastric ulceration in foals and mature horses. Equine Vet. J. Suppl. 29:30–33.

Andrews, F. M., B. R. Buchanan, S. B. Elliot, N. A. Clariday, and L. H. Edwards. 2005. Gastric ulcers in horses. J. Anim. Sci. 83 (E. Suppl.):E18–E21.

Annandale, E. J., S. J. Valberg, J. R. Mickelsen, and E. R. Seaquist. 2004. Insulin sensitivity and skeletal muscle glucose transport in horses with polysaccharide storage myopathy. Neuromusc. Dis. 14:666–674.

Árnason, T., and Bjarnason, T. 1994. Growth, development and size of Icelandic toelter horses. Búvísindi 8:73–83.

Art, T., N. Kirschvink, N. Smith, and P. Lekeux. 1999. Indices of oxidative stress in blood and pulmonary epithelium lining fluid in horses suffering from recurrent airway obstruction. Equine Vet. J. 31:397–401.

Art, T., B. C. McGorum, and P. Lekeux. 2002. Environmental control of respiratory diseases. In Equine Respiratory Diseases, P. Lekeux, ed. Document No. B0334.0302. Ithaca, NY: International Veterinary Information Services.

Bailey, S. R., C. M. Marr, and J. Elliott. 2004. Current research and theories on the pathogenesis of acute laminitis in the horse. Vet. J. 167:129–142.

Barneveld, A., and P. R. van Weeren, 1999. Conclusions regarding the influence of exercise on the development of the equine musculoskeletal system with special reference to osteochondrosis. Equine Vet. J. Suppl. 31:112–119.

Barneveld A., R. van Weeren, J. Knaap. 1999. Influence of early exercise on the locomotion system. 50th Annual Meeting of the European Association for Animal Production, Zurich.

Bell, R. A., B. D. Neilsen, K. Waite, D. Rosenstein, and M. Orth. 2001. Daily access to pasture turnout prevents loss of mineral in the third metacarpus of Arabian weanlings. J. Anim. Sci. 79:1142–1150.

Benamou, A. E., T. Art, D. J. Marlin, C. A. Roberts, and P. Lekeux. 1998. Variations in systemic and pulmonary endothelin-1 in horses with recurrent airway obstruction (heaves). Pulm. Pharmacol. Therap. 11:231–235.

Benders, N. A., K. Junker, T. H. Wensing, S. G. A. M. van den Ingh, and J. H. van der Kolk. 2001. Diagnosis of secondary hyperparathyroidism in a pony using intact parathyroid hormone radioimmunoassay. Vet. Rec. 149:185–187.

Beneus, L. 2005. Lokalisation av osteochondrosforandrengar hos Svenska havhodshastar. Ph.D. Thesis. Uppsala University, Sweden.

Bertone, J. J. 1992. Nutritional secondary hyperparathyroidism. Pp. 119–122 in Current Therapy in Equine Medicine, 3rd ed., N. E. Robinson, ed. Philadelphia: W. B. Saunders.

Beynen, A. C., and J. M. Hallebeek 2002. High-fat diets for horses. Pp 1–13 in Proc. 1st Europ. Equine Nutr. Health Cong., Antwerp Zoo, Belgium. Available at http://www.equine-congress.com. Accessed April 15, 2006.

Blackman, M., and M. J. S. Moore-Colyer. 1998. Hay for horses: the effects of three different wetting treatments on dust and nutrient content. Anim. Sci. 66:745–750.

Blaney, B. J., R. J. W. Gartner, and R. A. McKenzie. 1981. The effects of oxalate in some tropical grasses on the availability to horses of calcium, phosphorus and magnesium. J. Agric. Sci. 97:507–514.

Blikslager, A. T., and S. L. Jones. 2004. Obstructive disorders of the gastrointestinal tract. P. 922 in Equine Internal Medicine, 2nd ed., S. M. Reed, W. M. Bayly, and D. C. Sellon, eds. St. Louis: Saunders.

Blue, M. G., and R. W. Wittkopp. 1981. Clinical and structural features of equine enteroliths in equidae. J. Am. Vet. Med. Assoc. 179:79–82.

Boren, S. R., D. R. Topliff, C. W. Freeman, R. J. Bahr, D. G. Wagner, and C. V. Maxwell. 1987. Growth of weanling Quarter horses fed varying energy and protein levels. Pp. 43–48 in Proc. 10th Equine Nutr. Physiol. Soc. Symp., Ft. Collins, CO.

Bosy-Westphal, A., C. Eichhorn, D. Kutzner, I. Illner, M. Heller, and M. J. Muller. 2003. The age-related decline in resting energy expenditure in humans is due to the loss of fat-free mass and to alterations in its metabolically active components. J. Nutr. 133:2356–2362.

Bowles, K. S., R. E. Beadle, S. Mouch, S. S. Pourciau, M. A. Littlefield-Chabaud, C. LeBlanc, L. Mistric, D. Fermaglich, and D. W. Horohov. 2002. A novel model for recurrent airway obstruction. Vet. Immunol. Immunopathol. 87:385–389.

Brama, P. A. J., R. A. Bank, J. M. TeKoppele, and P. R. van Weeren. 2001. Training affects the collagen framework of subchondral bone in foals. Vet. J. 162:24–32.

Brama, P. A. J., J. M. TeKoppele, R. A. Bank, A. Barneveld, and P. R. van Weeren. 2002. Biochemical development of subchondral bone from birth until age eleven months and the influence of physical activity. Equine Vet. J. 34:143–149.

Brosnahan, M. M., and M. R. Paradis. 2003. Demographic and clinical characteristics of geriatric horses: 467 cases (1989–1999). J. Am. Vet. Med. Assoc. 223:93–98.

Buffa, E. A., S. S. Vandenberg, F. J. M. Verstraete, and N. G. N. Swart. 1992. Effect of dietary biotin supplement on equine hoof horn growth-rate and hardness. Equine Vet. J. 24:472–474.

Bureau, F., G. Bonizzi, N. Kirschvink, S. Delhalle, D. Desmecht, M. P. Merville, V. Bours, and P. Lekeux. 2000. Correlation between nuclear factor-kappaB activity in bronchial brushing samples and lung dysfunction in an animal model of asthma. Amer. J. Resp. Crit. Care Med. 161:1314–1321.

Bush, J. A., D. E. Freeman, K. H. Kline, N. R. Merchen, and G. C. Fahey, Jr. 2001. Dietary fat supplementation effects on in vitro nutrient disappearance and in vivo nutrient intake and total digestibility by horses. J. Anim. Sci. 79:232–239.

Butler, K. D., and H. F. Hintz. 1977. Effect of feed intake and gelatin supplementation on growth and quality of hoofs of ponies. J. Anim. Sci. 44:257–261.

Capen, C. C. 1983. Nutritional secondary hyperparathyroidism, Horses. Pp. 160–163 in Current Therapy in Equine Medicine, N. E. Robinson, ed. Philadelphia: W. B. Saunders.

Cargile, J. L., J. A. Burrows, I. Kim, N. D. Cohen, and A. M. Merritt. 2004. Effect of dietary corn oil supplementation on equine gastric fluid acid, sodium, and prostaglandin E2 content before and during pentagastrin infusion. J. Vet. Int. Med. 18:545–549.

Carr, E. A., S. J. Spier, G. D. Kortz, and E. P. Hoffman. 1996. Laryngeal and pharyngeal dysfunction in horses homozygous for Hyperkalemic Periodic Paralysis. J. Am. Vet. Med. Assoc. 209:798–803.

Carson, K., and D. G. M. Wood-Gush. 1983. Behavior of Thoroughbred foals during nursing. Equine Vet. J. 15:257–262.

Clarke, A. F., and T. Madelin. 1987. Technique for assessing respiratory health hazards from hay and other source materials. Equine Vet. J. 19:442–447.

Clarke, C. J., P. L. Roeder, and P. M. Dixon. 1996. Nasal obstruction caused by nutritional osteodystrophia fibrosa in a group of Ethiopian horses. Vet. Rec. 139:568–570.

Clarke, L. L., M. C. Roberts, and R. A. Argenzio. 1990. Feeding and digestive problems in horses—physiological responses to a concentrated meal. Vet. Clin. North Am. Equine Pract. 6:433–450.

Cohen, N. D. 1997. Epidemiology of colic. Vet. Clin. North Am. Equine Pract. 13:191–201.

Cohen, N. D., P. G. Gibbs, and A. M. Woods. 1999. Dietary and other management factors associated with colic in horses. J. Am. Vet. Med. Assoc. 215:53–60.

Cohen, N. D., C. A. Vontur, and P. C. Rakestraw. 2000. Risk factors for enterolithiasis among horses in Texas. J. Am. Vet. Med. Assoc. 216:1787–1794.

Coleman, R. J., G. W. Mathison, and L. Burwash. 1999. Growth and condition at weaning of extensively managed creep-fed foals. J. Equine Vet. Sci. 19:45–50.

Costa, L. R., T. L Seahorn, R. M. Moore, H. W. Taylor, S. D. Gaunt, and R. E. Beadle. 2000. Correlation of clinical score, intrapleural pressure, cytologic findings of bronchoalveolar fluid, and histopathologic lesions of pulmonary tissue in horses with summer pasture associated-obstructive pulmonary disease. Am. J. Vet. Res. 61:167–173.

Couetil, L. L., and M. P. Ward. 2003. Analysis of risk factors for recurrent airway obstruction in North American horses: 1,444 cases (1990–1999). J. Am. Vet. Med. Assoc. 223:1645–1650.

Crawford, C., A. Dobson, S. R. Bailey, P. A. Harris, and J. Elliott. 2005. Changes in hindgut pH of ponies following feeding with fructan carbohydrate in the form of inulin. Pferdeheilkunde 21:71–72.

Cymbaluk, N. F. 1989. Effects of dietary energy source and level of feed intake on growth of weanling horses. Equine Pract. 11:29–33.

Cymbaluk, N. F. 1990. Cold housing effects on growth and nutrient demand of young horses. J. Anim. Sci. 68:3152–3162.

Cymbaluk, N. F., and G. I. Christison. 1989a. Effects of diet and climate on growing horses. J. Anim. Sci. 67:48–59.

Cymbaluk, N. F., and G. I. Christison. 1989b. Effects of dietary energy and phosphorus content on blood chemistry and development of growing horses. J. Anim. Sci. 67:951–958.

Cymbaluk, N. F., and G. I. Christison. 1990. Environmental effects on thermoregulation and nutrition of horses. Vet. Clin. North Am. Equine Pract. 6:355–372.

Cymbaluk, N. F., J. D. Millar, and D. A. Christensen. 1986. Oxalate concentration in feeds and its metabolism by ponies. Can. J. Anim. Sci. 66:1107–1116.

Cymbaluk, N. F., M. E. Smart, F. Bristol, and V. A. Pouteaux. 1993. Importance of milk replacer intake and composition in rearing orphan foals. Can. Vet. J. 34:479–486.

David, J. B., N. D. Cohen, and R. Nachreiner. 1997. Equine nutritional secondary hyperparathyroidism. Comp. Cont. Ed. Pract. Vet. 19:1380–1387.

De La Corte, F. D., S. J. Valberg, J. M. MacLeay, S. E. Williamson, and J. R. Mickelsen. 1999a. Glucose uptake in horses with polysaccharide storage myopathy. Am. J. Vet. Res. 60:458–462.

De La Corte, F. D., S. J. Valberg, J. R. Mickelsen, and M. Hower-Moritz. 1999b. Blood glucose clearance after feeding and exercise in polysaccharide storage myopathy. Equine Vet. J. Suppl. 30:324–328.

De La Corte, F. D., S. J. Valberg, J. M. MacLeay, and J. R. Mickelsen. 2002. Developmental onset of polysaccharide storage myopathy in 4 Quarter Horse foals. J. Vet. Intern. Med. 16:581–587.

Deaton, C. M. 2006. The role of oxidative stress in an equine model of human asthma. Redox. Rep. 11:46–52.

Deaton, C. M., D. J. Marlin, C. A. Roberts, N. Smith, P. A. Harris, F. J. Kelly, and R. C. Schroter. 2002. Antioxidant supplementation and pulmonary function at rest and exercise. Equine Vet. J. Suppl. 34:58–65.

Deaton, C. M., D. J. Marlin, N. C. Smith, P. A. Harris, C. A. Roberts, R. C. Schroter, and F. J. Kelley. 2004. Pulmonary epithelial lining fluid and plasma ascorbic acid concentrations in horses affected by recurrent airway obstruction. Am. J. Vet. Res. 65:80–87.

Deaton, C. M., D. J. Marlin, N. C. Smith, C. A. Roberts, P. A. Harris, R. C. Schroter, and F. J. Kelly. 2005a. Antioxidant and inflammatory responses of healthy horses and horses affected by recurrent airway obstruction. Equine Vet. J. 37:243–249.

Deaton, C. M., D. J. Marlin, N. C. Smith, P. A. Harris, M. P. Dagleish, R. C. Schroter, and F. J. Kelly. 2005b. Effect of acute airway inflammation on the pulmonary antioxidant status. Exp. Lung Res. 31:653–670.

Dik, K. J. 1999. The radiographic development of osteochondral abnormalities in the hock and stifle of Dutch Warmblood foals from 1 to 11 months of age. Vet. Radiol. Ultrasound 40: Abstr. 183.

Dik, K. J., E. E. Enzerink, and P. R. van Weeren. 1999. Radiographic development of osteochondral abnormalities in the hock and stifle of Dutch Warmblood foals from age 1 to 11 months. Equine Vet. J. Suppl. 31:9–15.

DiMauro, S., and C. Lamperti. 2001. Muscle glycogenoses. Muscle Nerve 24:984–999.

Dionne, R. M., A. Vrins, M. Y. Doucet, and J. Pare. 2003. Gastric ulcers in Standardbred racehorses: prevalence, lesion description, and risk factors. J. Vet. Intern. Med. 17:218–222.

Donoghue, S. 1980. Nutritionally-related bone diseases. Proc. Am. Assoc. Equine Pract. 26:65–68.

Dulphy, J. P., W. Martin-Rosset, H. Duroeucq, J. M. Ballet, A. Detour, and M. Jailler. 1997. Compared feeding patterns in ad libitum intake of dry forages by horses and sheep. Livest. Prod. Sci. 52:49–56.

Estepa, J. C., B. Garfia, P. R. Gao, T. Cantor, M. Rodriguez, and E. Aguilera-Tejero. 2003. Validation and clinical utility of a novel immunoradiometric assay exclusively for biologically active whole parathyroid hormone in the horse. Equine Vet. J. 35:291–295.

Fackelman, G. E. 1980. Equine flexural deformities of developmental origin. Proc. Am. Assoc. Equine Pract. 26:97–105.

Fadel, J. G. 1992. In vitro buffering capacity changes of seven commodities under controlled moisture and heating conditions. J. Dairy Sci. 75:1287–1295.

Finkler-Schade, C., H. Enbergs, and L. Ahlswede. 1999. Wachstumsverlauf und ernahrungssituation von saugfohlen. Prak. Tierarzt. 11:980–991.

Firshman, A. M., S. J. Valberg, J. B. Bender, and C. J. Finno. 2003. Epidemiologic characteristics and management of polysaccharide myopathy in Quarter Horses. Am. J. Vet. Res. 64:1319–1327.

Firshman, A. M., J. D. Baird, and S. J. Valberg. 2005. Prevalence and clinical signs of polysaccharide storage myopathy and shivers in Belgian draft horses. J. Am. Vet. Med. Assoc. 227:1958–1964.

Firth, E. C., and H. Hodge. 1997. Physeal form of the longbones of the foal. Res. Vet. Sci. 62(3):217–221.

Firth, E. C., P. R. van Weeren, D. U. Pfeiffer, J. Delahunt, and A. Barneveld. 1999. Effect of age, exercise and growth rate on bone mineral density (BMD) in third carpal bone and distal radius of Dutch Warmblood foals with osteochondrosis. Equine Vet. J. Suppl. 31:74–78.

Frank, N., J. F. Hawkins, L. L. Couetil, and J. T. Raymond. 1998. Primary hyperparathyroidism with osteodystrophia fibrosa of the facial bones in a pony. J. Am. Vet. Med. Assoc. 212(1):84–86.

French, K. R., and C. C. Pollitt. 2004. Equine laminitis: loss of hemidesmosomes in hoof secondary epidermal lamellae correlates to dose in an oligofructose induction model: an ultrastructural study. Equine Vet. J. 36:230–235.

Fujimoto, Y., K. Matsukawa, H. Inubushi, M. Nakamatsu, H. Satoh, and S. Yamagiwa. 1967. Electron microscopic observations of the equine parathyroid glands with particular reference to those of equine osteodystrophia fibrosa. Jap. J. Vet. Res.15:37–52.

Furr, M., L. Taylor, and D. Kronfeld. 1994. The effects of exercise training on serum gastrin responses in the horse. Cornell Vet. 84:41–45.

Gabel, A. 1986. Incidence of developmental bone problems. Pp. 13–15 in Proc. Panel on Developmental Orthopedic Disease, Am. Quarter Horse Assoc., Dallas, TX.

Garcia M. C., and J. Beech. 1986. Endocrinologic, hematologic, and heart rate changes in swimming horses. Am. J. Vet. Res. 47:2004–2006.

Garner, H. E., D. P. Hutcheson, J. R. Coffman, A. W. Hahn, and C. Salem. 1977. Lactic-acidosis–factor associated with equine laminitis. J. Anim. Sci. 45:1037–1041.

Garner, H. E., J. N. Moore, J. H. Johnson, L. Clark, J. F. Amend, L. G. Tritschler, J. R. Coffmann, R. F. Sprouse, D. P. Hutcheson, and C. A. Salem. 1978. Changes in cecal flora associated with onset of laminitis. Equine Vet. J. 10:249–252.

Gee, E. K., N. D. Grace, E. C. Firth, and P. F. Fennessy. 2000. Changes in liver copper concentration of Thoroughbred foals from birth to 160 days of age and the effect of prenatal copper supplementation of their dams. Austral. Vet. J. 78:347–353.

Gee, E. K., E. C. Firth, P. C. Morel, P. F. Fennessy, N. F. Grace, and T. D. Mogg. 2005a. Enlargements of the distal third metacarpus and metatarsus in Thoroughbred foals at pasture from birth to 160 days of age. N. Z. Vet. J. 53:438–447.

Gee, E. K., E. C. Firth, P. C. Morel, P. F. Fennessy, N. F. Grace, and T. D. Mogg. 2005b. Articular / epiphyseal osteochondrosis in Thoroughbred foals at 5 months of age: influences of growth of the foal and prenatal copper supplementation of the dam. N. Z. Vet. J. 53:448–456.

Gee, E. K., M. Davies, E. Firth, L. Jeffcott, P. Fennessy, and T. Mogg. 2006. Osteochondrosis and copper: histology of articular cartilage from foals out of copper supplemented and non-supplemented dams. Vet. J. In press.

Geor, R. J., L. J. McCutcheon, and M. I. Lindinger. 1996. Adaptations to daily exercise in hot and humid ambient conditions in trained Thoroughbred horses. Equine Vet. J. Suppl. 22:63–68.

Gerber, V., N. E. Robinson, P. J. Venta, J. Rawson, A. M. Jefcoat, and J. A. Hotchkiss. 2003. Mucin genes in horse airways: MUC5AC but no MUC2, may play a role in recurrent airway obstruction. Equine Vet J. 35:252–257.

Gerber, V., A. Lindberg, C. Berney, and N. E. Robinson. 2004. Airway mucus in recurrent airway obstruction–short-term response to environmental challenge. J. Vet. Intern. Med. 18:92–97.

Gibbs, P. G., and N. D. Cohen. 2001. Early management of race-bred weanlings and yearlings on farms. J. Equine Vet. Sci. 21:279–283.

Goncalves, S., V. Julliand, and A. Leblond. 2002. Risk factors associated with colic in horses. Vet. Res. 33:641–652.

Grace, N. D., E. K. Gee, E. C. Firth, and H. L. Shaw. 2002. Digestible energy intake, dry matter digestibility and mineral status of grazing New Zealand Thoroughbred yearlings. N. Z. Vet. J. 50:63–69.

Graham, B. P. 2002. Dental care in the older horse. Vet. Clin. North Am. Equine Pract.. 18:509–522.

Graham, P. M., E. A. Ott, J. H. Brendemuhl, and S. H. TenBroeck. 1994. The effect of supplemental lysine and threonine on growth and development of yearling horses. J. Anim. Sci. 72:380–386.

Graham-Thiers, P. M., and D. S. Kronfeld. 2005. Amino acid supplementation improves muscle mass in aged and young horses. J. Anim. Sci. 83:2783–2788.

Grondahl, A. M., and N. I. Dolvik. 1993. Heritability estimations of osteochondrosis in the tibiotarsal joint and of bony fragments in the palmar/plantar portion of the metacarpo- and metatarsophalangeal joints of horses. J. Am. Vet. Med. Assoc. 203:101–104.

Hacklander, R., H. Enbergs, E. Niess, and L. Ahlswede. 1996. Analyse der Futterung von warmblutfohlen im zweiten lebenshalbjahr. Pferdeheilkunde 12:307–311.

Harper, E. J. 1998a. Changing perspectives on aging and energy requirements: aging and energy intakes in humans, dogs and cats. J. Nutr. 128:2623S–2626S.

Harper, E. J. 1998b. Changing perspectives on aging and energy requirements: aging and digestive function in humans, dogs and cats. J. Nutr. 128:2632S–2635S.

Harris, P., W. Staniar, and A. D. Ellis. 2005. Effect of exercise and diet on the incidence of DOD. Pp. 273–290 in The Growing Horse: Nutrition and Prevention of Growth Disorders, V. Juliand and W. Martin-Rosset, eds. EAAP Scientific Series No. 114. Wageningen, Netherlands: Wageningen Acad. Pub.

Hassel, D. M., D. L. Langer, J. R. Snyder, C. M. Drake, M. L. Goodell, and A. Wyle. 1999. Evaluation of enterolithiasis in equids: 900 cases (1973–1996). J. Am. Vet. Med. Assoc. 214:233–237.

Hassel, D. M., P. S. Schiffman, and J. R. Snyder. 2001. Petrographic and geochemic evaluation of enteroliths. Am. J. Vet. Res. 62:350–358.

Hassel, D. M., P. C. Rakestraw, I. A. Gardner, S. J. Spier, and J. R. Snyder. 2004. Dietary risk factors and colonic pH and mineral concentrations in horses with enterolithiasis. J. Vet. Intern. Med. 18:346–349.

Heilbronn, L. K., and E. Ravussin. 2003. Calorie restriction and aging: review of the literature and implications for studies in humans. Am. J. Clin. Nutr. 78:361–369.

Herthel, D., and D. M. Hood. 1999. Clinical presentation, diagnosis, and prognosis of chronic laminitis. Vet. Clin. North Am. Equine Pract. 15:375–394.

Hinckley, K. A., and I. W. Henderson. 1996. The epidemiology of equine laminitis in the UK. P. 62 in Proc. 35th Cong. Br. Equine Vet. Cong., Warwick, UK.

Hiney, K. M., B. D. Nielsen, and D. Rosenstein. 2004. Short duration exercise and confinement alters bone mineral content and shape in weanling horses. J. Anim. Sci. 82:2313–2320.

Hintz, H. F., H. F. Schryver, and J. E. Lowe. 1976. Delayed growth response and limb conformation in young horses. Pp. 94–96 in Proc. Cornell Nutr. Conf., Ithaca, NY.

Hintz, H. F., H. F. Schryver, J. Doty, C. Lakin, and R. A. Zimmerman. 1984. Oxalic acid content of alfalfa hays and its influence on the availability of calcium, phosphorus and magnesium to ponies. J. Anim. Sci. 58:939–942.

Hintz, H. F., J. E. Lowe, and P. Livesay-Wilkins. 1988. Studies on equine enterolithiasis. Pp. 116–118 in Proc. Equine Assoc. Equine Pract.

Hintz, H. F., T. Hernandez, and V. Soderholm. 1989. Effect of vinegar supplementation on pH of colonic fluid. Pp. 116–118 in Proc. 11th Equine Nutr. Physiol. Soc. Symp., Stillwater, OK.

Hoffman, R. M., D. S. Kronfeld, J. L. Holland, and K. M. Greiwe-Crandell. 1995. Preweaning diet and stall weaning method influences on stress response in foals. J. Anim. Sci. 73:2922–2930.

Hoffman, R. M., L. A. Lawrence, D. S. Kronfeld, W. L. Cooper, D. J. Sklan, J. J. Dascanio, and P. A. Harris. 1999. Dietary carbohydrates and fat influence radiographic bone mineral content of growing foals. J. Anim. Sci. 77:3330–3338.

Hoffman, R. M., J. A. Wilson, D. S. Kronfeld, W. L. Cooper, L. A. Lawrence, D. Sklan, and P. A. Harris. 2001. Hydrolyzable carbohydrates in pasture, hay, and horse feeds: direct assay and seasonal variation. J. Anim. Sci. 79:500–506.

Holbrook, T. C., R. D. Simmons, M. E. Payton, and C. G. MacAllister. 2005. Effect of repeated oral administration of hypertonic electrolyte solution on equine gastric mucosa. Equine Vet. J. 37:501–504.

Hood, D. M. 1999a. Laminitis in the horse. Vet. Clin. North Am. Equine Pract. 15:287–294.

Hood, D. M. 1999b. The pathophysiology of developmental and acute laminitis. Vet. Clin. North Am. Equine Pract. 15:321–343.

Hood, D. M. 1999c. Laminitis as a systemic disease. Vet. Clin. North Am. Equine Pract. 15:481–494.

Hudson, J. M., N. D. Cohen, P. G. Gibbs, and J. A. Thompson. 2001. Feeding practices associated with colic in horses. J. Am. Vet. Med. Assoc. 219:1419–1425.

Hughes, S. J., G. D. Potter, L. W. Greene, T. W. Odom, and M. Murray-Gerzik. 1995. Adaptation of Thoroughbred horses in training to a fat supplemented diet. Equine Vet. J. 18:349–352.

Hunt, E., and J. T. Blackwelder. 2002. Nutritional secondary hyperparathyroidism (big head, brain disease, osteodystrophia fibrosa). Pp. 1252–1253 in Large Animal Internal Medicine, B. P. Smith, ed. St. Louis: Mosby.

Hunt, L. M., S. J. Valberg, K. Steffenhagen, and J. B. Bender. 2005. A retrospective study of myopathies and associated gait abnormalities in 65 Warmblood horses. J. Vet. Intern. Med. 19:428 (Abstr.).

Hurtig, M., S. L. Green, H. Dobson, Y. Mikuni-Takagaki, and J. Choi. 1993. Correlative study of defective cartilage and bone growth in foals fed a low-copper diet. Equine Vet. J. Suppl. 16:66–73.

Jackson, B. F., A. E. Goodship, R. Eastell, and J. S. Price. 2003. Evaluation of serum concentrations of biochemical markers of bone metabolism and insulin-like growth factor I associated with treadmill exercise in young horses. Am. J. Vet. Res. 64:1549–1556.

Jackson, C. A., C. Berney, A. M. Jefcoat, and N. E. Robinson. 2000. Environment and prednisone interactions in the treatment of recurrent airway obstruction (heaves). Equine Vet. J. 32:432–438.

Jansen, W. L., J. Van der Kuilen, S. N. J. Neelen, and A. C. Beynen. 2001. The apparent digestibility of fiber in Trotters when dietary soybean oil is substituted for an isoenergetic amount of glucose. Arch. Anim. Nutr. 54:297–304.

Jeffcott, L. B. 1972. Passive immunity and its transfer with special reference to the horse. Biol. Rev. 47:439–464.

Jeffcott, L. B., and M. D. Henson. 1998. Studies on growth cartilage in the horse and their application to aetiopathogenesis of dyschondroplasis (osteochondrosis). Vet. J. 156:177–192.

Jeffcott, L. B., and C. J. Savage. 1996. Nutrition and the development of osteochondrosis. Pferdeheilkunde 12:338–342.

Jeffcott, L. B., J. R. Field, J. G. Mclean, and K. Odea. 1986. Glucose-tolerance and insulin sensitivity in ponies and Standardbred horses. Equine Vet. J. 18:97–101.

Jelan, Z. A., L. B. Jeffcott, N. Lundheim, and M. Osborne. 1996. Growth rates in Thoroughbred foals. Pferdeheilkunde 12:291–295.

Johnson, P. J., N. T. Messer, D. K. Bowles, S. H. Slight, V. K. Ganjam, and J. M. Kreeger. 2004a. Glucocorticoids and laminitis in horses. Comp. Cont. Ed. Pract. Vet. 26:547–558.

Johnson, P. J., N. T. Messer, and V. K. Ganjam. 2004b. Cushing's syndromes, insulin resistance and endocrinopathic laminitis. Equine Vet. J. 36:194–198.

Jones, S. L. 2004. Inflammatory diseases of the gastrointesintal tract causing diarrhea. P. 884 in Equine Internal Medicine, 2nd ed., S. M. Reed, W. M. Bayly, and D. C. Sellon, eds. St. Louis: Saunders.

Joyce, J. R., K. R. Pierce, W. M. Romane, and J. M. Baker. 1971. Clinical study of nutritional secondary hyperparathyroidism in horses. J. Am. Vet. Med. Assoc. 158:2033–2042.

Julen, T. R., G. D. Potter, L. W. Greene, and G. G. Stott. 1995. Adaptation to a fat-supplemented diet by cutting horses. Pp. 56–61 in Proc. 14th Equine Nutr. Physiol. Soc. Symp, Ontario, CA.

Kaneene, J. B., R. Miller, W. A. Ross, K. Gallagher, J. Marteniuk, and J. Rook. 1997. Risk factors for colic in the Michigan (USA) equine population. Prev. Vet. Med. 30:23–36.

Kidd, J. A., and A. R. S. Barr. 2002. Flexural deformities of foals. Equine Vet. Educ. 14:311–321.

Kienzle, E., C. Kaden, P. P. Hoppe, and B. Opitz. 2003. Nutrient digestion coefficients. J. Anim. Physiol. Anim. Nutr. 87:174–180.

Kirschvink, N., and P. Lekeux. 2005. Oxidants and airway inflammation. In Third World Equine Airways Symp., D. E. Ainsworth, B.C. McGorum, L. Viel, N. E. Robinson, and N.G. Ducharme, eds. Document No. P 2111.0705. Ithaca, NY: International Veterinary Information Service.

Kirschvink, N., N. Smith, L. Fievez, V. Bougnet, T. Art, D. Marlin, C. Roberts, B. Genicot, P. Lindsey, and P. Lekeux. 2002a. Effect of chronic airway inflammation and exercise on pulmonary and systemic antioxidant status of healthy and heaves-affected horses. Equine Vet. J. 34:563–571.

Kirschvink, N., L. Fievez, V. Bougnet, T. Art, G. Degand, N. Smith, D. Marlin, C. Roberts, P. Harris, and P. Lekeux. 2002b. Effect of nutritional antioxidant supplementation on systemic and pulmonary antioxidant status, airway inflammation and lung function in heaves-affected horses. Equine Vet. J. 34:705–712.

Kirschvink, N., F. di Silvestro, I. Sbai, S. Vandenput, T. Art, C. Roberts, and P. Lekeux. 2002c. The use of cardboard bedding material as part of an environmental control regime for heaves-affected horses: In vitro assessment of airborne dust and aeroallergen concentration and in vivo effects on lung function. Vet. J. 163:319–325.

Knight, D. A., A. A. Gabel, S. M. Reed, L. M. Bramlage, W. J. Tyznik, and R. M. Embertson. 1985. Correlation of dietary mineral to incidence and severity of metabolic bone disease in Ohio and Kentucky. Proc. Am. Assoc. Equine Pract. 31:445–461.

Knight, D. A., S. E. Weisbrode, L. M. Schmall, S. M. Reed, A. A. Gabel, L. R. Bramlage, and W. I. Tyznik. 1990. The effects of copper supplementation on the prevalence of cartilage lesions in foals. Equine Vet. J: 22:426–432.

Koenen, E. P. C., A. E. van Veldhuizen, and E. W. Brascamp. 1995. Genetic parameters of linear scored conformation traits and their relation to dressage and show-jumping performance in the Dutch Warmblood Riding Horse population. Livest. Prod. Sci. 43:85–94.

Kristula, M. A., and S. M. McDonnell. 1994. Drinking water temperature affects consumption of water during cold weather in ponies. Appl. Anim. Behav. Sci. 41:155–160.

Kronfeld, D. S. 1996. Dietary fat affects heat production and other variables of equine performance, under hot and humid conditions. Equine Vet. J. 22:24–34.

Kronfield, D. S., T. N. Meacham, and S. Donoghue. 1990. Dietary aspects of developmental orthopedic disease in young horses. Vet. Clin. North Am. Equine Pract. 6:451–455.

Kronfeld, D. S., S. E. Custalow, P. L. Ferrante, L. E. Taylor, J. A. Wilson, and W. Tiegs. 1998. Acid-base responses of fat-adapted horses: relevance to hard work in the heat. Appl. Anim. Behav. Sci. 59:61–72.

Lanyon, L. E. 1992. Control of bone architecture by functional load bearing. Journal of Bone and Mineral Research 7(Suppl.):S369-S375.

Larson, B. T., D. F. Lawler, E. L. Spitznagel, and R. D. Kealy. 2003. Improved glucose tolerance with lifetime diet restriction favorably affects disease and survival in dogs. J. Nutr. 133:2887–2892.

Lehmann-Horn, F., K. Jurkat-Rott, and R. Rudel. 2002. Periodic paralysis: understanding channelopathies. Curr. Neurol. Neurosci. Rep. 2:61–69.

Leibsle, S. R., M. A. Prichard, J. P. Morehead, N. S. Keuler, and E. M. Santschi. 2005. Forelimb conformation of the growing Thoroughbred and the impact of birth weight and parental conformation. Am. Assoc. Equine Pract. 51:297–298.

Lester, G. D. 2004. Gastrointestinal diseases of performance horses. Pp. 1037–1048 in Equine Sports Medicine and Surgery, K. W. Hinchcliff, A. J. Kaneps, and R. J. Geor, eds. London: Elsevier.

Lewis, L. D. 1995. Equine Clinical Nutrition. Feeding and Care. Philadelphia: Williams & Wilkins.

Li, X., J. E. Owen, A. J. Murdoch, and C. C. Pearson. 1993. Respirable dust from animal feeds. Pp. 747–753 in Livestock Environment IV, E. Collins and C. Boon, eds. University of Warwick, Coventry, England: Am. Soc. Ag. Eng.

Lloyd, K., H. F. Hintz, J. D. Wheat, and H. F. Schryver. Enteroliths in horses. 1987. Cornell Vet. 77:172–186.

Longland, A. C., and A. J. Cairns. 2000. Fructans and their implications in the aetiology of laminitis. Pp. 52–55 in Third International Conference on Feeding Horses, T. Hollands, ed. Dodson and Horrell.

Longland, A. C., A. J. Cairns, and M. O. Humphreys. 1999. Seasonal and diurnal changes in fructan concentration in Lolium perenne: implication for the grazing management of equines pre-disposed to laminitis. P. 258 in Proc. 16th Equine Nutr. Physiol. Soc. Symp., Raleigh, NC.

Lorenzo-Figueras, M., and A. M. Merritt. 2002. Effects of exercise on gastric volume and pH in the proximal portion of the stomach of horses. Am. J. Vet. Res. 63:1481–1487.

Lorenzo-Figueras, M., T. Preston, E. A. Ott, and A. M. Merritt. 2005. Meal-induced gastric relaxation and emptying in horses after ingestion of high-fat versus high-carbohydrate diets. Am. J. Vet. Res. 66:897–906.

MacCormack, J. A. D., and J. M. Bruce. 1991. The horse in winter–shelter and feeding. Farm Building Progress. 105:10–13.

MacLeay, J. M, S. J. Valberg, C. J. Geyer, S. A. Sorum, and M. D. Sorum. 1999. Heritable basis for recurrent exertional rhabdomyolysis in Thoroughbred racehorses. Am. J. Vet. Res. 60:250–256.

Malinowski, K., R. A. Christensen, A. Konopka, C. G. Scanes, and H. D. Hafs. 1997. Feed intake, body weight, body condition score, musculation, and immunocompetence in aged mares given equine somatotropin. J. Anim. Sci. 75:755–760.

Marlin, D. J., R. C. Schroter, S. L. White, P. Maykuth, G. Matthesen, P. C. Mills, N. Waran, and P. Harris. 2001. Recovery from transport and acclimatisation of competition horses in a hot humid environment. Equine Vet. J. 33:371–379.

Marti, E. 2001. Genetics of equine chronic airway disease. N. E. Robinson, chairperson. Inter. Workshop on Equine Chronic Airway Disease, Michigan State University. Equine Vet. J. 33:9–10.

Marti, E., and B. Ohnesorge. 2002. Genetic basis of respiratory disorders. P. 7 in Equine Respiratory Disease, P. Lekeux, ed. Ithaca, NY: International Veterinary Information Services.

Mase, C. A. 1987. Observations on radial maturation in foals as they relate to skeletal pathology. Proc. Am. Assoc. Equine Prac. 33:439–450.

Matera, M. G., L. Calzetta, A. Peli, A. Scagliarini, C. Matera, and M. Cazzola. 2005. Immune sensitization of equine bronchus: glutathione, IL – 1β expression and tissue responsiveness. Resp. Res. 6:104–111.

Mathiason-Kochan, K. J., G. D. Potter, S. Caggiano, and E. M. Michael. 2001. Ration digestibility, water balance and physiologic responses in horses fed varying diets and exercised in hot weather. Pp. 262–268 in Proc. 17th Equine Nutr. Physiol. Soc. Symp., Lexington, KY.

Mazan, M. R., E. F. Deveney, S. DeWitt, D. Bedenice, and A. Hoffman. 2004. Energetic cost of breathing, body composition, and pulmonary function in horses with recurrent airway obstruction. J. Appl. Physiol. 97:91–97.

McBride, G. E., R. J. Christopherson, and W. Sauer. 1985. Metabolic rate and plasma thyroid hormone concentrations of mature horses in response to changes in ambient temperature. Can. J. Anim. Sci. 65:375–382.

McCall, C. A., G. D. Potter, and J. L. Kreider. 1985. Locomoter, vocal and other behavioral responses to varying methods of weaning foals. Appl. Anim. Behav. Sci. 14:27–35.

McClure, S. R., L. T. Glickman, and N. W. Glickman. 1999. Prevalence of gastric ulcers in show horses. J. Am. Vet. Med. Assoc. 215:256–259.

McCue, P. M. 2002. Equine Cushing's disease. Vet. Clin. North Am. Equine Pract. 18:533–543.

McCutcheon, L. J., and R. J. Geor. 1996. Sweat fluid and ion losses in horses during training and competition in cool vs hot ambient conditions: implications for ion supplementation. Equine Vet. J. Suppl. 22:54–62.

McCutcheon, L. J., R. J. Geor, M. J. Hare, G. L. Ecker, and M. I. Lindinger. 1995. Sweating rate and sweat composition during exercise and recovery in ambient heat and humidity. Equine Vet. J. Suppl. 20:153–157.

McCutcheon, L. J., R. J. Geor, G. L. Ecker, and M. I. Lindinger. 1999. Equine sweating responses to submaximal exercise during 21 days of heat acclimation. J. Appl. Physiol. 87:1843–1851.

McDonnell, S. M., and M. A. Kristula. 1996. No effect of drinking water temperature (ambient vs chilled) on consumption of water during hot summer weather in ponies. Appl. Anim. Behav. Sci. 49:159–163.

McGorum, B. C., P. M. Dixon, and R. E. Halliwell. 1993. Responses of horses affected with chronic obstructive pulmonary disease to inhalation challenges with mould antigens. Equine Vet. J. 25:261–267.

McGorum, B., J. Ellison, and R. Cullen 1998. Total and respirable airborne dust endotoxins concentrations in three equine management systems. Equine Vet. J. 30:430–434.

McIlwraith, C. W. 2004. Developmental orthopedic disease: problems of limbs in young horses. J. Equine Vet. Sci. 24:475–479.

McKenzie, R. A. 1988. Purple pigeon grass (Setaria incrassata): a potential cause of nutritional secondary hyperparathyroidism of grazing horses. Austral. Vet. J. 65:329–330.

McKenzie, R. A., B. J. Blaney, and R. J. W. Gartner. 1981a. The effect of dietary oxalate on calcium, phosphorus and magnesium balances in horses. J. Agric. Sci. 97:69–74.

McKenzie, R. A., R. J. W. Gartner, B. J. Blaney, and R. J. Glanville. 1981b. Control of nutritional secondary hyperparathyroidism in grazing horses with calcium plus phosphorus supplementation. Austral. Vet. J. 57:554–557.

McKenzie, E. C., S. J. Valberg, and J. D. Pagan. 2003. Nutritional management of exertional rhabdomyolysis. Pp. 727–734 in Current Therapy in Equine Medicine, 5th ed., N. E. Robinson, ed. Philadelphia: W. B. Saunders.

Metayer, N., M. Lhote, A. Bahr, N. D. Cohen, I. Kim, A. J. Roussel, and V. Julliand. 2004. Meal size and starch content affect gastric emptying in horses. Equine Vet. J. 36:436–440.

Meyer, H., M. Coenen, and C. Gurer. 1985. Investigations of saliva production and chewing in horses fed various feeds. Pp. 38–41 in Proc. 9th Eq. Nutr. Physiol. Soc. Symp, East Lansing, MI.

Meyer, T. S., M. R. Fedde, J. H. Cox, and H. H. Erickson. 1999. Hyperkalemic Periodic Paralysis in horses: a review. Equine Vet. J. 31:362–367.

Meyers, M. C., G. D. Potter, L. W. Greene, S. F. Crouse, and J. W. Evans. 1987. Physiological and metabolic response of exercising horses to added dietary fat. Pp. 107–113 in Proc. 10th Equine Nutr. Physiol. Soc. Symp., Ft. Collins, CO.

Millward, D. J., A. Fereday, N. Gibson, and P. J. Pacy. 1997. Aging, protein requirements, and protein turnover. Am. J. Clin. Nutr. 66:774–786.

Minnick, P. D., C. M. Brown, W. E. Braselton, G. L. Meerdink, and M. R. Slanker. 1987. The induction of equine laminitis with an aqueous extract of the heartwood of black-walnut (Juglans Nigra). Vet. Human Toxicol. 29:230–233.

Minson, D. J. 1990. Forage in Ruminant Nutrition. New York: Academic Press.

Mohammed, H. O. 1990. Factors associated with the risk of developing osteochondrosis in horses: a case-control study. Prev. Vet. Med. 10:63–71.

Molina, A., M. Valera, R. Dos Santos, and A. Rodero. 1999. Genetic parameters of morphofunctional traits in andalusian horse. Livest. Prod. Sci. 60:295–303.

Moore, J. N., D. Allen, and E. S. Clark. 1989. Patho-physiology of acute laminitis. Vet. Clin. North Am. Equine Pract. 5:67–72.

Moore, R. M., S. C. Eades, and A. M. Stokes. 2004. Evidence for vascular and enzymatic events in the pathophysiology of acute laminitis: which pathway is responsible for initiation of this process in horses? Equine Vet. J. 36:204–209.

Moore-Colyer, M. J. 1996. Effect of soaking hay fodder for horses on dust and mineral content. Anim. Sci. 63:337–342.

Morgan, K., P. Funkquist, and G. Nyman. 2002. The effect of coat clipping on thermoregulation during intense exercise in trotters. Equine Vet. J. Suppl. 34:564–567.

Murray, M. J., and G. F. Schusser. 1993. Measurement of 24-hr gastric pH using an indwelling pH electrode in horses unfed, fed, and treated with ranitidine. Equine Vet. J. 25:417–421.

Murray, M. J., and E. S. Eichorn. 1996. Effect of intermittent feed deprivation, intermittent feed deprivation with ranitidine administration, and stall confinement with ad libitum access to hay on gastric ulceration in horses. Am. J. Vet. Res. 57:1599–1603.

Murray, R. C., G. M. Constantineau, and E. M. Green. 1992. Equine enterolithiasis. Comp. Cont. Educ. Pract. Vet. 14:1104–1113.

Murray, M. J., G. F. Schusser, F. S. Pipers, and S. J. Gross. 1996. Factors associated with gastric lesions in Thoroughbred racehorses. Equine Vet. J. 28:368–374.

Nadeau, J. A., F. M. Andrews, A. G. Mathews, R. A. Argenzio, J. T. Blackford, M. Sohtell, and A. M. Saxton. 2000. Evaluation of diet as a cause of gastric ulcers in horses. Am. J. Vet. Res. 61:784–790.

Nadeau, J. A., F. M. Andrews, C. S. Patton, R. A. Argenzio, A. G. Mathew, and A. M. Saxton. 2003a. Effects of hydrochloric, acetic, butyric, and propionic acids on pathogenesis of ulcers in the nonglandular portion of the stomach of horses. Am. J. Vet. Res. 64:404–412.

Nadeau, J. A., F. M. Andrews, C. S. Patton, R. A. Argenzio, A. G. Mathew, and A. M. Saxton. 2003b. Effects of hydrochloric, valeric, and other volatile fatty acids on pathogenesis of ulcers in the nonglandular portion of the stomach of horses. Am. J. Vet. Res. 64:413–417.

Naylor, J. M. 1979. Colostral immunity in the calf and the foal. Vet. Clin. North Am. Large Anim. Pract. 1:331–361.

Naylor, J. M., and R. Bell. 1985. Raising the orphan foal. Vet. Clin. North Am. Equine Pract. 1:169–178.

Nicol, C. J., H. P. Davidson, P. A. Harris, A. J. Waters, and A. D. Wilson. 2002. Study of crib-biting and gastric inflammation and ulceration in young horses. Vet. Rec. 151:658–662.

Nieto, J. E., J. R. Synder, P. Beldomenico, M. Aleman, J. W. Kerr, and S. J. Spier. 2004. Prevalence of gastric ulcers in endurance horses–a preliminary report. Vet. J. 167:33–37.

Nogueira, G. P., R. C. Barnabe, and I. T. N. Verreschi. 1997. Puberty and growth rate in Thoroughbred fillies. Theriogenology 48:518–588.

NRC (National Research Council). 1989. Nutrient Requirements of Horses, 5th rev. ed. Washington, DC: National Academy Press.

O'Donohue, D. D., F. H. Smith, and K. L. Strickland. 1992. The incidence of abnormal limb development in the Irish thoroughbred from birth to 18 months. Equine Vet. J. 24:305–309.

Olsson, S. E. 1978. Osteochondrosis in domestic animals. Acta Radiol. Suppl 358:139–179.

Orth, M. W. 1999. The regulation of growth plate cartilage turnover. J. Anim. Sci. Suppl. 77:183–189.

Orton, R. K., I. D. Humes, and R. A. Leng. 1985. Effects of exercise and level of dietary protein on digestive function in horses. Equine Vet. J. 17:386–390.

Osborne, C. A., J. J. Sanna, and L. K. Unger. 1989. Analyzing the mineral composition of uroliths from dogs, cats, horses, cattle, sheep, goats and pigs. Vet. Med. 84:750–764.

Ott, E. A., and R. L. Asquith. 1989. The influence of mineral supplementation on growth and skeletal abnormalities of yearling horses. J. Anim. Sci. 67:2831–2840.

Ott, E. A., and J. Kivipelto. 2002. Growth and development of yearling horses fed either alfalfa or coastal Bermudagrass: hay and a concentrate formulated for Bermudagrass hay. J. Equine Vet. Sci. 22:311–322.

Ott, E. A., M. P. Brown, G. D. Roberts, and J. Kivipelto. 2005. Influence of starch intake on growth and skeletal development of weanling horses. J. Anim. Sci. 83:1033–1043.

Ousey, J. C., N. Holdstock, P. D. Rossdale, and A. J. McArthur. 1996. How much energy do sick neonatal foals require compared to healthy foals? Pferdeheilkunde 12:231–237.

Ousey, J. C., S. Prani, J. Zimmer, N. Holdstock, and P. D. Rossdale. 1997. Effects of various feeding regimens on the energy balance of neonates. Am. J. Vet. Res. 58:1243–1251.

Pagan, J. 2003. The relationship between glycemic response and the incidence of OCD in Thoroughbred weanlings: a field study. Pp. 119–124 in Kentucky Equine Res. Nutr. Conf., Versailles, KY.

Pagan, J. D., R. J. Geor, P. A. Harris, K. Hoekstra, S. Gardner, C. Hudson, and A. Prince. 2002. Effects of fat adaptation on glucose kinetics and substrate oxidation during low-intensity exercise. Equine Vet. J. Suppl. 34:33–38.

Paradis, M. R. 2002. Demographics of health and disease in the geriatric horse. Vet. Clin. North Am. Equine Pract. 18:391–401.

Paragon, B. M., J. P. Valette, G. Blanchard, and J. M. Benoix. 2003. Nutrition and developmental orthopedic disease in horses: results of a survey on 76 yearlings from 14 breeding farms in Basse Normandie (France). European Zoo Nutr. Centre, Antwerp. Abstr. Article 34.

Pearce, S. G., E. C. Firth, N. D. Grace, J. J. Wichtel, and P. F. Fennessy. 1998a. Effect of copper supplementation on the copper status of pregnant mares and their neonates. Equine Vet. J. 30:200–203.

Pearce, S. G., N. D. Grace, E. C. Firth, J. J. Wichtel, S. A. Holle, and P. F. Fennessy. 1998b. Effect of copper supplementation on the copper status of pasture-fed young Thoroughbreds. Equine Vet. J. 30:204–210.

Pearce, S. G., E. C. Firth, N. D. Grace, and P. F. Fennessy. 1998c. Effect of copper supplementation on the evidence of developmental orthopaedic disease in pasture-fed New Zealand Thoroughbreds. Equine Vet. J. 30:211–218.

Pearson, R. A., and J. B. Merritt. 1991. Intake, digestion and gastrointestinal transit time in resting donkeys and ponies and exercised donkeys given ad libitum hay and straw diets. Equine Vet. J. 23:339–343.

Peauroi, J. R., D. J. Fisher, F. C. Mohr, and S. L. Vivrette. 1998. Primary hyperparathyroidism caused by a functional parathyroid adenoma in a horse. J. Am. Vet. Med. Assoc. 212:1915–1918.

Peterson, C. J., L. Lawrence, R. Coleman, D. Powell, L. White, A. Reinowski, S. Hayes, and L. Harbour. 2003. Effect of diet quality on growth during weaning. Pp. 326–327 in Proc. 18th Equine Nutr. Physiol. Soc. Symp., East Lansing, MI.

Pieramati, C., M. Pepe, M. Sivestrelli, and A. Bolla. 2003. Heritability estimation of osteochondrosis dissecans in Maremmano horses. Livest. Prod. Sci. 79:249–255.

Pirie, R. S., P. M. Dixon, and B. C. McGorum. 2003. Endotoxin contamination contributes to the pulmonary inflammatory and functional response to aspergillus fumigatus extract inhalation in heaves horses. Clin. and Exp. Allergy 33:1289–1296.

Pollitt, C. C., M. Kyaw-Tanner, K. R. French, A. W. Van Eps, J. K. Hendrikz, and M. Daradka. 2003. Equine laminitis. Proc. 49th Ann. Conv. Am. Assoc. of Equine Pract. Ithaca, NY: International Veterinary Information Service.

Pool, R. R. 1987. Developmental orthopedic disease in the horse: normal and abnormal bone formation. Proc. Am. Assoc. Equine Pract. 33: 143–158.

Pool, R. R. 1993. Difficulties in definition of equine osteochondrosis; differentiation of developmental and acquired lesions. Equine Vet. J. Suppl. 16:5–12.

Potter, G. D., F. F. Arnold, D. D. Householder, D. H. Hansen, and K. M. Brown. 1992. Digestion of starch in the small or large intestine of the equine. P. 107 in First Europaische Konferenz uber die Ernahrung des Pferdes. Institut fur Tierernahrung, Tierazliche Hochschule, Hanover, Germany.

Preisinger, R., J. Wilkens, and E. Kalm. 1991. Estimation of genetic parameters and breeding values for conformation traits for foals and mares in the Trakehner population and their practical implications. Livest. Prod. Sci. 29:77–86.

Price, J. S., B. F. Jackson, J. A. Gray, I. M. Wright, P. E. Harris, R. G. Russell, C. W. McIlwraith, S. W. Ricketts, and L. E. Lanyon. 1997. Serum levels of molecular markers in growing horses: the effects of age, season and orthopedic disease. Trans. Orthoped. Res. Soc. 22:587.

Price, J. S., B. F. Jackson, J. A. Gray, P. A. Harris, I. M. Wright, D. U. Pfeiffer, S. P. Robins, R. Eastell, and S. W. Ricketts. 2001. Biochemical markers of bone metabolism in growing Thoroughbreds: a longitudinal study. Res. Vet. Sci. 71:37–44.

Proudman C. J. 1991. A two years survey of equine colic in general practice. Equine Vet. J. 24:90–93.

Pugh, D. G., and J. T. Thompson. 1992. Impaction colics attributed to decreased water intake and feeding coastal bermuda grass hay in a boarding stable. Equine Pract. 14:9–14.

Pugh, D. G., and M. A. Williams. 1992. Feeding foals from birth to weaning. Comp. Cont. Educ. Pract. Vet. 14:526–532.

Rabuffo, T. S., J. A. Orsini, E. Sullivan, J. Engiles, T. Norman, and R. Boston. 2002. Associations between age or sex and prevalence of gastric ulceration in Standardbred racehorses in training. J. Am. Vet. Med. Assoc. 221:1156–1159.

Ralston, S. L. 1996. Hyperglycemia/hyperinsulinemia after feeding a meal of grain to young horses with osteochondritis dissecans (OCD) lesions. Pferdeheilkunde 3:320–322.

Ralston, S. L., and L. H. Breuer. 1996. Field evaluation of a feed formulated for geriatric horses. J. Equine Vet. Sci. 16:334–338.

Ralston, S. L., C. F. Nockels, and E. L. Squires. 1988. Differences in diagnostic-test results and hematologic data between aged and young horses. Am. J. Vet. Res. 49:1387–1392.

Ralston, S. L., E. L. Squires, and C. F. Nockels. 1989. Digestion in the aged horse. J. Equine Vet. Sci. 9:203–205.

Ramirez, S., and T. L. Seahorn. 1997. How to manage nutritional secondary hyperparathyroidism in horses. Vet. Med. 92:978, 980–985.

Raymond, S. L., E. F. Curtis, and A. F. Clarke. 1994. Comparative dust challenges faced by horses when fed alfalfa cubes or hay. Equine Pract. 16:4–47.

Reeves, M. J., M. D. Salman, and G. Smith. 1996. Risk factors for equine acute abdominal disease (colic): results from a multi-center case-control study. Prev. Vet. Med. 26:285–301.

Reilly, J. D., D. F. Cottrell, R. J. Martin, and D. J. Cuddeford. 1998. Effect of supplementary dietary biotin on hoof growth and hoof growth rate in ponies: a controlled trial. Equine Vet. J. Suppl. 26:51–57.

Reynolds, J. A. 1997. Genetic-diet interactions in the Hyperkalemic Periodic Paralysis syndrome in Quarter Horses fed varying amounts of potassium. Ph.D. Dissertation. Texas A&M University, College Station.

Reynolds, J. A., E. L. Morris, D. S. Senor, K. S. Frey, D. Reagan, V. A. Weir, J. Elslander and G. D. Potter. 1992. The incidence of bone lesions and the rate of physeal closure in the carpal and tarsal regions of weanling Quarter Horses. J. Equine Vet. Sci. 12:114-117.

Reynolds, J. A, G. D. Potter, and L. W. Greene. 1998a. Genetic-diet interactions in the Hyperkalemic Periodic Paralysis syndrome in Quarter Horses fed varying amounts of potassium: II. Symptoms of HYPP. J. Equine Vet. Sci. 18:655–661.

Reynolds J. A., G. D. Potter, and L. W. Greene. 1998b. Genetic-diet interactions in the Hyperkalemic Periodic Paralysis syndrome in Quarter Horses fed varying amounts of potassium: III. The relationship between plasma potassium concentration and HYPP Symptoms. J. Equine Vet. Sci. 18:731–735.

Ribeiro, W. P., S. J. Valberg, J. D. Pagan, and B. Essen-Gustavsson. 2004. The effect of varying dietary starch and fat content on serum creatine kinase activity and substrate availability in equine polysaccharide storage myopathy. J. Vet. Intern. Med. 18:887–894.

Rijnen, K. E., and J. H. van der Kolk. 2003. Determination of reference range values of glucose metabolism and insulin resistance by use of glucose clamp techniques in horses and ponies. Am. J. Vet. Res. 64: 1260–1264.

Riley, C. B., W. M. Scott, J. P. Caron, P. B. Fretz, J. V. Bailey, and S. M. Barber. 1998. Osteochondritis dessicans and subchondral cystic lesions in draft horses: a retrospective study. Can. Vet. J. 39:627–633.

Robinson, N. E. (Chairperson). 2001. Workshop conclusions. In Inter. Workshop on Equine Chronic Airway Disease, Michigan State University. Equine Vet. J. 33:13–19.

Robinson, N. E., F. J. Derksen, M. A. Olszewski, and V. A. Buechner-Maxwell. 1996. The pathogenesis of chronic obstructive pulmonary disease of horses. Br. Vet. J. 152:283–306.

Robinson, N. E., C. Berney, S. Eberhart, H. L. deFeijter-Rupp, A. M. Jefcoat, C. J. Cornelisse, V. M. Gerber, and F. J. Derksen. 2003. Coughing, mucus accumulation, airway obstruction, and airway inflammation in control horses and horses affected with recurrent airway obstruction. Am. J. Vet. Res. 64:550–557.

Ronen, N., J. van Heerden, and S. R. van Amstel. 1992. Clinical and biochemistry finding, and parathyroid hormone concentrations in three horses with secondary hyperparathyroidism. J. S. Afr. Vet. Assoc. 63:134–136.

Rooney, J. R. 1984. Weather factors and the growth of young Thoroughbred horses. J. Equine Vet. Sci. 4:106–107.

Ropp, J. K., R. H. Raub, and J. E. Minton 2003. The effect of dietary energy source on serum concentration of insulin-like growth factor-I, growth hormone, insulin, glucose, and fat metabolites in weanling horses. J. Anim. Sci. 81:1581–1589.

Roubenoff, R. 1999. The pathophysiology of wasting in the elderly. J. Nutr. 129:256S–259S.

Roussel, A. J., Y. C. Lin, J. R. Strait, and P. D. Modransky. 1987. Radioimmunoassay for parathyroid hormone in equids. Am. J. Vet. Res. 48:1621–1623.

Rowe, J. B., M. J. Lees, and D. W. Pethick. 1994. Prevention of acidosis and laminitis associated with grain feeding in horses. J. Nutr. 124:2742S–2744S.

Russell, R. M. 2000. The aging process as a modifier of metabolism. Am. J. Clin. Nutr. 72:529S–532S.

Saastamoinen, M. 1990. Heritabilities for body size and growth rate and phenotypic correlations among measurements in young horses. Acta Agric. Scand. 40:377–386.

Sandberg, B. 1993. Osteochondrosis in the tarsocrural joint and osteochondral fragments in the metacarpo/metatarsophalangeal joints in young Standardbreds. Ph.D. Thesis. Swedish University of Agricultural Sciences, Uppsala.

Sandgren, B. 1993. Osteochondrosis in the tarsocrural joint and osteochondral fragments in the metacarpo/metatarsophalangeal joints in young Standardbreds. Dissertation. Sveriges Lantbruksuniversitet, Uppsala, Sweden.

Savage, C. J., R. N. McCarthy, and L. B. Jeffcott. 1993a. Effects of dietary energy and protein on the induction of dyschondroplasia in foals. Equine Vet. J. Suppl. 16:74–79.

Savage, C. J., R. N. McCarthy, and L. B. Jeffcott. 1993b. Effects of dietary phosphorus and calcium on induction of dyschondroplasia in foals. Equine Vet. J. Suppl. 16:80–83.

Savage, C. J., R. N. McCarthy, and L. B. Jeffcott. 1993c. Histomorphometric assessment of bone biopsies from foals fed diets high in phosphorus and digestible energy. Equine Vet. J. Suppl. 16:89–93.

Schmidt, O., E. Deegen, H. Fuhrmann, R. Duhlmeier, and H. P. Sallmann. 2001. Effects of fat feeding and energy level on plasma metabolites and hormones in Shetland ponies. J. Vet. Med. A. 48:39–49.

Seahorn, T. L., and R. E. Beadle. 1993. Summer pasture-associated obstructive pulmonary disease in horses: 21 cases (1983–1991). J. Am. Vet. Med. Assoc. 202:779–782.

Sloet Van Oldruitenborgh-Oosterbaan, M. M. S., J. A. Mol, and A. Barneveld. 1999. Hormones, growth factors and other plasma variables in relation to osteochondrosis. Equine Vet. J. Suppl. 31:45–54.

Sondergaard, E. 2003. Activity, feed intake and physical development of young Danish Warmblood horses in relation to the social environment. Ph.D. Thesis. Danish Institute of Agricultural Sciences, Tjele. Pp. 55–75.

Spier S. J., J. Beech, J. Zhou, and H. Hoffman. 1994. Pathophysiology of sodium channelopathies: correlation of normal/mutant mRNA ratios with clinical phenotype in dominantly inherited periodic paralysis. Hum. Mol. Genet. 3:1599–1603.

Staniar, W. B. 2002. Growth and the somatotropic axis in young Thoroughbreds. Ph.D. Thesis. Virginia Polytechnic Institute and State University, Blacksburg.

Staun, H., F. Linnemann, B. Hansen, H. Schougaard, and L. Eriksen. 1989. The influence of two different calcium-phosphorus relationships on bone development in the young horse. Beretning fra Statens Husdyrbrugsforsog, #656, pp. 32.

Stoneham, S. J. 2005. How to feed the sick neonatal foal. Pp. 33–37 in The 1st BEVA and Waltham Nutrition Symposia, P. A. Harris, T. S. Mair, J. D. Slater, and R. E. Green, eds. Cambridge, England: Equine Veterinary Journal Ltd.

Stratton-Phelps, M., and A. J. Fascetti. 2003. Nutritional therapy in gastrointestinal disease. Pp. 722–726 in Current Therapy in Equine Medicine, 5th ed., N. E. Robinson, ed. Philadelphia: W. B. Saunders.

Stromberg, B. 1979. A review of the salient features of osteochondrosis in the horse. Equine Vet. J. 11:211–214.

Stromberg, B., and S. Rejno. 1978. Osteochondrosis in the horse. I. A clinical and radiologic investigation of osteochondritis dissecans of the knee and hock joint. Acta Radioll. Suppl. 358:159–152.

Swanson, T. D. 1999. Clinical presentation, diagnosis, and prognosis of acute laminitis. Vet. Clin. North Am. Equine Pract. 15:311–319.

Swartzman, J. A., H. F. Hintz, and H. F. Schryver. 1978. Inhibition of calcium absorption in ponies fed diets containing oxalic acid. Am. J. Vet. Res. 39:1621–1623.

Thompson, J. R., and E. A. McPherson. 1984. Effect of environmental control on pulmonary function of horses affected with chronic obstructive pulmonary disease. Equine Vet. J. 16:35–38.

Thompson, K. N. 1995. Skeletal growth rates of weanling and yearling Thoroughbred horses. J. Anim. Sci. 73:2513–2517.

Thompson, K. N., S. G. Jackson, and J. P. Baker. 1988a. The influence of high planes of nutrition on skeletal growth and development of weanling horses. J. Anim. Sci. 66:2459–2467.

Thompson, K. N., S. G. Jackson, and J. R. Rooney. 1988b. The effect of above average weight gains on the incidence of radiographic bone aberrations and epiphysitis in growing horses. Equine Vet. Sci. 8:383–385.

Tinker, M. K., N. A. White, P. Lessard, C. D. Thatcher, K. D. Pelzer, B. Davis, and D. K. Carmel. 1997a. Prospective study of equine colic incidence and mortality. Equine Vet. J. 29:448–453.

Tinker, M. K., N. A. White, P. Lessard, C. D. Thatcher, K. D. Pelzer, B. Davis, and D. K. Carmel. 1997b. Prospective study of equine colic risk factors. Equine Vet. J. 29:454–458.

Traub-Dargatz, J. L., C. A. Kopral, A. H. Seitzinger, L. P. Garber, K. Forde, and N. A. White. 2001. Estimate of the national incidence of and operation-level risk factors for colic among horses in the United States, spring 1998 to spring 1999. J. Am. Vet. Med. Assoc. 219:67–71.

Treiber, K. H., T. M. Hess, D. S. Kronfeld, R. C. Boston, R. Geor, and P. A. Harris. 2005. Insulin resistance and compensation in laminitis-predisposed ponies characterized by the Minimal Model. Pferdeheilkunde 21:91–92.

Treiber, K. H., D. S. Kronfeld, T. M. Hess, B. M. Byrd, R. K. Splan, and W. B. Staniar. 2006. Evaluation of genetic and metabolic predispositions and nutritional risk factors for pasture-associated laminitis in ponies. J. Am. Vet. Med. Assoc. 228:1538–1545.

Turner, A. S., and P. B. Fretz. 1977. A comparison of surgical techniques and associated complications of transphyseal bridging in foals. Proc. Am. Assoc. Equine Pract. 23:275–287.

Ueki, H., M. Akagami, T. Oyamada, H. Yoshikawa, Y. Katayama, M. Oikawa, and T. Yoshikawa. 2003. Effect of exercise on thyroid, parathyroid and bone in very young Thoroughbreds. J. Equine Sci. 14:51–58.

USDA (U.S. Department of Agriculture). 1998. Baseline Reference of 1998 Equine Health and Management. USDA: Animal and Plant Health Inspection Service: Veterinary Sciences, Centers for Epidemiology and Animal Health, National Animal Health Monitoring System, Fort Collins, CO.

USDA. 2000. Lameness and Laminitis in U.S. Horses. USDA: Animal and Plant Health Inspection Service: Veterinary Sciences, Centers for Epidemiology and Animal Health, National Animal Health Monitoring System, Fort Collins, CO.

USDA. 2001. Incidence of Colic in U.S. Available at http://www.aphis.usda.gov/vs/ceah/ncahs/nahms/equine/equine98/colic.PDF. Accessed July 25, 2006.

Valberg, S. J., G. H. Cardinet, 3rd, G. P. Carlson, and S. DiMauro. 1992. Polysaccharide storage myopathy associated with recurrent exertional rhabdomyolysis in horses. Neuromusc. Dis. 2:351–359.

Valberg, S. J., D. Townsend, and R. Mickelsen. 1998. Skeletal muscle glycolytic capacity and phosphofructokinase regulation in horses with polysaccharide storage myopathy. Am. J. Vet. Res. 59:782–785.

Valberg, S. J., J. R. Mickelsen, E. M. Gallant, J. M. MacLeay, L. Lentz, and F. de la Corte. 1999a. Exertional rhabdomyolysis in quarter horses and thoroughbreds: one syndrome, multiple aetiologies. Equine Vet. J. Suppl. 30:533–538.

Valberg, S. J., J. M. MacLeay, J. A. Billstrom, M. A. Hower-Moritz, and J. R. Mickelsen. 1999b. Skeletal muscle metabolic response to exercise in horses with "tying-up" due to polysaccharide storage myopathy. Equine Vet. J. 31:43–47.

Valentine, B. A., K. M. Credille, J. P. Lavoie, S. Fatone, C. Guard, J. F. Cummings, and B. J. Cooper. 1997. Severe polysaccharide storage myopathy in Belgian and Perceron draft horses. Equine Vet. J. 29:220–225.

Valentine, B. A., S. P. McDonough, Y. F. Chang, and A. J. Vonderchek. 2000. Polysaccharide storage myopathy in Morgan, Arabian, and Standardbred related horses and Welsh-cross ponies. Vet. Pathol. 37:193–196.

Valentine, B. A., P. L. Habecker, J. S. Patterson, B. L. Njaa, J. Shapiro, H. J. Holshuh, R. J. Bildfell, and K. E. Bird. 2001a. Incidence of polysaccharide storage myopathy in draft horse-related breeds: a necropsy study of 37 horses and a mule. J. Vet. Diagn. Invest. 13:63–68.

Valentine, B. A., R. J. Van Saun, K. N. Thompson, and H. F. Hintz. 2001b. Role of dietary carbohydrate and fat in horses with equine polysaccharide storage myopathy. J. Am. Vet. Med. Assoc. 219:1537–1544.

Van den Hoogen, B. M., C. H. van de Lest, P. R. van Weeren, L. M. van Golde, and A. Barneveld. 1999. Changes in proteoglycan metabolism in osteochondrotic articular cartilage of growing foals. Equine Vet J. Suppl. 31:38–44.

Van der Harst, M. R., C. H. van de Lest, J. Degroot, G. H. Kiers, P. A. Brama, and P. R. van Weeren. 2005. Study of cartilage and bone layers of the bearing surface of the equine metacarpophalangeal joint relative to different time scales of maturation. Equine Vet. J. 37: 200–206.

Vandenput, S., L. Istasse, B. Nicks, and P. Lekeux. 1997. Airborne dust and aeroallergen concentrations in different sources of feed and bedding for horses. Vet. Quart. 19:154–158.

Vandenput, S., D. H. Duvivier, D. Votion, T. Art, and P. Lekeux. 1998. Environmental control to maintain stabled COPD horses in clinical remission: effects on pulmonary function. Equine Vet. J. 30:93–96.

Van Weeren, P. R., M. M. S. van Oldruitenborgh-Oosterbaan, and A. Barneveld. 1999. The influence of birth weight, rate of weight gain and final achieved height and sex on the development of osteochondrotic lesions in a population of genetically predisposed Warmblood foals. Equine Vet. J. Suppl. 31:26–30.

Van Weeren, P. R., J. Knaap, and E. C. Firth. 2003. Influence of liver copper status of mare and newborn foal on the development of osteochondrotic lesions. Equine Vet. J. 35:67–71.

Vatistas, N., J. R. Synder, G. Carlson, B. Johnson, R. M. Arthur, M. Thurmond, H. Zhou, and K. L. K. Lloyd. 1999a. Cross-sectional study of gastric ulcers of the squamous mucosa in Thoroughbred racehorses. Equine Vet. J. Suppl. 29:34–39.

Vatistas, N., R. L. Sifferman, J. Holste, J. L. Cox, G. Pinalto, and K. T. Schultz. 1999b. Induction and maintenance of gastric ulceration in horses in race training. Equine Vet. J. Suppl. 29:40–44.

Vervuert, I., M. Coenen, A. Borchers, M. Granel, S. Winkelsett, L. Christmann, O. Distl, E. Bruns, and B. Hertsch. 2003. Growth rates and the incidence of osteochondrotic lesions in Hanoverian Warmblood foals–Preliminary data. E. European Zoo Nutr. Centre, Antwerp. Abstr. Article 34.

Vervuert, I., M. Coenen, S. Dahlhoff, and W. Sommer. 2005. Fructan concentrations in grass, silages and hay. P. 309 in 19th Symp. Proc. Equine Sci. Soc., May 31–June 3, Tucson, AZ.

Wagner, P. 1986. Incidence of developmental orthopaedic lesions. Pp. 8–9 in Proc. Panel on Developmental Orthopedic Disease, Am. Quarter Horse Assoc., Dallas, TX.

Walthall, J. C., and R. A. McKenzie. 1976. Osteodystrophia fibrosa in horses at pasture in Queensland: Field and laboratory observations. Austral. Vet. J. 52:11–16.

Ward, M. P., and L. L. Couetil. 2005. Climatic and aeroallergen risk factors for chronic obstructive pulmonary disease in horses. Am. J. Vet. Res. 66:818–824.

Ward, P. L., J. E. Wohlt, and S. E. Katz. 2001. Chemical, physical, and environmental properties of pelleted newspaper compared to wheat straw and wood shavings as bedding for horses. J. Anim. Sci. 79:1359–1369.

Webster, A. J. F., A. F. Clarke, T. M. Madelin, and C. M. Wathers. 1987. Air hygiene in stables 1. Effects of stable design, ventilation and management on the concentration of respirable dust. Equine Vet. J. 19:448–453.

White N. A. 1990. Epidemiology and etiology of colic. Pp. 53–56 in The Equine Acute Abdomen, N. A. White, ed. Philadelphia: Lea & Febiger.

White, N. A. 1999. Definition and causes of colic. P. 1 in Handbook of Equine Colic, N. A. White and G. B. Edwards, eds. Boston: Butterworth Heinemann.

Whitton, R. C. 1998. Equine developmental osteochondral lesions: the role of biomechanics. Vet. J. 156:167–168.

Wisniewski, E., W. Krumrych, M. Gehrke, and P. Mazurek. 1999. Fibrotic osteodystrophy in the horse. Medycyna-Weterynaryjna 55:84–88.

Wittenberg, K. M., S. A. Moshtaghi-Nia, P. A. Mills, and R. G. Platford. 1989. Chitin analysis of hay as a means of determining fungal invasion during storage. Anim. Feed Sci. Technol. 27:101–110.

Worth, M. J., J. P. Fontenot, and T. N. Meacham. 1987. Physiological effects of exercise and diet on metabolism in the equine. P. 145 in Proc. 10th Equine Nutr. Physiol. Soc. Symp., Ft. Collins, CO.

Zechner, P., F. Zohman, J. Solkner, I. Bodo, F. Habe, E. Marti, and G. Brem. 2001. Morphological description of the Lipizzan horse population. Livest. Prod. Sci. 69:163–177.

Zeyner, A., H. Kirbach, and M. Fürll. 2002. Effects of substituting starch with fat on the acid-base and mineral status of female horses. Equine Vet. J. Suppl. 34:85–91.

13

Donkeys and Other Equids

DONKEYS (ASSES, BURROS, *EQUUS ASINUS*)

Feeding Behavior

The donkey is a unique equid of special qualities, an evolutionary relative of the horse that will forever be compared with the horse (Burnham, 2002). However, the donkey is morphologically and behaviorally distinct, and presumably evolved in a hot semi-arid environment (Mueller et al., 1994a). Most likely, the domestic donkey originated from the African wild donkey (*Equus africanus,* Nubian or Somali subspecies; Groves, 1974). Mules (a cross between the mare and the jack) and hinnies (the reciprocal cross between jennets and stallions, but that are seldom found) are major sources of power in many regions of the world because of their astounding strength, endurance, and heat tolerance (Cole and Ronning, 1974).

Feral donkeys are known to be highly adaptable feeders that will consume a variety of grasses, browse, and forbs in order to obtain sufficient nutrients. In Botswana, donkeys consume browse such as *Boscia foetida* and *Acacia* species during the long dry season when the nutritive value and the quantity of the grasses are poor (Aganga and Tsopito, 1998). Donkeys will peel the bark off and consume the bark and the succulent layers underneath. Donkeys use different feeding strategies, depending on the quality of the feed. Thus, they will use a selective feeding strategy targeting high-quality bites when foraging over a mixed pasture or rangeland, but when fed homogenous hay, donkeys will maximize intake as an alternative feeding strategy (Mueller et al., 1998).

It is generally accepted that the donkey can exist with less feed than the horse. Donkeys and mules can utilize more mature, less digestible, woodier plant material than a horse (Svendsen, 1997). A report by Yousef (1985) indicated that two donkeys maintained good health during 12 years on a diet consisting only of grass hay. In confinement in tropical countries, a donkey diet will consist of crop residues and mature grasses of poor nutrient quality, high in fiber and low in nitrogen (Pearson et al., 2001). Suhartanto and Tisserand (1996) showed that the donkey was more able than the pony to use forages, even poor-quality forages. The authors indicated that the superiority of the donkey results from a higher feed intake, higher capacity to sort feed, lower water need, and more developed system to recycle blood urea.

Dry Matter Intake

Mediterranean miniature donkeys fed a diet consisting mainly of Bermudagrass hay (80 percent of total diet) plus supplements (electrolytes and chelated minerals) at 1.5 percent of body weight (BW) maintained good health status and an average target BW of 111 ± 1.3 kg for a long period of time (e.g., more than 2 years: Schlegel et al., 2004). Some studies that have compared feed intakes of donkeys and ponies fed moderate- to low-quality roughage have shown that donkeys generally consume less dry matter/day than ponies. On the contrary, some authors have suggested that dry matter intake (DMI) of donkeys is high compared to other large herbivores, at about 3.1 percent of body weight (Maloiy, 1973). Pearson (1991) and Pearson et al. (2001) reported voluntary dry matter intakes (VDMI) that ranged from 0.83 to 2.6 percent of BW, depending on the type of feed and physiological stage of the animal. Svendsen (1997) indicated that DMI of feed as a percentage of body weight should be 1.75–2.25 percent to meet the metabolic demands for maintenance for most donkeys and mules. When donkeys and ponies were fed moderate- and/or poor-quality forage diets, donkeys consumed less dry matter per day (Pearson and Merritt, 1991). The authors found that the digestibility coefficients of organic matter and fiber fractions (acid detergent fiber, ADF, and neutral detergent fiber, NDF) were higher ($P < 0.05$) for the donkeys than for the ponies, and higher for the alfalfa hay than for the oat-straw diet. Greater DMI by ponies ($P < 0.01$) compensated for the lower digestibility coefficients, suggesting that both species obtain similar quantities of nutrients if diets were fed ad libitum. Studies by Pearson et al. (2001) reported intake of dehydrated alfalfa by donkeys of 27 g/kg BW, higher than previously reported values for donkeys consuming grass and grass-legume hay mixtures (18–23 g/kg BW: Pearson and Merritt, 1991; Tisserand et al., 1991; Mueller et al., 1994b). Donkeys fed 1 kg of concentrate plus ad libitum dry chopped sorghum fodder consumed 23 g/kg BW (resting donkeys) and 29 g/kg BW (working donkey), respectively (Ram et al., 2004). For donkeys fed straw-type diets, reports indicated consumptions of 20 g/kg BW of oat straw and 9.8 g/kg BW of barley straw (Pearson et al., 1992; Pearson and Merritt, 1991). Donkeys (mean BW of 243 kg) showed higher ($P < 0.01$) DMI (14.7–16.5 g/kg) than ponies (9.7–11.14 g/kg, mean BW of 200 kg) of wheat-straw-based diets (Suhartanto et al., 1992). However, comparative studies of voluntary DMI of donkeys and ponies fed moderate- to low-quality forage have shown that donkeys generally consumed less dry matter per day than ponies (Pearson and Merritt, 1991; Tisserand and Pearson, 2003). Intake of cocksfoot/alfalfa hay by donkeys was 87 percent lower than that observed in ponies (Tisserand et al., 1991). Summer and winter DMI of grass/straw mixed diets were 64 and 69 percent of those calculated for ponies (Wood et al., 2005).

When donkeys (n = 18, mean BW: 150 kg for males and 142 kg for females) had ad libitum access to water, or were offered water every 48, or every 72 hours, DMI of a poor-quality diet (6 percent crude protein [CP], 78 percent NDF, 46 percent ADF) were 3.1 ± 0.2, 2.8 ± 0.1, and 2.7 ± 0.1 kg/d, respectively, indicating that water restriction did not affect DMI considerably (Nengomasha et al., 1999). Gross energy consumption was 81 ± 17 kcal/kg BW/d for donkeys (BW ranging between 117–129 kg BW), which was 67 percent lower than when the animals received an alfalfa hay diet (Izraely et al., 1989a).

Apparent Digestibility of Nutrients

It has been suggested that because of the differences in the ways in which donkeys and ponies consume and digest feeds, the donkey cannot be regarded as a small horse when considering its nutrition (Tisserand and Pearson, 2003). Thus, Izraely et al. (1989a) reported that the energy digestibility of low-quality forage in donkeys matched that recorded for the Bedouin goat and exceeded that when donkeys were fed an alfalfa hay diet (Brosh et al., 1986). Izraely et al. (1989a) reported digestible energy (DE) coefficients for donkeys of 49 ± 4 and 67 ± 3 percent for wheat-straw and alfalfa diets, respectively.

The digestibility coefficients of the main dietary components of forages measured in donkeys were higher than those measured when the same feeds were fed to ponies and horses (Araujo et al., 1997). When donkeys were fed an alfalfa or oat-straw diet, donkeys showed higher digestibility coefficients (percent) than ponies for DM, organic matter (OM), gross energy (GE), CP, ADF, and NDF ($P < 0.05$). The differences were greater on the oat-straw diet than on the alfalfa diet (Pearson et al., 2001). Similar observations have been previously reported in comparative studies with straw and alfalfa diets (Pearson and Merritt, 1991; Pearson et al., 1992; Cuddeford et al., 1995). Pearson and Merritt (1991) found that at rest, when ponies and donkeys had ad libitum access to a hay or a barley-straw diet, ponies consumed more ($P < 0.01$) on a g/kg BW/d basis than donkeys, but donkeys showed higher digestibility coefficients for dry matter, organic matter, and energy.

The mean retention time (MRT) of alfalfa and straw-type diets is shorter in the donkey (BW range 117–129 kg) than in the Bedouin goat, consistent with its capacity to compensate for a lower quality diet by increasing its intake rate (Izraely et al., 1989b). Mean retention time of digesta particle markers by the digestive tract of donkeys fed a wheat-straw or alfalfa-based diet were 37.7 ± 1.7 hours and 36.4 ± 3.2 hours, respectively. Furthermore, the transit time (marker first appearance in feces) was 16.8 ± 3.7 hours and 17.5 ± 2.6 hours when fed the wheat straw or alfalfa hay, respectively (Izraely et al., 1989b). Gastrointestinal transit time was significantly ($P < 0.01$) slower in the donkeys than in the ponies on both meadow hay and barley-straw diets (Pearson and Merritt, 1991). Similar results have been reported by Cuddeford et al. (1995), who found consistently slower rates of passage of the solid-phase marker for all diets given to donkeys compared to other equids ($P < 0.01$). The level of feeding and the forage type influenced the digestibility of forages by donkeys and ponies. Dry matter digestibility was higher when offered ad libitum access to an oat-straw diet compared to when it was restricted, especially in the donkey, which might be explained by improved selection of more digestible components in the oat-straw diet by this species (Pearson et al., 2001). The relatively narrow muzzle of the donkey as compared to the horse would indicate selectivity to be a characteristic of its feeding strategy (Van Soest, 1994). Tisserand et al. (1991) also indicated that donkeys tended to have higher digestibility coefficients of the dietary components (e.g., crude protein, crude fiber, and organic matter) than ponies. Digestive coefficients for ADF and NDF when donkeys were fed a wheat-straw diet were 42 ± 4.1 and 50.9 ± 4.9 percent, respectively, and 46.8 ± 4.8 and 54.2 ± 1.4 for ADF and NDF, respectively, when donkeys were fed an alfalfa hay diet (Izraely et al., 1989b).

More effective microbial digestion in the hindgut of the donkey compared to the pony might be the reason for the higher digestibility coefficients. The microbial cellulolytic activity in the cecum was higher by 13 percent in donkeys than in ponies when animals were fed a mixed cocksfoot/alfalfa hay or wheat straw hay (Suhartanto et al., 1992). When wheat straw was fed with or without concentrate, the authors observed higher ($P < 0.001$) volatile fatty acids (VFA) production (mmol/L) in donkeys (47–67.1) than in ponies (33.6–41.9). Furthermore, the authors found that the proportion of VFA (percent molar) indicated that the concentrations of butyric, isobutyric, valeric, and isovaleric acids were higher (P < 0.01) in donkeys than in ponies. In contrast, acetic acid values were not significantly different (69.3 vs. 72.8 mol percent) between donkeys and ponies, respectively. Dry matter intake, dry matter digestibility (DMD), and MRT of a poor-quality diet were not significantly different for working or nonworking donkeys (Nengomasha et al., 1999).

Energy

Guerouali et al (2003) and Tisserand and Pearson (2003) indicated that a donkey's resting metabolism is 20 percent lower (P < 0.05) than that of a horse and that donkeys require less feed over the working year than horses or cattle due to their small size. On a mass specific basis, oxygen consumption at rest were 3 ± 0.2 and 3.2 ± 0.3 ml/kg BW/min for horses and donkeys, respectively (Guerouali et al., 2003). Donkeys altered resting metabolic rate in response to diet quality. Thus, the resting oxygen consumption of donkeys fed wheat straw was 4 ± 0.2 L/kg BW/d, half the value recorded when donkeys were fed alfalfa hay (Izraely et al., 1989a). Walking for 8 h/d increased the daily energy expenditures by 60–70 percent in donkeys and horses (Guerouali et al., 2003).

There is a lack of information on the DE requirements specific for donkeys. However, recent reports by Wood et al. (2005) indicated that donkeys (n = 20, BW ranged from 133–217 kg) fed hay:straw mixed diets required considerably less DE intake for maintenance than ponies when using NRC (1989) equations. Their results indicated that DE intake was 54 and 74 percent of recommendations for summer and winter diets, respectively (Wood et al., 2005).

Researchers have applied equations developed for horses to estimate DE requirements of donkeys. However, these equations might overestimate requirements as indicated above. Pearson et al. (2001), has applied the following equations to estimate DE requirements:

(a) Maintenance requirements
(Equation 13-1): DE Mcal/d = $(0.975 + 0.021 \times M)$, where M = live body weight in kg (NRC, 1989)
(b) Maintenance requirements for ponies
(Equation 13-2): DE Mcal/d = $(465) \times M^{0.75}/4184$, where M = live body weight (Ellis and Lawrence, 1980, original units in MJ)

When Pearson et al. (2001) applied Equation 13-2 to calculate DE intake, the authors reported that intake of straw-based diets fed ad libitum exceeded pony energy requirements by 34 to 51 percent (9.6 Mcal/d), but energy requirements of donkeys were only just met (5.6 Mcal/d). In their study, the estimated DE requirements were 7 Mcal/d and 5.7 Mcal/d for ponies and donkeys, respectively. Miniature Mediterranean donkeys fed a diet of 3.94 Mcal/d (35.5 kcal/kg BW) maintained a healthy average body weight (111 ± 1 kg; range: 110–112 kg) for 3 years (Schlegel et al., 2004). However, the DE maintenance requirements were overestimated by 16.7 percent (4.73 Mcal/d) based on the Pagan and Hintz (NRC, 1989) formula for horses weighing 600 kg or less (DE (Mcal/d) = $1.4 + 0.03 \times BW$). Thus, the original Pagan and Hintz (1986a) formula to estimate DE maintenance requirements might be adjusted for these miniature donkeys as: DE (Mcal/d) = $0.61 + 0.03 \times BW$ (in kg). If Equation 13-1 above is applied to these miniature donkeys, the DE requirements are underestimated by 13 percent. Taylor (1997) suggested that the energy requirements of donkeys are of the order of 75 percent of those published for horses per unit body weight.

Energy Cost of Work

Walking with a load averaging 40 percent of their body weight 8 h/d increased the daily energy consumption by 60–70 percent for both donkeys and horses (Guerouali et al., 2003). Oxygen consumption (V_{O_2}) in donkeys running at a maximal speed on a 9.8 percent slope was 110 ± 2 ml × min^{-1} × kg^{-1}, 22 times pre-exercise V_{O_2} (Mueller et al., 1994a). Donkeys are more efficient at using energy for pulling and carrying loads, but their small size restricts the size of the load (Pearson et al., 1996). Average energy for donkeys under 0 or –15 percent slope were 0.23 and 0.16 for walking, 0.26 and 0.79 for carrying a load, and 6.3 and 1.5 cal/m/kg for pulling loads, respectively (Dijkman, 1992).

Vall (1996, as reported by Tisserand and Pearson, 2003), working with donkeys (150 kg BW) and ponies (250 kg BW) that were subjected to work for 10 km on level ground at a draught force of 200 Newtons (N) (light cart, LC) or 350 N (cultivator for weeding, CW), found that the daily net energy requirement (DNER, Mcal/d) and net energy used for work (NEW, Mcal/d) for donkeys on a LC and CW load were 4.6 Mcal and 1.7 Mcal, and 5.6 Mcal and 2.6 Mcal for DNER and NEW, respectively. The values for LC and CW reported for the ponies were 6.7 Mcal and 3.1 Mcal and 5.6 Mcal and 2.0 Mcal for DNER and NEW, respectively. The authors reported the net energy cost of work as a multiple of the maintenance energy requirements. For the donkey, these values were 0.57 and 0.91 for the LC and CW loads; for the pony, these values were 0.56 and 0.85, respectively (Vall, 1996, as reported by Tisserand and Pearson, 2003). In studies conducted by Yousef and Dill (1969) and Yousef et al. (1972), in which donkeys were compared to men, the energy cost of walking with or without a load and up and down grades, in terms of units body weight and unit distance, was significantly lower in the donkey. The low energy cost of walking and the associated economy in food and water requirements appear to be key mechanisms for the donkey to thrive in arid regions (Yousef, 1985). Table 13-1 summarizes information on energy expenditures on horses and donkeys (adapted from Guerouali et al., 2003).

TABLE 13-1 Comparative Energy Expenditures in Horses and Donkeys (adapted from Guerouali et al., 2003)[a]

	Resting (R)	Resting with Load	Walking	Walking with Load
Horses (kcal/kg BW[b])	21 ± 0.8	29.4 ± 1.8	35.3 ± 2.1	42.0 ± 0.6
Multiple of R	—	1.4	1.7	2.0
Donkeys (kcal/kg BW[c])	22 ± 1.3	26.4 ± 3.3	39.6 ±2.6	46.2 ± 0.3
Multiple of R	—	1.2	1.8	2.1

[a]Donkey's average BW: 120 kg; horses average BW: 310 kg; original units in kJ/kg$^{0.75}$ (1 kJ = 0.239 kcal); load weight corresponds to an average 40 percent of BW; horses and donkeys fed a diet of 1 kg barley and 2 kg straw/100 kg BW; donkeys: n = 4; horses: n = 2. Experimental design based on the measurement of oxygen consumption during four successive periods of 15 minutes each (resting, resting with load, walking, walking with load).
[b]Original data for resting energy expenditure in horses was 15.18 ± 0.57 kJ/kg$^{0.75}$/h.
[c]Original data for resting energy expenditure in donkeys was 12.64 ± 0.73 kJ/ kg$^{0.75}$/h (Guerouali et al. 2003).

Protein

There is a lack of information on the protein requirements for donkeys, but apparently donkeys are very efficient in the utilization of dietary protein. Izraely et al. (1989a) found that donkeys fed a wheat-straw diet containing less than 3 percent crude protein maintained body weights for a prolonged period of time and their capacity to recycle urea matched that showed by ruminants. Furthermore, when fed a wheat-straw diet, the amount of nitrogen recycled exceeded that consumed in the diet (Izraely et al., 1989a). The donkey reabsorbed 82 percent and 48 percent of the urea filtered by the kidney when fed a wheat-straw or alfalfa hay diet, respectively. Expressed as percentage of the entry rate, the urea nitrogen recycled when on wheat-straw averaged 76 percent of the urea nitrogen entry rate (Izraely et al., 1989b), matching Bedouin goats living in desert environments (Brosh et al., 1986, 1987). The efficient utilization of dietary protein, a high true nitrogen digestibility of 86–90 percent, and the high capacity to retain and recycle urea creates the ability for the donkey to subsist on low-protein forage (Izraely et al., 1989a,b). Pearson (1991) used the formula digestible crude protein (DCP)(g/d) = 2.7 BW$^{0.75}$ (NRC, 1978) to estimate digestible protein requirements for donkeys ranging from 160–190 kg BW. Miniature donkeys that consumed 1.2 g CP/kg BW (133 g of protein/d) fed an 8 percent crude protein diet (DM basis), comprised nearly entirely of Bermudagrass (80 percent), maintained body weights for a prolonged period of time (Schlegel et al., 2004). Mueller et al. (1994b) suggested that crude protein requirements of donkeys lies between 3.8 and 7.4 percent of the diet (DM basis).

Environmental Stress: Heat Stress and Dehydration

In Somali donkeys, complete deprivation of water under an environmental temperature of 22 ± 2°C depressed food intake by 83–90 percent by the end of 8–12 days (Maloiy, 1973). In the same study, a 15 percent level of dehydration at 22 ± 2°C depressed feed intake by 30.4 percent (P < 0.001) to 2.13 kg/100 kg BW/d of a low-quality hay diet that simulated the natural diet available during the dry season in the desert of Eastern Africa. However, the apparent digestibility of DM at 22 ± 2°C increased on dehydration from 41 percent to 51 percent in Somali donkeys. Dehydration under simulated desert conditions (22–40°C) had no effect on apparent digestibility (51 percent), although feed intake was depressed by 26.8 percent to 2.24 kg/100 kg BW (Maloiy, 1973). The donkey has an exceptional tolerance to dehydration that in part can be explained by its ability to conserve blood volume. This helps maintain circulation, dissipation of heat, and salivary flow (Yousef et al., 1970). This might explain the well-being of donkeys after a degree of dehydration that would cause dehydration exhaustion in many other mammals. El-Nauty et al. (1978) indicated that dehydration significantly decreased resting metabolic rate (Vo$_2$) in donkeys at environmental temperatures ranging from 20 to 35°C. The low resting metabolic rate in dehydrated animals is an adaptive mechanism to reduce water need for thermoregulation. Donkeys exposed to environmental temperatures ranging from 7 to 45°C increased skin evaporative water loss significantly at temperatures above 30°C (Maloiy, 1971). Yousef (1991) reported that the adaptation of donkeys to arid conditions are due to (1) its economy in the use of water such as reducing sweating and water excretion; (2) the ability to support dehydration, within limits, without negative effect; and (3) its capacity to fully rehydrate within a few minutes of availability of water. The donkey has an impressive capacity for rehydration. One study indicated that burros ingested water at a rate of about 17–20 percent of body weight within 5 minutes, without ill effects (Yousef et al., 1970). The donkey's capacity to fully rehydrate within 1.5 hours (recovery period) after being subjected to 36 hours of water deprivation has been also reported by Mueller and Houpt (1991). The same authors reported that ponies deprived of water during 36 hours, when offered water, undercompensated for the water deficit. The donkey's long ears, relatively small body, long legs, and short hair help its adaptation to hot climates (Cole and Ronning, 1974).

Water Consumption

The donkey is credited with the ability to continue eating for several days when deprived of drinking water (Dill et al., 1980). Maloiy (1970) suggested that donkeys can conserve body water and avoid thirst by reducing sweating for thermoregulation and reduced fecal water loss via increased intestinal sodium resorption. Donkeys have lower water requirements per unit of BW than other domesticated animals, with the exception of camels (Aganga et al., 2000). Water turnover rates of 88 ± 18 ml/kg BW/d and 115 ± 9 ml/kg BW/d were reported in donkeys (average BW 123 kg) fed wheat-straw or alfalfa hay, respectively (Izraely et al., 1989a). It seems reasonable to attribute this ability of the donkey to its desert inheritance. Dill et al. (1980) suggested that donkeys might be able to store water in their gastrointestinal tract that will help buffer against decreased water intake. However, in more recent studies by Mueller and Houpt (1991), in which comparisons were made between donkeys and ponies subjected to 36 hours of water deprivation, no differences were found between the two species when blood variables (packed cell volume, plasma protein, plasma osmolality) were used to assess dehydration. When water was offered ad libitum, donkeys (n = 18) fed a low-quality diet (6 percent CP, 78 percent NDF, 46 percent ADF/DM basis) drank an average of 8.5 ± 0.64 L/d (Nengomasha et al., 1999). In the same study, if donkeys were offered water every 48 or 72 h, water intakes were 4.9 ± 0.41 and 5.1 ± 0.4 L/d, lower (P < 0.001) if water was offered on an ad libitum basis. Ponies (BW: 266 kg) consumed (P < 0.001) more water than donkeys (BW: 197 kg) when fed an alfalfa-based diet (4.35 vs. 3.21 L/kg DM). Similar results were found when ponies (BW: 254 kg) and donkeys (BW: 182 kg) were fed an oat-straw diet (3.77 vs. 3.18 L/kg DM, for ponies and donkeys, respectively: Pearson et al., 2001). When donkeys (BW: 185–250 kg) were offered water on ad libitum basis, they consumed 8.3 ± 0.6 L/d when fed a mixed hay diet, but if donkeys were deprived of water for 36 hours, the water consumption dropped to 6.8 ± 0.6 L/d (Mueller and Houpt, 1991). Vall et al. (2003a) recommended that resting donkeys in Cameroon (average BW: 125 kg) be offered 12 liters per day of water in the cool season and 15 liters per day in the hot dry season. Ram et al. (2004) reported water intakes between 8.4 ± 0.47 L/d (resting donkeys) and 13.25 ± 0.64 L/d (working donkeys) for animals that ranged in weight from 130–154 kg BW and under environmental temperatures that varied between 28 and 32°C and relative humidity of 64–70 percent. Donkeys had lower (P < 0.05) water intakes (1.93 L/kg DM) than Shetland ponies (2.4 L/kg DM), and both ponies and donkeys had lower water intakes (P < 0.01) than Thoroughbreds (3.87 L/kg DM) or Highland ponies (4.22 L/kg DM: Cuddeford et al., 1995). Mueller et al. (1994b) reported that under conditions of high ambient temperature (25–37°C), donkeys consumed water at a rate of 9 percent of BW/d compared to donkeys in temperate regions that consumed water at a rate of 4–5 percent of BW/d even if fed high amounts of DM and NDF.

Body Condition Score in Donkeys

Obesity is the biggest challenge facing nonworking donkeys kept in temperate areas of the world where food sources are abundant and of good quality. In contrast, emaciation is the biggest problem facing donkeys in tropical areas where food is scarce and of poor quality and where donkeys are required to work (Svendsen, 1997; Pearson and Quassat, 2000). Body condition scoring (BCS) systems have been developed by Vall et al. (2003b) and Pearson and Quassat (2000), the latter modeled on a 9-point system (1-emaciated, 2-thin, 3-less thin, 4-less than moderate, 5-moderate, 6-more than moderate, 7-less fat, 8-fat, 9-obese) developed originally for zebu cattle. The BCS described by Vall et al. (2003b) has been developed for working donkeys and the score is given for the donkey's back and flank on a scale of 1 to 4 (1-emaciated, 2-thin, 3-average, and 4-good). Donkeys tend to accumulate fat on the neck, on either side of the chest wall giving a saddlebag appearance, and around the buttocks (Svendsen, 1997). Estimation of body weight in working donkeys (n = 500) from body measurements have been developed by Quassat et al. (1994):

$$\text{Weight (kg)} = \frac{(\text{heart girth, cm})^{2.12} \times (\text{length, cm})^{0.688}}{3,801}$$

where length = length of the body from the pin bone (tuber ischii) to elbow in a straight line in centimeters (cm) and girth is the measurement around the body just behind the front legs, in centimeters (cm). Donkeys used in this study ranged from 74–252 kg BW, height from 82–129 cm, length from 64–106 cm, and body condition from 2–7, as indicated above.

Chemical Composition of Donkey's Milk

The composition of donkey's milk is given in Table 13-2.

Blood Variables

There are not much published data on mineral and vitamin concentrations in the serum or plasma of donkeys. Schlegel et al. (2004) found plasma levels of 2.53 ± 0.61 μg/ml of α-tocopherol (average of three samples collected between 1999 and 2004) in miniature donkeys (n = 2) that fell within the recommended values for domestic equids (2–10 μg/ml: Puls, 1994). The same authors reported an average (n = two samples) plasma concentration value of 0.169 ± 0.046 μg/ml for vitamin A (retinol) that was marginally lower than reference values for domestic horses (0.175–0.35 μg/ml: Puls, 1994).

Practical Diets

Donkeys are fed different diets based on their geographical location. Thus, in tropical and arid regions, they are fed on crop residues and mature grasses consisting of low-protein and high-fiber contents for most of the year. Maintenance requirements can be met from forage alone for most

TABLE 13-2 Chemical Composition (g/100 ml) of Milk of Donkeys and Other Animal Species[a]

Milk Source	Lipid	Protein	Lactose	Total Solids	Ash
Donkey	0.38 (1.34)	1.72 (1.94)	6.88 (6.29)	8.84 (10.24)	0.39 (0.43)
Horse	1.36	2.10	6.16	10.04	0.42
Horse[b]	0.74	2.16	6.62	10.44	0.44
Cow	3.70	3.20	5.00	12.70	0.80
Goat	4.00	3.10	4.25	12.05	0.80

[a]Adapted from Miraglia et al. (2003). Figures in parentheses represent numbers for donkeys reported by Salimei et al. (2000, as reported by Miraglia et al. 2003).
[b]Adapted from Pagan and Hintz (1986b).

donkeys and concentrate feeds are offered only in situations where donkeys cannot eat sufficient forage to meet nutrient requirements, such as those in work and those that are pregnant, lactating, growing, or elderly (Taylor, 1997). Table 13-3 indicates recommended forage:concentrate ratios and daily DMI for adult donkeys as reported by Pearson (2005).

Applying the DMI and forage:concentrate ratios values from Table 13-3, nutrient intakes for adult donkeys can be estimated (Table 13-4).

However, the calculated DE intakes indicated in Table 13-4 are much higher than the recommended values for horses determined using the Pagan and Hintz equation (NRC, 1989). For example, miniature donkeys weighing an average of 111 kg, as previously indicated, can be maintained on a diet of 35.5 kcal/kg BW (3.94 Mcal/d). The adjusted Pagan and Hintz equation (1986a) for miniature donkeys under maintenance conditions as reported above (DE: Mcal/d = $0.61 + 0.03 \times BW$) can be used for better predict-

TABLE 13-3 Daily Rations for Adult Donkeys[a]

State	Body Weight kg	Total DMI[b] kg	Forage Poor, kg	Forage Good, kg	Concentrate kg
Mature idle	200	5	4.5	—	0.5
Mature idle	200	5	—	5.0	—
Work 4 h/d	200	4	1.6	—	2.4
Work 4 h/d	200	4	—	2.0	2.0
Lactation[c]	200	4	1.2	—	2.8
Lactation[c]	200	4	—	1.6	2.4

[a]Adapted from Pearson (2005).
[b]DMI = Dry matter intake.
[c]First 3 months.

TABLE 13-4 Estimated Nutrient Intakes for Adult Donkeys Consuming Diets Based on Poor or Good Quality Forage (dry matter basis)

Forage Quality	BW[a] kg	DMI kg[b]	DE Mcal/d	DE kcal/kg BW	Protein g	Calcium g	Phosphorus g
Good[c]	100	2.5	5.15	51.5	270	12.5	7.25
	200	5.0	10.30	51.5	540	25.0	14.50
Poor[d]	100	2.5	4.71	47.1	168	7.60	6.05
	200	5.0	9.43	47.1	336	15.2	12.1

[a]BW = Body weights of mature idle donkeys.
[b]DMI = Dry matter intake, Donkeys fed a good-forage quality, 100 percent of the diet is comprised by forage; donkeys fed a poor-quality forage received 90 percent of the diet as forage and 10 percent as concentrate.
[c]Good-quality forage: Timothy hay (early bloom), DE (Digestible energy): 2.1 Mcal/kg, Crude protein: 10.8 percent, Calcium: 0.51 percent, and Phosphorus: 0.29 percent (Dry matter basis).
[d]Poor-quality forage: Brome hay (mature), DE (Digestible energy): 1.7 Mcal/kg, Crude protein: 6 percent, Calcium: 0.26 percent, and Phosphorus: 0.22 percent (Dry matter basis). The composition of the concentrate used to estimate nutrient intakes (e.g., poor-forage-quality diet) is given in Table 14-1.

ing their energy requirements. Furthermore, protein intake based on the recommended DMI values by Pearson (2005) and the composition data indicated in Table 13-4 also show higher values than recommended levels. A daily protein intake of 133 g/d was adequate to maintain miniature donkeys weighing an average of 111 kg BW (Schlegel et al., 2004). Applying the equation for determining the crude protein requirements for a horse under maintenance conditions (BW × 1.26 g/kg BW/d, see Chapter 4, Protein and Amino Acids), the crude protein requirements will be 126 and 252 g, for 100 or 200 kg BW, respectively. Thus, the calculated values based on the information given on the above tables should be taken with caution.

FEEDING MANAGEMENT OF WILD EQUIDS IN CAPTIVITY

The family Equidae is comprised of some eight wild species within the genus *Equus*. International Species Inventory Systems (ISIS, 2002) lists eight wild species of horses with several subspecies (Table 13-5).

Like their domestic relatives, wild equids are bulk-feeding grazers. The anatomy and physiology of the wild horse species have not received special attention and are presumed similar to that of domestic horses and asses (Nelson, 1986). In captive environments, wild horses do not have special feeding requirements, and the domestic horse is used as a model to determine nutritional requirements. Many zoological institutions will feed wild equids good-quality grass hay in the summer and mixed hay in the winter. Ad libitum access to trace mineral block salts is offered. The Nutrition Advisory Group of the American Zoo and Aquarium Association (AZA) proposed general dietary nutrient concentrations for feeding zebras and other ungulates in captivity. The recommendations are based on the National Research Council requirements for domestic horses (NRC, 1989). The authors suggest offering a diet with a range of dietary crude protein between 12–14 percent. The latter can be achieved by offering a diet (DM basis) of a 25–40 percent low-protein pellet plus 60–75 percent of grass hay (Lintzenich and Ward, 1997). Maintenance requirements of wild equids are easily achieved on a high-fiber diet consisting of free-choice grass hay (10–12 percent crude protein) plus a balanced pelleted feed (12 percent crude protein) fed at a rate of 1 percent of BW per day (Reindl, 1997). Zoos will feed a variety of diets to wild horses depending on the institution or geographical location. Practical diets for wild equids fed in zoological institutions were reported by Schlegel et al. (2004). The crude protein, ADF, and DE content for these diets ranged between 9 and 15 percent, 30 and 35 percent, and 2 and 2.8 kcal/g, respectively. The proportion of hay fed ranged between 50 and 92 percent of the total diet DM and the pellet between 7.5 and 51 percent of the diet DM (Table 13-6).

Applying the formula (DE = 1.4 + 0.03 × BW) to estimate DE (Mcal/d) for maintenance requirements in domestic horses (Pagan and Hintz, 1986a), all zoo diets showed average energy levels above requirements (Table 13-6). The DE maintenance requirements for wild horses at the Zoological Society of San Diego and Disney's Animal Kingdom were calculated to be 9.92 and 10.43 Mcal/d, respectively. The calculated DE maintenance requirements for Toronto Zoo's Przewalski's horses and Grevy's zebras were 10.2 and 12.4 Mcal/d, respectively. With the exception of diet C, crude protein content was also above NRC requirements for maintenance (NRC, 1989). However, diets in Table 13-6 represent offered amounts and not necessarily consumed amounts.

Because obesity is a problem in captive equids, many institutions will not offer concentrate feeds. Furthermore, recent reports indicated that protein, calcium, phosphorus, magnesium, and potassium were fed in excessive amounts to Grevy's zebras (NRC, 2004) based on the NRC (1989) recommendations.

TABLE 13-5 Wild Equids Found in Zoological Parks[a]

Latin Name	Common Name	Occurrence
Equus przewalski[b]	Przewalski's or Asian wild horse	In the wild presumably extinct. Reintroduced in Mongolia in the 1990s.
Equus quagga (Six subspecies)	Plains zebras, Common or Burchell's	Most commonly found. Certain subspecies are rare.
Equus zebra	Mountain zebra	Extremely endangered (Hartman's)
Equus grevyi	Grevy's zebra	Endangered
Equus africanus	African wild ass	Highly endangered
Equus onager[c]	Onager (two subspecies)	Endangered
Equus kiang[c]	Kiang	Not threatened
Equus hemionus	Asiatic wild ass (Kulan, Khur)	Extremely endangered

[a]Reindl (1997).
[b]Average body weight: *Equus przewalski*: 350 kg, *Equus quagga*: 300 kg, *Equus zebra*: 320 kg, *Equus grevyi*: 450 kg, *Equus africanus*: 275 kg, *Equus hemoniuos*: 290 kg (Klingel, 1989).
[c]Average body weight: *Equus onager*: 254 kg (female), *Equus kiang*: 275 kg (female), 255 kg (male) (Edwards, 2004).

TABLE 13-6 Diet Ingredients and Nutrient Composition (dry matter basis) of Typical Diets Fed to Wild Equids in Zoological Parks[a]

Nutrient	A	B	C
Estimated dry matter %	90.0	86.4	90.6
Crude protein %	15.2	12.5	9.5
Crude fat %	2.9	3.0	1.9
ADF %	29.7	31.7	33.2
NDF %	49.3	60.1	60.4
NFC %	36.3	—	—
Ash %	6.98	6.46	6.83
Horse DE Mcal/kg	2.77	2.33	2.10
Mcal/d	15.0	16.5	16.7
Calcium %	1.09	0.70	0.40
Phosphorus %	0.51	0.40	0.30
Potassium %	1.69	1.59	2.00
Magnesium %	0.32	0.20	0.15
Vitamin E IU/kg	170.0	34.0	28.0

[a]**Diet A:** Zoological Society of San Diego (ZSSD) typical diet offered to a variety of wild horses including Eastern kiang, Somali wild ass, Przewalski's horse, Persian onager, Damara zebra, Grevy's zebra, and Hartmann's Mountain zebra (Edwards, 2004); **Diet B:** Toronto Zoo (TZ) diet offered to Przewalski's horse and Grevy's zebra (Schlegel et al., 2004); **Diet C:** Disney's Animal Kingdom (DAK) diet offered to Grant's zebra (Schlegel et al., 2004). The animals on diet C have free access to pastures. Average body weight (BW) for ZSSD horses across species (n = 43) was 284 ± 33 kg. Average body weight for TZ Przewalski's horses (n = 6) was 293 ± 38 kg and for Grevy's zebra (n = 3) 367 ± 29 kg. Average body weight for DAK common zebras (n = 6) was 301 ± 26 kg. Pelleted feed: **Diet A:** pellet approximately 25% ADF, 14% crude protein; **Diet B:** pellet approximately 22% ADF, 30% NDF, 14% crude protein; **Diet C:** pellet approximately 32% ADF, 50% NDF, 16.4% crude protein, 52% horse total digestible nutrients, 2.32 kcal/g horse digestible energy, 5.6% starch. Carrots and/or apples not included on the percentage of the total diet. **Diet A:** offered approximately 2% (as fed) of total diet; **Diet B:** offered at 3.5% (as fed) of total diet; **Diet C:** offered at 0.4% (as fed) of total diet.

Preliminary studies reported by Hintz et al. (1976) showed that onagers (*Equus hemionus onager*) digested dry matter, crude protein, and cellulose from a pelleted diet more efficiently than the Przewalski's horse (*Equus przewalski*) and Grevy's zebra (*Equus grevyi*).

Studies conducted in zoological institutions showed that wild captive zebras and other wild hindgut fermenters consumed more organic matter per unit time than wild ruminants. The higher rates of food intake compensate for their lesser ability to digest plant material. The differences were greater for grass than for alfalfa-hay diets (Foose, 1982; Duncan et al., 1990). Consequently, compared to wild ruminants of the same size, wild equids extract more nutrients per day from a whole range of forages (Table 13-7).

FEEDING THE YOUNG WILD CAPTIVE EQUID

Orphaned foals of many wild equine species are hand-reared only if there is maternal neglect or for medical reasons. A newborn should be fed equine or bovine colostrum for the first 24 hours of nursing. A common formula used to hand-rear many species of wild horses consists of commercial, fresh, nonfat, and 1 percent low-fat cow's milk, powdered edible-grade lactose, and tap water in a ratio of 9:9:1:3 (Blakeslee and Zuba, 2002). The authors recommended seven feedings per day, as foals do not need to be fed around the clock. The daily amount of formula offered is based on body weight beginning at 10 percent, divided equally among the seven feedings. The amount of formula offered is assessed every day and increased gradually to account for daily weight gains and appetite until the foal is consuming 16–18 percent of its body weight (around 2 weeks of age). Stomach capacity should be taken into consideration during feeding, and foals should be fed no more than 80 percent of their stomach capacity (Blakeslee and Zuba, 2002). After 3 weeks of age, the foal's appetite may dictate decreasing the percentage of daily intake to approximately 11–14 percent of its body weight, assuming its weight remains constant. Weight gains should be constantly monitored. At approximately 4 weeks of age, the feeding frequency should be reduced to five per day, four times per day at 2 months, and three times per day at 3 months of age, continuing until weaning. Formula increases are discontinued around 2 months of age, when the foal starts eating solids. Wild equids may be weaned as early as 4 or 5 months of age. Early studies by Schryver et al. (1986) showed that milk from the Przewalski's horse, Hartmann's zebra, and domestic horse had similar mineral composition. The authors reported that the milk of equids taken as a group had certain similarities such as a low content of total solids.

NUTRITIONAL DISORDERS IN WILD EQUIDS

The wild horse, being similar in anatomy and physiology to the domestic horse, might show similar medical nutritional related problems.

Colic

Colic in captive wild horses is not as common as in the domestic horse and is normally associated with sand impaction. Sand colic is best managed by providing concrete pads around feeding areas (Walzer, 2003).

Enterolithiasis

Domestic equids in the western and southwestern United States appear more likely to develop enteroliths than horses in other regions (Lloyd et al., 1987). This might also be true for wild horses. A report by McDuffee et al. (1994) indicated the presence of enteroliths in Grant's zebras; the elements forming the enteroliths were primarily magnesium, ammonium, and phosphates, similar to those found in domestic horses. The authors suggested that the higher magnesium content (5 to 7 times above maintenance requirements

TABLE 13-7 Digestibility Coefficients, Organic Matter (OM) Intake, OM Extraction, and Cell Wall Extraction by Wild Equids[a]

Item	Grevy's Zebra	Mountain Zebra	Plains Zebra	Asian Wild Ass
	Timothy Hay[b]			
Number of Animals	5	2	4	4
Body weight (kg)	354	272	329	174
Metabolic body weight ($W^{0.75}$)	82	67	85	50
OM matter digestibility (%)	50	49	48	51
OM intake (g $kg^{-1}W^{0.75}$)	101	119	105	104
OM extraction (g $kg^{-1}W^{0.75}$)	51	59	51	52
Cell wall digestibility (%)	46	42	45	46
Cell wall intake (g $kg^{-1}W^{0.75}$)	73	83	79	63
Cell wall extraction (g $kg^{-1}W^{0.75}$)	34	35	36	31
	Alfalfa Hay[c]			
Number of Animals	2	3	4	3
OM matter digestibility (%)	66	59	62	58
OM intake (g $kg^{-1}W^{0.75}$)	104	111	110	127
OM extraction (g $kg^{-1}W^{0.75}$)	69	64	68	74
Cell wall digestibility (%)	52	47	45	47
Cell wall intake (g $kg^{-1}W^{0.75}$)	49	58	56	70
Cell wall extraction (g $kg^{-1}W^{0.75}$)	26	27	25	32

[a]Adapted from Foose (1982).
[b]*Phleum pretense* (4–7 percent crude protein; 21–28 percent cell contents; 67–75 percent cell wall).
[c]*Medicago sativa* (18–22 percent crude protein; 3–60 percent cell contents; 31–56 percent cell wall).

according to Lloyd et al., 1987) in California alfalfa fed to the zebras might have contributed to the regional prevalence of enteroliths. Enterolithiasis was observed on necropsy of a Hartman's mountain zebra (Decker et al., 1975). The drinking water pH may also have an effect on the formation of stones. The Zoological Society of San Diego has reported several cases of enteroliths in captive wild equids that included 15 cases between 1996 and 2003, predominantly in kiangs, Somali wild asses, Przewalski's horses, a Persian onager, and a Grant's zebra (Gaffney et al., 1999; Howard et al., 2004).

Vitamin E Deficiency/Myelopathy

Degenerative myelopathy has been diagnosed in Przewalski's horses and related to vitamin E deficiency (Liu et al., 1983). The authors reported mean plasma α–tocopherol values in the affected horses of 0.04 ± 0.01 mg/dl (range: < 0.03 – 0.08 mg/dl). Vitamin E values of normal wild horses have been reported by Brush and Anderson (1986). The authors found mean values of plasma α-tocopherol of 2.6, 3, and 3.5 μmol/L for Przewalski's horses (n = 27), onagers (n = 2), and Grant's and Hartmann's zebras (n = 5), respectively. More recent reports on Przewalski's horses inhabiting the steppes of Ukraine (n = 19) showed mean α-tocopherol values of 4.7 and 6.6 μg/ml for foals and adult horses, respectively (Dierenfeld et al., 1997). Myodegenerative disorders in zebras (*Equus burchelli* spp.) caused by vitamin E deficiency were reported by Wallach (1970). Equine degenerative myeloencephalopathy (EDM) has been described in many occasions in Przewalski's horses, zebras, and kulans (Walzer, 2003), and vitamin E deficiencies in the first year of life have been implicated in the development of EDM. Foals showing EDM symptoms may be treated with oral vitamin E (1,500–2,000 IU daily: Blythe and Craig, 1997). Single serum α-tocopherol values are nondiagnostic for EDM as vitamin E can vary considerably (Walzer, 2003). Early reports on myodegenerative disorders and cardiac myopathies, as well as impaired reproductive capacity (Blaxter, 1962; Trinder et al., 1969), have been linked to vitamin E deficiencies.

Laminitis

Laminitis occurs rarely in wild equids but, more recently, there have been reports of the disease in Przewalski's horses maintained in semi-natural conditions (Budras et al., 2001). The authors reported that the cause of laminitis in three mares was the consumption of large amounts of carbohydrate-rich feed in the form of rich pasture and under certain climatic conditions. Previously, there had been only one report of laminitis in a Przewalski's horse (Kuntze, 1992).

Obesity/Starvation

Obesity is a common problem in most wild horse species maintained in captivity with free access to feed. Restricting pellets is a common practice in some institutions (Schlegel et al., 2004). Because obesity is a primary concern in captive wild horses, body scoring systems have been applied. Bray and Edwards (1999) applied a modified version of the scoring system for domestic horses (Henneke et al., 1983) to Przewalski's horses (*Equus przewalski*), Grevy's zebras (*Equus grevyi*), Eastern kiangs (*Equus kiang holdereri*), and Somalia wild asses (*Equus africanus somalicus*). Body condition scoring methods have been also developed for donkeys (Vall et al., 2003b; Pearson and Quassat, 2000), as described earlier in this chapter.

Poor body condition and death of one Grevy's zebra due to hypothermia and starvation has been reported in a zoological institution (NRC, 2004).

REFERENCES

Aganga, A. A., and C. M. Tsopito. 1998. A note on the feeding behavior of domestic donkeys: a Botswana case study. Appl. Anim. Behav. Sci. 60:235–239.

Aganga, A. A., M. Letso, and O. Aganga. 2000. Feeding donkeys. Livest. Res. Rural Dev. 12:1–7.

Araujo, L. O. D., L. C. Goncalves, A. S. C. Rezende, N. M. Rodriguez, and R. M. Mauricio. 1997. Digistibilidade aparente em equideos submetidos a dieta composta de concentrado e volumosos, fornecido com diferentes intervalos de tempo (Apparent digestibility in equids of diets differing in concentration and volume when fed over different time periods). Arquivo Brasileiro de Medicina Veterinaria Zootecnia 49: 225–237.

Blakeslee, T., and J. R. Zuba. 2002. Nondomestic equids. Pp. 229–235 in Hand-Rearing Wild and Domestic Mammals, L. J. Gage, ed. Ames: Iowa State University Press.

Blaxter, K. 1962. Vitamin E in health and disease of cattle and sheep. Vitam. Horm. 20:633–643.

Blythe, L. L., and A. M. Craig. 1997. Degenerative myeloencephalopathy. Pp. 319–320 in Current Therapy in Equine Medicine, 4th ed., N. E. Edwards, ed. Philadelphia: W. B. Saunders.

Bray, R. E., and M. S. Edwards. 1999. Body condition scoring of captive (Zoo) equids. Proceedings, Nutrition Advisory Group, American Zoo and Aquarium Assoc.

Brosh, A., A. Shkolnik, and I. Chosniak. 1986. Metabolic effects of infrequent drinking and low quality feed on Bedouin goats. Ecology 67:1086–1090.

Brosh, A., A. Shkolnik, and I. Chosniak. 1987. Effect of infrequent drinking on the nitrogen metabolism of Bedouin goats maintained on different diets. J. Agric. Sci. Camb. 109:165–169.

Brush, P. J., and P. H. Anderson. 1986. Levels of plasma alpha-tocopherol (vitamin E) in zoo animals. The Zoological Society of London, Int. Zoo Year Book. 24/25:316–321.

Budras, K. D., K. Sheibe, B. Patan, W. Streich, and K. Kim. 2001. Laminitis in Przewalski horses kept in a semireserve. J. Vet. Sci. 2:1–7.

Burnham, S. L. 2002. Anatomical differences of the donkey and mule. Pp. 102–108 in Proc. 48th Annual Convention Am. Assoc. of Equine Pract. Orlando, FL.

Cole, H. H., and M. Ronning. 1974. Horses, mules and asses. Pp. 201–217 in Animal Agriculture–The Biology of Domestic Animals and Their Use by Man. New York: W. H. Freeman and Company.

Cuddeford, D., R. A. Pearson, R. F. Archibald, and R. H. Muirhead. 1995. Digestibility and gastro-intestinal transit time of diets containing different proportions of alfalfa and oat-straw given to Thoroughbreds, Shetland ponies, Highland ponies and donkeys. Anim. Sci. 61:407–417.

Decker, R. A., T. L. Randall, and J. W. Prideaux. 1975. Enterolithiasis in a confined Hartman's Mountain zebra. J. Wildlife Dis. 11:357–359.

Dierenfeld, E. S., P. P. Hoppe, M. H. Woodford, N. P. Krilov, V. V. Klimov, and N. L. Yasinetskaya. 1997. Plasma-tocopherol, -carotene, and lipid levels in semi-free-ranging Przewalski horses (*Equus Przewalskii*). J. Zoo Wildlife Med. 28:144–147.

Dijkman, J. T. 1992. A note on the influence of negative gradients on the energy expenditure of donkeys walking, carrying and pulling loads. Anim. Prod. 54:153–156.

Dill, D. B., M. K. Yousef, C. R. Cox, and R. B. Barton. 1980. Hunger vs. thirst in the burro (*Equus asinus*). Physiol. Behav. 24:975–978.

Duncan, P., T. J. Foose, I. J. Gordon, C. G. Gakahu, and M. Lloyd. 1990. Comparative nutrient extraction from forages by grazing bovids and equids: a test of the nutritional model of equid/bovid competition and coexistence. Oecologia 84:411–418.

Edwards, M. S. 2004. Aspects of equine nutrition and management at the Zoological Society of San Diego. Pp. 30–38 in Proc. 5th Comparative Nutrition Society Symp., Michigan, C. L. Kirk Baer, ed. Silver Spring, MD.

Ellis, R. N. W., and T. L. J. Lawrence. 1980. The energy and protein requirement of the light horse. Br. Vet. J. 136:116–121.

El-Nauty, F. D., M. K. Yousef, A. B. Magdub, and H. D. Johnson. 1978. Thyroid hormones and metabolic rate in burros. *Equus asinus* and llamas, *Lama glama*: effects of environmental temperature. Comp. Biochem. Physiol. 60A:235–237.

Foose, T. J. 1982. Trophic strategies of ruminant versus non-ruminant ungulates. Ph.D. Dissertation University of Chicago.

Gaffney, M., R. E. Bray, and M. S. Edwards. 1999. Association of enterolith formation relative to water source pH consumed by wild equids under captive conditions. Pp. 51–54 in Proceedings of the 3rd Conf., Nutrition Advisory Group, Am. Zoo Aquarium Assoc., Columbus, OH.

Groves, C. P. 1974. Horses, Asses and Zebras in the Wild. Hollywood, FL: Ralph Curtis Books.

Guerouali, A., H. Bouayard, and M. Taouil. 2003. Estimation of energy expenditures in horses and donkeys at rest and when carrying a load. Pp. 75–78 in Working Animals in Agriculture and Transport. A collection of some current research and development observations, R. A. Pearson, P. Lhoste, M. Saastamoinen, and W. Martin-Rosset, eds. EAAP Technical Series No. 6. Wageningen, Netherlands: Wageningen Academic Publishers.

Henneke, D. R., G. D. Potter, J. L. Kreider, and B. F. Yeates, 1983. Relationship between condition score, physical measurements and body fat percentages in mares. Equine Vet. J. 15:371–372.

Hintz, H. F., C. J. Sedgewick, and H. F. Schryer. 1976. Some observations on digestion of pelleted diet by ruminants and non-ruminant. International Zoo Yearbook 16:54–57.

Howard, L. L., J. A. Allen, J. R. Zuba, and G. L. Richardson. 2004. Management of enterolithiasis in a Somali wild ass (*Equus africansus somalicus*) at the San Diego Wild Animal Park. Pp. 116–120 in Proc. Am. Assoc. of Zoo Veterinarians, Am. Assoc. of Wildlife Veterinarians, and Wildlife Disease Assoc., August 28–September 3, 2004, San Diego, CA.

ISIS (International species information system). 2002. International Species Inventory Systems No. 130. Eagan, MN: International Species Information System.

Izraely, H., I. Choshniak, C. E. Stevens, and A. Shkolnik. 1989a. Energy digestion and nitrogen economy of the domesticated donkey (*Equus asinus asinus*) in relation to food quality. J. Arid Environ. 17:97–101.

Klingel, H. 1989. Odd-Toed Ungulates. Pp. 550–596 in Grzimek's Encyclopedia of Mammals, vol 4, S. P. Parker, ed. New York: McGraw-Hill.

Kuntze, A. 1992. Auswertung von 505 Lahmheiten bei Zoo-Saugetieren. Verh. Ber. Erkrg. Zootiere. 34:187–193.

Lintzenich B. A., A. M. Ward. 1997. Hay and Pellet Ratios: Considerations in Feeding Ungulates. NAG Handbook Fact Sheet 006. Silver Spring, MD: Nutrition Advisory Group, Am. Zoo Aquarium Assoc.

Liu, Si-Kwang, E. P. Dolensek, C. R. Adams, and J. P. Tappe. 1983. Myolopathy and vitamin E deficiency in six Mongolian wild horses. J. Am. Vet. Med. Assoc. 11:1266–1268.

Lloyd, K., H. F. Hintz, J. D. Wheat, and H. F. Schryver. 1987. Enteroliths in horses. Cornell Vet. 77:172–186.

Maloiy, G. M. O. 1970. Water economy of the Somali donkey. Am. J. Physiol. 219:1522–1527.

Maloiy, G. M. O. 1971. Temperature regulation in the Somali donkey, Equus asinus. Comp. Biochem. Physiol. 39A:403–405.

Maloiy, G. M. O. 1973. The effect of dehydration and heat stress on intake and digestion of food in the Somali donkey. Environ. Physiol. Biochem. 3:36–39.

McDuffee, L. A., A. J. Dart, P. Schiffman, and J. J. Parrot. 1994. Enterolithiasis in two zebras. J. Am. Vet. Med. Assoc. 204:430–432.

Miraglia, N., M. Polidori, and E. Salimei. 2003. A review of feeding strategies, feeds and management of equines in Central-Southern Italy. Pp.103–112 in Working Animals in Agriculture and Transport. A collection of some current research and development observations, R. A. Pearson, P. Lhoste, M. Saastamoinen, and W. Martin-Rosset, eds. EAAP Technical Series No. 6. Wageningen, Netherlands: Wageningen Academic Publishers.

Mueller, P. J., and K. A. Houpt. 1991. A comparison of the responses of donkeys (Equus asinus) and ponies (Equus caballus) to 36 h of water deprivation. Pp. 86–95 in Donkeys, Mules and Horses in Tropical Agricultural Development, A. A. Pearson and D. Fielding, eds. Edinburgh: University of Edinburgh Press.

Mueller, P. J., M. T. Jones, R. E. Rawson, P. J. Van Soest, and H. F. Hintz. 1994a. Effect of increasing work rate on metabolic responses of the donkey (Equus asinus) J. Appl. Physiol. 77:1431–1438.

Mueller, P. J., H. F. Hintz, R. A. Pearson, P. Lawrence, and P. J. Van Soest. 1994b. Voluntary intake of roughage diets by donkeys. Pp. 137–148 in Working Equines, M. Bakkoury and A. Prentis, eds. Rabat, Morocco: Actes Editions.

Mueller, P. J., P. Protos, K. A. Houpt, and P. Van Soest. 1998. Chewing behaviour in the domestic donkey (Equus asinus) fed fibrous forage. Appl. Anim. Behav. Sci. 60:241–251.

Nelson, L. 1986. Equidae. Pp. 926–931 in Zoo and Wild Animal Medicine, 2nd ed., M. E. Fowler, ed. Philadelphia: W. B. Saunders.

Nengomasha, E. M., R. A. Pearson, and T. Smith. 1999. The donkey as a draught power resource in smallholder farming in semi-arid western Zimbabwe. Anim. Sci. 69:297–304.

NRC (National Research Council). 1978. Nutrient Requirements of Horses, 4th rev. ed. Washington, DC: National Academy Press.

NRC. 1989. Nutrient Requirements of Horses, 5th rev. ed. Washington, DC: National Academy Press.

NRC. 2004. Animal Care and Management at the National Zoo: Interim Report. Washington, DC: The National Academies Press.

Pagan, J. D., and H. F. Hintz. 1986a. Equine energetics I. Relationship between body weight and energy requirements in horses. J. Anim. Sci. 63:815–822.

Pagan, J. D., and H. F. Hintz. 1986b. Composition of milk from pony mares fed various levels of digestible energy. Cornell Vet. 76:139–148.

Pearson, R. A. 1991. Effects of exercise on digestive efficiency in donkeys given ad libitum hay and straw diets. Pp. 79–85 in Donkeys, Mules and Horses in Tropical Agricultural Development, A. A. Pearson and D. Fielding, eds. Edinburgh: University of Edinburgh Press.

Pearson, R. A. 2005. Nutrition and feeding of donkeys in Veterinary Care of Donkeys, N. S. Mathews and T. S. Taylor, eds. Ithaca, NY: International Veterinary Information Service (http://www.ivis.org).

Pearson, R. A., and J. B. Merritt. 1991. Intake, digestion and gastrointestinal transit time in resting donkeys and ponies and exercised donkeys given ad libitum hay and straw diets. Equine Vet. J. 23:339–343.

Pearson, R. A., and M. Quassat. 2000. A Guide to Live Weight Estimation and Body Condition Scoring of Donkeys. Edinburgh: University of Edinburgh Press.

Pearson, R. A., D. Cuddeford, R. F. Archibald, and R. H. Muirhead. 1992. Digestibility of diets containing different proportions of alfalfa and oat straw in thoroughbreds, Shetland ponies, Highland ponies and donkeys. Proceedings of the 1st European Conference on Equine Nutrition Pferdeheilkunde Sondergabe:153–157.

Pearson, R.A., P. R. Lawrence, and A. J. Smith. 1996. The centre for tropical veterinary medicine (CTVM) pulling its weight in the field of draught animal research. Trop. Anim. Health Prod. 28:49–59.

Pearson, R. A., R. F. Archibald, and R. H. Muirhead. 2001. The effect of forage quality and level of feeding on digestibility and gastrointestinal transit time of oat straw and alfalfa given to ponies and donkeys. Br. J. Nutr. 85:599–606.

Puls, R. 1994. Vitamin Levels in Animal Health: Diagnostic Data and Bibliographies. Clearbrook, British Columbia: Sherpa Int.

Quassat, M., R. A. Pearson, and M. Bakkoury. 1994. Pp. 374–377 in Working Equines—2nd International Colloquium, M. Bakkoury, R. A. Prentis, eds.. Rabat, Morocco: Actes Editions.

Ram, J. J, R. D. Padalkar, B. Anuraja, R. C. Hallikeri, J. B. Deshmanya, G. Neelkanthayya, and V. Sagar. 2004. Nutritional requirements of adult donkeys (Equus asinus) during work and rest. Trop. Anim. Health Prod. 36:407–412.

Reindl, N. J. 1997. American Zoo and Aquarium Association's (AZA's) Minimum Husbandry Guidelines for Mammals. Equids. Bethesda, MD: Am. Zoo Aquarium Assoc.

Salimei, E., R. Belli Blanes, A. Marano, E. Ferretti, G. Varisco, and D. Casamassima. 2000. Produzione quail-quantitativa di latte d'asina: risultati di due lattazioni. Pp. 315–322 in 35th Simp. Int. Zoot., May 25, Ragusa, Italy.

Schlegel, M. L., M. Miller, G. Crawshaw, M. Shaw, D. Barney, and E. V. Valdes. 2004. Practical diets and blood mineral and vitamin concentrations of captive exotic equids housed at Disney's Animal Kingdom and the Toronto Zoo. Second Annual Crissey Zoological Nutrition Symposium, December 10–11, Raleigh, North Carolina, pp. 39–46.

Schryver, H. F., O. T. Oftedal, J. Williams, N. F. Cymbaluk, D. Antczak, and H. F. Hintz. 1986. A comparison of the mineral composition of milk of domestic and captive wild equids (Equus Przewalski, E. Zebra, E. Burchelli, E. Caballus, E. Assinus). Comp. Biochem. Physiol. 85A: 233–235.

Suhartanto, B., and J. L. Tisserand. 1996. A comparison of the utilization of hay and straw by ponies and donkeys. 47th EAAP meeting, Lillehammer.

Suhartanto, B., V. Julliand, F. Faurie, and J. L. Tisserand. 1992. Comparison of digestion in donkey and ponies. Proceedings of the 1st European Conference on Equine Nutrition. Pferdeheilkunde Sondergabe: 158–161.

Svendsen, E. D. 1997. The Professional Handbook of the Donkey, 3rd ed. London: Whittet Books.

Taylor, F. 1997. Nutrition. Pp. 93–105 in The Professional Handbook of the Donkey, 3rd ed., E. D. Svendsen, ed. London: Whittet Books.

Tisserand, J. L., and R. A. Pearson. 2003. Nutritional requirements, feed intake and digestion in working donkeys: a comparison with other work animals. Pp. 63–73 in Working Animals in Agriculture and Transport. A collection of some current research and development observations, R. A. Pearson, P. Lhoste, M. Saastamoinen, and W. Martin-Rosset, eds. EAAP Technical Series No 6. Wageningen, Netherlands: Wageningen Academic Publishers.

Tisserand, J. L., F. Faurie, and M. Toure. 1991. A comparative study of donkey and pony digestive physiology. Pp. 67–72 in Donkeys, Mules and Horses in Tropical Agricultural Development, A. A. Pearson and D. Fielding, eds. Edinburgh: University of Edinburgh Press.

Trinder, N., C. D. Woodhouse, and C. P. Renton. 1969. The effect of vitamin E and selenium on the incidence of retained placentae in dairy cows. Vet. Rec. 85:550–553.

Vall, E. 1996. Capacités de travail, comportement â l'effort et réponses physiologuiques du zébu, de l'âne et du cheval au Nord-Cameroun. Thèse de doctorat. ENSAM, Montpellier, France. 418 pp.

Vall, E., O. Abakar, and P. Lhoste. 2003a. Adjusting the feed supply of draught donkeys to the intensity of their work. Pp. 79–91 in Working Animals in Agriculture and Transport. A collection of some current research and development observations, R. A. Pearson, P. Lhoste, M. Saastamoinen, and W. Martin-Rosset, eds. EAAP Technical Series No. 6. Wageningen, Netherlands: Wageningen Academic Publishers.

Vall, E., A. L. Ebangi, and O. Abakar. 2003b. A method of estimating body condition score (BCS) in donkeys. Pp. 93–102 in Working Animals in Agriculture and Transport. A collection of some current research and development observations, R. A. Pearson, P. Lhoste, M. Saastamoinen, and W. Martin-Rosset, eds. EAAP Technical Series No. 6. Wageningen, Netherlands: Wageningen Academic Publishers.

Van Soest, P. J. 1994. Nutritional Ecology of the Ruminant. Ithaca, NY: Comstock-Cornell University Press.

Wallach, J. D. 1970. Nutritional diseases of exotic animals. J. Am. Vet. Med. Assoc. 157: 583–599.

Walzer, C. 2003. Equidae. Pp. 578–586 in Zoo and Wild Animal Medicine, 5th ed. M. E. Fowler, ed. New York: Elsevier.

Wood, S. J., D. G. Smith, and C. J. Morris. 2005. Seasonal variation of digestible energy requirements of mature donkeys in the UK. Pferdeheilkunde 21:39–40.

Yousef, M. K. 1985. Physiological adaptations of less well-known types of livestock in arid zones: donkeys. Pp. 81–97 in Stress Physiology in Livestock, Volume II Ungulates, M. K. Yousef, ed. Boca Raton, FL: CRC Press.

Yousef, M. K. 1991. Physiological responses of the donkey to heat stress. P. 96 (Abstract) in Donkeys, Mules and Horses in Tropical Agricultural Development, A. A. Pearson and D. Fielding, eds. Edinburgh: University of Edinburgh Press.

Yousef, M. K., and D. B. Dill. 1969. Energy expenditures in desert walks: man and burro, *Equus asinus*. J. Appl. Physiol. 27:681–683.

Yousef, M. K., D. B. Dill, and M. G. Mayes. 1970. Shifts in body fluids during dehydration in the burro, *Equus asinus*. J. Appl. Physiol. 29: 345–349.

Yousef, M. K., D. B. Dill, and D. V. Freeland. 1972. Energetic costs of grade walking in man and burro, *Equus asinus*: desert and mountain. J. Appl. Physiol. 33:337–340.

14

Ration Formulation and Evaluation

The goal of feeding management is to provide nutrients that efficiently maintain a horse's body and well-being, and support functions related to growth, production, and work. The process of formulation aligns types and amounts of feedstuffs with nutrient requirements and needs for feeding management. Evaluation of rations allows for measurement of how well the formulation process meets feeding management goals. To be conducted correctly, ration formulation and evaluation requires knowledge of feedstuffs, feed manufacturing processes, feeding management practices, and the nutritional requirements and physiology of the horse.

Ration balancing involves mathematical procedures that align nutrient composition of feedstuffs with nutrient and intake needs of a horse. Methods range from simply accounting for nutrient profiles when combining certain feedstuffs to methods that impose limits of use to certain feeds, costs, feeding plans, and manufacturing methods. Individuals with limited experience in balancing rations or with limited knowledge of nutritional science of horses are cautioned. Mere mathematical manipulation of feedstuff nutrient values may fall short of effectively meeting dietary requirements. Successful diet formulation must take into account feed palatability, feeding behavior, and physiology of horses and feeding management practices.

IDENTIFYING REQUIREMENTS AND SELECTION OF FEEDS

Nutrient needs of horses within classes of production and use vary because of individual differences in the ability to utilize feeds and differing responses to environmental and management conditions. These individual variations enforce the need to individually manage the feeding of horses, especially those with heightened requirements imposed by rapid growth, heavy states of production, or intense work. Application of nutrient requirements may vary between different sources of information, partially because some nutrients may have wide ranges of what is considered to be optimal intake. Optimal ranges of nutrient intake have been defined as levels between amounts that are marginally adequate or deficient and upper levels that approach toxicities (Kronfeld, 1998).

Horses have and continue to be fed a wide variety of feedstuffs with varying levels of processing. Many horses receive nutrition solely from forages. Others receive mixed diets composed of concentrates, supplements, and forages. Some consume complete mixes, which are processed to visually resemble concentrates but contain nutrient profiles more like mixed rations of concentrates and forages.

One uniformly recommended guideline is for use of "high-quality" feedstuffs. Feeds should be free of irritants that cause ill effects and supply a nutrient profile that is aligned with requirements. Nutrients must be palatable and be safely fed through the intended feeding management routine. Digestible feedstuffs increase the efficiency of use and decrease waste. Feed-related factors that affect the use of specific ingredients include cost, availability, and palatability. Horse and management-related factors include the access to growing forage, the need for energy-dense rations, the use of the horse, and feeding management practices. Decisions to utilize specific feeds or feeding practices are also influenced by the decision maker's previous experience with particular feeds or rations, current trends in feed manufacturing, and the effects of marketing on purchaser preferences.

DETERMINING THE NUTRIENT CONTENT OF FEEDS

Methods used to estimate the nutritional value of feeds include information from feed tags, nutrient databases, and nutrient analyses via testing laboratories.

The feed tag of commercially prepared feeds provides minimum and maximum concentrations of certain nutrients. Requirements for feed tags in the United States include specified formats for listing product and brand names, inclusion statements of drugs, purpose and use statements, guarantees of limits to concentrations of certain nutrients, ingredient lists, directions for use, warning or caution statements, quantity statements, and contact information for the manufacturer or person responsible for distributing the feed (AAFCO, 2005).

Nutrient content of feedstuffs can also be estimated from feed composition tables or databases. Most of these sources report average values of nutrient composition. Averages are of limited value when the nutrient composition of similarly labeled feedstuffs is highly variable or if the average represents a small number of samples. Variation is expected as nutrient content of feedstuffs is affected by agronomic practices, environmental influences, and feedstuff variety.

Use of byproduct feeds has prompted reporting of nutrient variability of these feedstuffs. Arosemena et al. (1995) related the extent of nutrient variability of several byproduct feedstuffs to values listed in the Nutrient Requirements for Dairy Cattle (NRC, 2001). Comparison of average nutrients of the analyzed byproduct feeds differed more than 20 percent from values in the NRC (2001) table for most nutrients. Largest variations within sources of the sampled feedstuffs tended to be within mineral levels. Others have noted similar variability in the composition between different sources of byproduct feeds (DePeters et al., 2000) and differences in nutrient composition reported by commercial laboratories compared to those reported in NRC feedstuff composition tables (Berger, 1996).

These reports reinforce the need to consider the potential variability of the chemical composition of different sources of all feedstuffs when using estimates from nutrient tables and databases. The accuracy of use of values in nutrient databases is increased when sample sizes are large; when specific information is known about agronomic practices, environmental influences, and manufacturing conditions; and when the nutrient level variation between sources of the feedstuff is low.

Nutrient content of feedstuffs can be determined by near infrared reflectance and various wet chemistry procedures as described in Chapter 10. Testing can provide more accurate information on nutrient composition of a specific feed source as compared with other sources of information.

SAMPLE EXERCISES IN RATION FORMULATION AND EVALUATION

There are numerous methods used to formulate and evaluate rations, ranging from methods similar to these simple examples to more complex procedures that involve more nutrients, have more controls, and require higher degrees of accuracy. To be conducted correctly, ration formulation and evaluation require knowledge of feedstuffs, feed manufacturing processes, routine feeding management practices, and the nutritional requirements and physiology of the horse. Individuals with limited experience in balancing rations or with limited knowledge of nutritional science of horses are cautioned, as mere mathematical manipulation of feedstuff nutrient values may fall short of effectively meeting the dietary requirements.

Example A: Ration Evaluation Using Known Quantities of Two Feed Sources

Evaluate the nutrient profile of a ration containing 9 kg of forage and 1 kg of concentrate on an as-fed basis. Use the nutrient compositions for forage and concentrate in Table 14-1 and the example estimates for nutrient requirements in Table 14-2.

Check the units of the nutrient composition analysis. These units will be listed on a dry matter (DM) or as-fed basis. To convert as-fed to dry matter amounts, multiply the amount of feedstuff on an as-fed basis by the dry matter percentage of the feedstuff. To convert the amount on a dry matter basis to the amount as fed, divide the amount of feedstuff on a dry matter basis by the dry matter percentage of the feedstuff.

In this example, the composition data are presented on a dry matter basis. For accurate accounting, the amount fed must be converted to a dry matter basis, or the composition analysis must be converted to an as-fed basis. In this example, the amounts fed will be converted to a dry matter basis:

9 kg forage as fed × 89 percent dry matter = 8.01 kg forage DM
1 kg concentrate as fed × 90 percent dry matter = 0.9 kg concentrate DM

Calculate the amount of nutrients supplied in the ration by multiplying the amounts of dry matter for each feed source by the nutrient concentration in that feed source. For example, 8.01 kg DM forage × 9% crude protein = 0.721 kg × 1,000 g/kg = 721 g of crude protein. Calculate the total amount of each nutrient of concern, and compare the amounts to the example nutrient requirements (Table 14-3).

TABLE 14-1 Feed Ingredient Nutrient Composition (dry matter basis)

	DM (%)	CP (%)	Ca (%)	P (%)
Forage	89	9	0.3	0.2
Concentrate	90	10	0.5	0.4

TABLE 14-2 Example Estimates of Nutrient Requirements

Nutrient	g/d
Crude protein	630
Calcium	20
Phosphorus	14

In this example, the level of crude protein, calcium, and phosphorus are above the estimated requirement when feeding 10 kg of total ration per day on an as-fed basis.

Example B: Ration Evaluation Using Predetermined Forage to Concentrate Ratio

Evaluate the nutrient profile of a 90:10 (as-fed) forage to concentrate ratio, using the nutrient compositions for forage and concentrate in Table 14-4, and the upper intake limit and estimated requirements in Table 14-5.

The amount of ration is determined by meeting the estimated digestible energy requirement.

Digestible Energy Density of a 90:10 Ratio of Forage to Concentrate
(energy density of forage × percent forage in ration) + (energy density of concentrate × percent concentrate in ration)
1.7 Mcal/kg (0.90) + 3.3 Mcal/kg (0.10) = 1.86 Mcal DE per kg

Determine the amount needed to meet the estimated digestible energy (DE) requirement using the energy concentration of the combined forage and concentrate.

Amount of total ration: 16.7 Mcal DE ÷ 1.86 Mcal DE per kg = 8.98 kg

In this example, the total intake (as fed) is estimated at 8.98 kg to meet the estimated digestible energy requirement of 16.7 Mcal per day. This level of intake is well below the example upper intake limit of 12 kg per day. As such, total intake should be consumable, thus allowing for further evaluation.

Compare the nutrients provided by the forage and concentrate with the estimated requirements. Once an estimated amount of total ration is determined, the amount of forage and concentrate can be determined by multiplying the total amount by the percent of feed source. In this example, forage is 90 percent and concentrate is 10 percent of the ration.

Amount of forage: 8.98 kg (0.90) = 8.08 kg
Amount of concentrate: 8.98 kg (0.10) = 0.90 kg

Table 14-6 shows the total amount of crude protein (CP), calcium (Ca), and phosphorus (P) are higher than the example requirements when feeding this ration at levels to meet the estimated digestible energy requirement of 16.7 Mcal per day. If levels are unacceptable, the ratio of forage to concentrate or feed sources should be altered to provide a lower density of protein, calcium, and phosphorus in relation to the density of digestible energy.

Example C: Formulation of a Concentrate

Formulation methods were modified from procedures identified in Frape (1998) and Lewis (1995). The example uses a limited number of nutrients. Formulation methods for commercially prepared feed for horses will balance for specific energetic compounds, amino acids, vitamins, and additional minerals. This example formulates a concentrate with the specifications listed in Table 14.7 from feedstuffs with nutrient compositions provided in Table 14.8.

Determine the combination of grains needed to meet the targeted energy density of the concentrate. Note that if meet-

TABLE 14-3 Comparison of Nutrient Intake and Estimated Requirements

	DM Intake kg	CP (g)	Ca (g)	P (g)
Forage	8.01	721	24.0	16.0
Concentrate	0.90	90	4.5	3.6
Total	8.91	811	28.5	19.6
Requirement		630	20.0	14.0

TABLE 14-4 Feed Ingredient Nutrient Composition (as-fed basis)

	DM (%)	DE (Mcal/kg)	CP (%)	Ca (%)	P (%)
Forage	89	1.7	11	0.3	0.2
Concentrate	90	3.3	12	0.6	0.4

TABLE 14-5 Example Intake Limit (as-fed basis) and Estimated Nutrient Requirements

Upper Intake Limit (kg/d)	DE (Mcal)	CP (g)	Ca (g)	P (g)
12	16.7	630	20	14

TABLE 14-6 Comparison of Nutrient Intake and Estimated Requirements

	Intake (as fed) (kg/d)	DE (Mcal)	CP (g)	Ca (g)	P (g)
Forage	8.08	13.7	889	24.2	16.2
Concentrate	0.90	3.0	108	5.4	3.6
Total ration	8.98	16.7	997	29.6	19.8
Requirement		16.7	630	20.0	14.0

TABLE 14-7 Targeted Nutrient Concentration of the Example Concentrate (dry matter)

	DE Intake (Mcal/kg)	CP (%)	Ca (%)	P (%)
Concentrate	3.5	14	0.5	0.4

TABLE 14-8 Nutrient Composition of Feedstuffs (100% dry matter basis)

	DM (%)	DE (Mcal/kg)	CP (%)	Ca (%)	P (%)
Grain one	90	3.7	10	0.05	0.20
Grain two	90	3.2	12	0.09	0.38
Protein supplement	90	3.5	50	0.40	0.70
Mineral one	97			16.00	21.00
Mineral two	97			39.00	

ing or exceeding the minimal energy density of the final mix is critical, solving for a slightly higher energy density may be necessary to offset subsequent additions of ingredients lower in energy density, i.e., minerals. Ensuring or exceeding minimal energy densities is most important when balancing rations to be fed at intakes near maximal voluntary levels. In this example, the target energy density for the combination of the two grains will be adjusted to 3.6 Mcal/kg DE.

Assign one of the grains a value of x, the other y which equals $1 - x$, as $x + y = 1$.
x = grain one, $1 - x$ = grain two
(Energy density of grain one)x +
(Energy density of grain two)$1 - x$ =
Target energy density
$3.7x + 3.2(1 - x) = 3.6$
$3.7x + 3.2 - 3.2x = 3.6$
$0.5x = 0.4$
$x = 0.8$

A ratio of 80:20 of grain one to grain two would exceed the targeted energy density of 3.5 Mcal/kg DE. The resulting nutrient densities for crude protein, calcium, and phosphorus are calculated by summing the relative contributions from each of the grains. For example, crude protein (%) = $(10 \times 0.8) + (12 \times 0.2) = 10.4$. The nutrient concentration of the mix of grains one and two is presented in Table 14-9.

Add feedstuffs that supply large concentrations of deficient nutrients starting with crude protein. Rounding up the percent crude protein needed for the final concentrate to 14.5 percent will assist with maintaining a minimal density of crude protein as feedstuffs without protein are subsequently added. Balance the previously mixed grains with the protein supplement by methods similar to those used to balance energy density:

TABLE 14-9 Nutrient Concentration of an 80:20 Mix of Grain One and Grain Two

	DE (Mcal/kg)	CP (%)	Ca (%)	P (%)
Grain mix	3.6	10.4	0.06	0.24

x = grain, $1 - x$ = protein supplement
$10.4x + 50(1 - x) = 14.5$
$10.4x - 50x = -35.5$
$-39.6x = -35.5$
$x = 89.6$

Adjusting the ratio to a 90:10 grain mix to protein supplement will slightly exceed the targeted crude protein density of 14 percent. The subsequent nutrient densities are displayed in Table 14-10. The totals indicate that digestible energy and crude protein are at or slightly above the targeted densities for the final concentrate.

Calcium and phosphorus are below the targeted densities identified in Table 14-7. Solve for phosphorus first, as the available source of phosphorus, mineral one, also contains calcium.

x = grain mix with protein supplement, $1 - x$ = mineral one
$0.29x + 21(1 - x) = 0.4$
$0.29x - 21x = -20.6$
$x = 0.995$

Adjusting the ratio to 99.4:0.6 grain mix with protein supplement to mineral, one will increase the level of phosphorus slightly above the targeted phosphorus density of the concentrate (Table 14-11).

The calcium density of the mixture is less than the targeted level of the concentrate, so mineral two will need to be balanced into the mix.

x = grain mix, protein supplement and mineral one,
$1 - x$ = mineral two
$0.19x + 39(1 - x) = 0.5$
$0.19x - 39x = -38.5$
$x = 0.992$

TABLE 14-10 Comparison of the Grain Mix and Protein Supplement with the Targeted Nutrient Densities for the Concentrate

	% in mix	DE (Mcal/kg)	CP (%)	Ca (%)	P (%)
Grain mix	90	3.24	9.36	0.05	0.22
Protein supplement	10	0.35	5.00	0.04	0.07
Total	100	3.59	14.36	0.09	0.29
Difference		+0.09	+0.36	−0.41	−0.11

TABLE 14-11 Comparison of the Grain Mix, Protein Supplement, and Mineral One with the Targeted Nutrient Densities for the Concentrate

	% in mix	DE (Mcal/kg)	CP (%)	Ca (%)	P (%)
Grain mix	89.5	3.22	9.31	0.05	0.22
Protein supplement	9.9	0.35	4.95	0.04	0.07
Mineral one	0.6	0.00	0.00	0.10	0.13
Total	100.0	3.57	14.26	0.19	0.42
Difference		+0.07	+0.26	−0.31	+0.02

A ratio of 99.2:0.8 grain with protein supplement and mineral one to mineral two will increase the calcium density to the targeted level of the concentrate. The comparison of the final formulation to the targeted nutrient densities of the concentrate are presented in Table 14-12.

If values are acceptable, the final step is to convert the percentage contribution of feedstuffs in the concentrate from a dry matter to an as-fed basis. First, obtain an overall dry matter for the concentrate mix by summing the products of each feedstuff's contribution on a dry matter basis (Table 14-12) and its percent dry matter (Table 14-8):

Grain one	Grain two	Protein Supplement	Mineral one	Mineral two	Concentrate % DM
(71.0×0.90)	$+ (17.8 \times 0.90)$	$+ (9.8 \times 0.90)$	$+ (0.6 \times 0.97)$	$+ (0.8 \times 0.97)$	$= 90.1$

Multiply the percentage contribution of each feedstuff on a dry matter basis by the ratio of its percent dry matter to percent dry matter of the concentrate to obtain the contribution on an as-fed basis (Table 14-13):

Grain one	$71.0 \times (90/90.1) =$	70.9
Grain two	$17.8 \times (90/90.1) =$	17.8
Protein supplement	$9.8 \times (90/90.1) =$	9.8
Mineral one	$0.6 \times (97/90.1) =$	0.6
Mineral two	$0.8 \times (97/90.1) =$	0.9

TABLE 14-12 Comparison of the Final Formulation with the Targeted Nutrient Densities for the Concentrate

	% in mix	DE (Mcal/kg)	CP (%)	Ca (%)	P (%)
Grain mix	88.8	3.20	9.23	0.05	0.21
Grain one	71.0	2.63	7.10	0.03	0.14
Grain two	17.8	0.57	2.13	0.02	0.07
Protein supplement	9.8	0.34	4.90	0.04	0.07
Mineral one	0.6	0.00	0.0	0.10	0.13
Mineral two	0.8	0.00	0.0	0.31	0.00
Total	100.0	3.54	14.13	0.50	0.41
Difference		+0.04	+0.13	+0.00	+0.01

TABLE 14-13 Formulated Concentrate Constituents on a Dry Matter and As-Fed Basis

Feedstuff	% Dry Matter	% As-Fed
Grain one	71.0	70.9
Grain two	17.8	17.8
Protein supplement	9.8	9.8
Mineral one	0.6	0.6
Mineral two	0.8	0.9
Total	100.0	100.0

REFERENCES

AAFCO (Association of American Feed Control Officials, Inc.). 2005. Official Publication. Oxford, IN: Association of American Feed Control Officials.

Arosemena, A., E. J. DePeters, and J. G. Fadel. 1995. Extent of variability in nutrient composition within selected by-product feedstuffs. Anim. Feed Sci. Technol. 54:103–120.

Berger, L. L. 1996. Variation in the trace mineral content of feedstuffs. Prof. Anim. Scientist 12:1–5.

DePeters, E. J., J. G. Fadel, M. J. Arana, N. Ohanesian, M. A. Etchebarne, C. A. Hamilton, R. G. Hinders, M. D. Maloney, C. A. Old, T. J. Riordan, H. Perez-Monti, and J. W. Pareas. 2000. Variability in the chemical composition of seventeen selected by-product feedstuffs used by the California dairy industry. Prof. Anim. Scientist 16:69–99.

Frape, D. 1998. Equine Nutrition and Feeding, 2nd ed. Malden, MA: Blackwell Science.

Kronfeld, D. 1998. A practical method for ration evaluation and diet formulation: an introduction to sensitivity analysis. Pp. 77–88 in Advances in Equine Nutrition, vol. II. Lexington: Kentucky Equine Research.

Lewis, L. D. 1995. Equine Clinical Nutrition: Feeding and Care. Media, PA: Williams & Wilkins.

NRC (National Research Council). 2001. Nutrient Requirements of Dairy Cattle, 7th rev. ed. Washington, DC: National Academy Press.

15

Computer Model to Estimate Requirements

As discussed throughout the text of this publication, nutrient requirements of horses are often best described by a series of equations based on an understanding of the biology of the horse. Incorporation of these equations into a computer model provides a convenient way to calculate requirements for horses in specific situations (e.g., for a specific weight of horse and for a specific stage of the lifecycle). The values in the tables for horses of specific weights (200, 400, 500, 600, and 900 kg) given in this publication were generated by a computer program that uses equations and other information described in previous chapters. Users can access the program at the National Academies Press website (www.nap.edu). By using the software at that site, estimates of nutrient requirements can be tailored to specific horses more precisely than can be achieved by looking up values in the tables. The computer code used in the program is listed in this chapter.

Warning: Knowledge of nutritional constraints and limitations is essential for the proper use of nutrient requirements in tables and especially those generated by computer programs. Because of the many variables involved and judgments that must be made in choosing inputs and interpreting outputs, the NRC makes no claim for the accuracy of this software and the user is solely responsible for risk of use.

COMPUTER CODE

```
Required Inputs
    AnimalType - valid values: MAINTENANCE, STALLION, GROWING, PREGNANT, LACTATING, EXERCISE
        MAINTENANCE
        STALLION
        GROWING
        PREGNANT
        LACTATING
        EXERCISE

    MatureWeight - kg
    IntakeLevel - percent of actual bodyweight

    Age - months
    MonthOfGest - Months (integer)
    MonthOfLact - Months (integer)

    MaintLevel - valid values: 1, 2, 3
        1 - Low Maintenance
        2 - Average Maintenance
        3 - High Maintenance

    StallionMaintLevel - valid values: 0, 1
        0 - Not Breeding
        1 - Breeding
```

```
    WorkLoadGrow - valid values: 0, 1, 2, 3, 4
        0 - None
        1 - Low
        2 - Moderate
        3 - Heavy
        4 - Very Heavy

    WorkLoad - valid values: 1, 2, 3, 4
        1 - Low
        2 - Moderate
        3 - Heavy
        4 - Very Heavy

Outputs
    DM_req                              - kg/d
    DE_req                              - Mcal/d
    CP_req                              - g/d
    LYS_req                             - g/d
    Ca_req                              - g/d
    P_req                               - g/d
    Mg_req                              - g/d
    K_req                               - g/d
    VitA_req                            - IUx1000/d
    Na_req                              - g/d
    Cl_req                              - g/d
    S_req                               - g/d
    Co_req                              - mg/d
    Cu_req                              - mg/d
    I_req                               - mg/d
    Fe_req                              - mg/d
    Mn_req                              - mg/d
    Zn_req                              - mg/d
    Se_req                              - mg/d
    VitD_req                            - IU/d
    VitE_req                            - IU/d
    Thi_req                             - mg/d
    Ribo_req                            - mg/d

    SweatLoss                           - kg/d

_____*/

switch (AnimalType)
{
case "MAINTENANCE":
// Adult Horse at maintenance
    BodyWeight = MatureWeight;
    DM_req = (IntakeLevel/100) * BodyWeight;
    if (MaintLevel == 1) {
        // Minimum requirement
        DE_req = 0.0303 * BodyWeight;
        CP_req = 1.08 * BodyWeight;
    }
    if (MaintLevel == 2) {
        // Average requirement
        DE_req = 0.0333 * BodyWeight;
        CP_req = 1.26 * BodyWeight;
    }
    if (MaintLevel == 3) {
        // Elevated requirement
        DE_req = 0.0363 * BodyWeight;
        CP_req = 1.44 * BodyWeight;
    }
    LYS_req = 0.043 * CP_req;
    Ca_req = 0.04 * BodyWeight;
    P_req = 0.028 * BodyWeight;
```

COMPUTER MODEL TO ESTIMATE REQUIREMENTS

```
        Mg_req = 0.015 * BodyWeight;
        K_req = 0.05 * BodyWeight;
        Na_req = 0.02 * BodyWeight;
        Cl_req = 0.08 * BodyWeight;
        S_req = DM_req * 1000 * 0.0015;
        Co_req = DM_req * 0.05;
        Cu_req = 0.2 * BodyWeight;
        I_req = DM_req * 0.35;
        Fe_req = DM_req * 40;
        Mn_req = DM_req * 40;
        Zn_req = DM_req * 40;
        Se_req = DM_req * 0.1;
        VitA_req = 30 * BodyWeight;
        VitD_req = 6.6 * BodyWeight;
        VitE_req = 1.0 * BodyWeight;
        Thi_req = 0.06 * BodyWeight;
        Ribo_req = 0.04 * BodyWeight;
break;

case "EXERCISE":
    BodyWeight = MatureWeight;
    DM_req = (IntakeLevel/100) * BodyWeight;
    if (WorkLoad == 1) {
        // Light
        SweatLoss = 0.0025 * BodyWeight;
        DE_req = (0.0333 * BodyWeight )*1.2;
        CP_req = (1.26 * BodyWeight) + (0.089 * BodyWeight)+ (SweatLoss * 7.8 * 2.0 / 0.79);
        Ca_req = (0.06 * BodyWeight);
        P_req = (0.036 * BodyWeight);
        Mg_req = (0.019 * BodyWeight);
        VitE_req = 1.6 * BodyWeight;
        Thi_req = 0.06 * BodyWeight;
        Ribo_req = 0.04 * BodyWeight;
    }
    if (WorkLoad == 2) {
        // Moderate
        SweatLoss = 0.005 * BodyWeight;
        DE_req = (0.0333 * BodyWeight )*1.4;
        CP_req = (1.26 * BodyWeight) + (0.177 * BodyWeight) + (SweatLoss * 7.8 * 2.0 / 0.79);
        Ca_req = (0.07 * BodyWeight);
        P_req = (0.042 * BodyWeight);
        Mg_req = (0.023 * BodyWeight);
        VitE_req = 1.8 * BodyWeight;
        Thi_req = 0.113 * BodyWeight;
        Ribo_req = 0.04 * BodyWeight;
    }
    if (WorkLoad == 3) {
        // Heavy
        SweatLoss = 0.01 * BodyWeight;
        DE_req = (0.0333* BodyWeight )*1.6;
        CP_req = (1.26 * BodyWeight) + (0.266 * BodyWeight) + (SweatLoss * 7.8 * 2.0 / 0.79);
        Ca_req = (0.08 * BodyWeight);
        P_req = (0.058 * BodyWeight);
        Mg_req = (0.03 * BodyWeight);
        VitE_req = 2.0 * BodyWeight;
        Thi_req = 0.125 * BodyWeight;
        Ribo_req = 0.05 * BodyWeight;
    }
    if (WorkLoad == 4) {
        // Very Heavy
        SweatLoss = 0.02 * BodyWeight;
        DE_req = (0.0363* BodyWeight )*1.9;
        CP_req = (1.26 * BodyWeight) + (0.354 * BodyWeight) + (SweatLoss * 7.8 * 2.0 / 0.79);
        Ca_req = (0.08 * BodyWeight);
        P_req = (0.058 * BodyWeight);
        Mg_req = (0.03 * BodyWeight);
```

```
            VitE_req = 2.0 * BodyWeight;
            Thi_req = 0.125 * BodyWeight;
            Ribo_req = 0.05 * BodyWeight;
        }
        LYS_req = 0.043 * CP_req;
        K_req = (0.05 * BodyWeight) + ((1.4/0.5) * SweatLoss);
        Na_req = 0.02 * BodyWeight + 3.1 * SweatLoss;
        Cl_req = 0.08 * BodyWeight + 5.3 * SweatLoss;
        S_req = DM_req * 1000 * 0.0015;
        Co_req = DM_req * 0.05;
        Cu_req = DM_req * 10.0;
        I_req = DM_req * 0.35;
        Fe_req = DM_req * 40;
        Mn_req = DM_req * 40;
        Zn_req = DM_req * 40;
        Se_req = DM_req * 0.1;
        VitA_req = 45 * BodyWeight;
        VitD_req = 6.6 * BodyWeight;
break;

case "STALLION":
// Stallion
        BodyWeight = MatureWeight;
        DM_req = (IntakeLevel/100) * BodyWeight;
        if (StallionMaintLevel == 0)
        // Not Breeding
        {
            DE_req = 0.0363 * BodyWeight;
            CP_req = 1.44 * BodyWeight;
            Ca_req = 0.04 * BodyWeight;
            P_req = 0.028 * BodyWeight;
            Mg_req = 0.015 * BodyWeight;
            K_req = 0.05 * BodyWeight;
            Na_req = 0.02 * BodyWeight;
            Cl_req = 0.08 * BodyWeight;
            Cu_req = 0.2 * BodyWeight;
            VitA_req = 30 * BodyWeight;
            VitE_req = 1.0 * BodyWeight;
        }
        if (StallionMaintLevel == 1)
        // Breeding
        {
            SweatLoss = 0.0025 * BodyWeight; // - (Assumes light workload)
            DE_req = 0.0363 * BodyWeight * 1.2;
            CP_req = 1.44 * BodyWeight + (SweatLoss * 7.8 * 2 / 0.79) + 0.089 * BodyWeight;
            Ca_req = 0.06 * BodyWeight;
            P_req = 0.036 * BodyWeight;
            Mg_req = 0.019 * BodyWeight;
            K_req = 0.05 * BodyWeight +(1.4 / 0.5) * SweatLoss;
            Na_req = 0.02 * BodyWeight + 3.1 * SweatLoss;
            Cl_req = 0.08 * BodyWeight + 5.3 * SweatLoss;
            Cu_req = DM_req * 10.0;
            VitA_req = 45 * BodyWeight;
            VitE_req = 1.6 * BodyWeight;
}
        LYS_req = 0.043 * CP_req;
        S_req = DM_req * 1000 * 0.0015;
        Co_req = DM_req * 0.05;
        I_req = DM_req * 0.35;
        Fe_req = DM_req * 40;
        Mn_req = DM_req * 40;
        Zn_req = DM_req * 40;
        Se_req = DM_req * 0.1;
        VitD_req = 6.6 * BodyWeight;
break;
```

```
case "PREGNANT":
    // Pregnancy
    DM_req = (IntakeLevel/100) * MatureWeight;
    BodyWeight = MatureWeight;
    if (MonthOfGest < 5)
    {
        DE_req = 0.0333 * BodyWeight;
        CP_req = 1.26 * BodyWeight;
        Ca_req = 0.04 * BodyWeight;
        P_req = 0.028 * BodyWeight;
        Mg_req = 0.015 * BodyWeight;
        K_req = 0.05 * BodyWeight;
        Na_req = 0.02 * BodyWeight;
        Cl_req = 0.08 * BodyWeight;
        Cu_req = 0.2 * BodyWeight;
        I_req = DM_req * 0.35;
        Fe_req = DM_req * 40;
    }
    else
    {
        GestDay = MonthOfGest * 30.4;
        BirthWeight = 0.097 * MatureWeight;
        FetalMass = (0.0000001 * Math.pow(GestDay, 3.5512)) * 0.01 * BirthWeight;
        PUMass = (-0.0135 + (0.00009 * GestDay)) * BodyWeight;
        FetalGain = (0.00000035512 * Math.pow(GestDay, 2.5512)) * 0.01 * BirthWeight + 0.00009 *
            BodyWeight;
        DE_req = (0.0333 * BodyWeight ) + (0.0333 * 2 * (FetalMass+PUMass))
                                        + ((0.03 * FetalGain * 9.4)+(0.2*FetalGain*5.6))/0.6;
        CP_req = (1.26 * BodyWeight) + (FetalGain * 1000* 2.0 * 0.2 /0.79);
        if (MonthOfGest < 7)
        {
            Ca_req = 0.04 * BodyWeight;
            P_req = 0.028 * BodyWeight;
            Mg_req = 0.015 * BodyWeight;
            K_req = 0.05 * BodyWeight;
            Na_req = 0.02 * BodyWeight;
            Cl_req = 0.08 * BodyWeight;
            Cu_req = 0.2 * BodyWeight;
            I_req = DM_req * 0.35;
            Fe_req = DM_req * 40;
        }
        else if (MonthOfGest < 9)
        {
            Ca_req = 0.056 * BodyWeight;
            P_req = 0.04 * BodyWeight;
            Mg_req = 0.0152 * BodyWeight;
            K_req = 0.05 * BodyWeight;
            Na_req = 0.02 * BodyWeight;
            Cl_req = 0.08 * BodyWeight;
            Cu_req = 0.2 * BodyWeight;
            I_req = DM_req * 0.35;
            Fe_req = DM_req * 40;
        }
        else
        {
            Ca_req = (0.072 * BodyWeight);
            P_req = (0.0525 * BodyWeight);
            Mg_req = (0.0153 * BodyWeight);
            K_req = (0.0517 * BodyWeight);
            Na_req = 0.022 * BodyWeight;
            Cl_req = 0.082 * BodyWeight;
            Cu_req = 0.25 * BodyWeight;
            I_req = DM_req * 0.4;
            Fe_req = DM_req * 50;
        }
        BodyWeight = BodyWeight + (FetalMass + PUMass)*1.25;
```

```
        }
        LYS_req = 0.043 * CP_req;
        S_req = DM_req * 1000 * 0.0015;
        Co_req = DM_req * 0.05;
        Mn_req = DM_req * 40;
        Zn_req = DM_req * 40;
        Se_req = DM_req * 0.1;
        VitA_req = 60 * BodyWeight;
        VitD_req = 6.6 * BodyWeight;
        VitE_req = 1.6 * BodyWeight;
        Thi_req = 0.06 * BodyWeight;
        Ribo_req = 0.04 * BodyWeight;
        DailyGain = FetalGain*1.25;
break;

case "LACTATING":                                        // Lactating
        BodyWeight = MatureWeight;
        DM_req = (IntakeLevel/100) * BodyWeight;

        var MilkVals;
        var MilkProd;
        MilkVals = new Array(6);
        MilkVals[0] = 0.0326;
        MilkVals[1] = 0.0324;
        MilkVals[2] = 0.0299;
        MilkVals[3] = 0.0271;
        MilkVals[4] = 0.0244;
        MilkVals[5] = 0.0218;

        MilkProd = MilkVals[MonthOfLact-1] * BodyWeight;
        if (BodyWeight > 700) {
            DE_req = (0.0333 * BodyWeight ) + ((MilkProd * 10 * 50)/ (1000 * .6));
        } else {
            DE_req = (0.0363 * BodyWeight ) + ((MilkProd * 10 * 50)/ (1000 * .6));
        }
        CP_req = (1.44 * BodyWeight ) + (MilkProd * 50);
        LYS_req = (0.043 * 1.44 * BodyWeight) + (MilkProd * 3.3);
        if (MonthOfLact < 4)                              // Lactation - 'early lact'
        {
            Na_req = 0.02 * BodyWeight + (MilkProd * 0.17);
            Ca_req = (0.04 * BodyWeight) + ((MilkProd * 1.2)/0.5);
            P_req = (0.01/0.45 * BodyWeight) + ((MilkProd * 0.75)/0.45);
            Mg_req = (0.015 * BodyWeight) + ((MilkProd * 0.09)/0.4);
            K_req = (0.05 * BodyWeight) + ((MilkProd * 0.7)/0.5);
        }
        else if (MonthOfLact < 6)
        {
            Na_req = 0.02 * BodyWeight + (MilkProd * 0.14);
            Ca_req = (0.04 * BodyWeight) + ((MilkProd * 0.8)/0.5);
            P_req = (0.01/0.45 * BodyWeight) + ((MilkProd * 0.5)/0.45);
            Mg_req = (0.015 * BodyWeight) + ((MilkProd * 0.09)/0.4);
            K_req = (0.05 * BodyWeight) + ((MilkProd * 0.4)/0.5);
        }
        else
        {
            Na_req = 0.02 * BodyWeight + (MilkProd * 0.14);
            Ca_req = (0.04 * BodyWeight) + ((MilkProd * 0.8)/0.5);
            P_req = (0.01/0.45 * BodyWeight) + ((MilkProd * 0.5)/0.45);
            Mg_req = (0.015 * BodyWeight) + ((MilkProd * 0.045)/0.4);
            K_req = (0.05 * BodyWeight) + ((MilkProd * 0.4)/0.5);
        }
        Cl_req = 0.091 * BodyWeight;
        S_req = DM_req * 1000 * 0.0015;
        Co_req = DM_req * 0.05;
        Cu_req = 0.25 * BodyWeight;
        I_req = DM_req * 0.35;
        Fe_req = DM_req * 50;
```

```
        Mn_req = DM_req * 40;
        Zn_req = DM_req * 40;
        Se_req = DM_req * 0.1;
        VitA_req = 60 * BodyWeight;
        VitD_req = 6.6 * BodyWeight;
        VitE_req = 2.0 * BodyWeight;
        Thi_req = 0.075 * BodyWeight;
        Ribo_req = 0.05 * BodyWeight;
break;

case "GROWING":                                                              // Growing Animal
    BodyWeight = MatureWeight * (9.7 + (90.3 * (1.0 - (Math.exp(-0.0772 * Age)))))/100.0;
    DailyGain = MatureWeight * ( 6.97121 * Math.exp(-0.0772 * Age))/(30.4 * 100);
    DM_req = (IntakeLevel/100) * BodyWeight;
    if (WorkLoadGrow == 0)
    {
        DE_req=((56.5*Math.pow(Age,-0.145))/1000)*BodyWeight+(1.99+1.21*Age-0.021*Age*Age)*DailyGain;
        if (Age < 6.5) {
                CP_req = 1.44*BodyWeight+((DailyGain*1000*0.2)/0.5)/0.79;
                Cl_req = 0.093 * BodyWeight;
                VitD_req = 22.2 * BodyWeight;
        } else if (Age < 8.5) {
                CP_req = 1.44*BodyWeight+((DailyGain*1000*0.2)/0.45)/0.79;
                Cl_req = 0.085 * BodyWeight;
                VitD_req = 17.4 * BodyWeight;
        } else if (Age < 10.5) {
                CP_req = 1.44*BodyWeight+((DailyGain*1000*0.2)/0.40)/0.79;
                Cl_req = 0.085 * BodyWeight;
                VitD_req = 17.4 * BodyWeight;
        } else if (Age < 11.5) {
                CP_req = 1.44*BodyWeight+((DailyGain*1000*0.2)/0.35)/0.79;
                Cl_req = 0.085 * BodyWeight;
                VitD_req = 17.4 * BodyWeight;
        } else {
                CP_req = 1.44*BodyWeight+((DailyGain*1000*0.2)/0.3)/0.79;
                Cl_req = 0.0825 * BodyWeight;
        }
        Mg_req = (0.015 * BodyWeight) + (1.25 * DailyGain);
        K_req = (0.05 * BodyWeight) + (3.0 * DailyGain);
        Na_req = 0.02 * BodyWeight + (1.0 * DailyGain);
    }
    if (WorkLoadGrow == 1)
    {
        // Only applied to animals > 12 mo of age
        SweatLoss = 0.0025 * BodyWeight;
        DE_req = ((56.5*Math.pow(Age,-0.145))/1000)*1.2*BodyWeight+(1.99+1.21*Age-0.021*Age*Age)
            *DailyGain;
        CP_req = 1.44*BodyWeight+((DailyGain*1000*0.2)/0.3)/0.79 + (SweatLoss* 7.8 * 2 / 0.79)+0.089*Body
            Weight;
        Mg_req = (0.03 * BodyWeight);
        K_req = (0.05 * BodyWeight) + (3.0 * DailyGain) +(1.4/0.5)*SweatLoss;
        Na_req = 0.02 * BodyWeight + (1.0 * DailyGain) + 3.1 * SweatLoss;
        Cl_req = 0.0825 * BodyWeight + 5.3 * SweatLoss;
    }
    if (WorkLoadGrow == 2)
    {
        // Only applied to animals > 12 mo of age
        SweatLoss = 0.005 * BodyWeight;
        DE_req = ((56.5*Math.pow(Age,-0.145))/1000)*1.4*BodyWeight+(1.99 + 1.21*Age - 0.021*Age*Age)*
            DailyGain;
        CP_req = 1.44*BodyWeight+((DailyGain*1000*0.2)/0.3)/0.79 + (SweatLoss* 7.8 * 2 / 0.79)+0.177*
            BodyWeight;
        Mg_req = (0.03 * BodyWeight);
        K_req = (0.05 * BodyWeight) + (3.0 * DailyGain) +(1.4/0.5)*SweatLoss;
        Na_req = 0.02 * BodyWeight + (1.0 * DailyGain) + 3.1 * SweatLoss;
        Cl_req = 0.0825 * BodyWeight + 5.3 * SweatLoss;
```

```
        }
        if (WorkLoadGrow == 3)
        {
            // Only applied to animals > 12 mo of age
            SweatLoss = 0.01 * BodyWeight;
            DE_req = ((56.5*Math.pow(Age,-0.145))/1000)*1.6*BodyWeight+(1.99 + 1.21*Age - 0.021*Age*Age )*
                DailyGain;
            CP_req = 1.44*BodyWeight+((DailyGain*1000*0.2)/0.3)/0.79 + (SweatLoss* 7.8 * 2 / 0.79)+0.266*
                BodyWeight;
            Mg_req = (0.03 * BodyWeight);
            K_req = (0.05 * BodyWeight) + (3.0 * DailyGain) +(1.4/0.5)*SweatLoss;
            Na_req = 0.02 * BodyWeight + (1.0 * DailyGain) + 3.1 * SweatLoss;
            Cl_req = 0.0825 * BodyWeight + 5.3 * SweatLoss;
        }
        if (WorkLoadGrow == 4)
        {
            // Only applied to animals > 12 mo of age
            SweatLoss = 0.02 * BodyWeight;
            DE_req = ((56.5*Math.pow(Age,-0.145))/1000)*1.9*BodyWeight+(1.99 + 1.21*Age - 0.021*Age*Age )*
                DailyGain;
            CP_req = 1.44*BodyWeight+((DailyGain*1000*0.2)/0.3)/0.79 + (SweatLoss* 7.8 * 2 / 0.79)+0.354*
                BodyWeight;
            Mg_req = (0.03 * BodyWeight);
            K_req = (0.05 * BodyWeight) + (3.0 * DailyGain) +(1.4/0.5)*SweatLoss;
            Na_req = 0.02 * BodyWeight + (1.0 * DailyGain) + 3.1 * SweatLoss;
            Cl_req = 0.0825 * BodyWeight + 5.3 * SweatLoss;
        }
        LYS_req = 0.043 * CP_req;
        Ca_req = (0.072 * BodyWeight) + (32 * DailyGain);
        P_req = (0.04 * BodyWeight) + (17.8 * DailyGain);
        S_req = DM_req * 1000 * 0.0015;
        Co_req = DM_req * 0.05;
        Cu_req = 0.25 * BodyWeight;
        I_req = DM_req * 0.35;
        Fe_req = DM_req * 50;
        Mn_req = DM_req * 40;
        Zn_req = DM_req * 40;
        Se_req = DM_req * 0.1;
        VitA_req = 45 * BodyWeight;
        VitD_req = 20 * BodyWeight;
        VitE_req = 2.0 * BodyWeight;
        Thi_req = 0.075 * BodyWeight;
        Ribo_req = 0.05 * BodyWeight;
break;

default:
    alert("Undefined Animal Type");
    }
```

16

Nutrient Requirements, Feedstuff Composition, and Other Tables

TABLE 16-1 Daily Nutrient Requirements of Horses (Mature Body Weight of 200 kg)[a]

Type	Wt kg	ADG/Milk kg/d	DE Mcal	CP g	Lys g	Ca g	P g	Mg g	K g	Na g
Adult—no work[b]										
Minimum	200		6.1	216	9.3	8.0	5.6	3.0	10.0	4.0
Average	200		6.7	252	10.8	8.0	5.6	3.0	10.0	4.0
Elevated	200		7.3	288	12.4	8.0	5.6	3.0	10.0	4.0
Working[c]										
Light exercise	200		8.0	280	12.0	12.0	7.2	3.8	11.4	5.6
Moderate exercise	200		9.3	307	13.2	14.0	8.4	4.6	12.8	7.1
Heavy exercise	200		10.7	345	14.8	16.0	11.6	6.0	15.6	10.2
Very heavy exercise	200		13.8	402	17.3	16.0	11.6	6.0	21.2	16.4
Stallions										
Nonbreeding	200		7.3	288	12.4	8.0	5.6	3.0	10.0	4.0
Breeding	200		8.7	316	13.6	12.0	7.2	3.8	11.4	5.6
Pregnant Mares										
Early (< 5 months)	200		6.7	252	10.8	8.0	5.6	3.0	10.0	4.0
5 months	201	0.05	6.8	274	11.8	8.0	5.6	3.0	10.0	4.0
6 months	203	0.07	7.0	282	12.1	8.0	5.6	3.0	10.0	4.0
7 months	206	0.10	7.2	291	12.5	11.2	8.0	3.0	10.0	4.0
8 months	209	0.13	7.4	304	13.1	11.2	8.0	3.0	10.0	4.0
9 months	214	0.16	7.7	319	13.7	14.4	10.5	3.1	10.3	4.4
10 months	219	0.21	8.1	336	14.5	14.4	10.5	3.1	10.3	4.4
11 months	226	0.26	8.6	357	15.4	14.4	10.5	3.1	10.3	4.4
Lactating Mares										
1 months	200	6.52	12.7	614	33.9	23.6	15.3	4.5	19.1	5.1
2 months	200	6.48	12.7	612	33.8	23.6	15.2	4.5	19.1	5.1
3 months	200	5.98	12.2	587	32.1	22.4	14.4	4.3	18.4	5.0
4 months	200	5.42	11.8	559	30.3	16.7	10.5	4.2	14.3	4.8
5 months	200	4.88	11.3	532	28.5	15.8	9.9	4.1	13.9	4.7
6 months	200	4.36	10.9	506	26.8	15.0	9.3	3.5	13.5	4.6
Growing animals										
4 months	67	0.34	5.3	268	11.5	15.6	8.7	1.4	4.4	1.7
6 months	86	0.29	6.2	270	11.6	15.5	8.6	1.7	5.2	2.0
12 months	128	0.18	7.5	338	14.5	15.1	8.4	2.2	7.0	2.8
18 months	155	0.11	7.7	320	13.7	14.8	8.2	2.5	8.1	3.2
18 light exercise	155	0.11	8.8	341	14.7	14.8	8.2	4.6	9.2	4.4
18 moderate exercise	155	0.11	10.0	362	15.6	14.8	8.2	4.6	10.3	5.6
24 months	172	0.07	7.5	308	13.2	14.7	8.1	2.7	8.8	3.5
24 light exercise	172	0.07	8.7	332	14.3	14.7	8.1	5.2	10.0	4.8
24 moderate exercise	172	0.07	9.9	355	15.3	14.7	8.1	5.2	11.2	6.2
24 heavy exercise	172	0.07	11.2	387	16.7	14.7	8.1	5.2	13.6	8.8
24 very heavy exercise	172	0.07	13.0	436	18.8	14.7	8.1	5.2	18.4	14.1

[a]The daily requirements listed in this table for S, Co, I, Fe, Mn, Se, and Zn are calculated using assumed feed intakes of 2.5% of BW for heavy and very heavy exercise, lactating mares, and growing horses; 2.25% of BW for moderate exercise; and 2% of BW for all other classes. Daily requirements for Cu are also calculated from assumed feed intakes for adult horses (no work) and exercising horses.

[b]Minimum maintenance applies to adult horses with a sedentary lifestyle, due either to confinement or to a docile temperament. Average maintenance applies to adult horses with alert temperaments and moderate voluntary activity. Elevated maintenance applies to adult horses with nervous temperaments or high levels of voluntary activity.

[c]Examples of the type of regular exercise performed by horses in each category are described in Chapter 1. These categories are based on average weekly exercise. Four categories are given but users should recognize that the nutrient requirements are more accurately described by a continuous function than by discrete groups.

Cl g	S g	Co mg	Cu mg	I mg	Fe mg	Mn mg	Se mg	Zn mg	A kIU	D IU	E IU	Thiamin mg	Riboflavin mg
16.0	6.0	0.2	40.0	1.4	160.0	160.0	0.40	160.0	6.0	1320	200	12.0	8.0
16.0	6.0	0.2	40.0	1.4	160.0	160.0	0.40	160.0	6.0	1320	200	12.0	8.0
16.0	6.0	0.2	40.0	1.4	160.0	160.0	0.40	160.0	6.0	1320	200	12.0	8.0
18.7	6.0	0.2	40.0	1.4	160.0	160.0	0.40	160.0	9.0	1320	320	12.0	8.0
21.3	6.8	0.2	45.0	1.6	180.0	180.0	0.45	180.0	9.0	1320	360	22.6	9.0
26.6	7.5	0.3	50.0	1.8	200.0	200.0	0.50	200.0	9.0	1320	400	25.0	10.0
37.2	7.5	0.3	50.0	1.8	200.0	200.0	0.50	200.0	9.0	1320	400	25.0	10.0
16.0	6.0	0.2	40.0	1.4	160.0	160.0	0.40	160.0	6.0	1320	200	12.0	8.0
18.7	6.0	0.2	40.0	1.4	160.0	160.0	0.40	160.0	9.0	1320	320	12.0	8.0
16.0	6.0	0.2	40.0	1.4	160.0	160.0	0.40	160.0	12.0	1320	320	12.0	8.0
16.0	6.0	0.2	40.0	1.4	160.0	160.0	0.40	160.0	12.0	1320	320	12.0	8.0
16.0	6.0	0.2	40.0	1.4	160.0	160.0	0.40	160.0	12.0	1320	320	12.0	8.0
16.0	6.0	0.2	40.0	1.4	160.0	160.0	0.40	160.0	12.0	1320	320	12.0	8.0
16.0	6.0	0.2	40.0	1.4	160.0	160.0	0.40	160.0	12.0	1320	320	12.0	8.0
16.4	6.0	0.2	50.0	1.6	200.0	160.0	0.40	160.0	12.0	1320	320	12.0	8.0
16.4	6.0	0.2	50.0	1.6	200.0	160.0	0.40	160.0	12.0	1320	320	12.0	8.0
16.4	6.0	0.2	50.0	1.6	200.0	160.0	0.40	160.0	12.0	1320	320	12.0	8.0
18.2	7.5	0.3	50.0	1.8	250.0	200.0	0.50	200.0	12.0	1320	400	15.0	10.0
18.2	7.5	0.3	50.0	1.8	250.0	200.0	0.50	200.0	12.0	1320	400	15.0	10.0
18.2	7.5	0.3	50.0	1.8	250.0	200.0	0.50	200.0	12.0	1320	400	15.0	10.0
18.2	7.5	0.3	50.0	1.8	250.0	200.0	0.50	200.0	12.0	1320	400	15.0	10.0
18.2	7.5	0.3	50.0	1.8	250.0	200.0	0.50	200.0	12.0	1320	400	15.0	10.0
18.2	7.5	0.3	50.0	1.8	250.0	200.0	0.50	200.0	12.0	1320	400	15.0	10.0
6.3	2.5	0.1	16.8	0.6	84.2	67.4	0.17	67.4	3.0	1496	135	5.1	3.4
8.0	3.2	0.1	21.6	0.8	107.9	86.4	0.22	86.4	3.9	1917	173	6.5	4.3
10.6	4.8	0.2	32.1	1.1	160.6	128.5	0.32	128.5	5.8	2236	257	9.6	6.4
12.8	5.8	0.2	38.7	1.4	193.7	155.0	0.39	155.0	7.0	2464	310	11.6	7.7
14.8	5.8	0.2	38.7	1.4	193.7	155.0	0.39	155.0	7.0	2464	310	11.6	7.7
16.9	5.8	0.2	38.7	1.4	193.7	155.0	0.39	155.0	7.0	2464	310	11.6	7.7
14.2	6.4	0.2	42.9	1.5	214.6	171.7	0.43	171.7	7.7	2352	343	12.9	8.6
16.4	6.4	0.2	42.9	1.5	214.6	171.7	0.43	171.7	7.7	2352	343	12.9	8.6
18.7	6.4	0.2	42.9	1.5	214.6	171.7	0.43	171.7	7.7	2352	343	12.9	8.6
23.3	6.4	0.2	42.9	1.5	214.6	171.7	0.43	171.7	7.7	2352	343	12.9	8.6
32.4	6.4	0.2	42.9	1.5	214.6	171.7	0.43	171.7	7.7	2352	343	12.9	8.6

TABLE 16-2 Daily Nutrient Requirements of Horses (Mature Body Weight of 400 kg)[a]

Type	Wt kg	ADG/ Milk kg/d	DE Mcal	CP g	Lys g	Ca g	P g	Mg g	K g	Na g
Adult—no work[b]										
Minimum	400		12.1	432	18.6	16.0	11.2	6.0	20.0	8.0
Average	400		13.3	504	21.7	16.0	11.2	6.0	20.0	8.0
Elevated	400		14.5	576	24.8	16.0	11.2	6.0	20.0	8.0
Working[c]										
Light exercise	400		16.0	559	24.1	24.0	14.4	7.6	22.8	11.1
Moderate exercise	400		18.6	614	26.4	28.0	16.8	9.2	25.6	14.2
Heavy exercise	400		21.3	689	29.6	32.0	23.2	12.0	31.2	20.4
Very heavy exercise	400		27.6	804	34.6	32.0	23.2	12.0	42.4	32.8
Stallions										
Nonbreeding	400		14.5	576	24.8	16.0	11.2	6.0	20.0	8.0
Breeding	400		17.4	631	27.1	24.0	14.4	7.6	22.8	11.1
Pregnant Mares										
Early (< 5 months)	400		13.3	504	21.7	16.0	11.2	6.0	20.0	8.0
5 months	403	0.11	13.7	548	23.6	16.0	11.2	6.0	20.0	8.0
6 months	407	0.15	13.9	563	24.2	16.0	11.2	6.0	20.0	8.0
7 months	412	0.19	14.3	583	25.1	22.4	16.0	6.1	20.0	8.0
8 months	419	0.26	14.8	607	26.1	22.4	16.0	6.1	20.0	8.0
9 months	427	0.33	15.4	637	27.4	28.8	21.0	6.1	20.7	8.8
10 months	439	0.42	16.2	673	28.9	28.8	21.0	6.1	20.7	8.8
11 months	453	0.52	17.1	714	30.7	28.8	21.0	6.1	20.7	8.8
Lactating Mares										
1 months	400	13.04	25.4	1228	67.8	47.3	30.6	8.9	38.3	10.2
2 months	400	12.96	25.3	1224	67.5	47.1	30.5	8.9	38.1	10.2
3 months	400	11.96	24.5	1174	64.2	44.7	28.8	8.7	36.7	10.0
4 months	400	10.84	23.6	1118	60.5	33.3	20.9	8.4	28.7	9.5
5 months	400	9.76	22.7	1064	57.0	31.6	19.7	8.2	27.8	9.4
6 months	400	8.72	21.8	1012	53.5	30.0	18.6	7.0	27.0	9.2
Growing animals										
4 months	135	0.67	10.6	535	23.0	31.3	17.4	2.9	8.8	3.4
6 months	173	0.58	12.4	541	23.3	30.9	17.2	3.3	10.4	4.0
12 months	257	0.36	15.0	677	29.1	30.1	16.7	4.3	13.9	5.5
18 months	310	0.23	15.4	639	27.5	29.6	16.5	4.9	16.2	6.4
18 light exercise	310	0.23	17.7	682	29.3	29.6	16.5	9.3	18.4	8.8
18 moderate exercise	310	0.23	20.0	725	31.2	29.6	16.5	9.3	20.5	11.2
24 months	343	0.14	15.0	616	26.5	29.3	16.3	5.3	17.6	7.0
24 light exercise	343	0.14	17.4	663	28.5	29.3	16.3	10.3	20.0	9.7
24 moderate exercise	343	0.14	19.9	710	30.6	29.3	16.3	10.3	22.4	12.3
24 heavy exercise	343	0.14	22.3	775	33.3	29.3	16.3	10.3	27.2	17.7
24 very heavy exercise	343	0.14	26.0	873	37.5	29.3	16.3	10.3	36.8	28.3

[a] The daily requirements listed in this table for S, Co, I, Fe, Mn, Se, and Zn are calculated using assumed feed intakes of 2.5% of BW for heavy and very heavy exercise, lactating mares, and growing horses; 2.25% of BW for moderate exercise; and 2% of BW for all other classes. Daily requirements for Cu are also calculated from assumed feed intakes for adult horses (no work) and exercising horses.

[b] Minimum maintenance applies to adult horses with a sedentary lifestyle, due either to confinement or to a docile temperament. Average maintenance applies to adult horses with alert temperaments and moderate voluntary activity. Elevated maintenance applies to adult horses with nervous temperaments or high levels of voluntary activity.

[c] Examples of the type of regular exercise performed by horses in each category are described in Chapter 1. These categories are based on average weekly exercise. Four categories are given but users should recognize that the nutrient requirements are more accurately described by a continuous function than by discrete groups.

Cl	S	Co	Cu	I	Fe	Mn	Se	Zn	A	D	E	Thiamin	Riboflavin
g	g	mg	mg	mg	mg	mg	mg	mg	kIU	IU	IU	mg	mg
32.0	12.0	0.4	80.0	2.8	320.0	320.0	0.80	320.0	12.0	2640	400	24.0	16.0
32.0	12.0	0.4	80.0	2.8	320.0	320.0	0.80	320.0	12.0	2640	400	24.0	16.0
32.0	12.0	0.4	80.0	2.8	320.0	320.0	0.80	320.0	12.0	2640	400	24.0	16.0
37.3	12.0	0.4	80.0	2.8	320.0	320.0	0.80	320.0	18.0	2640	640	24.0	16.0
42.6	13.5	0.5	90.0	3.2	360.0	360.0	0.90	360.0	18.0	2640	720	45.2	18.0
53.2	15.0	0.5	100.0	3.5	400.0	400.0	1.00	400.0	18.0	2640	800	50.0	20.0
74.4	15.0	0.5	100.0	3.5	400.0	400.0	1.00	400.0	18.0	2640	800	50.0	20.0
32.0	12.0	0.4	80.0	2.8	320.0	320.0	0.80	320.0	12.0	2640	400	24.0	16.0
37.3	12.0	0.4	80.0	2.8	320.0	320.0	0.80	320.0	18.0	2640	640	24.0	16.0
32.0	12.0	0.4	80.0	2.8	320.0	320.0	0.80	320.0	24.0	2640	640	24.0	16.0
32.0	12.0	0.4	80.0	2.8	320.0	320.0	0.80	320.0	24.0	2640	640	24.0	16.0
32.0	12.0	0.4	80.0	2.8	320.0	320.0	0.80	320.0	24.0	2640	640	24.0	16.0
32.0	12.0	0.4	80.0	2.8	320.0	320.0	0.80	320.0	24.0	2640	640	24.0	16.0
32.0	12.0	0.4	80.0	2.8	320.0	320.0	0.80	320.0	24.0	2640	640	24.0	16.0
32.8	12.0	0.4	100.0	3.2	400.0	320.0	0.80	320.0	24.0	2640	640	24.0	16.0
32.8	12.0	0.4	100.0	3.2	400.0	320.0	0.80	320.0	24.0	2640	640	24.0	16.0
32.8	12.0	0.4	100.0	3.2	400.0	320.0	0.80	320.0	24.0	2640	640	24.0	16.0
36.4	15.0	0.5	100.0	3.5	500.0	400.0	1.00	400.0	24.0	2640	800	30.0	20.0
36.4	15.0	0.5	100.0	3.5	500.0	400.0	1.00	400.0	24.0	2640	800	30.0	20.0
36.4	15.0	0.5	100.0	3.5	500.0	400.0	1.00	400.0	24.0	2640	800	30.0	20.0
36.4	15.0	0.5	100.0	3.5	500.0	400.0	1.00	400.0	24.0	2640	800	30.0	20.0
36.4	15.0	0.5	100.0	3.5	500.0	400.0	1.00	400.0	24.0	2640	800	30.0	20.0
36.4	15.0	0.5	100.0	3.5	500.0	400.0	1.00	400.0	24.0	2640	800	30.0	20.0
12.5	5.1	0.2	33.7	1.2	168.5	134.8	0.34	134.8	6.1	2992	270	10.1	6.7
16.1	6.5	0.2	43.2	1.5	215.9	172.7	0.43	172.7	7.8	3834	345	13.0	8.6
21.2	9.6	0.3	64.2	2.3	321.2	257.0	0.64	257.0	11.6	4471	514	19.3	12.8
25.6	11.6	0.4	77.5	2.7	387.5	310.0	0.77	310.0	13.9	4929	620	23.2	15.5
29.7	11.6	0.4	77.5	2.7	387.5	310.0	0.77	310.0	13.9	4929	620	23.2	15.5
33.8	11.6	0.4	77.5	2.7	387.5	310.0	0.77	310.0	13.9	4929	620	23.2	15.5
28.3	12.9	0.4	85.8	3.0	429.2	343.4	0.86	343.4	15.5	4704	687	25.8	17.2
32.9	12.9	0.4	85.8	3.0	429.2	343.4	0.86	343.4	15.5	4704	687	25.8	17.2
37.4	12.9	0.4	85.8	3.0	429.2	343.4	0.86	343.4	15.5	4704	687	25.8	17.2
46.5	12.9	0.4	85.8	3.0	429.2	343.4	0.86	343.4	15.5	4704	687	25.8	17.2
64.7	12.9	0.4	85.8	3.0	429.2	343.4	0.86	343.4	15.5	4704	687	25.8	17.2

TABLE 16-3 Daily Nutrient Requirements of Horses (Mature Body Weight of 500 kg)[a]

Type	Wt kg	ADG/Milk kg/d	DE Mcal	CP g	Lys g	Ca g	P g	Mg g	K g	Na g
Adult—no work[b]										
Minimum	500		15.2	540	23.2	20.0	14.0	7.5	25.0	10.0
Average	500		16.7	630	27.1	20.0	14.0	7.5	25.0	10.0
Elevated	500		18.2	720	31.0	20.0	14.0	7.5	25.0	10.0
Working[c]										
Light exercise	500		20.0	699	30.1	30.0	18.0	9.5	28.5	13.9
Moderate exercise	500		23.3	768	33.0	35.0	21.0	11.5	32.0	17.8
Heavy exercise	500		26.6	862	37.1	40.0	29.0	15.0	39.0	25.5
Very heavy exercise	500		34.5	1004	43.2	40.0	29.0	15.0	53.0	41.0
Stallions										
Nonbreeding	500		18.2	720	31.0	20.0	14.0	7.5	25.0	10.0
Breeding	500		21.8	789	33.9	30.0	18.0	9.5	28.5	13.9
Pregnant Mares										
Early (< 5 months)	500		16.7	630	27.1	20.0	14.0	7.5	25.0	10.0
5 months	504	0.14	17.1	685	29.5	20.0	14.0	7.5	25.0	10.0
6 months	508	0.18	17.4	704	30.3	20.0	14.0	7.5	25.0	10.0
7 months	515	0.24	17.9	729	31.3	28.0	20.0	7.6	25.0	10.0
8 months	523	0.32	18.5	759	32.7	28.0	20.0	7.6	25.0	10.0
9 months	534	0.41	19.2	797	34.3	36.0	26.3	7.7	25.9	11.0
10 months	548	0.52	20.2	841	36.2	36.0	26.3	7.7	25.9	11.0
11 months	566	0.65	21.4	893	38.4	36.0	26.3	7.7	25.9	11.0
Lactating Mares										
1 months	500	16.30	31.7	1535	84.8	59.1	38.3	11.2	47.8	12.8
2 months	500	16.20	31.7	1530	84.4	58.9	38.1	11.1	47.7	12.8
3 months	500	14.95	30.6	1468	80.3	55.9	36.0	10.9	45.9	12.5
4 months	500	13.55	29.4	1398	75.7	41.7	26.2	10.5	35.8	11.9
5 months	500	12.20	28.3	1330	71.2	39.5	24.7	10.2	34.8	11.7
6 months	500	10.90	27.2	1265	66.9	37.4	23.2	8.7	33.7	11.5
Growing animals										
4 months	168	0.84	13.3	669	28.8	39.1	21.7	3.6	10.9	4.2
6 months	216	0.72	15.5	676	29.1	38.6	21.5	4.1	13.0	5.0
12 months	321	0.45	18.8	846	36.4	37.7	20.9	5.4	17.4	6.9
18 months	387	0.29	19.2	799	34.4	37.0	20.6	6.2	20.2	8.0
18 light exercise	387	0.29	22.1	853	36.7	37.0	20.6	11.6	22.9	11.0
18 moderate exercise	387	0.29	25.0	906	39.0	37.0	20.6	11.6	25.7	14.0
24 months	429	0.18	18.7	770	33.1	36.7	20.4	6.7	22.0	8.8
24 light exercise	429	0.18	21.8	829	35.7	36.7	20.4	12.9	25.0	12.1
24 moderate exercise	429	0.18	24.8	888	38.2	36.7	20.4	12.9	28.0	15.4
24 heavy exercise	429	0.18	27.9	969	41.7	36.7	20.4	12.9	34.0	22.1
24 very heavy exercise	429	0.18	32.5	1091	46.9	36.7	20.4	12.9	46.0	35.4

[a]The daily requirements listed in this table for S, Co, I, Fe, Mn, Se, and Zn are calculated using assumed feed intakes of 2.5% of BW for heavy and very heavy exercise, lactating mares, and growing horses; 2.25% of BW for moderate exercise; and 2% of BW for all other classes. Daily requirements for Cu are also calculated from assumed feed intakes for adult horses (no work) and exercising horses.

[b]Minimum maintenance applies to adult horses with a sedentary lifestyle, due either to confinement or to a docile temperament. Average maintenance applies to adult horses with alert temperaments and moderate voluntary activity. Elevated maintenance applies to adult horses with nervous temperaments or high levels of voluntary activity.

[c]Examples of the type of regular exercise performed by horses in each category are described in Chapter 1. These categories are based on average weekly exercise. Four categories are given but users should recognize that the nutrient requirements are more accurately described by a continuous function than by discrete groups.

Cl g	S g	Co mg	Cu mg	I mg	Fe mg	Mn mg	Se mg	Zn mg	A kIU	D IU	E IU	Thiamin mg	Riboflavin mg
40.0	15.0	0.5	100.0	3.5	400.0	400.0	1.00	400.0	15.0	3300	500	30.0	20.0
40.0	15.0	0.5	100.0	3.5	400.0	400.0	1.00	400.0	15.0	3300	500	30.0	20.0
40.0	15.0	0.5	100.0	3.5	400.0	400.0	1.00	400.0	15.0	3300	500	30.0	20.0
46.6	15.0	0.5	100.0	3.5	400.0	400.0	1.00	400.0	22.5	3300	800	30.0	20.0
53.3	16.9	0.6	112.5	4.0	450.0	450.0	1.13	450.0	22.5	3300	900	56.5	22.5
66.5	18.8	0.6	125.0	4.4	500.0	500.0	1.25	500.0	22.5	3300	1000	62.5	25.0
93.0	18.8	0.6	125.0	4.4	500.0	500.0	1.25	500.0	22.5	3300	1000	62.5	25.0
40.0	15.0	0.5	100.0	3.5	400.0	400.0	1.00	400.0	15.0	3300	500	30.0	20.0
46.6	15.0	0.5	100.0	3.5	400.0	400.0	1.00	400.0	22.5	3300	800	30.0	20.0
40.0	15.0	0.5	100.0	3.5	400.0	400.0	1.00	400.0	30.0	3300	800	30.0	20.0
40.0	15.0	0.5	100.0	3.5	400.0	400.0	1.00	400.0	30.0	3300	800	30.0	20.0
40.0	15.0	0.5	100.0	3.5	400.0	400.0	1.00	400.0	30.0	3300	800	30.0	20.0
40.0	15.0	0.5	100.0	3.5	400.0	400.0	1.00	400.0	30.0	3300	800	30.0	20.0
40.0	15.0	0.5	100.0	3.5	400.0	400.0	1.00	400.0	30.0	3300	800	30.0	20.0
41.0	15.0	0.5	125.0	4.0	500.0	400.0	1.00	400.0	30.0	3300	800	30.0	20.0
41.0	15.0	0.5	125.0	4.0	500.0	400.0	1.00	400.0	30.0	3300	800	30.0	20.0
41.0	15.0	0.5	125.0	4.0	500.0	400.0	1.00	400.0	30.0	3300	800	30.0	20.0
45.5	18.8	0.6	125.0	4.4	625.0	500.0	1.25	500.0	30.0	3300	1000	37.5	25.0
45.5	18.8	0.6	125.0	4.4	625.0	500.0	1.25	500.0	30.0	3300	1000	37.5	25.0
45.5	18.8	0.6	125.0	4.4	625.0	500.0	1.25	500.0	30.0	3300	1000	37.5	25.0
45.5	18.8	0.6	125.0	4.4	625.0	500.0	1.25	500.0	30.0	3300	1000	37.5	25.0
45.5	18.8	0.6	125.0	4.4	625.0	500.0	1.25	500.0	30.0	3300	1000	37.5	25.0
45.5	18.8	0.6	125.0	4.4	625.0	500.0	1.25	500.0	30.0	3300	1000	37.5	25.0
15.7	6.3	0.2	42.1	1.5	210.6	168.5	0.42	168.5	7.6	3740	337	12.6	8.4
20.1	8.1	0.3	54.0	1.9	269.9	215.9	0.54	215.9	9.7	4793	432	16.2	10.8
26.5	12.0	0.4	80.3	2.8	401.5	321.2	0.80	321.2	14.5	5589	642	24.1	16.1
32.0	14.5	0.5	96.9	3.4	484.4	387.5	0.97	387.5	17.4	6161	775	29.1	19.4
37.1	14.5	0.5	96.9	3.4	484.4	387.5	0.97	387.5	17.4	6161	775	29.1	19.4
42.2	14.5	0.5	96.9	3.4	484.4	387.5	0.97	387.5	17.4	6161	775	29.1	19.4
35.4	16.1	0.5	107.3	3.8	536.5	429.2	1.07	429.2	19.3	5880	858	32.2	21.5
41.1	16.1	0.5	107.3	3.8	536.5	429.2	1.07	429.2	19.3	5880	858	32.2	21.5
46.8	16.1	0.5	107.3	3.8	536.5	429.2	1.07	429.2	19.3	5880	858	32.2	21.5
58.2	16.1	0.5	107.3	3.8	536.5	429.2	1.07	429.2	19.3	5880	858	32.2	21.5
80.9	16.1	0.5	107.3	3.8	536.5	429.2	1.07	429.2	19.3	5880	858	32.2	21.5

TABLE 16-4 Daily Nutrient Requirements of Horses (Mature Body Weight of 600 kg)[a]

Type	Wt kg	ADG/Milk kg/d	DE Mcal	CP g	Lys g	Ca g	P g	Mg g	K g	Na g
Adult—no work[b]										
Minimum	600		18.2	648	27.9	24.0	16.8	9.0	30.0	12.0
Average	600		20.0	756	32.5	24.0	16.8	9.0	30.0	12.0
Elevated	600		21.8	864	37.2	24.0	16.8	9.0	30.0	12.0
Working[c]										
Light exercise	600		24.0	839	36.1	36.0	21.6	11.4	34.2	16.7
Moderate exercise	600		28.0	921	39.6	42.0	25.2	13.8	38.4	21.3
Heavy exercise	600		32.0	1034	44.5	48.0	34.8	18.0	46.8	30.6
Very heavy exercise	600		41.4	1205	51.8	48.0	34.8	18.0	63.6	49.2
Stallions										
Nonbreeding	600		21.8	864	37.2	24.0	16.8	9.0	30.0	12.0
Breeding	600		26.1	947	40.7	36.0	21.6	11.4	34.2	16.7
Pregnant Mares										
Early (< 5 months)	600		20.0	756	32.5	24.0	16.8	9.0	30.0	12.0
5 months	604	0.16	20.5	822	35.3	24.0	16.8	9.0	30.0	12.0
6 months	610	0.22	20.9	845	36.3	24.0	16.8	9.0	30.0	12.0
7 months	618	0.29	21.5	874	37.6	33.6	24.0	9.1	30.0	12.0
8 months	628	0.38	22.2	911	39.2	33.6	24.0	9.1	30.0	12.0
9 months	641	0.49	23.1	956	41.1	43.2	31.5	9.2	31.0	13.2
10 months	658	0.63	24.2	1009	43.4	43.2	31.5	9.2	31.0	13.2
11 months	679	0.78	25.7	1072	46.1	43.2	31.5	9.2	31.0	13.2
Lactating Mares										
1 months	600	19.56	38.1	1842	101.7	70.9	45.9	13.4	57.4	15.3
2 months	600	19.44	38.0	1836	101.3	70.7	45.7	13.4	57.2	15.3
3 months	600	17.94	36.7	1761	96.4	67.1	43.2	13.0	55.1	15.0
4 months	600	16.26	35.3	1677	90.8	50.0	31.4	12.7	43.0	14.3
5 months	600	14.64	34.0	1596	85.5	47.4	29.6	12.3	41.7	14.0
6 months	600	13.08	32.7	1518	80.3	44.9	27.9	10.5	40.5	13.8
Growing animals										
4 months	202	1.01	15.9	803	34.5	46.9	26.1	4.3	13.1	5.1
6 months	259	0.87	18.6	811	34.9	46.4	25.8	5.0	15.6	6.0
12 months	385	0.54	22.5	1015	43.6	45.2	25.1	6.5	20.9	8.3
18 months	465	0.34	23.1	959	41.2	44.5	24.7	7.4	24.3	9.6
18 light exercise	465	0.34	26.5	1023	44.0	44.5	24.7	13.9	27.5	13.2
18 moderate exercise	465	0.34	30.0	1087	46.7	44.5	24.7	13.9	30.8	16.9
24 months	515	0.22	22.4	924	39.7	44.0	24.4	8.0	26.4	10.5
24 light exercise	515	0.22	26.1	995	42.8	44.0	24.4	15.5	30.0	14.5
24 moderate exercise	515	0.22	29.8	1066	45.8	44.0	24.4	15.5	33.6	18.5
24 heavy exercise	515	0.22	33.5	1162	50.0	44.0	24.4	15.5	40.8	26.5
24 very heavy exercise	515	0.22	39.0	1309	56.3	44.0	24.4	15.5	55.2	42.4

[a]The daily requirements listed in this table for S, Co, I, Fe, Mn, Se, and Zn are calculated using assumed feed intakes of 2.5% of BW for heavy and very heavy exercise, lactating mares, and growing horses; 2.25% of BW for moderate exercise; and 2% of BW for all other classes. Daily requirements for Cu are also calculated from assumed feed intakes for adult horses (no work) and exercising horses.

[b]Minimum maintenance applies to adult horses with a sedentary lifestyle, due either to confinement or to a docile temperament. Average maintenance applies to adult horses with alert temperaments and moderate voluntary activity. Elevated maintenance applies to adult horses with nervous temperaments or high levels of voluntary activity.

[b]Examples of the type of regular exercise performed by horses in each category are described in Chapter 1. These categories are based on average weekly exercise. Four categories are given but users should recognize that the nutrient requirements are more accurately described by a continuous function than by discrete groups.

Cl g	S g	Co mg	Cu mg	I mg	Fe mg	Mn mg	Se mg	Zn mg	A kIU	D IU	E IU	Thiamin mg	Riboflavin mg
48.0	18.0	0.6	120.0	4.2	480.0	480.0	1.20	480.0	18.0	3960	600	36.0	24.0
48.0	18.0	0.6	120.0	4.2	480.0	480.0	1.20	480.0	18.0	3960	600	36.0	24.0
48.0	18.0	0.6	120.0	4.2	480.0	480.0	1.20	480.0	18.0	3960	600	36.0	24.0
56.0	18.0	0.6	120.0	4.2	480.0	480.0	1.20	480.0	27.0	3960	960	36.0	24.0
63.9	20.3	0.7	135.0	4.7	540.0	540.0	1.35	540.0	27.0	3960	1080	67.8	27.0
79.8	22.5	0.8	150.0	5.3	600.0	600.0	1.50	600.0	27.0	3960	1200	75.0	30.0
111.6	22.5	0.8	150.0	5.3	600.0	600.0	1.50	600.0	27.0	3960	1200	75.0	30.0
48.0	18.0	0.6	120.0	4.2	480.0	480.0	1.20	480.0	18.0	3960	600	36.0	24.0
56.0	18.0	0.6	120.0	4.2	480.0	480.0	1.20	480.0	27.0	3960	960	36.0	24.0
48.0	18.0	0.6	120.0	4.2	480.0	480.0	1.20	480.0	36.0	3960	960	36.0	24.0
48.0	18.0	0.6	120.0	4.2	480.0	480.0	1.20	480.0	36.0	3960	960	36.0	24.0
48.0	18.0	0.6	120.0	4.2	480.0	480.0	1.20	480.0	36.0	3960	960	36.0	24.0
48.0	18.0	0.6	120.0	4.2	480.0	480.0	1.20	480.0	36.0	3960	960	36.0	24.0
48.0	18.0	0.6	120.0	4.2	480.0	480.0	1.20	480.0	36.0	3960	960	36.0	24.0
49.2	18.0	0.6	150.0	4.8	600.0	480.0	1.20	480.0	36.0	3960	960	36.0	24.0
49.2	18.0	0.6	150.0	4.8	600.0	480.0	1.20	480.0	36.0	3960	960	36.0	24.0
49.2	18.0	0.6	150.0	4.8	600.0	480.0	1.20	480.0	36.0	3960	960	36.0	24.0
54.6	22.5	0.8	150.0	5.3	750.0	600.0	1.50	600.0	36.0	3960	1200	45.0	30.0
54.6	22.5	0.8	150.0	5.3	750.0	600.0	1.50	600.0	36.0	3960	1200	45.0	30.0
54.6	22.5	0.8	150.0	5.3	750.0	600.0	1.50	600.0	36.0	3960	1200	45.0	30.0
54.6	22.5	0.8	150.0	5.3	750.0	600.0	1.50	600.0	36.0	3960	1200	45.0	30.0
54.6	22.5	0.8	150.0	5.3	750.0	600.0	1.50	600.0	36.0	3960	1200	45.0	30.0
54.6	22.5	0.8	150.0	5.3	750.0	600.0	1.50	600.0	36.0	3960	1200	45.0	30.0
18.8	7.6	0.3	50.5	1.8	252.7	202.1	0.51	202.1	9.1	4488	404	15.2	10.1
24.1	9.7	0.3	64.8	2.3	323.8	259.1	0.65	259.1	11.7	5751	518	19.4	13.0
31.8	14.5	0.5	96.4	3.4	481.8	385.5	0.96	385.5	17.3	6707	771	28.9	19.3
38.4	17.4	0.6	116.2	4.1	581.2	465.0	1.16	465.0	20.9	7393	930	34.9	23.2
44.5	17.4	0.6	116.2	4.1	581.2	465.0	1.16	465.0	20.9	7393	930	34.9	23.2
50.7	17.4	0.6	116.2	4.1	581.2	465.0	1.16	465.0	20.9	7393	930	34.9	23.2
42.5	19.3	0.6	128.8	4.5	643.8	515.0	1.29	515.0	23.2	7056	1030	38.6	25.8
49.3	19.3	0.6	128.8	4.5	643.8	515.0	1.29	515.0	23.2	7056	1030	38.6	25.8
56.1	19.3	0.6	128.8	4.5	643.8	515.0	1.29	515.0	23.2	7056	1030	38.6	25.8
69.8	19.3	0.6	128.8	4.5	643.8	515.0	1.29	515.0	23.2	7056	1030	38.6	25.8
97.1	19.3	0.6	128.8	4.5	643.8	515.0	1.29	515.0	23.2	7056	1030	38.6	25.8

TABLE 16-5 Daily Nutrient Requirements of Horses (Mature Body Weight of 900 kg)[a]

Type	Wt kg	ADG/Milk kg/d	DE Mcal	CP g	Lys g	Ca g	P g	Mg g	K g	Na g
Adult—no work[b]										
Minimum	900		27.3	972	41.8	36.0	25.2	13.5	45.0	18.0
Average	900		30.0	1134	48.8	36.0	25.2	13.5	45.0	18.0
Elevated	900		32.7	1296	55.7	36.0	25.2	13.5	45.0	18.0
Working[c]										
Light exercise	900		36.0	1259	54.1	54.0	32.4	17.1	51.3	25.0
Moderate exercise	900		42.0	1382	59.4	63.0	37.8	20.7	57.6	32.0
Heavy exercise	900		48.0	1551	66.7	72.0	52.2	27.0	70.2	45.9
Very heavy exercise	900		62.1	1808	77.7	72.0	52.2	27.0	95.4	73.8
Stallions										
Nonbreeding	900		32.7	1296	55.7	36.0	25.2	13.5	45.0	18.0
Breeding	900		39.2	1421	61.1	54.0	32.4	17.1	51.3	25.0
Pregnant Mares										
Early (< 5 months)	900		30.0	1134	48.8	36.0	25.2	13.5	45.0	18.0
5 months	906	0.24	30.8	1233	53.0	36.0	25.2	13.5	45.0	18.0
6 months	915	0.33	31.4	1267	54.5	36.0	25.2	13.5	45.0	18.0
7 months	927	0.44	32.2	1311	56.4	50.4	36.0	13.7	45.0	18.0
8 months	942	0.57	33.3	1367	58.8	50.4	36.0	13.7	45.0	18.0
9 months	962	0.74	34.6	1434	61.7	64.8	47.3	13.8	46.5	19.8
10 months	987	0.94	36.4	1514	65.1	64.8	47.3	13.8	46.5	19.8
11 months	1019	1.17	38.5	1607	69.1	64.8	47.3	13.8	46.5	19.8
Lactating Mares										
1 months	900	29.34	54.4	2763	152.6	106.4	68.9	20.1	86.1	23.0
2 months	900	29.16	54.3	2754	152.0	106.0	68.6	20.1	85.8	23.0
3 months	900	26.91	52.4	2642	144.5	100.6	64.9	19.6	82.7	22.6
4 months	900	24.39	50.3	2516	136.2	75.0	47.1	19.0	64.5	21.4
5 months	900	21.96	48.3	2394	128.2	71.1	44.4	18.4	62.6	21.1
6 months	900	19.62	46.3	2277	120.5	67.4	41.8	15.7	60.7	20.7
Growing animals										
4 months	303	1.52	23.9	1204	51.8	70.3	39.1	6.4	19.7	7.6
6 months	389	1.30	28.0	1217	52.3	69.5	38.7	7.5	23.3	9.1
12 months	578	0.82	33.8	1522	65.5	67.8	37.7	9.7	31.4	12.4
18 months	697	0.51	34.6	1438	61.8	66.7	37.1	11.1	36.4	14.5
18 light exercise	697	0.51	39.8	1535	66.0	66.7	37.1	20.9	41.3	19.9
18 moderate exercise	697	0.51	45.0	1631	70.1	66.7	37.1	20.9	46.2	25.3
24 months	773	0.32	33.7	1386	59.6	66.0	36.7	12.0	39.6	15.8
24 light exercise	773	0.32	39.2	1492	64.2	66.0	36.7	23.2	45.0	21.8
24 moderate exercise	773	0.32	44.7	1599	68.7	66.0	36.7	23.2	50.4	27.7
24 heavy exercise	773	0.32	50.2	1744	75.0	66.0	36.7	23.2	61.2	39.7
24 very heavy exercise	773	0.32	58.4	1964	84.5	66.0	36.7	23.2	82.9	63.7

[a]The daily requirements listed in this table for S, Co, I, Fe, Mn, Se, and Zn are calculated using assumed feed intakes of 2.5% of BW for heavy and very heavy exercise, lactating mares, and growing horses; 2.25% of BW for moderate exercise; and 2% of BW for all other classes. Daily requirements for Cu are also calculated from assumed feed intakes for adult horses (no work) and exercising horses.

[b]Minimum maintenance applies to adult horses with a sedentary lifestyle, due either to confinement or to a docile temperament. Average maintenance applies to adult horses with alert temperaments and moderate voluntary activity. Elevated maintenance applies to adult horses with nervous temperaments or high levels of voluntary activity.

[c]Examples of the type of regular exercise performed by horses in each category are described in Chapter 1. These categories are based on average weekly exercise. Four categories are given but users should recognize that the nutrient requirements are more accurately described by a continuous function than by discrete groups.

Cl g	S g	Co mg	Cu mg	I mg	Fe mg	Mn mg	Se mg	Zn mg	A kIU	D IU	E IU	Thiamin mg	Riboflavin mg
72.0	27.0	0.9	180.0	6.3	720.0	720.0	1.80	720.0	27.0	5940	900	54.0	36.0
72.0	27.0	0.9	180.0	6.3	720.0	720.0	1.80	720.0	27.0	5940	900	54.0	36.0
72.0	27.0	0.9	180.0	6.3	720.0	720.0	1.80	720.0	27.0	5940	900	54.0	36.0
83.9	27.0	0.9	180.0	6.3	720.0	720.0	1.80	720.0	40.5	5940	1440	54.0	36.0
95.9	30.4	1.0	202.5	7.1	810.0	810.0	2.03	810.0	40.5	5940	1620	101.7	40.5
119.7	33.8	1.1	225.0	7.9	900.0	900.0	2.25	900.0	40.5	5940	1800	112.5	45.0
167.4	33.8	1.1	225.0	7.9	900.0	900.0	2.25	900.0	40.5	5940	1800	112.5	45.0
72.0	27.0	0.9	180.0	6.3	720.0	720.0	1.80	720.0	27.0	5940	900	54.0	36.0
83.9	27.0	0.9	180.0	6.3	720.0	720.0	1.80	720.0	40.5	5940	1440	54.0	36.0
72.0	27.0	0.9	180.0	6.3	720.0	720.0	1.80	720.0	54.0	5940	1440	54.0	36.0
72.0	27.0	0.9	180.0	6.3	720.0	720.0	1.80	720.0	54.0	5940	1440	54.0	36.0
72.0	27.0	0.9	180.0	6.3	720.0	720.0	1.80	720.0	54.0	5940	1440	54.0	36.0
72.0	27.0	0.9	180.0	6.3	720.0	720.0	1.80	720.0	54.0	5940	1440	54.0	36.0
72.0	27.0	0.9	180.0	6.3	720.0	720.0	1.80	720.0	54.0	5940	1440	54.0	36.0
73.8	27.0	0.9	225.0	7.2	900.0	720.0	1.80	720.0	54.0	5940	1440	54.0	36.0
73.8	27.0	0.9	225.0	7.2	900.0	720.0	1.80	720.0	54.0	5940	1440	54.0	36.0
73.8	27.0	0.9	225.0	7.2	900.0	720.0	1.80	720.0	54.0	5940	1440	54.0	36.0
81.9	33.8	1.1	225.0	7.9	1125.0	900.0	2.25	900.0	54.0	5940	1800	67.5	45.0
81.9	33.8	1.1	225.0	7.9	1125.0	900.0	2.25	900.0	54.0	5940	1800	67.5	45.0
81.9	33.8	1.1	225.0	7.9	1125.0	900.0	2.25	900.0	54.0	5940	1800	67.5	45.0
81.9	33.8	1.1	225.0	7.9	1125.0	900.0	2.25	900.0	54.0	5940	1800	67.5	45.0
81.9	33.8	1.1	225.0	7.9	1125.0	900.0	2.25	900.0	54.0	5940	1800	67.5	45.0
81.9	33.8	1.1	225.0	7.9	1125.0	900.0	2.25	900.0	54.0	5940	1800	67.5	45.0
28.2	11.4	0.4	75.8	2.7	379.0	303.2	0.76	303.2	13.6	6731	606	22.7	15.2
36.1	14.6	0.5	97.1	3.4	485.7	388.6	0.97	388.6	17.5	8627	777	29.1	19.4
47.7	21.7	0.7	144.5	5.1	722.7	578.2	1.45	578.2	26.0	10061	1156	43.4	28.9
57.5	26.2	0.9	174.4	6.1	871.9	697.5	1.74	697.5	31.4	11090	1395	52.3	34.9
66.8	26.2	0.9	174.4	6.1	871.9	697.5	1.74	697.5	31.4	11090	1395	52.3	34.9
76.0	26.2	0.9	174.4	6.1	871.9	697.5	1.74	697.5	31.4	11090	1395	52.3	34.9
63.7	29.0	1.0	193.1	6.8	965.7	772.6	1.93	772.6	34.8	10584	1545	57.9	38.6
74.0	29.0	1.0	193.1	6.8	965.7	772.6	1.93	772.6	34.8	10584	1545	57.9	38.6
84.2	29.0	1.0	193.1	6.8	965.7	772.6	1.93	772.6	34.8	10584	1545	57.9	38.6
104.7	29.0	1.0	193.1	6.8	965.7	772.6	1.93	772.6	34.8	10584	1545	57.9	38.6
145.6	29.0	1.0	193.1	6.8	965.7	772.6	1.93	772.6	34.8	10584	1545	57.9	38.6

TABLE 16-6 Nutrient Composition of Selected Feedstuffs
(NRC 2001, Nutrient Requirements of Dairy Cattle)
All values on a dry matter (DM) basis unless otherwise noted

Feed Name	Energy Class	IFN	DM % as Fed	DE[a] Mcal/kg DM	CP % DM	Lys % DM	Fat % DM	NDF % DM	ADF % DM	Ash % DM
Concentrates										
Bakery Byproduct Meal	Conc	4-00-466	84.7	3.71	12.5	0.36	9.5	13.9	6.5	3.8
Barley Grain, rolled	Conc	4-00-528	91.0	3.67	12.4	0.45	2.2	20.8	7.2	2.9
Barley Malt Sprouts	Conc	5-00-545	90.5	2.87	20.1	0.88	2.3	47.0	21.8	7.4
Beet Sugar Pulp, molassed (3%)	Conc	4-00-675	88.0	2.84	10.0	0.42	1.1	44.4	22.4	7.4
Beet Sugar Pulp, unmolassed	Conc	4-00-669	88.3	2.80	10.0	0.44	1.1	45.8	23.1	7.3
Bread, waste	Conc	4-00-466	68.3	3.90	15.0	0.44	2.2	8.9	3.1	2.8
Brewers' Grains, dried	Conc	5-12-024	90.7	2.85	29.2	1.19	5.2	47.4	22.2	4.3
Brewers' Grains, wet	Conc	5-00-517	21.8	2.80	28.4	0.97	5.2	47.1	23.1	4.9
Canola Meal, mech. extract	Conc	5-03-870	90.3	2.94	37.8	2.12	5.4	29.8	20.5	7.4
Cereal Byproduct	Conc	4-00-466	88.5	3.86	9.1	0.37	3.5	10.0	3.9	3.2
Citrus Pulp, dried	Conc	4-01-237	85.8	2.85	6.9	0.18	4.9	24.2	22.2	7.2
Cookie Byproduct	Conc	4-24-852	90.1	3.71	9.7	0.17	10.6	12.7	6.5	3.0
Corn Dry Distiller Grain+sol	Conc	5-28-236	90.2	2.99	29.7	0.67	10.0	38.8	19.7	5.2
Corn Gluten Feed, dried	Conc	5-28-243	89.4	3.40	23.8	0.65	3.5	35.5	12.1	6.8
Corn Gluten Meal, dried	Conc	5-28-242	86.4	3.62	65.0	1.10	2.5	11.1	8.2	3.3
Corn Grain, cracked, dry	Conc	4-02-854	88.1	3.88	9.4	0.27	4.2	9.5	3.4	1.5
Corn Grain, ground, dry	Conc	4-02-854	88.1	3.88	9.1	0.26	4.2	9.5	3.4	1.5
Corn Grain, steam-flaked	Conc	4-02-854	88.1	3.88	9.4	0.29	4.2	9.5	3.4	1.5
Corn Grain+cob, dry ground	Conc	4-02-849	89.2	3.63	8.6	0.22	3.9	21.5	8.0	1.7
Corn, Hominy	Conc	4-02-887	88.5	3.73	11.9	0.44	4.2	21.1	6.2	2.7
Cottonseed Meal, solvent	Conc	5-01-630	90.5	2.98	44.9	1.85	1.9	30.8	19.9	6.7
Fish Meal, anchovy	Conc	5-01-985	92.0	4.07	71.2	5.63	4.6	0.0	0.0	16.0
Fish Meal, menhaden	Conc	5-02-009	91.2	4.07	68.5	5.24	10.4	0.0	0.0	19.7
Linseed Meal, solvent	Conc	5-30-288	90.3	2.85	32.6	1.20	1.7	36.1	22.1	6.5
Molasses, beet sugar	Conc	4-00-668	77.9	4.06	8.5	0.09	0.2	0.1	0.1	11.4
Molasses, sugarcane	Conc	4-04-696	74.3	4.06	5.8	0.06	0.2	0.4	0.2	13.3
Oats, Grain, rolled	Conc	4-03-309	90.0	3.27	13.2	0.55	5.1	30.0	14.6	3.3
Oats, Grain, whole 32/lb per bu	Conc	4-03-318	91.0	3.23	13.6	0.55	4.9	42.0	13.5	5.0
Oats, Grain, whole 38/lb per bu	Conc	4-03-309	89.0	3.33	13.6	0.55	5.2	29.3	13.5	3.3
Peanut Meal, solvent	Conc	5-08-605	92.3	3.33	51.8	1.73	1.4	21.4	13.5	5.8
Potato Byproduct Meal	Conc	4-03-775	35.4	3.16	10.5	0.44	10.8	22.1	16.5	12.8
Rice Bran	Conc	4-03-928	90.6	3.35	15.5	0.72	15.2	26.1	13.1	10.4
Safflower Meal, solvent	Conc	5-04-110	93.5	1.92	29.0	0.92	2.4	53.8	39.1	4.7
Sorghum, Grain, dry rolled	Conc	4-04-380	88.6	3.75	11.6	0.28	3.1	10.9	5.9	2.0
Sorghum, Grain, steam-flaked	Conc	4-04-380	88.6	3.75	11.6	0.28	3.1	10.9	5.9	2.0
Soybean, Meal, expellers	Conc	5-12-820	89.6	3.50	46.3	2.90	8.1	21.7	10.4	5.5
Soybean, Meal, nonenz. brown	Conc	None	89.0	3.55	50.0	2.89	2.3	29.7	9.5	6.8
Soybean, Meal, solv. 44% CP	Conc	5-20-637	89.1	3.52	49.9	3.13	1.6	14.9	10.0	6.6
Soybean, Meal, solv. 48% CP	Conc	5-20-638	89.5	3.73	53.8	3.38	1.1	9.8	6.2	6.4
Soybean, Seeds, whole	Conc	5-04-610	90.0	3.35	39.2	2.34	19.2	19.5	13.1	5.9
Soybean, Seeds, whole heated	Conc	5-04-597	91.0	3.26	43.0	2.57	19.0	22.1	14.7	5.0
Sunflower Meal, solvent	Conc	5-30-032	92.2	2.42	28.4	1.01	1.4	40.3	30.0	7.7
Wheat Bran	Conc	4-05-190	89.1	3.22	17.3	0.70	4.3	42.5	15.5	6.3
Wheat Grain, rolled	Conc	4-13-245	89.4	3.83	14.2	0.40	2.3	13.4	4.4	2.0
Wheat Middlings	Conc	4-05-205	89.5	3.40	18.5	0.67	4.5	36.7	12.1	5.0
Forages										
Alfalfa Meal, 17% CP	Forage	1-00-023	90.3	2.43	19.2	0.83	2.5	41.6	32.8	11.0
Almond Hulls	Forage	4-00-359	86.9	2.89	6.5	0.18	2.9	36.8	28.7	6.1
Barley Silage, headed	Forage	3-00-512	35.5	2.28	12.0	0.28	3.5	56.3	34.5	7.5
Bermudagrass hay, Coastal	Forage	1-20-900	87.1	1.87	10.4	0.36	2.7	73.3	36.8	8.1
Bermudagrass hay, Tifton-85	Forage	1-28-254	87.3	1.86	13.7	0.48	2.7	76.9	36.2	6.5
Corn Silage, immature	Forage	3-28-247	23.5	2.45	9.7	0.25	2.5	54.1	34.1	4.8
Corn Silage, mature	Forage	3-28-249	44.2	2.78	8.5	0.21	3.2	44.5	27.5	4.0
Corn Silage, normal	Forage	3-28-248	35.1	2.75	8.8	0.22	3.2	45.0	28.1	4.3
Corn, Yellow, cobs	Forage	1-28-234	90.8	1.76	3.0	0.08	0.6	86.2	42.2	2.2
Cottonseed, hulls	Forage	1-01-599	89.0	1.69	6.2	0.29	2.5	85.0	64.9	2.8
Cottonseed, whole with lint	Forage	5-01-614	90.1	2.89	23.5	1.02	19.3	50.3	40.1	4.2

Ca % DM	P % DM	Mg % DM	Cl % DM	K % DM	Na % DM	S % DM	Cu mg/kg	I mg/kg	Fe mg/kg	Mn mg/kg	Se mg/kg	Zn mg/kg	Co mg/kg	Vit A	Vit D	Vit E
0.20	0.36	0.13	1.20	0.42	0.72	0.14	5.0		273	30	0.29	46	1.05	7.7		44.9
0.06	0.39	0.14	0.13	0.56	0.02	0.12	6.0	0.05	70	22	0.11	38	0.35			
0.24	0.51	0.18	0.39	1.19	0.04	0.29	9.0		353	49	0.67	65				
0.89	0.09	0.23	0.17	1.11	0.35	0.31	11.3		625	62	0.14	22				
0.91	0.09	0.23	0.18	0.96	0.31	0.30	11.0		642	62	0.14	22				
0.14	0.20	0.05	0.94	0.23	0.85	0.17	4.0		140	10	0.00	16				
0.30	0.67	0.26	0.07	0.50	0.04	0.38	11.0		224	45	1.06	85				
0.35	0.59	0.21	0.12	0.47	0.01	0.33	9.0		247	49	1.06	91				
0.75	1.10	0.53	0.04	1.41	0.07	0.73	5.0		296	62	1.09	61				
0.17	0.29	0.10	0.69	0.33	0.59	0.10	4.0		252	26		80				
1.92	0.12	0.12	0.08	1.10	0.06	0.10	8.0		151	9		11				
0.23	0.29	0.13	1.20	0.46	0.68	0.13	5.0		235	27		38				
0.22	0.83	0.33	0.26	1.10	0.30	0.44	8.0		178	27	0.39	65				
0.07	1.00	0.42	0.20	1.46	0.13	0.44	6.0		196	23	0.19	75				
0.06	0.60	0.14	0.11	0.46	0.05	0.86	4.0		138	15	0.34	49				
0.04	0.30	0.12	0.08	0.42	0.02	0.10	3.0		54	11	0.07	27				
0.04	0.30	0.12	0.08	0.42	0.02	0.10	3.0		54	11	0.07	27				
0.04	0.30	0.12	0.08	0.42	0.02	0.10	3.0		54	11	0.07	27				
0.06	0.29	0.13	0.07	0.49	0.03	0.10	3.0		91	10	0.07	27				
0.03	0.65	0.26	0.10	0.82	0.01	0.12	3.0		87	14	0.10	49				
0.20	1.15	0.61	0.07	1.64	0.07	0.40	14.0		149	24	0.30	67				
4.06	2.69	0.27	0.80	0.79	0.96	0.78	10.0	3.41	234	12	1.47	114				
5.34	3.05	0.20	0.80	0.74	0.68	1.16	7.0	1.19	562	32	2.26	112				
0.40	0.83	0.55	0.00	1.22	0.09	0.37	19.0		369	39	1.05	69				
0.15	0.03	0.29	0.00	6.06	1.48	0.60	22.0		87	66		18				
1.00	0.10	0.42	0.00	4.01	0.22	0.47	66.0	2.10	263	59		21				
0.11	0.40	0.16	0.00	0.52	0.03	0.19	8.0		106	43	0.48	41	0.06			
0.07	0.30	0.16	0.10	0.45	0.06	0.23	6.7	0.13	80	40	0.24	39	0.06	0.2		15
0.01	0.41	0.16	0.10	0.51	0.02	0.21	8.6	0.13	94	40	0.24	41	0.06	0.2		15
0.20	0.64	0.32	0.10	1.32	0.03	0.32	13.0	0.07	302	33	0.21	54				
0.49	0.29	0.11	0.19	1.04	0.26	0.11	11.0		1006	26		25				
0.07	1.78	0.81	0.09	1.57	0.03	0.19	10.0		239	186	0.17	71				
0.38	0.72	0.39	0.00	1.21	0.04	0.32	22.0		319	30		77				
0.07	0.35	0.17	0.06	0.47	0.01	0.11	6.0		89	21	0.46	25				
0.07	0.35	0.17	0.06	0.47	0.01	0.11	6.0		89	21	0.46	25				
0.36	0.66	0.30	0.10	2.12	0.04	0.34	17.0	0.12	169	39		72				
0.39	0.75	0.30	0.00	2.32	0.10	0.40	15.0		111	38		54				
0.40	0.71	0.31	0.13	2.22	0.04	0.46	22.0		185	35	0.14	57				
0.35	0.70	0.29	0.13	2.41	0.03	0.39	16.0		206	40	0.13	58				
0.32	0.60	0.25	0.04	1.99	0.01	0.31	13.0		148	29	0.11	49				
0.26	0.64	0.25	0.06	1.99	0.01	0.32	15.0		142	29	0.28	48				
0.48	1.00	0.63	0.12	1.50	0.04	0.39	32.0		298	45	0.50	88				
0.13	1.18	0.53	0.16	1.32	0.04	0.21	11.0		157	122	0.50	85				
0.05	0.43	0.15	0.11	0.50	0.01	0.15	5.0		72	42	0.28	40				
0.16	1.02	0.42	0.10	1.38	0.03	0.18	10.0		158	125	0.46	91				
1.47	0.28	0.29	0.65	2.37	0.10	0.26	9.0	0.16	619	44	0.36	28	0.31			
0.28	0.13	0.13	0.03	2.62	0.02	0.04	7.0		247	22	0.07	22				
0.48	0.30	0.18	0.72	2.43	0.13	0.17	7.0		343	43	0.12	30	0.72			
0.49	0.27	0.19	0.67	1.80	0.17	0.48	8.0		224	62		32				
0.39	0.22	0.15	0.54	1.40	0.14	0.38	8.0		224	62		32				
0.29	0.24	0.19	0.30	1.30	0.01	0.14	6.2		157	46	0.04	29				
0.26	0.25	0.16	0.17	1.10	0.01	0.10	5.5		92	36	0.04	23				
0.28	0.26	0.17	0.29	1.20	0.01	0.14	5.7		104	36	0.04	24				
0.10	0.06	0.06	0.00	0.90	0.04	0.07	6.0		254	5	0.08	11				
0.18	0.12	0.17	0.06	1.16	0.02	0.07	5.0		68	22	0.00	17				
0.17	0.60	0.37	0.06	1.13	0.02	0.23	7.0		94	18	0.14	37				

TABLE 16-6 continued

Feed Name	Energy Class	IFN	DM % as Fed	DE(1) Mcal/kg DM	CP % DM	Lys % DM	Fat % DM	NDF % DM	ADF % DM	Ash % DM
Grass Hay, cool season, mature	Forage	1-02-244	84.4	2.04	10.8	0.38	2.0	69.1	41.6	7.0
Grass Hay, cool season, immature	Forage	1-02-212	84.0	2.36	18.0	0.63	3.3	49.6	31.4	9.2
Grass Hay, cool season, mid-mat.	Forage	1-02-243	83.8	2.18	13.3	0.46	2.5	57.7	36.9	8.8
Grass Pasture, cool season, veg.	Forage	2-02-260	20.1	2.39	26.5	0.92	2.7	45.8	25.0	9.8
Grass Silage, cool season, immature	Forage	3-02-217	36.2	2.30	16.8	0.55	2.8	51.0	32.9	9.9
Grass Silage, cool season, mature	Forage	3-02-219	38.7	1.98	12.7	0.43	3.0	66.6	41.1	8.0
Grass Silage, cool season, mid-mat.	Forage	3-02-218	42.0	2.16	16.8	0.55	2.4	58.2	35.2	8.7
Legume Forage Hay, immature	Forage	1-07-792	84.2	2.62	20.5	1.05	2.1	36.3	28.6	9.5
Legume Forage Hay, mature	Forage	1-07-789	83.8	2.21	17.8	0.89	1.6	50.9	39.5	9.2
Legume Forage Hay, mid-mat.	Forage	1-07-788	83.9	2.43	20.8	1.06	2.0	42.9	33.4	9.4
Legume Forage Pasture, veg.	Forage	2-29-431	21.4	2.71	26.5	1.37	3.7	33.1	23.9	10.0
Legume Forage Silage, mid-mat.	Forage	3-07-797	42.9	2.35	21.9	0.97	2.2	43.2	35.2	10.8
Legume Forage Silage, immat.	Forage	3-07-795	41.2	2.52	23.2	1.04	2.3	36.7	30.2	11.1
Legume Forage Silage, mature	Forage	3-07-798	42.6	2.19	20.3	0.87	2.1	50.0	40.9	10.3
Mix Grass+Leg. Hay, mid-mat.	Forage	1-02-277	85.3	2.30	18.4	0.79	2.3	50.8	35.8	9.3
Mix Grass+Leg. Sil., immature	Forage	3-02-302	45.9	2.39	20.3	0.78	2.3	45.3	30.8	9.8
Mix Grass+Leg. Sil., mature	Forage	3-02-266	42.8	2.07	17.4	0.67	2.3	57.4	42.1	9.6
Mix Grass+Leg. Sil., mid-mat.	Forage	3-02-265	44.1	2.25	19.1	0.74	2.5	50.4	35.4	10.1
Mix Grass+Legume Hay, mature	Forage	1-02-280	89.7	2.11	18.2	0.77	2.0	56.0	40.1	9.9
Mix Grass+Legume Hay, immat.	Forage	1-02-275	83.1	2.46	19.7	0.85	2.5	45.4	30.8	8.8
Mostly Grass Hay, immature	Forage	1-02-275	84.3	2.35	18.4	0.72	2.4	49.6	31.5	9.2
Mostly Grass Hay, mature	Forage	1-02-280	84.7	2.08	13.3	0.51	2.3	62.5	42.1	7.9
Mostly Grass Hay, mid-mat.	Forage	1-02-277	87.3	2.19	17.4	0.68	2.6	55.1	36.4	9.5
Mostly Grass Silage, mid-mat.	Forage	3-02-265	44.5	2.19	17.6	0.63	2.9	54.5	35.7	9.5
Mostly Grass Silage, immat.	Forage	3-02-302	47.1	2.34	18.0	0.64	2.9	49.9	31.8	9.1
Mostly Grass Silage, mature	Forage	3-02-266	38.5	2.01	15.4	0.55	2.6	61.7	42.2	9.0
Mostly Legume Hay, immature	Forage	1-02-275	83.8	2.49	20.5	0.97	2.0	41.7	30.5	9.2
Mostly Legume Hay, mature	Forage	1-02-280	84.3	2.20	17.2	0.80	1.7	53.6	41.5	8.7
Mostly Legume Hay, mid-mat.	Forage	1-02-277	84.2	2.35	19.1	0.90	2.0	47.2	35.4	9.1
Mostly Legume Silage, immature	Forage	3-02-302	43.2	2.38	20.0	0.84	2.2	42.2	31.1	11.5
Mostly Legume Silage, mid-mat.	Forage	3-02-265	43.3	2.27	19.0	0.78	2.1	47.0	35.4	10.8
Mostly Legume Silage, mature	Forage	3-02-266	42.9	2.11	18.3	0.74	2.0	53.7	41.6	10.2
Oats, Hay, headed	Forage	1-09-099	85.0	2.16	9.1	0.32	2.2	58.0	36.4	8.5
Oats, Silage, headed	Forage	3-21-843	34.6	2.04	12.9	0.46	3.4	60.6	38.9	9.8
Rye, Annual, Silage, veg.	Forage	3-21-853	29.7	2.12	16.1	0.38	3.8	57.8	34.9	9.6
Sorghum, Grain Type, Silage	Forage	3-22-371	28.8	2.17	9.1	0.24	2.9	60.7	38.7	7.5
Sorghum, Sudan Type, Hay	Forage	1-04-480	86.5	2.00	9.4	0.33	2.3	64.8	40.0	8.7
Sorghum, Sudan Type, Silage	Forage	3-04-499	28.8	1.95	10.8	0.36	3.6	63.3	40.7	10.9
Soybean, hulls	Forage	1-04-560	90.9	2.25	13.9	0.87	2.7	60.3	44.6	4.8
Soybean, Silage, early mat.	Forage	3-04-579	40.4	2.26	17.4	0.78	5.7	46.6	36.9	12.2
Triticale Silage, headed	Forage	3-26-208	32.0	2.07	13.8	0.25	3.8	59.7	39.6	9.7
Wheat Hay, headed	Forage	1-05-170	86.1	2.14	9.4	0.40	1.7	61.1	38.1	6.7
Wheat Silage, early head	Forage	3-21-865	33.3	2.11	12.0	0.51	3.2	59.9	37.6	8.6
Fats and oils										
Hydrol. Tallow Fatty Acids	High-fat	4-00-376	99.8	9.12	0.0	0.00	99.2	0.0	0.0	0
Partial Hydrogenated Tallow	High-fat	None	100.0	9.15	0.0	0.00	99.5	0.0	0.0	0
Tallow	High-fat	4-25-306	99.8	9.18	0.0	0.00	99.8	0.0	0.0	0
Vegetable Oil	High-fat	4-05-077	100.0	9.19	0.0	0.00	99.9	0.0	0.0	0

[a]Calculations of energy values are dependent on energy class and are detemined as follows:

Concentrates: DE = 4.07 − 0.055 ADF

Forages: DE = 2.118 + 0.01218 CP − 0.00937 ADF − 0.00383 (NDF − ADF) + 0.04718 EE + 0.02035 NFC − 0.0262 Ash (where NFC = 100 − %NDF − %CP − %EE − %Ash)

Fats and oils: DE = (−3.6 + 0.211 CP + 0.421 EE + 0.015 CF) / 4.184.

Ca % DM	P % DM	Mg % DM	Cl % DM	K % DM	Na % DM	S % DM	Cu mg/kg	I mg/kg	Fe mg/kg	Mn mg/kg	Se mg/kg	Zn mg/kg	Co mg/kg	VitA	VitD	VitE
0.47	0.26	0.18	0.66	1.97	0.02	0.17	8.0		180	90	0.06	25				
0.72	0.34	0.23	0.42	2.57	0.03	0.24	9.0		199	84	0.06	27				
0.66	0.29	0.23	0.92	2.13	0.08	0.24	9.0		194	72	0.06	25				
0.56	0.44	0.20	0.56	3.36	0.02	0.20	10.0		275	75		36				
0.57	0.36	0.22	0.67	3.11	0.05	0.21	9.0		280	56	0.09	31				
0.56	0.31	0.20	0.89	2.42	0.05	0.20	9.0		327	90	0.09	30				
0.60	0.36	0.21	0.67	2.78	0.05	0.21	9.0		275	79	0.09	31				
1.56	0.31	0.33	0.55	2.56	0.03	0.33	10.0		213	49	0.20	26	0.65			
1.22	0.28	0.27	0.48	2.38	0.02	0.23	9.0		250	44	0.20	24	0.65			
1.37	0.30	0.30	0.61	2.45	0.02	0.31	9.0		207	46	0.20	24	0.65			
1.31	0.37	0.28	0.60	3.21	0.01	0.31	10.0		215	54	0.20	33	0.44			
1.36	0.35	0.28	0.61	3.00	0.02	0.28	9.0		395	64	0.18	30	0.65			
1.39	0.36	0.30	0.55	3.03	0.03	0.30	9.0		401	67	0.18	31	0.65			
1.30	0.33	0.26	0.48	2.87	0.02	0.28	9.0		403	63	0.18	29	0.65			
1.04	0.32	0.25	0.80	2.59	0.03	0.24	9.0		197	59	0.12	25				
1.08	0.35	0.28	1.77	2.89	0.01	0.16	9.0		328	71	0.14	29				
1.06	0.33	0.24	0.52	2.70	0.02	0.31	9.0		262	72	0.14	30				
1.09	0.35	0.27	1.10	2.80	0.01	0.26	9.0		252	71	0.14	31				
0.97	0.37	0.26	0.93	2.24	0.01	0.28	9.0		403	75	0.12	27				
1.20	0.31	0.29	0.50	3.06	0.07	0.27	10.0		160	59	0.12	24				
1.01	0.31	0.26	0.74	2.83	0.03	0.28	9.0		117	53	0.09	25				
0.73	0.27	0.21	0.71	2.09	0.10	0.29	8.0		124	74	0.09	24				
0.88	0.36	0.25	0.77	2.45	0.01	0.27	9.0		358	75	0.09	26				
0.89	0.36	0.26	0.45	2.64	0.01	0.25	9.0		264	78	0.11	30				
1.02	0.34	0.25	0.74	2.88	0.03	0.27	9.0		234	74	0.11	27				
0.85	0.33	0.23	0.90	2.50	0.10	0.34	9.0		241	73	0.11	28				
1.30	0.30	0.30	0.60	2.41	0.03	0.20	10.0		167	58	0.15	24				
1.09	0.28	0.25	0.21	2.23	0.01	0.26	8.0		141	43	0.15	24				
1.17	0.30	0.27	0.43	2.34	0.08	0.26	9.0		141	49	0.15	24				
1.16	0.36	0.30	0.60	2.95	0.01	0.32	11.0		279	70	0.17	36				
1.14	0.34	0.28	0.60	2.88	0.01	0.25	9.0		244	64	0.17	28				
1.17	0.33	0.26	0.60	2.77	0.03	0.26	9.0		339	66	0.17	29				
0.37	0.22	0.17	1.08	2.01	0.33	0.14	8.0		250	59		23				
0.52	0.31	0.20	1.34	2.89	0.24	0.19	9.0		500	66		29				
0.43	0.42	0.16	0.90	3.34	0.05	0.20	9.0		373	63		32				
0.50	0.21	0.27	0.60	1.75	0.02	0.12	9.0		392	65	0.03	31				
0.54	0.20	0.32	1.16	2.36	0.03	0.13	10.0		284	44		34				
0.64	0.24	0.31	0.56	2.57	0.03	0.15	11.0		990	79		33				
0.63	0.17	0.25	0.05	1.51	0.01	0.12	10.0		604	26	0.21	35	0.12			
1.07	0.37	0.35	0.00	2.25	0.01	0.22	14.0		656	75		42				
0.57	0.33	0.19	0.00	3.01	0.05	0.21	7.0		404	66		37				
0.31	0.20	0.13	0.38	1.71	0.06	0.13	8.0		319	62		25				
0.38	0.29	0.16	0.83	2.28	0.07	0.17	7.0		391	72		27				
0.00	0.00	0.00	0.00	0.00	0.00	0.00										
0.00	0.00	0.00	0.00	0.00	0.00	0.00										
0.00	0.00	0.00	0.00	0.00	0.00	0.00										
0.00	0.00	0.00	0.00	0.00	0.00	0.00										

TABLE 16-7 Compositions of Inorganic Mineral Sources on a 100% Dry Matter Basis

Mineral Element Content	International Feed No.[a]	Dry Matter[b]	Crude Protein Equivalent (CPE) = N% × 6.25	Primary Mineral Element Source
Calcium Sources		(DM%)	(CPE%)	Ca (%)
Bone meal, steamed, fg[c]	6-00-400	97	13.2	30.71
Calcium carbonate, $CaCO_3$, fg	6-01-069	100	—[d]	39.39
Calcium chloride anhydrous, $CaCl_2$, cp[e] *	NA[f]	100	—	36.11
Calcium chloride dihydrate, $CaCl_2 \cdot 2H_2O$, cp *	NA	100	—	27.53
Calcium hydroxide, $Ca(OH)_2$, cp	NA	100	—	54.09
Calcium oxide, CaO, cp *	NA	100	—	71.47
Calcium phosphate (monobasic), $Ca(H_2PO_4)_2$, from defluorinated phosphoric acid, fg	6-01-082	97	—	16.40
Calcium sulfate dihydrate, $CaSO_4 \cdot 2H_2O$, cp	6-01-089	97	—	23.28
Curacao, phosphate, fg	6-05-586	99	—	34.34
Dicalcium phosphate (dibasic), $CaHPO_4$, from defluorinated phosphoric acid, fg	6-01-080	97	—	22.00
Dolomitic limestone (magnesium), fg	6-02-633	99	—	22.30
Limestone, ground, fg	6-02-632	100	—	34.00
Magnesium oxide, MgO, fg	6-02-756	98	—	3.07
Oystershell, flour (ground), fg	6-03-481	99	—	38.00
Phosphate, defluorinated, fg	6-01-780	100	—	32.00
Phosphate rock, fg	6-03-945	100	—	35.00
Phosphate rock, low-fluorine, fg	6-03-946	100	—	36.00
Soft rock phosphate colloidal clay, fg	6-03-947	100	—	17.00
Phosphorus Sources		(DM%)	(CPE%)	P (%)
Ammonium phosphate (dibasic), $(NH_4)_2HPO_4$, fg	6-00-370	97	115.9	20.60
Ammonium phosphate (monobasic), $(NH_4)H_2PO_4$, fg	6-09-338	97	70.9	24.74
Bone meal, steamed, fg	6-00-400	97	13.2	12.86
Calcium phosphate (monobasic), $Ca(H_2PO_4)_2$, from defluorinated phosphoric acid, fg	6-01-082	97	—	21.60
Curacao, phosphate, fg	6-05-586	99	—	14.14
Dicalcium phosphate (dibasic), $CaHPO_4$, from defluorinated phosphoric acid, fg	6-01-080	97	—	19.30
Phosphate, defluorinated, fg	6-01-780	100	—	18.00
Phosphate rock, fg	6-03-945	100	—	13.00
Phosphate rock, low-fluorine, fg	6-03-946	100	—	14.00
Phosphoric acid, $-H_3PO_4$, fg *	6-03-707	75	—	31.60
Sodium phosphate (monobasic) monohydrate, $NaH_2PO_4 \cdot H_2O$, fg	6-04-288	97	—	22.50
Sodium tripolyphosphate (meta- and pyro-phosphate), $Na_5P_3O_{10}$, fg	6-08-076	96	—	25.00
Soft rock phosphate, colloidal clay, fg	6-03-947	100	—	9.00
Sodium Sources		(DM%)	(CPE%)	Na (%)
Bone meal, steamed, fg	6-00-400	97	13.2	5.69
Phosphate, defluorinated, fg	6-01-780	100	—	4.90
Potassium chloride, KCl, fg	6-03-755	100	—	1.00
Sodium bicarbonate, $NaHCO_3$, fg	6-04-272	100	—	27.00
Sodium carbonate monohydrate, $Na_2CO_3 \cdot H_2O$, cp	NA	100	—	37.08
Sodium chloride, NaCl, fg	6-04-152	100	—	39.34
Sodium phosphate (monobasic) monohydrate, $NaH_2PO_4 \cdot H_2O$, fg	6-04-288	97	—	16.68
Sodium selenate decahydrate, $Na_2SeO_4 \cdot 10H_2O$, cp	NA	100	—	12.46
Sodium selenite, Na_2SeO_3, fg	6-26-013	98	—	26.60
Sodium sesquicarbonate dihydrate, $Na_2CO_3 + NaHCO_3 \cdot 2H_2O$, fg	NA	100	—	30.50
Sodium sulfate decahydrate, $Na_2SO_4 \cdot 10H_2O$, cp	6-04-292	97	—	14.27
Sodium tripolyphosphate (meta- and pyro-phosphate), $Na_5P_3O_{10}$, fg	6-08-076	96	—	31.00
Chloride Sources		(DM%)	(CPE%)	Cl (%)
Ammonium chloride, cp	NA	100	163.63	66.28
Calcium chloride anhydrous, $CaCl_2$, cp *	NA	100	—	63.89
Calcium chloride dihydrate, $CaCl_2 \cdot 2H_2O$, cp *	NA	100	—	48.23
Cobalt dichloride hexahydrate, $CoCl_2 \cdot 6H_2O$, cp	NA	100	—	29.80
Cupric chloride dihydrate, $CuCl_2 \cdot 2H_2O$, cp	NA	100	—	41.65

TABLE 16-7 continued

Mineral Element Content	International Feed No.[a]	Dry Matter[b]	Crude Protein Equivalent (CPE) = N% × 6.25	Primary Mineral Element Source
Magnesium chloride hexahydrate, $MgCl_2 \cdot 6H_2O$, cp	NA	100	—	34.88
Manganese dichloride, $MnCl_2$, cp	NA	100	—	56.34
Manganese chloride tetrahydrate, $MnCl_2 \cdot 4H_2O$, cp	NA	100	—	35.80
Potassium chloride, KCl, fg	6–03–755	100	—	47.30
Sodium chloride, NaCl, fg	6–04–152	100	—	60.66
Zinc chloride, $ZnCl_2$, cp	NA	100	—	52.03
Potassium Sources		(DM%)	(CPE%)	K (%)
Potassium bicarbonate, $KHCO_3$, cp	6–29–493	99	—	39.05
Potassium carbonate, K_2CO_3, cp	NA	100	—	56.58
Potassium chloride, KCl, fg	6–03–755	100	—	50.00
Potassium iodide, KI, fg	6–03–759	100	—	21.00
Potassium sulfate, K_2SO_4, fg	6–06–098	98	—	41.84
Magnesium Sources		(DM%)	(CPE%)	Mg (%)
Dolomitic limestone (magnesium), fg	6–02–633	99	—	9.99
Limestone, ground, fg	6–02–632	100	—	2.06
Magnesium carbonate, $MgCO_3$, fg	6–02–754	98	—	30.81
Magnesium chloride hexahydrate, $MgCl_2 \cdot 6H_2O$, cp	NA	100	—	11.96
Magnesium hydroxide, $Mg(OH)_2$, cp	NA	100	—	41.69
Magnesium oxide, MgO, fg	6–02–756	98	—	56.20
Magnesium sulfate heptahydrate, $MgSO_4 \cdot 7H_2O$, fg	6–02–758	98	—	9.80
Sulfur Sources		(DM%)	(CPE%)	S (%)
Ammonium phosphate (dibasic), $(NH_4)_2HPO_4$, fg	6–00–370	97	115.9	2.16
Ammonium phosphate (monobasic), $(NH_4)H_2PO_4$, fg	6–09–338	97	70.9	1.46
Ammonium sulfate, $(NH_4)_2SO_4$, fg	6–09–339	100	134.1	24.10
Bone meal, steamed, fg	6–00–400	97	13.2	2.51
Calcium phosphate (monobasic), $Ca(H_2PO_4)_2$, from defluorinated phosphoric acid, fg	6–01–082	97	—	1.22
Calcium sulfate, dihydrate $CaSO_4 \cdot 2H_2O$, fg	6–01–089	97	—	18.62
Cupric sulfate pentahydrate, $CuSO_4 \cdot 5H_2O$	6–01–720	100	—	12.84
Dicalcium phosphate (dibasic), $CaHPO_4$, from defluorinated phosphoric acid, fg	6–01–080	97	—	1.14
Ferrous sulfate heptahydrate, $FeSO_4 \cdot 7H_2O$, fg	6–20–734	98	—	12.35
Magnesium sulfate heptahydrate, $MgSO_4 \cdot 7H_2O$, fg	NA	98	—	13.31
Manganese sulfate monohydrate, $MnSO_4 \cdot H_2O$, cp	NA	100	—	18.97
Manganese sulfate pentahydrate, $MnSO_4 \cdot 5H_2O$, cp	NA	100	—	13.30
Phosphoric acid, $-H_3PO_4$, fg *	6–03–707	75	—	1.55
Potassium sulfate, K_2SO_4, fg	6–06–098	98	—	17.35
Sodium sulfate decahydrate, $Na_2SO_4 \cdot 10H_2O$, cp	6–04–292	97	—	9.95
Zinc sulfate monohydrate, $ZnSO_4 \cdot H_2O$, fg	6–05–555	99	—	17.68
Cobalt Sources		(DM%)	(CPE%)	Co (mg/kg)
Cobalt carbonate, $CoCO_3$, fg	6–01–566	99	—	460,000
Cobalt carbonate hexahydrate, $CoCO_3 \cdot 6H_2O$, cp	NA	100	—	259,000
Cobalt dichloride hexahydrate, $CoCl_2 \cdot 6H_2O$, cp	NA	100	—	247,800
Copper (Cupric) Sources		(DM%)	(CPE%)	Cu (mg/kg)
Cupric chloride dihydrate, $CuCl_2 \cdot 2H_2O$, cp	NA	100	—	372,000
Cupric oxide, CuO, cp	NA	100	—	798,800
Cupric sulfate pentahydrate, $CuSO_4 \cdot 5H_2O$, cp	6–01–720	100	—	254,500
Iodine Sources		(DM%)	(CPE%)	I (mg/kg)
Ethylenediaminodihydroiodide (EDDI), fg	6–01–842	98	—	803,400
Potassium iodide, KI, fg	6–03–759	100	—	681,700
Iron Sources		(DM%)	(CPE%)	Fe (mg/kg)
Ammonium phosphate (dibasic), $(NH_4)_2HPO_4$, fg	6–00–370	97	115.9	12,400

TABLE 16-7 continued

Mineral Element Content	International Feed No.[a]	Dry Matter[b]	Crude Protein Equivalent (CPE) = N% × 6.25	Primary Mineral Element Source
Ammonium phosphate (monobasic), $(NH_4)H_2PO_4$, fg	6-09-338	97	70.9	17,400
Bone meal, steamed, fg	6-00-400	97	13.2	26,700
Calcium phosphate (monobasic), $Ca(H_2PO_4)_2$, from defluorinated phosphoric acid, fg	6-01-082	97	—	15,800
Dicalcium phosphate (dibasic), $CaHPO_4$, from defluorinated phosphoric acid, fg	6-01-080	97	—	14,400
Ferrous sulfate heptahydrate, $FeSO_4 \cdot 7H_2O$, fg	6-20-734	98	—	218,400
Phosphate rock, fg	6-03-945	100	—	16,800
Phosphoric acid, $-H_3PO_4$, fg *	6-03-707	75	—	17,500
Soft rock phosphate, colloidal clay, fg	6-03-947	100	—	19,000
Manganese (Manganous) Sources		(DM%)	(CPE%)	Mn (mg/kg)
Manganese carbonate, $MnCO_3$, cp	6-03-036	97	—	478,000
Manganese chloride, $MnCl_2$, cp	NA	100	—	430,000
Manganese chloride tetrahydrate, $MnCl_2 \cdot 4H_2O$, cp	NA	100	—	277,000
Manganese oxide, MnO, cp	6-03-056	99	—	774,500
Manganese sulfate monohydrate, $MnSO_4 \cdot H_2O$, cp	NA	100	—	325,069
Manganese sulfate pentahydrate, $MnSO_4 \cdot 5H_2O$, cp	NA	100	—	227,891
Selenium Sources		(DM%)	(CPE%)	Se(mg/kg)
Sodium selenate decahydrate, $Na_2SeO_4 \cdot 10H_2O$, cp	NA	100	—	213,920
Sodium selenite, Na_2SeO_3, cp	6-26-013	98	—	456,000
Zinc Sources		(DM%)	(CPE%)	Zn (mg/kg)
Zinc carbonate, $ZnCO_3$, cp	NA	100	—	521,400
Zinc chloride, $ZnCl_2$, cp	NA	100	—	479,700
Zinc oxide, ZnO, cp	6-05-533	100	—	780,000
Zinc sulfate monohydrate, $ZnSO_4 \cdot H_2O$, fg	6-05-555	99	—	363,600
Fluorine Sources			(CPE%)	Fl (mg/kg)
Ammonium phosphate (dibasic), $(NH_4)_2HPO_4$, fg	6-00-370	97	115.9	2,100
Ammonium phosphate (monobasic), $(NH_4)H_2PO_4$, fg	6-09-338	97	70.9	2,500
Calcium phosphate (monobasic), $Ca(H_2PO_4)_2$, from defluorinated phosphoric acid, fg	6-01-082	97	—	2,100
Curacao, phosphate, fg	6-05-586	99	—	5,550
Dicalcium phosphate (dibasic), $CaHPO_4$, from defluorinated phosphoric acid, fg	6-01-080	97	—	1,800
Phosphate, defluorinated, fg	6-01-780	100	—	1,800
Phosphate rock, fg	6-03-945	100	—	35,000
Phosphoric acid, H_3PO_4, fg *	6-03-707	75	—	3,100
Soft rock phosphate, colloidal clay, fg	6-03-947	100	—	15,000

NOTE: The compositions of hydrated mineral sources (e.g., $CaSO_4 \cdot 2H_2O$) are shown including the waters of hydration. Mineral element compositions of feed-grade sources vary by source, processing method, site of mining, and manufacturer. Sources should be analyzed or manufacturer's analyses should be used when available. Element composition of a source is listed if specific element concentration is ≥ 1.0 percent for macromineral elements, or ≥ 10,000 mg/kg for micromineral elements, except for fluorine concentrations, which are listed because of potential toxicity.

[a] First digit denotes the class of feed: 1, dry forages and roughages; 2, pastured, range plants, and forages fed green; 3, silages; 4, energy feeds; 5, protein supplement; 6, minerals; 7, vitamins; 8, additives. The other five digits identify the individual feed.
[b] Dry matter contents have been estimated for the sources; actual analysis will be more accurate.
[c] fg = Feed-grade source.
[d] None present.
[e] cp = Chemically pure form.
[f] NA = Not available.
*Use caution when handling and mixing, can be extremely hazardous.

TABLE 16-8 Research Findings on Composition of Mare's Milk (1989 NRC)

Time After Foaling	Number of Animals	Total Solids (%)	Energy (kcal/100 g)	Protein (%)	Fat (%)	Lactose (%)	Ca	P	Mg	K	Na	Cu	Zn	References
							\multicolumn{8}{c}{Concentrations (μg/g of fluid milk)}	
1–4 weeks	10	11.6	59	3.1	2.1	5.9	1,212	433	88	773	246	0.46	3.2	Ullrey et al. (1966, 1974)
5–8 weeks	10	11.1	55	2.5	1.9	5.9	1,008	305	56	505	196	0.24	2.5	
9–17 weeks	10	10.2	50	2.0	1.3	6.5	661	230	41	388	168	0.22	2.2	
1–4 weeks	5	11.1	56	2.3	1.6	6.8	1,223	811	101	586	194	0.62	2.6	Schryver et al. (1986a,b)
5–8 weeks	5	10.5	50	1.9	1.3	6.9	894	596	66	420	167	0.38	1.9	Oftedal et al. (1983)
9–17 weeks	2						786	557	49	370	137	0.21	1.8	
1–4 weeks	14	10.9		2.5	1.5									Gibbs et al. (1982)
5–8 weeks	14	10.5		2.1	1.4									
9–21 weeks	14	10.2		1.9	1.0									
2–12 weeks	22[a]	10.4	45	2.2	0.8	6.6	1,220	660						Pagan and Hintz (1986)
1–10 weeks	5[a]						857	418	77	380	127	0.37	1.7	Schryver et al. (1986a)
1–4 weeks	20											0.17	1.8	Breedveld et al. (1987)
5–8 weeks	20											0.17	1.8	
1–4 weeks	20	9.8					915	502	85			0.32	2.2	Baucus et al. (1987)
1 week	6[a]	9.8		3.1	1.6									Lukas et al. (1972)
6 weeks	6[a]	9.6		2.1	1.4									
18 weeks	6[a]	9.8		1.9	1.8									
1–4 weeks	5	11.6		2.5	2.0		1,240	780						Bouwman and van der Schee (1978)
1–12 weeks	28	10.4		2.0	1.6					887	203			Meadows et al. (1979)
	24	11.2	47	2.6	1.9	6.2	1,179	926						Neseni et al. (1958)
6–8 weeks	3[a]			2.1	1.4	6.9								Anwer et al. (1975)
	10			3.3	1.6	6.2								Doreau et al. (1986)
	Review[b]	10.0		2.1	1.3	6.2	1,050	715		685	170			Neuhaus (1959)
Day 10	26	11.0		3.1	1.9	6.4								Smoczynski and Tomczynski (1982)
Average of 6-month lactation	110			2.0	1.4	6.1		394	29			0.25	0.9	Kulisa (1986)
Average of 6-month lactation		10.2		1.9	1.6	6.6								Fedotov and Akimbekov (1983)
Average of 6-month lactation	25			2.0	1.6	6.4								Duisembaev and Akimbekov (1982)

continued

TABLE 16-8 continued

Time After Foaling	Number of Animals	Total Solids (%)	Energy (kcal/100 g)	Protein (%)	Fat (%)	Lactose (%)	Concentrations (µg/g of fluid milk)							References
							Ca	P	Mg	K	Na	Cu	Zn	
Summary														
1–4 weeks		10.7	58	2.7	1.8	6.2	1,200	725	90	700	225	0.45	2.5	
5–8 weeks		10.5	53	2.2	1.7	6.4	1,000	600	60	500	190	0.26	2.0	
9–21 weeks		10.0	50	1.8	1.4	6.5	800	500	45	400	150	0.20	1.8	

[a]Ponies.
[b]Review of many studies; values are averages obtained from Neuhaus (1959).

REFERENCES FOR MILK COMPOSITION TABLE

Anwer, M.S., R. Cronwall, W. E. Chapman, and R. D. Klenz. 1975. Glucose utilization and contribution to milk components in lactating ponies. J. Anim. Sci. 41:568–571.

Baucus, K. L., S. L. Ralston, G. Rich, and E. L. Squires. 1987. The effect of dietary copper and zinc supplementation on composition of mares milk. Pp. 179–184 in Proc. 10th Equine Nutr. Physiol. Soc. Symp., Fort Collins, CO.

Bouwman, H., and W. van der Schee. 1978. Composition and production of milk from Dutch warmblooded saddle horse mares. Z. Tierphysiol. Tierernaehr. Futtermittelk. 40:39–53.

Breedveld, L., S. G. Jackson, and J. P. Baker. 1987. The determination of a relationship between copper, zinc, and selenium levels in mares and those in the foals. Pp. 159–164 in Proc. 10th Equine Nutr. Physiol. Soc. Symp., Fort Collins, CO.

Doreau, M., S. Boulot, W. Martin-Rosset, and H. DuBroeucq. 1986. Milking lactating mares using oxytocin: milk volume and composition. Reprod. Nutr. Dev. 26:1–11.

Duisembaev, K. I., and B. R. Akimbekov. 1982. Variation of milk yield and its relationship with milk composition of mares at a koumiss farm. Sbornik Nauchnykh Trudov. Kazakhskii Nauchno-Issledovatel'skii Teknological Institut Ovtsevodstva (as cited in J. Dairy Sci. 46:1984) (Abstr.).

Fedotov, P., and B. Akimbekov. 1983. Increasing milk production of Kushum mares. Konevodstvo I KonnyiSport. (11):6–7 (as cited in J. Dairy Sci. 46:264) (Abstr.).

Gibbs, P. G., G. D. Potter, R. W. Bake, and W. C. McMullan. 1982. Milk production of quarter horse mares during 150 days of lactation. J. Anim. Sci. 54:496–499.

Kulisa, M. 1986. Some components of mare milk. Paper presented at 37th Annu. Meet. Eur. Asoc. Anim. Prod., Budapest, Hungary, September 1–4, 1986. Summaries, vol. 2. Commission on horse production (as cited in J. Dairy Sci. 49:806) (Abstr.).

Lukas, V. K., W. W. Albert, F. N. Owens, and A. Peters. 1972. Lactation of Shetland mares. J. Anim. Sci. 34:350 (Abstr.).

Meadows, D. G., G. D. Potter, W. B. Thomas, J. Hesby, and J. G. Anderson. 1979. Foal growth, milk production and milk composition from mares fed combinations of soybean meal and urea supplements. J. Anim. Sci. 49(Suppl. 1):247.

Neseni, R., E. Flade, G. Heidler, and H. Steger. 1958. Milcheistung und Milchzusammensetzung von Stuten im Verlaufe der Laktation. Arc. Tierzucht. 1:91–129.

Neuhaus, U. 1959. Milch und Milchgewinnung von Pferdestuten. Z. Tierzucht. 73:370.

Oftedal, O. T., H. F. Hintz, and H. F. Schryver. 1983. Lactation in the horse: milk composition and intake by foals. J. Nutr. 113:2096–2106.

Pagan, J. D., and H. F. Hintz. 1986. Composition of milk from pony mares fed various levels of digestive energy. Cornell Vet. 76:139–148.

Schryver, H. F., O. T. Oftedal, J. Williams, N. F. Cymbaluk, D. Antczak, and H. F. Hintz. 1986a. A comparison of the mineral composition of milk of domestic and captive wild equids (E. przewalski, E. zebra, E. burchelli, E. caballus, E. asinus). Comp. Biochem. Physiol. 85A:233–235.

Schryver, H. F., O. T. Oftedal, J. Williams, L. V. Soderholm, and H. F. Hintz. 1986b. Lactation in the horse: the mineral composition of mare milk. J. Nutr. 116:2142–2147.

Smoczynski, S., and R. Tomczynski. 1982. Composition of mare's milk. I. The first 10 days of lactation. Badania skladu chemicznego mleka klaczy. I. Pierwsze dziesiec dni laktacji. Zeszyty Naukowe Adademii. Rolniczo-Technicznej w Olsztynie, Technologia Zywnosci. 17:77–83 (as cited in J. Dairy Sci. 45:777) (Abstr.).

Ullrey, D. E., R. D. Struthers, D. G. Henricks, and B. E. Brent. 1966. Composition of mare's milk. J. Anim. Sci. 25:217–222.

Ullrey, D. E., E. T. Ely, and R. L. Covert. 1974. Iron, zinc, and copper in mare's milk. J. Anim. Sci. 38:1276–1277.

TABLE 16-9 Research Findings on Composition of Mare's Milk (Since 1989 NRC)

Time After Foaling	Number of Animals	Total Solids (%)	Energy (kcal/100 g)	Protein (%)	Fat (%)	Lactose (%)	Ca	P	Mg	K	Na	Cu	Zn	References
							\multicolumn{7}{c	}{Concentrations (μg/g of fluid milk)}	
2–5 d	29			4.1	2.1		953	638	86	709	177	0.25	2.1	Csapo et al. (1995);
8–45 d	29			2.3	1.3		823	499	66	517	167	0.23	2.0	Csapo-Kiss et al. (1995);
10 d	18	9.2		2.3	1.1									Davison et al. (1991)[a]
30 d	18	9.1		1.7	0.9									
60 d	18	8.8		1.5	0.6									
1 wk	11		61	2.4	2.5	6.3	1,350	460						Doreau et al. (1990)
4 wk	11		55	2.1	2.0	6.6	1,180	420						
8 wk	11		49	2.1	1.3	6.7	970	360						Doreau et al. (1992)[a]
1 wk	10			2.9	1.8									
2 wk	10			2.7	1.4									
4 wk	10			2.4	1.2									
8 wk	10			2.2	0.7									
1 wk	11		53	2.4	1.7	6.2								Doreau et al. (1993)[a]
4 wk	11		50	2.0	1.4	6.5								
8 wk	11		47	1.9	1.1	6.6								
2 wk	10		61	3.4	1.9									Glade (1991)[a]
4 wk	10		58	2.9	1.9									
6 wk	10		57	2.8	1.8									
8 wk	10		56	2.5	1.8									
30 d	18	9.9		1.7	0.4									Kubiak et al. (1991)[a]
60 d	18	9.6		1.5	0.3									
4 d	Review[b]		48	2.1	1.2	6.4								Malacarne et al. (2002)
	5		58	3.3	1.7	6.4								Mariani et al. (2001)
2 mo	5		44	1.8	0.7	6.8								
4 mo	5		42	1.6	0.6	6.9								
6 mo	5		41	1.6	0.4	6.9								
1–6 mo (Ass)				1.7	1.8	5.9	1,150	730						Oftedal and Jenness (1988)
3–12 mo (Mountain zebra)				1.6	1.0	6.9	840	550						
3–8 mo (Plains zebra)				1.6	2.2	7.0	750	530						
3–12 mo (Przewalski horse)				1.5	1.5	6.7	820	430						
1–6 mo (Pony)				1.8	1.5	6.7	840	530	117	1,036	355	0.50	3.2	
1 wk	18						1,156	848						Rook et al. (1999)

[a]Average of two dietary treatment means.
[b]Review of many studies; average values compiled by authors of citation.

continued

REFERENCES FOR MILK COMPOSITION TABLE

Csapo, J., J. Stefler, T. G. Martin, S. Makray, and Zs. Csapo-Kiss. 1995. Composition of mares' colostrum and milk. Fat content, fatty acid composition and vitamin content. Int. Dairy J. 5:393–402.

Csapo-Kiss, Zs., J. Stefler, T. G. Martin, S. Makray, and J. Csapo. 1995. Composition of mares' colostrum and milk. Protein content, amino acid composition and contents of macro- and micro-elements. Int. Dairy J. 5:403–415.

Davison, K. E., G. D. Potter, L. W. Greene, J. W. Evans, and W. C. McMullan. 1991. Lactation and reproductive performance of mares fed added dietary fat during late gestation and early lactation. Equine Vet. Sci. 11:111–115.

Doreau, M., S. Boulot, D. Bauchart, J. Barlet, and P. Patureau-Mirand. 1990. Yield and composition of milk from lactating mares: effect of lactation stage and individual differences. J. Dairy Res. 57:449–454.

Doreau, M., S. Boulot, D. Bauchart, J. Barlet, and W. Martin-Rosset. 1992. Voluntary intake, milk production and plasma metabolites in nursing mares fed two different diets. J. Nutr. 122:992–999.

Doreau, M., S. Boulot, and Y. Chilliard. Yield and composition of milk from lactating mares: effect of body condition at foaling. J. Dairy Res. 60:457–466.

Glade, M. J. 1991. Dietary yeast culture supplementation of mares during late gestation and early lactation. J. Equine Vet. Sci. 11:89–95.

Kubiak, J. R., J. W. Evans, G. D. Potter, P. G. Harms, and W. L. Jenkins. 1991. Milk yield and composition in the multiparous mare fed to obesity. J. Equine Vet. Sci. 11:158–162.

Malacarne, M., F. Martuzzi, A. Summer, and P. Mariani. 2002. Review: Protein and fat composition of mare's milk: some nutritional remarks with reference to human and cow's milk. Inter. Dairy J. 12:869–877.

Mariani, P., A. Summer, F. Martuzzi, P. Formaggioni, A. Sabbioni, A. L. Catalano. 2001. Physicochemical properties, gross composition, energy value and nitrogen fractions of Haflinger nursing mare milk throughout 6 lactation months. Anim. Res. 50:415–425.

Oftedal, O. T. and R. Jenness. 1988. Interspecies variation in milk composition among horses, zebras and asses. J. Dairy Res. 55:57–66.

Rook, J. S., W. E. Braselton, J. W. Lloyd, M. E. Shea, and J. E. Shelle. 1999. Comparison of element concentrations in Arabian mare's milk and commercial mare's milk replacement products. Vet. Clin. Nutr. 6:17–21.

NUTRIENT REQUIREMENTS, FEEDSTUFF COMPOSITION, AND OTHER TABLES

TABLE 16-10 Conversion Factors

Units	Multiplied by equals	Units	Multiplied by equals	Units
pound (lb)	0.4536	kilogram (kg)	2.205	pound (lb)
ounce (oz)	28.35	gram (g)	0.03527	ounce (oz)
gallon, U.S. liquid (gal)	3.785	liter (L)	0.2642	gallon, U.S. liquid (gal)
gallon, U.K. (gal)	4.546	liter (L)	0.2200	gallon, U.K. (gal)
bushel, U.S. (bu)	35.24	liter (L)	0.02838	bushel, U.S. (bu)
bushel, U.K. (bu)	36.37	liter (L)	0.02750	bushel, U.K. (bu)
calorie (cal)	4.184	joule (J)	0.2390	calorie (cal)
mile (mi)	1.609	kilometer (km)	0.6214	mile (mi)
acre (ac)	0.4047	hectare (ha)	2.471	acre (ac)
hectare (ha)	10,000	square meter (m^2)	0.0001	hectare (ha)
ppm	1	mg/kg	1	ppm
ppm	1	µg/g	1	ppm
ppm	0.0001	%	10,000	ppm

Prefixes for the International System of Units (SI)

Units Greater Than the Standard Unit

Item	Prefix	To convert from standard unit multiply by[a]
G	giga	1,000,000,000
M	mega	1,000,000
k	kilo	1,000

Units Less Than the Standard Unit

Item	Prefix	To convert from standard unit divide by[b]
d	deci	10
c	centi	100
m	milli	1,000
µ	micro	1,000,000
n	nano	1,000,000,000

[a]For example, 1 kg (kilogram) = 1 g multiplied by 1,000 = 1,000 g.
[b]For example, 1 mg (milligram) = 1 g divided by 1,000 = 1/1,000 g.

Fahrenheit to Celsius (Centigrade) Conversions

Fahrenheit	Celsius
110	43.3
105	40.6
100	37.8
95	35.0
90	32.2
85	29.4
80	26.7
75	23.9
70	21.1
65	18.3
60	15.6
55	12.8
50	10.0
45	7.2
40	4.4
35	1.7
30	−1.1
25	−3.9
20	−6.7
15	−9.4
10	−12.2
5	−15.0
0	−17.8
−5	−20.6
−10	−23.3
−15	−26.1
−20	−28.9
−25	−31.7
−30	−34.4
−35	−37.2
−40	−40.0

Appendix A

Committee Statement of Task

The objective of this project is to prepare a report that will evaluate the scientific literature on the nutrient requirements of horses and ponies in all stages of life and management techniques for feeding horses and ponies. The report will address all classes of horses and ponies during various physiological life phases, nutrient requirements, deficiencies, and general considerations for feeding equines. Updated information on the composition of feeds, feed additives, and other compounds routinely fed to horses will be included. Physiological factors affecting production and performance and various management circumstances will be addressed. A computer program will be developed to accompany the report and will function to predict nutrient requirements. All information contained in the report and computer model will be based on scientific input obtained from various sources, scientific literature, reports, and reviews.

The broad charge will include the following tasks:

- an update of the recommendations contained in the 1989 publication, which currently serves as the authoritative source of information (in the U.S. and internationally) for feeding horses;
- a comprehensive analysis of recent research on feeding horses, horse nutrition, nutrient requirements, and physiological and environmental factors affecting requirements; and
- development of a user-friendly, menu-driven computer model program incorporating new technologies.

Appendix B

Abbreviations and Acronyms

3MH	3-methylhistidine	CF	Crude fiber
AACC	American Association of Cereal Chemists	CFR	Code of Federal Regulations
		CHO-F	Fermentable carbohydrates
AAFCO	Association of American Feed Control Officials	$CHO\text{-}F_R$	Rapidly fermentable carbohydrates
		$CHO\text{-}F_S$	Slowly fermentable carbohydrates
ADF	Acid detergent fiber	CHO-H	Hydrolyzable carbohydrates measured by direct methods (sugars + starch)
ADFCP	Acid detergent insoluble protein		
ADFN	Acid detergent insoluble nitrogen	CK	Creatine kinase
ADG	Average daily gain	CP	Crude protein
ADICP	Acid detergent insoluble crude protein	CS	Condition score; citrate synthase
ADIN	Acid detergent insoluble nitrogen	CSM	Cottonseed meal
ADL	Acid detergent lignin	CSREES	Cooperative State Research, Education, and Extension Service
ADP	Adenosine diphosphate		
AEE	Acid ether extract	CT	Calcitonin
AIA	Acid insoluble ash	CTVM	Centre for Tropical Veterinary Medicine
ALD	Angular limb deformities	CV	Coefficient of variation
aNDF	Neutral detergent fiber treated with amylase and sulfite solutions	CW	Cultivator for weeding
		D_a	Apparent digestibility
ANZECC	Australian and New Zealand Environment and Conservation	DAK	Disney's Animal Kingdom
		DCAD	Dietary cation-anion difference
AOAC	Association of Official Analytical Chemists	DCP	Digestible crude protein
		DE	Digestible energy
AOCS	American Oil Chemists Society	DE_m	Digestible energy for maintenance
AP	Available protein	DFM	Direct fed microbials
ATP	Adenosine triphosphate	DHA	Docosahexaenoic acid
AVDMI	Average voluntary dry matter intake	DM	Dry matter
AZA	American Zoo and Aquarium Association	DMD	Dry matter digestibility
		DMI	Dry matter intake
BALF	Bronchoalveolar lavage fluid	DNER	Daily net energy requirement
BCAA	Branch chain amino acids	DOD	Developmental orthopedic disease
BCS	Body condition score	DON	Deoxynivalenol
BDG	Brewer's dried grains	DP	Digestible protein; degree of polymerization
BHA	Butylated hydroxyanisole		
BHT	Butylated hydroxytoluene	DSHEA	Dietary Supplement Health and Education Act
BW	Body weight		
CAST	Council for Agricultural Science and Technology	D_t	True digestibility
		EAAP	European Association for Animal Production
CCME	Canadian Council of Ministers of the Environment		

ECF	Extracellular fluid	HYPP	Hyperkalemic periodic paralysis
EDDI	Ethylenediaminedihydroiodide	ICF	Intracellular fluid
EDM	Equine degenerative myeloencephalopathy	IE	Intake energy
		IGF-I	Insulin-like growth factor I
EE	Ether extract	IgG	Immunoglobulin G
EFA	Essential fatty acid	INRA	L'Institut National de la Recherche Agronomique
EGUS	Equine gastric ulcer syndrome		
ELF	Epithelial lining fluid	ISIS	International Species Inventory Systems
EMND	Equine motor neuron disease	IU	International units
ENSAM	Ecole Supérieure d'Agronomie Agro Montpellier	IVDMD	In vitro dry matter digestibility
		JAVMA	Journal of the American Veterinary Medical Association
EPA	Eicosapentaenoic acid		
EPM	Equine protozoal myeloencephalitis	K_1	Phylloquinone
EPSM	Equine polysaccharide storage myopathy	K_2	Menaquinone
		K_3	Menadione
ER	Exertional rhabdomyolysis	LC	Light cart
EU	Enzyme units	LCT	Lower critical temperature
FAD	Flavin adenine dinucleotide	LD_{50}	Lethal dose that kills 50%
FAO/WHO	Food and Agriculture Organization/ World Health Organization	LE	Lactation energy
		LH	Luteinizing hormone
FDA	Food and Drug Administration	LPL	Lipoprotein lipase
FE	Fecal energy	LPS	Lipopolysaccharide
FE test	Urinary fractional electrolyte excretion test	MADC	Matières Azotées Digestibles Cheval
		MCT	Medium-chain triglycerides
FFA	Free fatty acids	ME	Metabolizable energy
FMN	Flavin mononucleotide	ME_m	Metabolizable energy for maintenance
FOS	Fructooligosaccharides		
FSH	Follicle stimulating hormone	MG	Muscle gain
FTU	Phytase unit	MRT	Mean retention time
GAG	Glycosaminoglycan	MSM	Methylsulfonylmethane
GC	Gas chromatography	MuFA	Monounsaturated fatty acid
GE	Gross energy	NAD	Nicotinamide adenine dinucleotide
GEH	Gesellschaft fur Ernahrungsphysiologie der Haustiere	NADP	Nicotinamide adenine dinucleotide phosphate
GH	Growth hormone	ND	Not detectable
GI	Glycemic index	NDF	Neutral detergent fiber
GLUT	Glucose transporter	NDICP	Neutral detergent insoluble crude protein
GLUT-4	Glucose transporter-4	NDIN	Neutral detergent insoluble nitrogen (protein)
GnRH	Gonadotropin releasing hormone		
GRAS	Generally recognized as safe	NDSC	Neutral detergent soluble carbohydrates
GSH-px	Glutathione peroxidase	NDSF	Neutral detergent soluble fiber
HAD	β-hydroxyacyl CoA dehydrogenase	NE	Net energy
H_cE	Heat of thermal regulation	NE_m	Net energy for maintenance
H_dE	Heat of digestion and absorption	NE_r	Recovered energy
HE	Heat energy	NEW	Net energy used for work
H_eE	Heat associated with basal metabolism	NFC	Nonfibrous carbohydrates
H_fE	Heat of fermentation	NFE	Nitrogen-free extract
H_iE	Heat increment	NFTA	National Forage Testing Association
H_jE	Heat associated with voluntary activity	NIR	Near infrared reflectance
HPLC	High performance liquid chromatography	NIRS	Near infrared reflectance spectroscopy
HR	Heart rate in beats per minute	NMD	Nutritional muscular dystrophy
H_rE	Heat associated with product formation	NPN	Nonprotein nitrogen
HSCAS	Hydrated sodium calcium aluminosilicate	NRC	National Research Council
		NSC	Nonstructural carbohydrates
HSL	Hormone sensitive lipase	NSH	Nutritional secondary hyperparathyroidism
H_wE	Heat associated with waste formation and excretion		

NSP	Nonstarch polysaccharides	SZA	Sodium zeolite A
OC	Osteochondrosis	T_3	Triiodothyronine
OCD	Osteochondrosis dissecans	T_4	Thyroxin
OM	Organic matter	TAG	Triglyceride (triacylglycerol)
OMD	Organic matter digestibility	TBAR	Thiobarbiturate reactive substances
PM 2.5	Particulate matter with fine particles less than 2.5 micrometers in diameter	TBHQ	Tertiary butyl hydroquinone
		TBW	Total body water
PMU	Pregnant mares' urine	TDF	Total dietary fiber
PSSM	Polysaccharide storage myopathy	TDN	Total digestible nutrients
PTH	Parathyroid hormone	TDS	Total dissolved solids
PUFA	Polyunsaturated fatty acid	TE	Tissue energy
PUN	Plasma urea nitrogen	TMR	Total mixed ration
PV	Plasma volume	TNC	Total nonstructural carbohydrates
RAO	Recurrent airway obstruction	TNZ	Thermoneutral zone
RBP	Retinol binding protein	TRH	Thyroid releasing hormone
RDR	Relative dose response test	TSH	Thyroid stimulating hormone
RE	Recovered energy	TSS	Total soluble salts
RER	Respiratory exchange ratio; recurrent exertional rhabdomyolysis	TZ	Toronto Zoo
		UCT	Upper critical temperature
RH	Relative humidity	UE	Urinary energy
ROS	Reactive oxygen species	UFC	Unite Fourragere Cheval (horse feed unit)
SAS	Statistical Analysis System		
SBM	Soybean meal	VDMI	Voluntary dry matter intake
SC	Structural carbohydrates	VE	Hair energy
SDF	Soluble dietary fiber	VFA	Volatile fatty acid
SE	Standard error	VFI	Voluntary feed intake
SET	Standard exercise test	V_{O_2}	Oxygen consumption
SFA	Saturated fatty acid	$V_{O_2}max$	Maximum volume of oxygen
SL	Sweat loss	WSC	Water soluble carbohydrates
SPAOPD	Summer pasture-associated obstructive pulmonary disease	YE	Conceptus energy
		ZSSD	Zoological Society of San Diego

Appendix C

Committee Member Biographies

Laurie M. Lawrence, Ph.D. *(Chair)* is professor in the Department of Animal Science at the University of Kentucky. Lawrence received a B.S. (1975) from Cornell University and an M.S. (1978) and Ph.D. (1982) in Animal Nutrition from Colorado State University. She is a past president of the Equine Nutrition and Physiology Society and a past director of the Kentucky Horse Council. She has received numerous awards for excellence in research and teaching. From 1992 to 1995, she served on the National Research Council's Committee on Animal Nutrition. Her research interests include equine nutrition, metabolism, and exercise physiology. Her most recent research has focused on the effect of exercise on the nutrition of horses and the effects of high- and low-fiber diets on water balance. She is currently on the Editorial Board of the *Journal of Animal Science* and a director of the Kentucky Equine Management Internship.

Nadia F. Cymbaluk, M.Sc., D.V.M. is director of veterinary research and field compliance at the Linwood Equine Ranch of Wyeth Canada in Manitoba. Cymbaluk received a B.Sc. (1968) from the University of Alberta, an M.Sc. (1970) from the University of Guelph, and a D.V.M. (1974) from the University of Saskatchewan. She has previously held positions at the University of Saskatchewan and has worked in a private veterinary practice. Cymbaluk's primary areas of expertise are water requirements and metabolism of horses and effects of cold conditions.

David W. Freeman, Ph.D. is professor and extension equine specialist in the Department of Animal Science at Oklahoma State University. Freeman received a B.S. (1979), an M.S. (1981), and a Ph.D. (1984) from Texas A&M University. Freeman is a past member of the Board of Directors of the Equine Nutrition and Physiology Society, associate editor of the *Professional Animal Scientist*, and a member of the Review Board of the *Journal of Equine Veterinary Science*. He is a registered professional equine Animal Scientist through the American Registry of Professional Animal Scientists and a Charter Diplomate of the American College of Animal Nutrition. He is also an officer and member of several horse sport and breed associations. Freeman has authored numerous bulletins, audiovisual materials, and manuals on horse feeding and management. Although Freeman is primarily an extension specialist, he conducts research on various topics of applied nutrition.

Raymond J. Geor, D.V.M., Ph.D. is the Paul Mellon Distinguished Professor in the College of Agriculture and Life Sciences, Virginia Polytechnic and State University. Geor received a B.V.Sc. (1982) from Massey University (NZ), an M.V.Sc. (1988) from the University of Saskatchewan, and a Ph.D. (1999) from Ohio State University. He was previously a faculty member in the College of Veterinary Medicine at the University of Minnesota and the Ontario Veterinary College at the University of Guelph. He is board certified in veterinary internal medicine, an associate editor of one scientific journal, and member of the review board of two other journals. He has conducted research on the effects of heat stress in exercising horses and on the effects of diet and exercise on carbohydrate metabolism. His primary area of research in recent years has been the dietary regulation of carbohydrate metabolism in horses.

Patricia M. Graham-Thiers, Ph.D. is professor in the Department of Equine Studies at Virginia Intermont College in Bristol, Virginia. Graham-Thiers received a B.S. (1990) from the University of Massachusetts, an M.S. (1992) from the University of Florida, and a Ph.D. (1998) from Virginia Polytechnic and State University. She has previous experience in the horse feed industry in the northeast United States. Her primary research program has been with the protein and amino acid nutrition of horses. She has worked both with young, exercising horses and with aged horses.

Annette C. Longland, Ph.D. is senior research scientist at the Institute of Grassland and Environmental Research in

Aberystwyth, United Kingdom. Longland received a B.Sc. (1978) from the University of Stirling (Scotland) and a Ph.D. (1986) from Imperial College, University of London (England). She has conducted research on dietary fiber and its utilization by pigs, ruminants, and horses. She has also been involved in investigations into the effects of processing on the utilization of starch by horses and various nutritional diseases in horses, including hindgut dysfunction, acidosis, and laminitis. Longland also contributes an international perspective and a focus on some of the environmental issues related to horse husbandry.

Brian D. Nielsen, Ph.D. is associate professor in the Department of Animal Science at Michigan State University. Nielsen received a B.S. (1990) from the University of Wisconsin (River Falls) and an M.S. (1992) and Ph.D. (1996), both from Texas A&M University. He is currently serving as a director of the Equine Nutrition and Physiology Society. The primary emphasis of Nielsen's research has been bone development and metabolism. He is also an expert in mineral metabolism and has experience in water loss and rehydration of horses during exercise.

Paul D. Siciliano, Ph.D. is associate professor in the Department of Animal Sciences at North Carolina State University. Siciliano received a B.S. (1987) from the Ohio State University and an M.S. (1992) and Ph.D. (1996), both from the University of Kentucky. He was previously a faculty member in the Department of Animal Science at Colorado State University. Siciliano is a past member of the Board of Directors (2000–2005) and current Secretary/Treasurer (2005–2007) of the Equine Science Society. He currently serves on the Editorial Review Board of the *Journal of Animal Science*. His primary area of research is vitamin and trace mineral nutrition of horses.

Donald R. Topliff, Ph.D. is professor and department head of the Division of Agriculture at West Texas A&M University. Topliff received a B.S. (1978) from Kansas State University and an M.S. (1981) and Ph.D. (1984), both from Texas A&M University. He has conducted research on the importance of dietary cation-anion balance on the performance of race horses. He has also published chapters in four different text books about horses and the horse industry. Topliff is a member of several horse-related organizations, including serving as current president of the Equine Nutrition and Physiology Society.

Eduardo V. Valdes, Ph.D. is a nutritionist at Disney's Animal Kingdom (DAK), Orlando, Florida. He received his B.Sc. (1972) from the University of Chile and M.Sc. (1981) and Ph.D. (1991) in animal nutrition from the University of Guelph in Ontario. He oversees DAK's Animal Nutrition Centers, where he is responsible for implementing and assessing the animal nutrition program for Walt Disney World, Animal Programs. Animals in the Disney programs include numerous horses and close relatives to the horse. His duties at DAK also include teaching basic applied zoo animal nutrition to DAK staff members. Before joining DAK, he was the nutritionist for the Toronto Zoo. He is an adjunct professor with the Department of Animal and Poultry Sciences, University of Guelph and also has courtesy appointments with the University of Central Florida and the University of Florida. He is involved in many nutrition research projects with wild captive species, in particular with endangered species. He was one of the founder members of the Nutrition Advisory Group (NAG) for the American Zoo and Aquarium (AZA). He has published many articles in the area of wildlife nutrition and evaluation of feedstuffs using near infrared spectroscopy.

Robert J. Van Saun, Ph.D., D.V.M. is extension veterinarian and associate professor in the Department of Veterinary Science at The Pennsylvania State University. Van Saun received a B.S. (1978), D.V.M. (1982), and M.S. (1988) from Michigan State University and a Ph.D. (1993) from Cornell University. Before his current position, he was a faculty member at Oregon State University, and he has spent time in private veterinary practice. He is a member of numerous animal science and veterinary medicine societies. Among his teaching assignments is a course on pathobiology of nutritional and metabolic disease. Van Saun has given numerous presentations on the health and nutrition of a wide variety of farm animals. He has conducted nutritional (primarily minerals and vitamins) research in beef and dairy cattle, horses, and llamas. He has developed several computer applications in animal nutrition, including development of the model in the NRC Nutrient Requirements of Horses (1989).

Appendix D

Board on Agriculture and Natural Resources Publications

POLICY AND RESOURCES

Agricultural Biotechnology and the Poor: Proceedings of an International Conference (2000)
Agricultural Biotechnology: Strategies for National Competitiveness (1987)
Agriculture and the Undergraduate: Proceedings (1992)
Agriculture's Role in K-12 Education: A Forum on the National Science Education Standards (1998)
Air Emissions from Animal Feeding Operations: Current Knowledge, Future Needs (2003)
Alternative Agriculture (1989)
Animal Biotechnology: Science-Based Concerns (2002)
Animal Care and Management at the National Zoo: Final Report (2005)
Animal Care and Management at the National Zoo: Interim Report (2004)
Animal Health at the Crossroads: Preventing, Detecting, and Diagnosing Animal Diseases (2005)
Biological Confinement of Genetically Engineered Organisms (2004)
Brucellosis in the Greater Yellowstone Area (1998)
California Agricultural Research Priorities: Pierce's Disease (2004)
Colleges of Agriculture at the Land Grant Universities: Public Service and Public Policy (1996)
Colleges of Agriculture at the Land Grant Universities: A Profile (1995)
Countering Agricultural Bioterrorism (2003)
Critical Needs for Research in Veterinary Science (2005)
Designing an Agricultural Genome Program (1998)
Designing Foods: Animal Product Options in the Marketplace (1988)
Diagnosis and Control of Johne's Disease (2003)
Direct and Indirect Human Contributions to Terrestrial Carbon Fluxes (2004)
Ecological Monitoring of Genetically Modified Crops (2001)
Ecologically Based Pest Management: New Solutions for a New Century (1996)
Emerging Animal Diseases—Global Markets, Global Safety: A Workshop Summary (2002)
Ensuring Safe Food: From Production to Consumption (1998)
Environmental Effects of Transgenic Plants: The Scope and Adequacy of Regulation (2002)
Exploring a Vision: Integrating Knowledge for Food and Health (2004)
Exploring Horizons for Domestic Animal Genomics: Workshop Summary (2002)
Forested Landscapes in Perspective: Prospects and Opportunities for Sustainable Management of America's Nonfederal Forests (1997)
Forestry Research: A Mandate for Change (1990)
Frontiers in Agricultural Research: Food, Health, Environment, and Communities (2003)
Future Role of Pesticides for U.S. Agriculture (2000)
Genetic Engineering of Plants: Agricultural Research Opportunities and Policy Concerns (1984)
Genetically Modified Pest-Protected Plants: Science and Regulation (2000)
Incorporating Science, Economics, and Sociology in Developing Sanitary and Phytosanitary Standards in International Trade: Proceedings of a Conference (2000)
Investing in Research: A Proposal to Strengthen the Agricultural, Food, and Environmental System (1989)
Investing in the National Research Initiative: An Update of the Competitive Grants Program in the U.S. Department of Agriculture (1994)
Managing Global Genetic Resources: Agricultural Crop Issues and Policies (1993)
Managing Global Genetic Resources: Forest Trees (1991)
Managing Global Genetic Resources: Livestock (1993)
Managing Global Genetic Resources: The U.S. National Plant Germplasm System (1991)
National Capacity in Forestry Research (2002)

National Research Initiative: A Vital Competitive Grants Program in Food, Fiber, and Natural Resources Research (2000)
New Directions for Biosciences Research in Agriculture: High-Reward Opportunities (1985)
Pesticide Resistance: Strategies and Tactics for Management (1986)
Pesticides and Groundwater Quality: Issues and Problems in Four States (1986)
Pesticides in the Diets of Infants and Children (1993)
Precision Agriculture in the 21st Century: Geospatial and Information Technologies in Crop Management (1997)
Predicting Invasions of Nonindigenous Plants and Plant Pests (2002)
Professional Societies and Ecologically Based Pest Management (2000)
Rangeland Health: New Methods to Classify, Inventory, and Monitor Rangelands (1994)
Regulating Pesticides in Food: The Delaney Paradox (1987)
Resource Management (1991)
Safety of Genetically Engineered Foods: Approaches to Assessing Unintended Health Effects (2004)
Scientific Criteria to Ensure Safe Food (2003)
Soil and Water Quality: An Agenda for Agriculture (1993)
Soil Conservation: Assessing the National Resources Inventory, Volume 1 (1986); Volume 2 (1986)
Sustainable Agriculture and the Environment in the Humid Tropics (1993)
Sustainable Agriculture Research and Education in the Field: A Proceedings (1991)
Toward Sustainability: A Plan for Collaborative Research on Agriculture and Natural Resource Management (1991)
Understanding Agriculture: New Directions for Education (1988)
The Scientific Basis for Estimating Air Emissions from Animal Feeding Operations: Interim Report (2002)
The Use of Drugs in Food Animals: Benefits and Risks (1999)
Water Transfers in the West: Efficiency, Equity, and the Environment (1992)
Wood in Our Future: The Role of Life Cycle Analysis (1997)

ANIMAL NUTRITION PROGRAM AND RELATED TITLES

Building a North American Feed Information System (1995)
Metabolic Modifiers: Effects on the Nutrient Requirements of Food-Producing Animals (1994)
Mineral Tolerance of Animals: Second Revised Edition (2005)
Nutrient Requirements of Beef Cattle, Seventh Revised Edition, Update (2000)
Nutrient Requirements of Dairy Cattle, Seventh Revised Edition (2001)
Nutrient Requirements of Dogs and Cats (2006)
Nutrient Requirements of Fish (1993)
Nutrient Requirements of Laboratory Animals, Fourth Revised Edition (1995)
Nutrient Requirements of Nonhuman Primates, Second Revised Edition (2003)
Nutrient Requirements of Poultry, Ninth Revised Edition (1994)
Nutrient Requirements of Small Ruminants (2007)
Nutrient Requirements of Swine, Tenth Revised Edition (1998)
Predicting Feed Intake of Food-Producing Animals (1986)
Role of Chromium in Animal Nutrition (1997)
Ruminant Nitrogen Uses (1985)
Scientific Advances in Animal Nutrition: Promise for the New Century (2001)
Vitamin Tolerance of Animals (1987)

Further information, additional titles (prior to 1984), and prices are available from the National Academies Press, 2101 Constitution Avenue, NW, Washington, DC 20418, 202-334-3313 (information only). To order any of the titles listed above, visit the National Academies Press bookstore at *http://www.nap.edu/bookstore*.

Index

A

Absorption of nutrients. *See also individual nutrients*
    diet and, 71, 72
    energy cost of, 7
    environment and, 77
    starch intake and, 141
Acacia spp., 268
Acclimation, 10, 84, 129-130, 271
Acetate, 6-7, 35, 37
Acetazolamide, 240
Acid-base balance, 48, 64, 65, 73, 81, 84, 86
Acid insoluble ash method, 190, 204
Acremonium coenophialum, 158
Adenosine diphosphate, 76
Adenosine triphosphate, 6, 76, 118, 119, 141, 225
Aeroallergens, 154, 156
Aflatoxins, 157, 185-186
Age. *See also* Foals; Mature horses; Old horses; Yearlings
    body condition score, 236
    body weight, 14
    chronologic, 236
    demographic, 236
    drinking behavior, 133
    energy requirements, 10, 12, 13, 14, 24
    growth rate, 16
    feeding behavior, 213, 214, 216, 218, 221
    heart rate, 24
    heat or cold stress, 10
    mineral requirements, 72, 75-76, 89, 97
    physiologic, 236
    protein requirements, 60
    total body water, 128
    vitamin C, 124, 237
Alanine, 207
Alfalfa (*Medicago sativa* L.)
    dehydrated, 269
    digestibility, 55, 72, 145, 152, 153, 189, 269
    dry matter intake by donkeys, 269
    and enterolithiasis, 256, 275-276
    feeding behavior on, 213-214, 215, 216, 269
    fungal contaminants, 157, 257
    and gastric ulcer syndrome, 253-254
    hays, 71, 72, 79, 80, 92, 113, 120, 129, 130, 132, 149, 150, 151, 152, 153, 156, 169, 213-214, 226, 251, 256, 257, 269, 271, 272
    meal, 118, 218
    nutrient content, 59, 71, 76, 79, 80, 88, 92, 111, 118, 119-120, 121, 128, 129, 143, 144, 145, 146, 156, 164, 226, 240, 252, 256, 271
    oxalates, 251
    pasture species for horses, 148, 212, 215
    pelleted or cubed, 88, 160, 169, 189-190, 259
    silage, 154, 155
    voluntary dry matter intake, 145, 151, 155
    and water intakes, 130, 131, 132
Algae, 137-138, 227
Alkali disease, 96
Alkaline phosphatase, 97, 97
Alkaloids, 190
Allergic respiratory disease, 154, 194
Almond hulls, 161
Alopecia, 92, 96, 97
α-Amylase, 224
α-Ketoglutarate dehydrogenase, 118
α-Linoleic acid, 44, 49, 50, 193-194
α-Lipoproteins, 46
Alsike clover (*Trifolium hybridum*), 156
Altai wildrye (*Leysum angustus* L.), 151, 212
Alternaria, 257
Aluminum, 76, 79, 99
American Association of Cereal Chemists, 203
American Horse Council, 1, 227
American Institute of Nutrition, 99
American Oil Chemists Association, 203
American Saddlebreds, 255
American Zoo and Aquarium Association, 274
Amino acids. *See also* Protein and amino acids; *individual amino acids*
    analytical methods, 207
    branched-chain, 64
    digestibilities, 56
    essential, 54
    free, 54
    metabolism, 120
    metal complexes and chelates, 194, 195
    sulfur-containing, 87
    supplementation, 64
Ammonia, 54, 149, 227, 228
Amprolium, 118
Amylopectin, 38
Amylose, 38
Anabaena, 137
Andalusians, 243
Anglo-Arab horses, 19
Animal Feeding Operations, 227
Anorexia/inappetance, 97, 118, 217, 219, 252
Anthelmintics, 192
Antimicrobial agents, 192-193
Antioxidants
    dietary application, 188-189, 258
    in fats and oils, 162, 184, 258
    health-enhancing additives, 186-189
    minerals, 187, 188, 189
    preservatives in feeds, 184
    vitamins, 114, 115, 119, 123
Aphanizomenon, 137
Appaloosas, 15, 240
Apple cider vinegar, 256, 257
Arabians, 14, 24, 48, 75, 97, 153, 162, 188, 189, 213, 240, 243, 247, 255
Arabinogalatan, 193
Arachidonic acid, 50
Arginine, 54, 56, 62, 65, 164-166, 207
Ascorbyl palmitate, 123, 187
Ascorbyl stearate, 187
Ash, feed composition tables, 304, 306
Aspartate aminotransferase, 95
Aspartic acid, 207
Aspartic-pyruvic tranaminase, 95
Aspergillus spp., 150, 157, 162, 196, 257
Assateague ponies, 217
Asses. *See* Donkeys; Wild asses
Association of American Feed Control Officials, 167, 183, 196
Association of Official Analytical Chemists, 203, 204, 205, 207, 208
Athletic performance, 48-49
Australia, water quality criteria, 134, 135, 136
Australian Stockhorses, 19, 130

B

B vitamins, 144. *See also individual vitamins*
Bacteria. *See also individual species*
    in forages, 154, 156-157
    human health concerns, 227-228
    probiotics, 192-193, 189, 196
    in water, 138
Bahiagrass (*Paspalum notatum*), 144, 148, 212
Bark chewing, 147, 158, 220, 268
Barley (*Hordeum vulgare*), 6, 36, 58, 110, 118, 119, 120, 121, 156, 159-160, 161, 162, 164, 168, 169, 170, 171, 172, 212, 214, 215, 269
Beans, 163, 164
Beet pulp, 4, 35, 36, 79, 131, 160, 161, 196, 218, 241
Behavior. *See also* Drinking behavior; Feeding behavior; *specific behaviors*
    aggression, 216, 217
    box/stall walking, 221
    compulsive, 25, 158, 221
    diet and, 49, 158
    fat supplementation and, 49
    fiber deficiency and, 158
    head pressing, 96
    herd social orders, 216, 223
    water restriction and, 134
    weaving, 221
Belgian horses, 14, 15, 28, 240-241
Bentonite, 185
Beriberi, 118
Bermudagrass, 55, 71, 76, 88, 143, 144, 148, 150, 151, 153, 166, 170, 171, 172, 189, 212, 240, 245, 247, 255, 268
β-Carotene, 110, 111, 112, 187, 189
β-Endorphins, 222
β-Glucans, 37
β-Hydroxyacyl CoA dehydrogenase activity, 46, 47
Bicarbonate, 135, 136
Bifidobacteria, 189, 193
Bioavailability. *See also individual nutrients*
    defined, 166
    form of nutrient and, 97, 98, 163, 166-167, 194-196
    interactions of nutrients and, 136
    processing effects, 172, 259
    protein, 56-57, 172
Biotin
    associations/interactions, 120
    deficiency, 120-121
    function, 120, 250
    requirements, 109, 121
    sources, 120
    supplements, 168, 250
    toxicity, 121
Bird's-foot trefoil (*Lotus corniculatus*), 148
Black walnut shavings, 249
Blind staggers, 96, 157, 161
Blister beetles (*Epicauta* spp.), 152, 156
Blue couch (*Digitaria didactyla*), 147, 212
Bluegrass, 146, 147
Bluestem (*Andropogon* spp.), 148, 151, 153, 212
Body composition, 7, 8, 215, 225, 243

Body condition
    aging signs, 236
    donkeys, 27, 272
    energy deficiency or excess and, 27-28
    exercise and, 225
    and heat or cold stress, 10, 238
    heat production and, 8
    and lactation, 20
    management, 225
    optimal, 27, 225
    and reproductive efficiency, 21-22, 27
    scoring systems, 21, 27
    and weight gain during pregnancy, 19
Body fluid compartments, 128
Body temperature, 25, 11, 238-239
Body weight
    age and, 14
    body condition score, 19, 27-28
    and energy requirement, 7, 12, 19, 27-28
    exercise and, 15, 226
    fat supplementation and, 51
    fiber intake and, 147
    gestation and, 19
    hard keeper horses, 51
    loss, 86, 156
    management, 225-226, 250
    predicting, 14, 18
    sweat losses estimated from, 84, 86, 133
    total body water, 128
    water requirements, 131, 132, 133
    yeast supplements, 197
Boerperd horses, 132
Bones. *See* Skeletal health
Boron, 99, 144
Boscia foetida, 268
Botryodiploidin, 157
Botulism, 154, 156
Bracken fern, 118
Bran, 110, 250
Breed differences. *See also individual breeds*
    developmental orthopedic disease, 243-244, 248
    feeding behavior, 213, 216, 221
    growth rate, 13-15
    heart rate, 24
    maintenance requirements, 21
    milk production, 19, 21
    water requirements, 132
Breeding. *See also* Broodmares; Pregnancy; Reproduction; Reproductive efficiency
    energy requirements, 6, 16-17, 21-22, 147, 216
    minerals, 70, 74
    nutrient requirement tables, 294-303
    protein, 147
    stallions, 16-17, 70, 116, 118, 119
    vitamins, 112, 116, 118, 119
Brewer's yeast, 98, 118, 165
Bromegrass, 55, 151, 153, 156, 212, 253
Bromus carinatus, 142
Broodmares, 6, 9, 21-22, 74, 85, 90, 91, 213. *See also* Gestation; Pregnancy
Buckwheat, 164
Buffel grass (*Cenchrus ciliaris*), 251
Burros. *See* Donkeys

Butylated hydroxyanisole (BHA), 184
Butylated hydroxytoluene (BHT), 167, 184
Butyrate, 35, 37
Byssochlamys nivea, 157

C

Cabbage, 92
Cadmium, 88, 92
Calcinosis, 71
Calcitonin, 251
Calcium
    absorption, 45, 71-72, 73, 74, 113, 167
    age and, 75-76
    associations/interactions, 65, 71, 72, 75, 77, 78, 79, 80, 81, 92, 93, 113, 152, 156, 160, 161, 186
    bioavailability, 186
    composition of inorganic sources, 308
    deficiency or excess, 70, 71, 72-73, 77, 113, 121, 156, 247, 250-252, 274
    feed composition, 144, 161, 305, 307
    function, 70-71, 239, 240, 246, 247, 251
    in mare milk, 311-314
    recommendations, 73-76
    requirement tables, 294, 296, 298, 300, 302
    sources, 71-72, 144, 152, 252
    supplements, 71, 72, 92, 160, 167, 253
    in water, 135
Calcium ascorbyl monophosphate, 123, 187
Calcium:phosphorus ratio, 72, 73, 77, 90, 161, 244, 246, 247, 235, 244, 248, 250-252
Camargue horses, 213, 217
Canada, water quality guidelines, 138
Canarygrass, 157
Canola meal, 58-59, 163, 164
Canola oil, 162, 163
Cantharidin, 152, 156
Carbohydrates. *See also* Fiber; *individual types of compounds*
    analysis of feeds, 34-35, 205-206, 207-208
    categories/classifications, 34-35, 207-208
    digestion/digestibility, 34, 35, 37-39, 141, 167-168, 189, 207-208
    energy value, 3, 6, 34, 35, 141, 189
    environmental factors, 143
    excess intakes, 248-249
    exercise and, 40-41, 47-48
    fat supplementation and, 46
    feed composition, 34-35, 36-37, 141-143, 149, 160, 161
    and fetal development, 40
    loading, 40
    maintenance requirement, 38
    metabolism and storage, 39-41, 45, 46, 47-48, 51, 87, 94, 98, 118, 122, 123, 143
    nonfibrous, 34-35, 149, 160, 161, 205, 224, 241
    nonstructural, 34, 35, 46, 141, 142, 143, 149, 154
    structural, 35, 37-38, 141
    water-soluble, 35, 142-143, 149, 154, 205, 206, 248-249

Carbonates, 136
Carbonic anhydrase, 97
Carboxylase enzymes, 120
Carboxypeptidase, 97
Carnitine, 123
Carotenoids, 109, 110, 144
Casein, 164
Cassava, 164
Catalases, 187
Catarrhal conjunctivitis, 119
Cellulose, 34, 37, 141, 142, 159, 189, 204
Ceruloplasmin, 187
Cestrum diurnum, 71
Chaff, 214-215
Chicory (*Cichorium intybus*), 212, 249
Chlorine
  absorption, 86
  associations/interactions, 76
  chlorides in water, 135, 136
  composition of inorganic sources, 308-309
  deficiency or excess, 70, 86
  feed composition tables, 305, 307
  function, 86
  recommendations, 86-87
  requirement tables, 295, 297, 299, 301, 303
  sources, 86
  supplements, 253
  sweat losses, 238
Chlortetracycline, 192
Cholesterol, 44, 46, 48, 120
Chondroitin sulfate, 87, 94, 190-192
Chromic oxide, 170
Chromium, 98-99
Citrate synthase, 46
Citrinin, 157, 162
Citrobacter, 138
Citrus pulp, 160-161, 164
Cladosporium, 257
Clamp grass, 154, 155, 156
Claviceps, 157, 162
Clays, 186
Clean Water Act, 227
Clostridium spp., 138, 154, 156, 228
Clovers, 119, 144, 145, 146, 147
Clydesdale, 243
Coastgrass, 153
Cobalt
  absorption, 88
  associations/interactions, 87-88, 92, 122
  composition of inorganic sources, 309
  deficiency or excess, 70, 88
  feed composition, 144, 305, 307
  function, 87-88
  recommendations, 88
  requirement tables, 295, 297, 299, 301, 303
  sources, 88, 144
Cocksfoot orchardgrass, 146, 269
Coconut, 164
Coconut oil, 162
Cod liver oil, 111
Cold temperatures and cold stress, 10, 11, 22, 128, 131-132, 133, 217, 238, 244
Colic, 96, 134, 143, 153-154, 157, 158, 189, 220, 224, 239, 254-255, 275
Colitis, 192
Concentrated Animal Feeding Operations, 227

Concentrates, 35, 38, 55, 132, 147
  defined, 173
  digestibility of nutrients, 56, 76
  and growth, 13
  and lactation, 19
  meal feeding, 223-224
  mixed, 160
  nutrient composition, 84, 304-305
  and polysaccharde torage myopathy, 241
  unusual oral behavior, 220, 221, 222
Concussion, 249
Congenital contracted tendon, 242
Constipation, 86
Copper
  absorption, 88-89, 167, 195
  associations/interactions, 87, 88, 89, 92, 93, 97, 136, 187
  composition of inorganic sources, 309
  deficiency or excess, 70, 88-89, 90, 97, 246-247, 235, 244, 248
  feed composition, 144, 305, 307
  function, 88, 187, 189, 246
  hepatic decay, 247
  in mare milk, 90-91, 311-314
  processing effects, 259
  recommendations, 89-91
  requirement tables, 295, 297, 299, 301, 303
  sources, 88, 144, 194, 195, 220, 227
  supplements, 90, 166, 167, 187, 189, 246-247
Coprophagy, 220
Corn and corn byproducts. *See also* Maize
  common feeds, 159
  contaminants, 156, 157, 161, 162
  digestibility, 37, 38, 86, 224
  distiller's dried grains, 159, 251
  gluten feed, 159, 251
  gluten meal, 35, 55, 57, 159
  ground, 37, 224
  hominy, 159
  nutrient composition, 35, 36, 38, 55, 57, 86, 110, 115, 118, 119, 120, 121, 159, 165, 251
  oil, 115, 162, 163, 194, 218, 226
  palatability, 162, 214
  processing effects, 169, 170, 171, 172
  screenings, 162
  silage, 166, 214
  starch digestibility, 169, 170, 171, 172
  steam flaked, 36, 169-170, 171
Cortisol, 49
Cottonseed meal, 55, 118, 162, 163
Cottonseed oil, 162, 163, 218
Crabgrass (*Digitaria* spp.), 148, 212
Creatine kinase, 95, 117, 187
Creatine phosphokinase, 189
Creep feed, 60, 76, 132, 212, 222, 235, 244, 248
Creeping red fescue (*Festuca rubra*), 147, 212
Crested wheatgrass (*Agropyron cristatum*), 151, 153, 212
Cribbing, 25, 158, 220, 221-223, 252
Crude protein, 4. *See also* Protein and amino acids
  acid detergent insoluble nitrogen, 57, 207
  digestibility, 45, 55, 57, 60, 154, 155

feed composition, 143, 150, 159, 160, 304, 306
  for gain, 59
  neutral detergent insoluble nitrogen, 207
  requirement tables, 294, 296, 298, 300, 302
Cryptosporidium, 137
Culicoides hypersensitivity, 50, 194
Cyanogenic glycosides, 156
Cyanophyceae (blue-green) algae, 137
Cysteine, 62, 87, 164-166
Cystine, 207
Cystitis, 156

D

Dallisgrass (*Paspalum* spp.), 148, 157, 251
Dandelion (*Taraxacum officinale*), 212
Danish Warmbloods, 216
Deficiency or toxicity signs and symptoms
  anemia or leukopenia, 93, 121, 190
  anorexia/inappetance, 97, 118
  blindness, 96
  calcification of soft tissue, 113
  cardiac problems, 82, 95, 96, 118
  coagulopathy, 115
  coat or hair abnormalities, 50, 65, 92, 96, 97, 119
  coma, 93
  constipation, 86
  convulsions, 87, 122
  corneal changes, 119
  dehydration, 86, 93
  diarrhea, 93, 96
  feeding/drinking behavior, 65, 85, 86
  fetal abnormalities, 50
  gastrointestinal problems, 96, 122, 158
  goiter, 91, 92
  growth impairment, 97, 110
  head pressing, 96
  hematological defects, 93, 110, 121, 122
  hoof changes, 65, 70, 96, 121
  icterus, 93
  immune depression, 92, 111, 123
  lacrimation, 119
  lactation changes, 65
  lethargy/listlessness, 87, 93, 96
  liver damage, 93
  locomotion disturbances, 89, 95, 97, 99, 114-115
  muscle weakness/degeneration, 86, 95, 97, 114, 115, 118
  neurological changes, 79, 85, 86, 87, 114-115
  night blindness, 110
  perspiration, 96
  photophobia, 119
  renal hypertrophy, 122
  reproductive problems, 50, 65, 91-92, 111
  respiratory problems, 87, 95, 96, 111, 119
  skeletal abnormalities, 72, 77, 89, 90, 91, 92, 94, 97, 99, 111, 113, 115, 242
  skin disorders, 50, 85, 92, 111, 119, 120
  suckling or swallowing difficulties, 95
  tooth discoloration, 99
  unthriftiness, 82, 99

weight changes, 65, 86
wound healing problems, 123
Dehydration, 86, 93, 129, 130, 136, 271
Deoxynivalenol (vomitoxin), 157, 161, 186, 219
Depression, 219
Dermatophilosis, 92
Developmental orthopedic disease
  bone growth disorders, 244-247
  breed differences, 243-244, 248
  energy, protein, and fat intake and, 245-246, 248
  exercise and training and, 247-248
  growth rates and, 147, 243-244, 248
  mineral intake and, 89, 246-247, 248
  nutrient intake effects, 89, 111, 244-247
  pathogenesis, 242-243, 248
  vitamin A and, 111
Diacetoxyscirpenol, 157
Diarrhea, 82, 93, 96, 128-129, 137, 189, 192, 193, 220, 228
Dicoumarol, 157
Diet. *See also* Feeding management; Forage
  and absorption of nutrients, 71, 72
  accommodation/adaptation, 45, 46, 47-48, 254
  and behavior, 49
  donkeys, 272-274
  and energy requirements, 7-8, 13
  environmental considerations, 11, 226-228
  and exercise, 40-41
  and feeding behavior, 214-215, 218, 219, 220, 221, 222
  high-concentrate, 13, 19, 35, 38, 55, 132, 147, 220, 221, 222, 223-224
  high-energy, 38, 223, 245-246
  high-fat, 11, 221, 238, 245, 254
  high-fiber, 38, 219, 221, 224, 254
  high-forage, 20, 35, 37, 132, 223
  high-grain, 192-193
  high-hay, 239
  high-protein, 246
  high-starch, 37, 39, 196, 197, 221, 223-224
  low-energy, 220, 250
  low-fiber, 158, 221, 222, 224
  low-forage, 196, 197
  low-protein, 220
  low-starch, 254
  and milk production, 19-20
  mixed, 56, 225
  and nutrient excretion, 227-228
  pelleted or processed feeds, 221
  and water balance, 128, 129, 131-132
Dietary cation-anion difference (DCAD), 73, 79, 129
Dietary Supplement Health and Education Act, 186
Digestible energy
  and body condition score, 27
  calculation of feed content, 3-6
  carbohydrates, 34
  conversion to ME, 5
  conversion to NE, 28
  dry matter intake and, 145, 155
  efficiency of use, 13, 25
  ensilaged forages, 155
  factors affecting, 4, 8, 10-11, 145, 238

feed composition, 146, 159, 160, 161, 304, 306
growth-related intakes, 11, 238
maintenance intakes, 7, 9, 10-11, 20, 238
requirements, 3-4, 14, 16, 20, 25, 28, 238, 294, 296, 298, 300, 302
Digestion/digestibility. *See also individual nutrients and feeds*
  associative effects of feeds, 4, 45, 225
  dry matter, 45, 55, 154, 155, 160, 237
  energy cost, 7
  exercise and, 4, 35, 60, 94
  feed processing and, 38, 152, 163, 168-169, 171-172, 206
  individual variation, 4
  microbial fermentation, 34, 35, 37, 38, 39, 44, 45, 141, 189, 196
  particle size effects, 38, 167
  probiotics and, 189, 196
  processing effects, 38, 169-171, 172
  silica and, 153
  species differences, 3
  starch, 37, 38-39, 169-171, 172, 223-224, 225
Disaccharides, 34, 35
Diuretics, 240
Docosahexanoic acid, 49, 50
Docosapentanoic acid, 49
Donkeys (*Equus asinus*)
  blood variables, 272
  body condition score, 27, 272
  calcium, 273
  digestibility of nutrients (apparent), 269-270
  dry matter intake, 213-214, 268-269, 273
  endolithiasis, 256
  energy cost of work, 270-271
  energy requirements, 28, 270
  feeding behavior, 213, 214, 268
  heat stress and dehydration, 271
  hyperlipidemia, 28
  lactation, 273
  milk composition, 272, 273
  nutrient intakes from forage, 273
  phosphorus, 273
  practical diets, 272-274
  protein, 271, 273
  vitamin A, 272
  water, 129, 131, 132, 271-272
Draft horses, 9, 15, 18-19, 21, 132, 145, 213, 216, 240-241, 243. *See also individual breeds*
Drinking behavior, 84, 133-134
Dry matter intake
  digestibility, 45, 55, 154, 155, 160, 237
  donkeys, 213-214, 268-269
  energy, 145, 155
  ensilaged forages, 154, 155, 156
  exercise and, 70, 154
  fat intake and, 70, 239
  feed composition, 142, 151, 304, 306
  growth, 70, 145, 225
  hay, 149, 150, 151, 156
  lactation, 70, 144, 145
  maintenance, 70, 154
  pasture, 144-145
  pregnancy, 70

and protein intake, 55, 62, 63, 155
race horses, 25, 48
voluntary, 144-145, 149, 150, 151, 213-214
and water balance, 128, 130, 132
Dust mites, 257, 258
Dutch Warmbloods, 243, 247

E

Eastern gammagrass (*Tripsacum dactyloides*), 151, 212
Eicosanoids, 44, 49, 50
Eicosapentanoic acid, 49, 50
Elephant grass (*Pennisetum purpureum*), 153, 212
Endophyte-free perennial ryegrass (*Lolium perenne*), 147
Endotoxins, 50, 249, 257
Endurance horses, 27, 147, 252. *See also* Racing
Energy cost
  of eating, 5
  of maintenance, 8
  of storing and mobilizing energy, 7
  of tissue accretion during pregnancy, 18
  of work/exercise, 23-25, 270-271
Energy intakes
  and bone growth disorders, 244, 245-246
  excess, 244, 245-246
  and milk production, 19
  and protein intake, 57
Energy requirements
  age and, 10, 12, 13, 14, 24
  body condition score and, 27-28
  body weight basis, 7, 12, 19, 27-28
  breeding, 6, 16-17, 21-22, 147
  deficiencies and excesses, 27-28
  diet composition and, 7-8, 13
  donkeys, 28, 270
  environment and, 8, 10-11, 12, 15, 25, 27
  estimating, 7-9
  exercising horses, 10, 17, 21, 23-27, 270-271
  and feeding behavior, 211-212
  gender and, 13
  growth (maintenance + gain), 6, 11-16, 216, 225
  growth rate and, 13-16
  individual variation, 8
  lactation, 19-21, 147, 216
  maintenance, 6, 7-11, 20, 21, 236
  old horses, 8, 236-237
  oxygen utilization and, 22-23
  pregnancy, 17-19, 28
  reproduction, 16-22
Energy sources, 6-7
Energy status, and reproductive efficiency, 21-22
Energy systems. *See also* Digestible energy; Gross Energy; Metabolizable energy; Net energy
  calculations of feed composition by, 3-6
  Unite Fourragere Cheval, 5-6
  units, 3
Energy value
  carbohydrates, 3, 6, 34, 35, 141, 189
  fats, 3, 4, 5, 6, 8, 44, 45-46, 51, 169

forages, 4, 13, 141, 142, 145, 189
mare milk, 311-314
Ensilaged forages
big bale, 155
clamp, 154, 155, 156
classification, 154
conservation process, 154
digestibility, 154-156
dry matter intake, 154, 155, 156
energy content, 155
high-DM-baled, 154
maize, 154, 155
palatability, 154
potential problems, 156, 157
soaking in water, 237
vitamins, 114, 121
voluntary dry matter intakes, 154, 155
Enterolithiasis
clinical signs, 255
nutritional factors, 255-256
nutritional management, 256-257
in wild equids in captivity, 275-276
Environment
and absorption of nutrients, 77
bedding, 257-258
and body condition, 10, 27
climatic factors, 10-11, 15, 81, 95, 143, 217, 222, 237-239; see also Temperature, ambient
Concentrated Animal Feeding Operations, 227
and diet, 11, 226-228
and drinking behavior, 133
and energy requirements, 8, 10-11, 12, 15, 25, 27
and exercise, 25, 81, 84, 85, 87, 129, 133
and feed intake, 217-218
and feeding behavior, 10, 216-217, 218, 221
and feeding management, 217, 237-239
and forage nutrient content, 142, 143
and growth rate, 15, 244
and maintenance requirements, 10-11, 238
physical modifications, 238
pollution concerns, 227-228
and recurrent airway obstruction, 257-258
stabling, 25, 93, 132, 134, 257-258
waste management considerations, 65, 76, 77, 148, 150, 195, 220, 226-228
and water requirements, 128, 129, 131-132, 133, 134
Epiphysitis, 89, 90, 97
Equine Cushing's disease, 237
Equine degenerative myeloencephalopathy, 114-115
Equine hyperlipemia, 28
Equine leucoencephalomalacia, 157, 161
Equine motor neuron disease, 115
Equine polysaccharide storage myopathy, 240-241
Equine protozoal myeloencephalitis, 122
Equitation horses, 27, 147
Ergotamine, 157, 160, 162, 186
Ergovaline, 158
Escherichia coli, 50, 138, 193, 227
Essential fatty acids, 44, 49, 50-51, 193. *See also* Fat and fatty acids

Estimating requirements, computer model, 285-292
Ether extract (crude fat), 45, 207, 169
Ethoxyquin, 167, 184
Ethylenediaminedihydroiodide, 91, 92
European grass, 157
European Warmbloods, 240
Exercise/work
acclimation, 10, 84, 129-130
acid-base response, 48, 64, 65
amino acid supplementation, 64
athletic performance, 49, 122
and body condition, 225
and bone health, 73, 74-75, 81, 247-248
calcium, 70, 72, 73, 74-76, 78, 81
carbohydrate utilization, 40-41, 47-48
categories, 25
chlorine, 70, 83, 87
chromium, 98
components of, 23
conditioning, 24, 63, 64, 116, 120, 124
copper, 88, 91, 189
cutting-type, 24, 27, 49
and developmental orthopedic disease, 247-248
and digestibility of nutrients and feeds, 4, 35, 60, 94
drinking behavior, 133
dry matter intake, 70, 154
duration and intensity, 22, 24, 26, 49, 63, 64, 75, 76, 79, 81, 83, 84, 129, 133, 147, 247
electrolyte losses in sweat, 70, 81, 82, 83-85, 86, 87
endurance-type, 27, 75, 82, 84, 85, 116, 117, 123, 124, 188
energy costs, 23-25, 270-271
energy requirements, 10, 17, 21, 23-27, 270-271
environment and, 25, 81, 84, 85, 87, 129, 133, 247
equitation-type, 27
fat supplementation and, 47-49, 81
and feeding behavior, 215-216, 221, 222
feeding management for, 40-41, 122
fiber intake and, 147, 158
folate, 122
and gastric ulcer syndrome, 158, 253, 252-253
and glycogen repletion, 41, 47, 48, 49, 64, 241
and heart rate, 23, 24-26
incline vs. flat surface, 23
iodine, 92
iron, 93, 94
and lipid metabolism, 41
magnesium, 79, 81
manganese, 94
metabolic response to, 47-48
niacin, 120
nutrient requirement tables, 294-303
old horses, 236, 237
oxidative stress, 116, 187, 188, 189
oxygen utilization, 22-23, 24, 25
pasture feeding, 122, 147
phosphorus, 75, 78-79, 81

and polysaccharide storage myopathy, 241, 242
potassium, 82, 83-84
protein, 58, 59-60, 62-64, 65, 150
reining-type, 24
riboflavin, 119
run time to fatigue, 49, 122
sand track, 24
selenium, 188, 189
silicon, 99
sodium and chloride, 82, 83, 84-86
tendon injuries, 113
thiamin, 118
three-day event, 24-25, 41, 84
training, 15, 24, 26, 41, 72, 75, 78, 81, 84, 85, 99, 113, 122, 129-130, 158, 252-253
treadmill, 23, 117, 122, 132, 188
vitamin A, 112-113, 189
vitamin C, 123, 124, 187, 188, 189
vitamin E, 116-117, 188, 189
water, 63, 64, 70, 84, 86, 87, 129, 130, 131, 132, 133
and weight, 15, 226
zinc, 97, 189
Exertional rhabomyolysis syndromes, 49, 95, 98-99, 116, 240
Exmoor ponies, 213, 217
Exudative dermatitis, 50

F

Fat and fatty acids. *See also* Lipid metabolism
accommodation/adaptation period, 45, 46, 47-48
acid-base responses, 48
adverse effects, 45-46
analysis of feeds, 207-208
associative or additive effects on other nutrients, 4, 45, 46, 48, 50, 72, 81, 115, 239
athletic performance, 48-49
and behavior, 49
benefits, 49-50, 240, 241, 242
bioavailability, 45
bone growth disorders, 245-246
carbohydrate metabolism, 45, 46-47, 48, 51
cell content of forages, 144
deficiencies and excesses, 50-51
digestibility and energy value, 3, 4, 5, 6, 8, 44, 45-46, 51, 169
disease management with, 240, 241, 242
and dry matter intake, 70, 239
ether extract (crude fat), 45, 161, 207
exercise, 47-49, 81
feed additives, 193-194
feed composition, 159, 160, 161, 162-163, 304, 306-307
and fiber digestion, 4, 45, 46, 239
function and structure, 44, 50, 162, 184
glycerol-based lipids, 44, 48
and glycogen storage and utilization, 46-47, 48, 49
growth, 49
health effects of n-3 and n-6 fatty acids, 49-50

lactation, 20, 49
in mare milk, 20, 49, 311-314
metabolic response, 47-48
nutrient composition, 306-307
oxidation, 162, 184, 187
palatability, 44, 162, 218
physiologic effects, 46-50
processing effects on, 169
and protein digestion, 48, 62, 239
reproductive performance, 49, 50
requirements, 50-51
sources, 44-45, 162-163
supplements, 8, 11, 20, 44, 45, 46-49, 51, 81, 221, 224, 226, 238-239, 240, 241, 245
synthesis, 120
and thermoregulation, 11, 238-239
Febendazole, 192
Feed. *See also* Concentrates; Forages; Fresh pasture; Grains and grain products; Hay
associative effects, 4, 45, 225
contaminants, 92, 156-158, 161-162, 219-220
determining nutrient content, 280-281; *see also* Feed analysis
effects on feeding behavior, 218-219, 220
fats and oils in, 4, 7, 162-163, 218
label claims, 184, 185, 186, 191-192
mineral supplements, 163, 166-167
moisture content, 208
palatability, 44, 154, 162, 185, 218-219
and pasture management, 148
protein supplements, 163, 164-166
selection of, 280
terminology, 173-174
vitamin supplements, 167, 168
Feed Additive Directive 70/524/EC, 95
Feed additives
AAFCO-approved, 183
anticaking agents, 162, 185-186
antioxidants, 162, 167, 184, 186-189
colors, 184
defined, 173, 183
direct fed microbials (probiotics), 189
dust reducers, 162, 186, 218
emulsifying agents, 186
enzymes, 189-190
flavors, 185, 190, 218
GRAS status, 184, 185, 190
health- and performance-promoting, 185, 186-197
herbs and botanicals, 190
interactions, 190
joint supplements, 190-192
lubricants, 186
medicinal compounds, 186, 192-193
oligosaccharides, 193
omega-3 fatty acids, 193-194
organic trace minerals, 194-196
pellet binders, 162, 185-186
physical enhancers of feed, 183-186
preservatives, 184
processing, 167
regulation, 183-184, 186, 190, 192
sequestrants, 186

stabilizers, 186
technical, 184
toxicity, 190, 192, 193
yeast culture or extract, 196-197
Feed analysis
carbohydrate analysis in horse nutrition, 34-35, 142, 205-206, 207-208
fat and fatty acids, 207-208
fiber, 142, 203-205
general considerations, 203
near infrared reflectance spectroscopy, 208
nonfiber carbohydrates, 205
protein and amino acids, 207
starch, 205
water-soluble carbohydrates, 205, 206
Feed composition
carbohydrates, 34-35, 36-37, 141-143, 149, 160, 161
cereal straw, 152
concentrates, 84, 304-305
conserved forages, 148-158
contaminants, 92, 156-158, 161-162, 219-220
dry matter intake, 142, 151, 304, 306
energy, 3-6, 146, 159, 160, 161, 304, 306
ensilaged forages, 114, 121, 154-156
fats and oils, 159, 160, 161, 162-163, 304, 306-307
forages, 69, 141-159, 304-307
fresh pastures, 144-148
grains and grain byproducts, 159-162
hays, 148-151, 152-154
minerals, 69, 89, 144, 161, 305, 307
moisture, 130
nitrates, 136
tables, 203, 304-307
Feed intakes. *See also* Dry matter intake; Feeding behavior
animal factors affecting, 216-217
decreased, 86
environment and, 217-218, 238
fat supplementation and, 49
forages, 144-145, 151, 154, 155
particle size effects, 38, 151-152, 223
transportation and, 133
water demand, 130, 133, 134
Feed processing and manufacturing, 167-168
additives, 167, 186
associative interactions, 170
benefits, 167, 172
and bioavailability of nutrients, 172
crimping, 172, 173
digestibility, 38, 152, 163, 168-169, 171-172, 206
and energy value, 4
extruded ingredients, 237
and fat digestibility, 169
and feeding behavior, 172
gelatinization, 170, 173
grinding, 167, 170, 171, 173
inactivation of anti-nutrients and toxins, 163, 167, 172
methods and systems, 167, 173-174
micronizing, 170, 171, 172
pellets, wafer, or cubes, 88, 151-152, 159, 160, 162, 167, 169, 173, 174, 185-186, 221

and protein digestibility, 163, 171-172, 206
rolling, 170, 171, 174
standards, 167
and starch digestibility, 38, 169-171, 172
steam flaking, 170, 174
terminology, 173-174
and total tract digestibility, 168-169
vitamin stability, 167
Feeding behavior. *See also* Feed intakes
age and, 213, 214, 216, 218
bark chewing, 147, 158, 220, 268
bolting feed, 223
breed differences, 213, 216, 221-222
confinement and, 216-217, 218, 220, 221, 222
coprophagy, 220
cribbing, 25, 158, 220, 221-223, 252
depraved appetite, 86
diet and, 214-215, 218, 219, 220, 221, 222
diurnal patterns, 217
donkeys, 213, 214, 268
energy balance and, 211-212
environment and, 10, 216-217, 218, 221
exercise and, 215-216, 221, 222
external parasites and, 217-218
fat supplementation and, 215-216, 221, 222
feed-related effects, 150, 151, 158, 172, 185, 218-219
fiber restriction and, 158, 221, 222, 224
foals, 82, 212, 216, 220, 222
gender difference, 213, 222
geophagia, 220
illness and, 65, 85, 86, 217, 221
latrine behavior, 219-220
mature horses on pasture, 212-216
preferred feeds, 213-213, 218-219
rate of intake, 152, 214
refusal to eat, 82, 85, 150
seasonal differences, 213, 217
sidedness or handedness, 218
taste aversion, 149, 150, 219-220
typical patterns, 212-216
unusual oral behavior, 152, 158, 220-223
water restriction and, 131
wood chewing, 152, 158, 220-221, 222, 224
Feeding management. *See also* Diet; Nutrition management
body condition management, 225
climate and, 217, 237-239
cold weather and, 217, 238
disease-specific nutrition management, 239-259
for exercise and performance, 40-41, 122
fat and fatty acids, 40-41, 122
foals, 77, 235-236, 244, 248, 275
forages, 223, 224-225
frequency of feeding, 224, 254
general considerations, 223-226
in group-fed situations, 216-217, 223
hot weather and, 238-239
meal feeding concentrates, 223-224
old horses, 237
pollution control considerations, 226-228
ration balancing, 223, 225, 280-284
refeeding starved horses, 226
regulations, 227, 228
size of meal, 254

transition to new environment/diet, 218, 223, 254-255
waste management considerations, 65, 76, 226-228
weight vs volume of feed, 223
weight management, 225-226, 250
wild equids in captivity, 274-275
Ferritin, 187
Ferrous fumarate, 93
Fertilizers and manure, 143, 145, 147, 156, 195, 227, 228
Fescue, 55, 143, 146, 147, 151, 153, 158, 212
Fetal development, 17-18, 40, 50, 60-61, 73-74, 80. See also Pregnancy
Fiber
    acid detergent fiber, 4, 45, 142, 159, 160, 161, 190, 204, 208, 304, 306
    analytical methods, 203-205, 208
    associative effects of fat, 4, 45, 46, 239
    cell wall phenolics (lignin), 204
    crude fiber, 205
    deficiency, 158
    defined, 203
    digestibility and energy value, 4, 37-38, 45, 154, 155, 189-190, 224, 239
    and exercise, 147, 158
    feed composition, 141, 145, 150, 159, 160, 161, 304, 306
    and feeding behavior, 158, 221, 222, 224
    and mineral absorption, 72
    neutral detergent fiber, 34, 35, 37-38, 45, 142, 151, 159, 160, 161, 190, 204, 224, 304, 306
    rations, 225
    restriction, 158, 221, 222, 224
    supplement, 46, 147, 190
    total dietary fiber, 204
    and water balance, 128, 131
Finnhorses, 244
Fish oils, 163
Fishmeal, 55, 56, 57, 163
Flavin adenine dinucleotide, 118
Flavin mononucleotide, 118
Flaxseed, 50, 164, 194
Fluorine, 99, 310
Fluorosis, 99
Foals. See also Growth
    amino acid digestibilities, 56
    birth weights, 17, 60, 193, 243
    bone health, 72
    calcium, 72, 73, 74, 235
    congenital defects, 122
    copper, 88-89, 90
    coprophagy, 220
    creep feed, 60, 76, 132, 212, 222, 235, 244, 248
    crooked-legged, 242
    developmental orthopedic disease, 242-248
    drinking behavior, 133
    energy requirements, 10, 12, 90
    fat supplementation, 49
    feeding behavior, 82, 212, 216, 220, 222
    feeding management, 77, 235-236, 275
    feral, 212
    fostering, 235-236
    gastric ulcer syndrome, 252

heat or cold stress, 10
iron, 92, 93
oligosaccharides, 193
orphans, 110, 112, 132, 235-236
peripartum asphyxia syndrome, 252
phosphorus, 235
probiotics, 189
protein requirements, 60, 61-62, 65, 90, 235
selenium, 96, 196
sepsis, 252
sucklings, 20, 61, 116, 132, 133, 212, 235-236, 244
vitamin A, 110, 112
vitamin E, 114, 115-116
water, 132, 133, 236
weaning, 49, 222, 235, 236
weight gain, 20, 197, 243, 244
wood chewing, 220
zinc, 97
Folate
    deficiency, 121-122
    dietary sources, 121
    function, 121
    requirements, 109, 122
    toxicity, 122
Folic acid, 121, 168
Follicle stimulating hormone, 22
Food and Drug Administration, 95, 161, 183, 186, 190, 192, 196
    Center for Veterinary Medicine, 162
Forages
    analysis, 203, 205, 207
    anti-quality factors, 156-158, 172
    bacteria, 154, 156-157
    carbohydrates, 37, 141, 142-143
    cell contents, 142-144
    chemical composition, 141-144
    conserved, 148-157; see Ensilaged forages; Hay; Straw
    dietary-fiber–cell wall carbohydrates, 141-142, 204
    digestion/digestibility, 13, 35, 37, 45, 55, 58, 141, 142, 143, 145-146, 152, 153, 154-156, 204, 208
    diurnal variations, 143
    dry matter, 142, 148
    endophyte contamination, 158, 215, 216
    energy value, 4, 13, 141, 142, 145, 189
    environmental influences, 142, 143
    feeding management, 223, 224-225
    fiber, 141-142
    harvesting consideration, 114
    inherent plant anti-nutrients, 71, 76, 77, 79, 118, 156
    insect contamination, 152, 156
    lipids, 144
    microbial contamination, 156-157
    minerals, 81, 82, 83, 92, 93, 94, 95, 99, 141, 144, 240
    nutrient composition, 304-307
    pastures, see Fresh pastures
    processing, 148
    protein, 55, 58, 60, 141, 143-144, 165-166
    requirements, 158-159
    seasonal variations, 143
    toxins, 152

vitamins, 110, 114, 119, 120, 144
    and water balance, 128, 131, 141
Founder, 224, 248
Foxtail millet (*Selaria italica*), 251
Free fatty acids, 46, 47, 48, 120, 161, 207
Fresh pastures
    carbohydrates, 36, 142, 145, 205, 249-250
    cell wall content, 142
    DE, 146
    digestibility, 145-146, 224-225
    dry matter intake, 144-145
    exercise and, 122, 147
    feed analysis, 142
    feeding behavior of mature horses, 144, 147, 158, 212-216
    feeding value, 112, 144, 145, 146-147
    fiber, 145, 147
    and laminitis, 205, 249-250
    management practices, 143-144, 145, 147-148, 220, 223
    and milk yields, 20
    and mineral deficiency or excess, 79-80
    protein, 145, 146
    species for horses, 147-148, 212-213
    stockpiling, 148
    toxic weeds and fungi, 148, 154, 219, 250
    and vitamin status, 112, 121, 122
    voluntary dry matter intakes, 144-145
    waste management, 148
    water content, 130, 132, 146
Fructans, 34, 35, 37, 38, 141, 142, 143, 203, 205, 249, 250
Fructooligosaccharides, 193, 204
Fumonisins, 157, 161-162
Fungi, 150, 157, 161-162, 257, 259
Furosemide, 84, 85
Fusaric acid, 219
Fusarium spp., 157, 161

G

Gait, 23, 24, 97, 114, 156
Galactan, 205
Gamma-glutamyltransferase, 95
Garlic supplements, 190, 218-219
Gastric ulcer syndrome
    antacid therapy, 222
    calcium and, 73
    clinical signs, 252
    in cribbing foals, 222, 252
    epidemiology and risk factors, 252-253
    exercise and, 158, 253
    nutritional factors (putative), 73, 84, 158, 253-254
    risk factors, 252
    sodium and, 84
    stall confinement and, 253
    temperament and, 253
Gastrointestinal health, water balance and, 129
Geldings, 9, 16, 27, 28, 73, 133, 167, 188, 189, 214
Gender differences
    energy requirements, 13
    feeding behavior, 213, 222
    growth rate, 14

Geophagia, 220
Geriatric horses, 98, 236, 248
Gestation. *See also* Fetal; Pregnancy
   length, 18, 19, 61
   tissue accretion rates, 17-18
   weight gain, 19, 61
Giardia, 137
Glucocorticoid, 249
Glucomannans, 193
Glucosamine, 190-192
Glucose
   metabolism, 5, 6, 7, 37, 38, 39-41, 47-48, 51, 98, 120, 241
   transporters, 41, 84
   vitamin C synthesis from, 123
Glutamic acid, 207
Glutathione peroxidase, 91, 94, 95, 96, 114, 115, 187, 196
Glycemic index, 39, 171
Glycemic response, 46, 171, 224
Glycine, 56, 207
Glycogen storage and utilization, 7, 39-40, 41, 46-47, 48, 49, 64, 240-241
Glycosaminoglycans, 190-192
Goiter, 91, 92
Goitrogens, 92
Gonadotrophin releasing hormone, 22
Gossypol, 163
Grains and grain byproducts. *See also individual grains*
   analytical methods, 204, 208
   brewer's/distillers, 55, 58, 59, 159, 160, 163, 164, 218
   byproduct feeds, 159, 160-161
   carbohydrates, 35, 36, 38, 169, 170, 241
   and colic, 255
   common feeds, 159-160
   digestion/digestibility, 45, 55, 159, 160, 161, 168, 170, 192-193, 224, 225
   energy content, 4, 38, 160, 161
   fat and fatty acids, 45, 161
   fiber, 161
   grading criteria, 159
   meal size, 254
   minerals, 81-82, 86, 92, 95, 99, 159, 160, 161, 240, 250-251
   mold-inhibiting agents, 184
   mycotoxins in, 160, 161-162
   palatability, 159, 160
   processing effects, 159, 169, 170, 214, 250-251
   protein, 160
   rancidification, 161
   starch digestibility, 169-171, 224
   straws, 129
   vitamins, 110, 114, 116, 118, 119, 121
   and water requirements, 128, 129, 130, 131, 132, 134, 160
Grasses, 142, 143, 144, 145, 148, 149, 150, 151, 152, 155, 165, 172, 212, 240, 241. *See also* Forages; Fresh pasture; *individual species*
Greasy feces (steatorrhea), 46
Green lipped mussel (*Perna canaliculus*) extract, 192
Gross energy, 3, 5, 20, 34, 236

Growth
   age and, 14
   calcium, 73, 75, 156
   chlorine, 86-87
   copper, 89-90
   critical period, 242
   daily DE for, 13, 16
   developmental orthopedic disease and, 242
   dry matter intake, 70, 145, 225
   energy requirements, 6, 11-16, 216, 225, 238
   environment and, 238
   fat supplementation and, 49
   fetal, 60-61
   iron, 93
   magnesium, 79, 80, 81
   manganese, 94
   mineral supplements, 167, 196
   nutrient requirement tables, 294-303
   pasture feeding and, 147
   phosphorus, 76, 77-78, 79, 156
   potassium, 82, 83
   protein, 58-61, 64, 150, 163
   sodium, 85
   thiamin, 118
   vitamin A, 110, 111-112
   vitamin D, 113-114
   vitamin E, 109, 115-116
   zinc, 97, 98
Growth hormone (GH), 22
Growth rate
   age and, 16
   antibiotics and, 192
   body weight and, 14-15
   breed differences, 13-15
   and developmental orthopedic disease, 147, 243-244
   dietary stress and, 244
   and energy requirements, 13-16
   environment and, 15, 244
   fetal, 18
   hormonal factors, 244
   mineral source and, 195
   predictions, 13-16
   seasonal differences, 244

H

Hanoverians, 14, 90, 243
Harness racing horses, 7
Hay. *See also* Straw
   allergic respiratory disease, 154
   baling/baled, 149-150, 157
   carbohydrates, 35, 36, 38, 149
   curing, 113, 148-149, 152
   defined, 174
   digestibility, 38, 56, 72, 149, 150, 152, 153, 196
   dipping in water, 134
   dry matter intake, 149, 150, 151, 156
   drying, 149
   energy source, 6, 7, 35, 153
   feeding behavior on, 221, 222
   fiber, 150, 153
   grasses, 119, 215
   heating/combustion, 150

high-moisture, 149, 150, 156
   leaf shatter, 149
   Maillard products, 149
   minerals, 71, 72, 80, 149, 151, 152, 154
   moldy, 149, 150
   nutrient and dry matter losses, 149-151
   palatability, 214
   particle size effects, 151-152
   poisons/toxins in, 152, 154, 157
   preferences of horses, 149, 215
   problems with, 149, 152-154, 157, 158
   protein and amino acids, 56, 59, 149, 153
   quality, 149-151
   rejection by horses, 149, 150
   soaking or steaming, 154, 259
   storage, 150
   sun-cured, 113
   vitamin content, 110, 112, 113, 119, 120, 121, 149
   voluntary dry matter intakes, 144-145, 149, 150, 151
   wafers, pellets, or cubes, 151-152, 160, 161
   and water requirements, 128, 129, 130, 131, 132, 134
Haylage, 154, 155, 157
Heart rate, 23, 24-26
Heat production (energy loss), 5, 7, 8, 11, 48, 84
Heat stress and high temperatures. *See also* Dehydration
   age and, 10
   donkeys, 271
   and energy requirements, 10, 11
   feeding management, 238-239
   and water balance, 132, 133
Heinz body anemia, 190, 219
Hemicellulose, 34, 37, 141, 142, 190
Hemoglobin, 123
Heparin, 87
Hepatotoxins, 137, 154, 156
Hexokinase, 46
Highland ponies, 272
Hindgut acidosis, 158
Hinnies, 268
Histidine, 54, 62, 65, 164-166, 207
Hominy feed, 159
Hoof health, 65, 70, 96, 121, 195, 242, 248, 250
Hordenine, 160
Hormone sensitive lipase, 28
Hyaluronan, 191
Hyaluronic acid, 99
Hydrated sodium calcium aluminosilicate (HSCAS), 185-186
Hydroxyl ions, 136
Hypercalcemia, 71
Hypercalcitonism, 72
Hyperglycemia, 237, 245
Hyperinsulinemia, 237, 245
Hyperkalemia, 82
Hyperkalemic periodic paralysis
   etiology and genetic basis, 239
   nutritional management, 239-240
   and potassium balance, 82
Hyperlipidemia, 28
Hyperostosis, 111
Hyperphosphatemia, 251-252
Hypertonic electrolyte solution, 253

Hypertriglyceridemia, 28
Hypocalcemia, 72, 80, 251
Hypochloremia, 86
Hypoglycemia, 41
Hypohydration, 133
Hypokalemia, 82
Hypomagnesemia, 79, 80
Hyponatremia, 84
Hypothyroidism, 91

I

Iatrogenic iodism, 92
Icelandic horses, 95-96, 216, 220
IGF-I (insulin-like growth factor I), 22
Immune function, 92, 96-97, 98, 109, 111, 115, 123, 193, 195
Immunoglobulin G, 116
India grass (*Sorgastrum nutans* L.), 151, 212
Industry economics, 1
Inflammatory diseases, 50
Insects, 152
Insulin, 22, 39, 41, 46, 51, 87, 98, 99, 143, 171, 226, 241, 245, 249
Insulin-like growth factor I, 245
Intake energy, 3
Iodine
  absorption, 91
  associations/interactions, 91
  composition of inorganic sources, 309
  deficiency or excess, 70, 91-92
  feed composition tables, 305, 307
  function, 91
  recommendations, 92
  requirement tables, 295, 297, 299, 301, 303
  supplementation, 91
  sources, 91
Iodothyronine-5-deiodinase I, 95
Ionophores, 192-193, 219
Iron
  absorption, 92
  associations/interactions, 88, 89, 92, 93, 163, 187
  composition of inorganic sources, 309-310
  deficiency or excess, 70, 93
  feed composition, 144, 305, 307
  function, 92, 187
  in mare milk, 93
  recommendations, 93-94
  requirement tables, 295, 297, 299, 301, 303
  sources, 92, 93, 144, 220
  supplements, 93
Iron ammonium citrate, 185
Isoleucine, 54, 56, 62, 64, 65, 164-166, 207

J

Johnson grass, 156

K

Kale, 92
Kentucky bluegrass (*Poa paratensis*), 147, 151, 153, 212, 215, 216

Keratan sulfate, 191
Keratin, 96
Kiangs, 274, 276
Kikuyu grass (*Pennisetum clandestinum*), 147, 156, 212, 251
Klebsiella, 138
Kulans, 276

L

Lactate, 35, 48, 64, 98, 171, 189
Lactate acidosis, 158
Lactation. *See also* Milk
  body condition and, 20
  breed differences, 19, 21
  calcium, 74, 156, 251
  chlorine, 87
  copper, 90-91
  diet composition and, 19-20
  drinking behavior, 133
  dry matter intake, 70, 144, 145, 251
  energy requirements, 19-21, 147, 216
  equine hyperlipemia, 28
  fat supplementation and, 20, 49
  feeding behavior, 213, 215, 216, 217
  fiber, 158
  iodine, 92
  iron, 93-94
  magnesium, 80-81
  nutrient requirement tables, 294-303
  pasture feeding, 144, 145, 146, 147
  phosphorus, 76, 78, 156
  potassium, 83
  protein, 19, 61-62, 147, 150, 163
  sodium, 85
  stage of, 20
  vitamin A, 112
  vitamin E, 109, 116
  water, 128, 130, 131, 132-133
  zinc, 98
Lactobacillus spp., 189
Lactose
  digestion, 38
  in mare milk, 20, 34, 311-314
Laminitis
  acute, 248, 249-250
  chronic, 248, 250
  etiology, 248-249
  nutritional management, 143, 158, 205, 225, 249-250
  pathogenesis, 249
  in wild equids in captivity, 276
Lasalocids, 192
Laxatives, 80, 154
Lead, 88
Lectins, 193
Legumes, 119, 142, 144, 147-148, 149, 150, 152, 161, 165-166, 212, 214, 215, 240, 251. *See also* Forages; individual species
Lentil, 164
Leptin, 22, 98
Leptospira, 119
Lespedeza (*Kummerowia* spp.), 148
Leucine, 54, 56, 62, 64, 65, 164-166, 207

Leukopenia, 121
Lignin, 141, 142, 150, 152, 204, 205, 207
Lignin sulfonate, 185
Lincomycin, 192
Linoleic acid, 44, 49, 50-51, 162, 193-194
Linseed meal, 55, 58, 59, 163, 164
Linseed oil, 162, 163, 194
Lipase, 47, 161
Lipid metabolism, 28, 41, 46-48, 94, 98, 119, 122, 123. *See also* Fat and fatty acids
Lipid oxidation, 116, 162, 184, 187
Lipizaners, 243
Lipoic acid, 187, 188
Lipoprotein lipase activity, 46
Listeria spp., 154, 156, 227
Listerosis, 156-157
Liver disease, 162
Locoweed, 219
Lolitrem B, 158
Lotonosis (*Lotonosis banessi*), 147
Lupin seed meal, 163
Lusitanos, 20
Lutein, 187
Luteinizing hormone (LH), 22
Lycopene, 187
Lysine, 48, 54, 56, 58, 59, 60, 61, 62, 64, 65, 159, 163, 164-166, 207, 237, 246, 294, 296, 298, 300, 302, 304, 306

M

Macrominerals. *See also* Calcium; Chlorine; Magnesium; Phosphorus; Potassium; Sodium; Sulfur
  defined, 69
MADC (Matières Azotées Digestibles Cheval), 56
Madurmycin, 192
Magnesium
  absorption, 45, 79, 197
  associations/interactions, 71, 75, 78, 79, 80, 81, 152, 186
  bioavailability, 186
  composition of inorganic sources, 309
  deficiency or excess, 70, 79-80, 274
  and enterolithiasis, 256
  feed composition, 144, 305, 307
  function, 79
  in mare milk, 80, 311-314
  medicinal applications, 80
  processing effects, 259
  recommendations, 80-81
  requirement tables, 294, 296, 298, 300, 302
  sources, 79, 80, 144, 152, 197
  supplements, 79, 253
  in water, 135
Maintenance
  breed differences, 21
  calcium, 71, 75
  carbohydrates, 38
  chlorine, 86
  copper, 89, 91
  donkeys, 272-273
  dry matter intake, 70, 154

energy cost of, 8
energy requirements, 6, 7-11, 20, 21, 236, 238
environment and, 10-11, 238
forage feeding, 147
iodine, 92
iron, 94
magnesium, 80
nutrient requirements table, 294-303
old horses, 236
phosphorus, 77, 78
potassium, 82-83
protein, 57-58
riboflavin, 119
sodium, 85, 86
thiamin, 118
vitamin A, 111
vitamin E, 115
water, 132-133
Maize silage, 154, 155
Maltose, 34
Manganese
absorption, 94, 167
associations/interactions, 92, 93, 94
composition of inorganic sources, 310
deficiency or excess, 70, 94
feed composition, 144, 305, 307
function, 94, 187
recommendations, 94
requirement tables, 295, 297, 299, 301, 303
sources, 94, 144
supplements, 167
Manganese ascorbate, 190, 192
Mannose, 193
Manure. *See* Fertilizers and manure
Maremmano Warmbloods, 243
Mares. *See also* Broodmares; Gestation; Pregnancy; Lactation
energy requirements, 16
Matua, 151, 153
Matua prairiegrass (*Bromus wildenowii*), 147, 212
Mature horses
coprophagy, 220
energy requirements for maintenance, 238
feeding behavior on pasture, 145, 147, 212-216
hay intakes and digestibilities, 151, 153
minerals, 195, 196
vitamin E, 115
water, 128, 131
zinc, 97
Meadow fescue (*Festuca pratensis*), 147, 212
Meadow hay, 151, 153, 155
Megaloblastic anemia, 121
Melanin, 88
Metabolic acidosis, 82
Metabolic alkalosis, 86
Metabolic bone disease, 72, 89-90, 98
Metabolizable energy (ME)
calculation, 4-5, 7
carbohydrates, 34
Metallic matrix metalloproteinases, 249
Metalloenzymes, 97
Metallothionein, 97
Methemoglobin, 136

Methionine, 54, 56, 62, 65, 87, 94, 121, 164-166, 207
Methylsulfonylmethane, 192
Microcystins, 137
Microcystis, 137
Microcytic hypochromic anemia, 93
Microfilaria (*Onchrocera cervicalis*), 119
Microminerals. *See also* Cobalt; Copper; Iodine; Iron; Manganese; Selenium; Zinc
antioxidants, 187
bioavailability of organic vs inorganic sources, 194-196
defined, 69, 174
Milk. *See also* Lactation
byproduct blends (cattle), 55, 58, 59, 163, 164
colostrum, 80, 95, 112, 123, 196, 235
composition, 20, 35, 49, 62, 65, 78, 80, 90-91, 93, 95, 98, 112, 116, 123, 196, 236, 272, 273, 311-314
digestibility, 235
donkeys, 272, 273
energy value, 311-314
immunoglobulin content, 235
mares, 19-21, 49, 74, 78, 90-91, 98, 116, 235, 273, 311-314
replacer, 60, 65, 89, 235, 236
yields, 19-20, 21, 61, 62, 74, 86, 197
Millet, 164
Mineral oil, 186
Minerals. *See* Macrominerals; Microminerals; *individual minerals*
absorption, 70
age and, 72, 75-76, 89, 97
analytical methods, 208
antioxidants, 187, 188, 189
associations/interactions, 69, 71, 72, 73, 75, 76, 77, 78, 79, 80, 81, 85, 87-88, 89, 91, 92, 93, 94, 95, 96, 97, 99, 113, 114, 115, 116, 122, 136, 187
balance studies, 69, 71
bioavailability, 163, 166-167
body weight basis for recommendations, 69, 70
and bone growth disorders, 89, 246-247
cell content of forages, 144
chelates, 165-166
determinants of feed content, 69, 144
digestibility, 70, 71, 72, 73, 77, 79, 85, 88, 89, 91, 94, 97, 98
endogenous losses, 70
environmental influences, 144
fetal deposition rate, 80
in forages, 141, 150
licks, 84, 95, 274
maximum tolerable concentration, 69
methodological limitations, 69-70
organic-trace-mineral feed additives, 194-196
for pregnancy, 69
in soil, 88, 93, 95, 144, 156, 220
supplements, 163, 166-167
urinary fractional electrolyte excretion test, 69
in water, 135-136, 256

Miniature donkeys, 268, 270, 271, 272, 273, 274
Miniature horses, 78, 195, 255
Molasses, 36, 86, 88, 160, 164
Molds, 149, 150, 156, 161-162, 184, 257, 259
Molybdenum, 88, 136, 144
Monensin, 192, 219
Monosaccharides, 34, 35, 205
Monounsaturated fatty acids, 44
Moon blindness, 119
Morgan horses, 14, 240, 255
Mules, 268
Mustard, 92
Mycotoxins, 150, 157, 158, 161-162, 185-186, 193, 219

N

Namib horses, 132
Napier (*Pennisetum* spp.), 251
Narasin, 192
National Animal Health Monitoring System, 162, 236
National Forage Testing Association, 203, 204
National Pollution Discharge Elimination System, 227
National Water Quality Network, 134
Navicular disease, 191
Neotyphodium spp., 157, 158
Net energy (NE), 5-6, 12, 28, 34, 39, 236
Neurotransmitters, 123
Neutral detergent solubles, 34
New Zealand, water quality criteria, 134, 135
Niacin
deficiency, 120
function, 119
requirements, 109, 120
sources, 119-120
supplements, 168
toxicity, 120
Nickel, 99, 144
Nicotinamide adenine dinucleotide, 119
Nicotinamide adenine dinucleotide phosphate, 119
Night blindness, 110, 111
Nitrates and nitrites, 136-137, 156, 227
Nitrogen. *See also* Crude protein; Protein and amino acids; Urea
balance studies, 56-57, 60
endogenous losses, 57, 58, 59, 63, 64
and enterolithiasis, 256
environmental burden, 150, 227, 228
fertilizer, 156
nonprotein sources, 54, 149, 154
Nitrogen-free extract, 45
Norepinephrine, 123
North Carolina State University, 157
Nostoc, 137
Nutrient requirements
computer model for estimating, 285-292
tables, 294-303
Nutritional management
of diseases, 50, 239-259
nursing and orphan foals, 235-236
old horses, 236-239

Nutritional muscular dystrophy, 96, 114, 115-116
Nutritional secondary hyperparathyroidism
    clinical signs, 250
    nutritional factors, 71, 77, 250-251
    nutritional management and prevention, 252
    pathogenesis, 251-252

O

Oat hay, 151, 153, 156, 166, 226, 241
Oat hulls, 4, 37, 159
Oat straw, 152, 214, 269
Oats (*Avena sativa*), 38-39, 76, 110, 118, 119, 120, 121, 131, 134, 152, 159, 160, 161, 164, 168, 169, 170, 172, 190, 212
Obesity, 28, 146, 154, 225-226, 249, 272, 274
Ochratoxins, 157, 162
Oilseeds and oilseed meals, 81, 120, 204, 208
Old horses
    caloric restriction, 237
    Cushing's disease, 237
    defined, 236
    energy requirements, 8, 236-237
    exercise, 236, 237
    feed form, 237
    feeding management, 252, 226
    micronutrient requirements, 237
    protein and amino acid requirements, 237
Oligosaccharides, 34, 35, 193, 205
Olive oil, 163
Onagers, 274-275, 276
Oral rehydration therapy, 82
Orchardgrass (*Dactylis* spp.), 77, 142, 143, 145, 146, 147, 153, 156, 212, 215, 217
Osteoarthritis, 190, 191, 192
Osteocalcin, 244
Osteochondrosis, 72, 77, 89, 90, 97, 242-243, 247, 248
Osteodysgenesis, 89
Osteodystrophia fibrosa, 156, 250
Osteomalacia, 77
Osteopenia, 72
Oxalates, 71, 76, 77, 79, 156, 251
Oxidative stress, 116, 187, 188, 189
Oxygen utilization, 22-23, 24, 25

P

Paints, 15
Palm oil, 163
Panic grasses, 251
Pangola grass (*Digitaria recumbens*), 251
Pantothenic acid, 109, 123
Paraffin, 186
Parakeratosis, 97
Parasites, 148, 192, 217-218, 219, 226
Parathyroid hormone, 71, 247, 251
Paspalum (*Paspalum dilantatum*), 212
Pasture. *See* Fresh pastures
Patulin, 157
Peanut meal, 118, 162, 163, 164
Peanut oil, 163, 218
Pearl millet (*Pennisetum glaucum*), 148, 212

Peas, 164
Pectins, 34, 37, 141, 142
Penicillium spp., 157, 162, 219, 257
Penitrim A, 157
Pentose phosphate pathway, 118
Percherons, 28, 110, 111, 118, 243
Performance horses, 9, 25-26, 27, 40, 190, 252
Periodic ophthalmia, 119
Petrolatum and petroleum jelly, 186
Phalaris aquatica, 142
Phenylalanine, 54, 62, 65, 164-166, 207
Phosphofructokinase, 46
Phospholipids, 46, 49, 50
Phosphorus
    absorption, 45, 76-77, 113, 189, 197
    associations/interactions, 76, 78, 79, 81, 92, 94, 113, 156, 160, 161
    calcium:phosphorus ratio, 71, 72, 77, 75, 161, 244, 246, 247, 235, 244, 248, 250-252
    composition of inorganic sources, 308
    deficiency or excess, 70, 77, 113, 156, 246, 247, 250-252, 274
    and enterolithiasis, 256
    environmental burden, 76, 219, 227, 228
    feed composition, 144, 149, 154, 160, 161, 305, 307
    function, 76, 246
    in mare milk, 311-314
    old horses, 237
    processing effects, 259
    protein intakes and, 65
    recommendations, 77-79
    requirements, 237, 294, 296, 298, 300, 302
    sources, 76-77, 144, 154, 197
    supplements, 92, 99
    in water, 137
Phytase, 76, 79, 189, 190
Phytates, 71, 76, 156, 160, 189
Phytochemicals, 190
Planktothrix/Oscillataria, 137
Pleasure horses, 221, 222
Polo ponies, 26-27
Polysaccharide storage myopathy
    clinical signs, 240-241
    nutritional factors, 241
    nutritional management, 99, 224, 241-242
    pathogenesis, 99, 241
Polysaccharides, 34, 194, 195, 204, 205
Polyunsaturated fatty acids, 44, 49-50, 114
Ponies
    carbohydrates, 37, 38, 39, 170, 171
    developmental orthopedic disease, 243, 247
    digestion/digestibility of nutrients, 152, 153, 170, 171, 269
    dry matter intake, 268
    energy cost of work, 270
    energy requirements, 8, 9, 11, 14, 15, 20, 23, 26-27, 28, 270
    enterolithiasis, 256
    fats and fatty acids, 45, 47, 50, 51, 245
    feeding behavior, 213, 214, 217, 218, 219
    forage intake, 144, 151, 155
    laminitis, 249
    listeriosis, 156-157
    maintenance requirements, 270

    minerals, 71, 80, 82, 86, 89, 93, 96, 97
    mycotoxicosis susceptibility, 161
    palatability of feeds, 154
    processed feeds, 170, 171
    protein, 54, 57, 60, 61
    ryegrass staggers, 158
    vitamins, 110, 112, 113, 121, 122, 247
    water, 130, 131, 132, 133, 271, 272
    wild, 144
Population of horses, 1
Porphyrin, 123
Potash, 149
Potassium
    absorption, 81-82, 83
    associations/interactions, 73, 79, 85, 95
    composition of inorganic sources, 309
    deficiency or excess, 70, 82, 83, 274
    and enterolithiasis, 256
    environment and, 82, 84, 219
    feed composition, 144, 154, 160, 305, 307
    and feeding behavior, 82
    function, 81, 239
    furosemide and, 84
    hyperkalemic periodic paralysis, 239-240
    in mare milk, 311-314
    parenteral administration, 82
    processing effects, 259
    recommendations, 82-84
    requirement tables, 294, 296, 298, 300, 302
    restricted diets, 240
    sources, 81-82, 83, 144, 154, 240
    supplementation, 82, 83, 84, 253
    sweat losses, 82, 83-84, 238
    and water balance, 129, 131
Potato, 165
Pregnancy. *See also* Gestation
    calcium, 73-74
    chlorine, 87
    copper, 90, 246-247, 248
    drinking behavior, 133
    dry matter intake, 70
    energy cost of, 18
    energy requirements, 17-19, 28
    equine hyperlipemia, 28
    fat supplementation, 49
    feeding behavior, 215
    feeding value of pastures, 146
    folate, 122
    iodine, 92
    iron, 93
    magnesium, 80
    nutrient requirement tables, 294-303
    oligosaccharides, 193
    phosphorus, 78
    potassium, 83
    protein, 56, 60-61
    protozoal myeloencephalitis, 122
    riboflavin, 119
    sodium, 85
    thiamin, 118
    vitamin A, 110, 112
    vitamin E, 112, 116
    water, 128, 129, 130, 131, 132, 133
    weight gain, 19
    yeast supplement, 197
    zinc, 98

Probiotics, 192-193, 189, 196
Progesterone, 60
Prolactin, 22
Proline, 207
Propionate, 7, 35, 37, 194, 195
Propionic acid, 149, 158, 184
Prostaglandins, 44, 50, 254
Proteases, 189
Protein and amino acids. *See also* Crude protein; Nitrogen
   and acid-base balance, 64, 65
   age and, 60, 237
   analysis of feeds, 57, 207, 208
   associations/interactions, 65, 120, 163, 239
   bioavailability, 56-57, 172
   and bone growth disorders, 244, 246
   catabolism, 6
   cell content of forages, 141, 143-144
   deficiency, 48, 54, 57, 60, 65, 121, 163, 244
   digestion and utilization, 45, 54-57, 59, 65, 120, 145-146, 149, 155, 163, 171-172, 196-197, 206
   donkeys, 271
   dry matter intake and, 55, 62, 63, 155
   energy value, 3, 4, 5, 6
   excess, 65, 244, 274
   for exercise, 58, 59-60, 62-64, 65
   fat supplementation and, 48, 62, 239
   feed composition, 145, 160
   and feeding behavior, 220
   feeding management, 65-66
   forages, 149, 155, 256
   French MADC system, 56
   function and structure, 54
   and glycogen utilization, 64
   for growth, 58-62, 65, 66
   ideal, 64-65
   for lactation, 19, 61-62
   Maillard products, 149, 172
   maintenance requirement, 57-58
   in mare milk, 20, 65, 311-314
   and mineral absorption, 72
   muscle turnover rate, 63
   nonprotein nitrogen sources, 54-55
   old horses, 237
   pregnancy, 56, 60-61
   in processed feeds, 163, 171-172, 206
   quality (amino acid profile), 54, 55-56, 59, 61, 62, 64-65, 66, 87, 163, 164-166, 207
   requirements, 19, 54, 56-66
   supplemental, 4, 55, 56, 58, 59, 61, 62, 64, 65, 118, 163, 164-166
   and water balance, 129, 131
Proteinates, 195
Protozoa, 37, 122, 137
Przewalski's horses, 216-217, 274, 275, 276, 277
Purine, 121
Purple pigeon grass (*Selaria incrassate*), 251
Pyrantel tartrate, 192
Pyrimethamine, 122
Pyruvate dehydrogenase, 118
Pythomyces, 157

Q

Quarter horses, 14, 15, 19, 21, 49, 73, 78, 130, 153, 192, 193, 239, 240, 241, 242, 243, 244, 245, 247

R

Racing and race horses, 25, 26, 48-49, 75, 78, 84, 96, 99, 113, 122, 123, 147, 158, 187, 189, 222, 252-253
Ragwort (*Sennecio* spp.), 148, 154
Rape, 156
Rare earth elements, 99
Ration formulation and evaluation
   determining nutrient content of feeds, 280-281
   examples, 281-284
   identifying requirements, 280
   selection of feeds, 280
Reactive oxygen species, 186-187, 258
Recovered energy, 5
Recurrent airway obstruction
   nutritional factors, 124, 257-258
   nutritional management and prevention, 187, 188, 194, 258-259
   pathogenesis and clinical symptoms, 257, 258
   prevalence and risk factors, 257
Recurrent seasonal pruritis (sweet itch), 50
Recurrent uveitis, 119
Red clover (*Trifolium pratense*), 145, 146, 148, 149, 150, 154, 155, 156, 157, 212
Reed canarygrass (*Phalaris arundinaceae*), 147, 151, 153, 160, 212
Reproduction. *See also* Breeding; Gestation; Pregnancy
   antibiotics and, 192
   energy requirement, 16-22
   external parasites and, 218
   mineral status and, 65, 91-92, 195
   plant toxins and, 156, 158, 162
Reproductive efficiency
   body condition and, 21-22, 27
   energy status and, 21-22
   fat supplementation and, 49, 50
   mineral source and, 195
   vitamin A and, 109, 111, 112
   vitamin E and, 116
Respiration and respiratory problems, 10, 25, 47, 250
Resting metabolic rate, 10
Retinol binding protein, 111
Retinyl-acetate, 110
Retinyl-palmitate, 110, 112
Rhinopneumonia, 123
Rhizoctonia, 157
Rhizomucor, 257
Rhodes grass (*Chloris gayana*), 147, 212
Ribgrass (*Plantago lanceolata*), 212
Riboflavin
   deficiency, 118-119
   function, 119
   requirements, 109, 119, 295, 297, 299, 301, 303
   sources, 119
   supplements, 168
   toxicity, 119
Rice bran, 118, 161, 165, 241, 250
Rice oil, 162
Rickets, 113
Rye, 160
Ryegrass, 130, 142, 143, 144, 145, 146, 147, 148, 150, 152, 157, 158, 212, 213, 249
Ryegrass staggers, 158, 219

S

Saccharomyces spp., 196, 197
Safflower meal, 165
Safflower oil, 162, 163, 218
Sainfoin (*Onobrychis viciifolia*), 148, 212
Salinomycin, 192
Salmonella, 189, 227-228
Satratoxins, 157
Scurvy, 123
Seasonal differences
   feeding behavior, 213, 217
   forage nutrient content, 143
   growth rate, 15, 244
   water quality, 137
Seaweed, 91, 92
Selenium
   absorption, 95
   associations/interactions, 88, 91, 95, 96, 114, 115, 116
   composition of inorganic sources, 95, 310
   deficiency or excess, 70, 95-96, 114, 116, 156
   feed composition tables, 305, 307
   function, 94-95, 96-97, 114, 187, 188, 189, 258
   in mare milk, 95
   recommendations, 96-97
   requirement tables, 295, 297, 299, 301, 303
   sources, 95, 195, 196
   supplementation, 95, 96, 187, 188, 189, 195, 258
   yeast, 195, 196
Selenocysteine, 96, 196
Selenocystine, 96
Selenomethionine, 96, 196
Selle Francais, 19
Serine, 207
Sesame meal, 165
Sesame oil, 163
Setaria (*Setaria* spp.), 156, 212, 251
Shetland ponies, 46, 51, 119, 123
Shivers, 241
Show horses, 25, 190, 222
Silage. *See* Ensilaged forages
Silicon/silica, 99, 153, 185, 204
Silver, 88
Skeletal health, 72, 74-75, 77, 81, 89, 90, 91, 92, 94, 97, 98, 99, 111, 113, 115, 195, 244-248
Slaframine, 157
Smelter smoke syndrome, 94
Smooth bromegrass (*Bromus inermis*), 147, 212

Smooth stalked meadow grass, 212
Sodium
    absorption, 84-85
    associations/interactions, 73, 76, 85
    composition of inorganic sources, 308
    deficiency or excess, 70, 84, 85
    from de-icing salt, 136
    and enterolithiasis, 256
    exercise and, 70, 82, 83
    feed composition, 144, 154, 305, 307
    function, 84, 239, 240
    furosemide and, 85
    in mare milk, 311-314
    processing effects, 259
    recommendations, 85-86
    requirement tables, 294, 296, 298, 300, 302
    sources, 84-85, 144, 154, 227
    supplements, 84, 253
    sweat losses, 84-85, 238
    and water balance, 129, 131, 132
    in water, 135, 136
Sodium bicarbonate, 86
Sodium zeolite A, 99
Soil erosion, 228
Somali donkeys, 271
Sorghum fodder, 269
Sorghum grain, 156, 160, 165, 170, 172
Sorghum hay, 93
Sorghum-Sudan grass hybrids, 156
Soybean hulls, 4, 35, 37, 160, 161
Soybean meal, 35, 37, 55, 57, 58, 59, 62, 86, 119, 120, 163, 165, 172, 246
Soybean oil, 45, 46, 47, 49, 51, 115, 162, 163, 218, 239
Soybeans, whole, 92, 161
Speed of travel, 22-23, 25
Stachybotrys spp., 157, 257
Stall confinement
    and compulsive behavior, 25, 220, 221, 222
    and enterolithiasis, 256
    and exercise, 247-248
    and feeding behavior, 216-217, 218, 220, 221, 222
    and gastric ulcer syndrome, 253
    and recurrent airway obstruction, 257-258
Stall-kicking, 25
Stallions
    breeding, 16-17
    energy requirements, 9, 16-17, 28
    feeding behavior, 213
    maintenance requirements, 16-17
    nutrient requirements table, 294-303
    ponies, 8
Standardbreds, 10, 19, 23, 25, 27, 47, 48, 75, 84, 96, 112, 129, 130, 132, 133, 134, 192, 221, 240, 253
Starches, 5, 34, 35, 37, 38-39, 45, 38-39, 46, 49, 141, 142, 143, 158, 159, 160, 161, 169-171, 205, 223-224, 225, 240, 241, 242, 249
Stargrass, 144
Starvation, 6, 28, 226
Steroid hormones, 123
Stock horses, 145. *See also* individual breeds
Strangles, 123
Strawberry clover (*Trifolium fragiferum*), 212

Straws
    bedding, 257-258
    feed, 88, 110, 116, 129, 152, 157, 158, 214, 215, 269
Sudan grass, 156
Sugar beets, 157, 160, 164
Sulfadiazine, 122
Sulfur
    absorption, 87
    associations/interactions, 87, 88, 96, 136
    composition of inorganic sources, 309
    deficiency or excess, 87
    and enterolithiasis, 256
    feed composition, 144, 305, 307
    function, 87, 192
    recommendations, 69, 87
    requirement tables, 295, 297, 299, 301, 303
    sources, 87, 144, 192
    sulphates in water, 135, 136
Summer-pasture-associated obstructive pulmonary disease, 257
Sunflower meal, 163, 165
Sunflower oil, 162, 163
Superoxide dismutase, 88, 187
Swainsone, 219
Swedish Standardbreds, 14, 243
Swedish Warmbloods, 14, 243
Sweet clover, 156, 157
Sweet feed, 46, 72, 76, 152, 158, 159, 162, 185, 190, 215, 241
Switchgrass (*Panicum virgatum* L.), 212

T

T-2 toxin, 161
Teeth, 99, 237
Temperament
    diet and, 49, 79
    and gastric ulcer syndrome, 253
    nervousness, 79, 98
Temperature, ambient. *See also* Cold; Heat
    acclimation, 10, 84, 129-130
    and body condition score, 10
    critical lower and upper, 11, 237-238
    and energy requirements, 10-11, 15
    and fat supplementation, 11, 238-239
    and feeding management, 81, 217, 237-239
    and forage nutrient content, 142
    and growth rate, 15
    hay storage, 150
    and maintenance requirements, 10-11
    and mycotoxin contamination of feed, 161
    and nutrient losses in sweat, 82, 84, 85, 238
    thermoneutral zone, 10
    and water balance, 128, 129, 131-132, 238
Teratogenesis, 111
Tertiary butyl hydroquinone (TBHQ), 184
Tetany, 79-80
Tetracycline, 192
Thiamin
    deficiency, 118
    dietary sources, 118
    function, 87, 118
    requirements, 109, 118, 295, 297, 299, 301, 303

supplements, 168
toxicity, 118
Thoroughbreds, 13, 14, 15, 17, 19, 21, 23, 24, 25, 27, 46, 47, 48, 49, 51, 61, 84, 113, 121, 122, 123, 124, 130, 132, 145, 146, 147, 187, 188, 189, 193, 212, 213, 220, 221, 222, 235, 240, 242, 243, 244, 245, 247, 252
Threonine, 48, 54, 56, 59, 62, 64, 65, 164-166, 207, 237, 246
Thromboxane, 50
Thyroid hormones, 22, 91, 94
Thyroid stimulating hormone, 22
Thyroxine, 91
Timothy (*Phleum pretense*), 120, 121, 143, 147, 151, 153, 158, 212, 240, 276
Tocopherols, 114, 184, 188. *See also* Vitamin E
Tocotrienols, 114
Toronto Zoo, 274
Total body water, 128
Total digestible nutrients, 9
Total Maximum Daily Load Standards, 228
Toxin- or endophyte-free tall fescue (*Festuca arundinacea*), 147
Training. *See* Exercise
Trakehners, 243
Transketolase, 118
Transportation of horses, water requirements, 130-131, 133, 135
Tricetum flavescens, 71
Tricothecenes, 157
Triglycerides, 6, 28, 44, 46, 47
Triiodothyronine, 91
Triticale, 165, 224
Trotters, 243
Trypsin, 161, 163, 172
Tryptophan, 54, 65, 120, 207
Tyrosine, 164-166
Tumor necrosis factor, 50

U

Unit conversion tables, 315
University of California–Davis, 255
University of Illinois, 64
Unthriftiness, 82, 99, 218
Urea, 54-55, 59, 61, 64, 65, 95, 163, 227. *See also* Nitrogen; Protein
Urinary fractional electrolyte excretion test, 69
U.S. Department of Agriculture, 208
    Cooperative State Research, Education, and Extension Service, 134
    National Animal Health Monitoring System, 162
U.S. Environmental Protection Agency, 227
U.S. Geological Survey, 134

V

Valine, 54, 62, 64, 65, 207
Vanadium, 99
Vetch (*Vicia atropurpurea*), 212
Virginiamycin, 192-193

Vitamin A
    absorption, 50, 110
    associations/interactions, 71, 112, 122, 187
    deficiency, 110-111, 247
    feed composition tables, 305, 307
    function, 71, 109, 187
    in mare milk, 112
    requirements, 109, 111-113, 272, 295, 297, 299, 301, 303
    sources, 109-110
    supplements, 109, 110, 112, 167, 168
    units, 109-110
    toxicity, 111
Vitamin B_6, 109, 123
Vitamin B_{12} (cyanocobalamin), 87-88, 109, 122-123
Vitamin C
    age and, 124, 237
    associations/interactions, 115, 187
    bioavailability, 187
    deficiency, 123
    function, 123, 187, 188, 258
    requirements, 109, 123-124
    sources, 123
    supplements, 168, 187-188, 258
    toxicity, 123, 187-188
Vitamin D
    absorption, 50
    associations/interactions, 113
    deficiency, 113, 247
    feed composition tables, 305, 307
    function, 113
    requirements, 109, 113-114, 295, 297, 299, 301, 303
    sources, 113
    supplements, 113, 167, 168
    toxicity, 113
Vitamin E
    absorption, 50
    associations/interactions, 95, 96, 112, 114, 115, 116, 187
    deficiency, 114-115, 276
    feed composition tables, 305, 307
    function, 114, 184, 187, 188, 258
    in mare milk, 116
    requirements, 109, 115-117, 295, 297, 299, 301, 303
    sources, 114
    supplements, 114, 116-117, 167, 168, 258
    toxicity, 115
Vitamin K
    absorption, 50
    deficiency, 117
    dietary sources, 117
    function, 117
    requirements, 109, 117-118
    supplements, 167, 168
    toxicity, 117
Vitamins. *See also individual vitamins*
    adaptive response, 110
    antioxidants, 114, 115, 119, 123
    associations/interactions, 95, 96, 112, 114, 115, 118, 120, 122
    and bone growth disorders, 246-247
    defined, 109
    drug interactions, 122
    estimating/determining requirements, 109
    microbial synthesis, 118, 119, 120, 121, 122, 123
    oxidation effects, 184
    relative dose response test, 111
    seasonal variations, 112
    supplements, 167, 168
    upper safe level, 109
Volatile fatty acids, 5, 6-7, 35, 37, 44, 46, 141, 189, 193, 253, 269-270

W

Warmblood horses, 14, 46, 51, 240, 241, 246, 257
Waste management, 65, 76, 77, 148, 150, 195, 220, 226-228
Water intake
    dietary effects, 82, 130-131
    donkeys, 271-272
    drinking patterns of horses, 133-134
    excessive, 157
    from feeds, 141
    measuring, 134
    restricted, 134
    sodium balance and, 85, 86
    temperature effects, 131-132, 135, 238
Water losses. *See also* Dehydration
    body weight as measure of, 84-86
    estimating, 84, 86, 133
    evaporative, 129, 271
    fecal, 128-129
    lactational, 128, 130
    nutrient losses in, 63, 64, 65, 70, 82, 83, 84, 87, 238
    respiratory, 130
    sweat, 63, 64, 70, 82, 83, 84, 86, 87, 129-130, 133, 238
    urine, 64, 129, 131
Water management, 134
Water quality
    adaptation to, 135
    algae, 137-138, 227
    bacteria, 138
    chemical criteria, 135-136
    hardness, 135, 136
    minerals, 135, 136, 227, 256
    nitrates and nitrites, 136-137
    pH, 135-136
    physical criteria, 135
    protozoa, 137
    standards, 134-135
    tap water, 86
    total soluble salts, 135
    waste management considerations, 227-228
Water requirements
    body weight and, 131, 132, 133
    breed differences, 132
    diet composition and, 128, 129, 131-132
    donkeys, 129, 131, 132, 271-272
    dry matter intake and, 128, 130, 132
    environment and, 128, 129, 131-132, 133, 134
    exercise and, 63, 64, 70, 84, 86, 87, 129, 130, 131, 132, 133
    for maintenance, 132-133
    pregnancy and lactation, 132-133
    protein intake and, 65
    suckling foals, 132
    work or exercise, 133
Weanling horses
    antibiotics, 192
    calcium, 72, 75
    copper, 88-89
    cribbing, 252
    dry matter intake, 145
    feeding behavior, 221
    feeding management, 225
    flavor preferences, 185
    growth requirements, 12, 59
    heat or cold stress, 10, 11
    minerals, 195
    pasture feeding, 147
    stress, 49, 222, 235, 252
    thiamin, 118
    vitamin A, 111
    water, 130
    yeast supplement, 197
Weaving, 25
Weight gain, 10
Welsh ponies, 155, 217, 240
Wheat bran, 118, 160, 165, 169, 194, 250, 256-257
Wheat grain, 118, 156, 165, 170
Wheat midds, 160, 165
Wheat straw, 129, 152, 166, 269, 271, 272
Whey, 165
White bent (*Agrostis gigantea*), 212
White clover (*Trifolium repens*), 145, 146, 147, 148, 212
White muscle disease, 95, 114
White sweet clover (*Melilotus alba*), 156, 157
Wild equids in captivity
    asses, 274, 276, 277
    body condition scoring, 277
    colic, 275
    enterolithiasis, 275-276
    feeding behavior, 144, 216
    feeding management, 216, 274-275
    kiangs, 274, 276
    laminitis, 276
    nutritional disorders, 275-277
    obesity/starvation, 274, 277
    onagers, 274-275, 276
    orphaned foals, 275
    Przewalski's horses, 216-217, 274, 275, 276, 277
    vitamin E deficiency/myelopathy, 276
    zebras, 80, 274, 275, 276, 277
Wood chewing, 152, 158, 220-221, 222, 224
Work. *See* exercise/work

X

Xylans, 159, 190

Y

Yearling horses, 10, 59, 72, 73, 75, 81, 88, 90, 94, 97, 131, 145, 147, 151, 153, 167, 193, 196, 213, 215, 238, 245. *See also* Growth

Yeast supplements, 197
Yellow prussiate of soda, 185
Yellow sweet clover (*Melilotus officinalis*), 157

Z

Zearalenone, 161, 186, 219
Zearolone, 157

Zebras, 80, 274, 275, 276, 277
Zeolites, 186
Zinc
    absorption, 97, 167
    associations/interactions, 88, 89, 92, 97, 186
    bioavailability, 186
    composition of inorganic sources, 310
    deficiency or excess, 70, 97, 247
    feed composition, 144, 305, 307
    function, 97, 187, 189
    in mare milk, 98, 311-314
    recommendations, 98
    requirement tables, 295, 297, 299, 301, 303
    sources, 97, 144, 227
    supplements, 167, 187, 189
Zinc:copper ratio, 97